# Heart Failure: An Issue of Cardiology Clinics

# Heart Failure: An Issue of Cardiology Clinics

Editor: Ellie Gibson

AMERICAN
MEDICAL PUBLISHERS
www.americanmedicalpublishers.com

AMERICAN
MEDICAL PUBLISHERS
www.americanmedicalpublishers.com

**Cataloging-in-Publication Data**

Heart failure : an issue of cardiology clinics / edited by Ellie Gibson.
p. cm.
Includes bibliographical references and index.
ISBN 978-1-63927-028-6
1. Heart failure. 2. Cardiac arrest. 3. Heart--Diseases. 4. Heart failure clinics. I. Gibson, Ellie.
RC685.C53 H43 2021
616.129--dc23



American Medical Publishers,
41 Flatbush Avenue,
1st Floor, New York,
NY 11217, USA

ISBN 978-1-63927-028-6 (Hardback)

# Contents

# Preface

This book was inspired by the evolution of our times; to answer the curiosity of inquisitive minds. Many developments have occurred across the globe in the recent past which has transformed the progress in the field.

Heart failure is the condition in which the heart cannot sustain the sufficient pumping of blood to meet the requirements of the body. Shortness of breath, swelling in the leg, and exhaustion are common signs of heart failure. Heart failure is generally caused due to coronary artery disease, high blood pressure, valvular heart disease, atrial fibrillation, cardiomyopathy, etc. The severity of the condition may be determined by the severity of symptoms during exercise. It can be diagnosed based on a review of symptoms, a medical examination and echocardiographic evaluation. Chest radiography and blood tests can aid in determining the underlying cause of heart failure. In cases of mild heart failure, lifestyle and dietary changes, and medications generally suffice to manage the problem. However for those with severe heart failure, drugs such as diuretics and aldosterone antagonist may be used. Devices like implantable cardiac defibrillator or pacemakers may also be used to aid cardiac activity. For cases that cannot be resolved by such measures, heart transplantation may be performed. This book aims to shed light on some of the unexplored aspects of heart failure. The various studies that are constantly contributing towards advancing technologies and therapeutic interventions in cardiology are examined in detail. The readers would gain knowledge that would broaden their perspective about heart failure.

This book was developed from a mere concept to drafts to chapters and finally compiled together as a complete text to benefit the readers across all nations. To ensure the quality of the content we instilled two significant steps in our procedure. The first was to appoint an editorial team that would verify the data and statistics provided in the book and also select the most appropriate and valuable contributions from the plentiful contributions we received from authors worldwide. The next step was to appoint an expert of the topic as the Editor-in-Chief, who would head the project and finally make the necessary amendments and modifications to make the text reader-friendly. I was then commissioned to examine all the material to present the topics in the most comprehensible and productive format.

I would like to take this opportunity to thank all the contributing authors who were supportive enough to contribute their time and knowledge to this project. I also wish to convey my regards to my family who have been extremely supportive during the entire project.

**Editor**

1

# Strategy to recognize and initiate treatment of chronic heart failure in primary care (STRETCH)

Evelien ES van Riet[1*], Arno W Hoes[1], Alexander Limburg[2], Henk van der Hoeven[2], Marcel AJ Landman[1] and Frans H Rutten[1]

**Abstract**

**Background:** Most patients with heart failure are diagnosed and managed in primary care, however, underdiagnosis and undertreatment are common. We assessed whether implementation of a diagnostic-therapeutic strategy improves functionality, health-related quality of life, and uptake of heart failure medication in primary care.

**Methods/Design:** A selective screening study followed by a single-blind cluster randomized trial in primary care. The study population consists of patients aged 65 years or over who presented themselves to the general practitioner in the previous 12 months with shortness of breath on exertion. Patients already known with established heart failure, confirmed by echocardiography, are excluded. Diagnostic investigations include history taking, physical examination, electrocardiography, and serum N-terminal pro B-type natriuretic peptide levels. Only participants with an abnormal electrocardiogram or an N-terminal pro B-type natriuretic peptide level exceeding the exclusionary cutpoint for non-acute onset heart failure (> 15 pmol/L (≈ 125 pg/ml)) will undergo open-access echocardiography. The diagnosis of heart failure (with reduced or preserved ejection fraction) is established by an expert panel consisting of two cardiologists and a general practitioner, according to the criteria of the European Society of Cardiology guidelines.
Patients with newly established heart failure are allocated to either the 'care as usual' group or the 'intervention' group. Randomization is at the level of the general practitioner. In the intervention group general practitioners receive a single half-day training in heart failure management and the use of a structured up-titration scheme. All participants fill out quality of life questionnaires at baseline and after six months of follow-up. A six-minute walking test will be performed in patients with heart failure. Information on medication and hospitalization rates is extracted from the electronic medical files of the general practitioners.

**Discussion:** This study will provide information on the prevalence of unrecognized heart failure in elderly with shortness of breath on exertion, and the randomized comparison will reveal whether management based on a half-day training of general practitioners in the practical application of an up-titration scheme results in improvements in functionality, health-related quality of life, and uptake of heart failure medication in heart failure patients compared to care as usual.

**Keywords:** Heart failure, Diagnosis, Treatment, Elderly, Primary care, Cluster randomized trial

* Correspondence: E.E.S.vanRiet@umcutrecht.nl
[1]Julius Center for Health Sciences and Primary care, University Medical Center Utrecht, PO Box 85500, 3508 AB, Utrecht, The Netherlands
Full list of author information is available at the end of the article

## Background

Heart failure (HF) is an emerging epidemic in the elderly, causing high mortality rates, substantial loss in quality of life, and high healthcare costs [1]. The last two decades, progress in patient management, including multiple drug therapies and implantable devices, has improved prognosis of patients with heart failure with reduced ejection fraction (HF-REF) [2,3]. Poor compliance to and insufficient up-titration of evidence-based medication is a major contributor to hospital (re)admissions and loss of life years in these patients [4]. Angiotensin converting enzyme (ACE) inhibitors, angiotensin receptor blockers (ARBs) and beta-blockers did not show a significant beneficial effect in patients with heart failure with preserved ejection fraction (HF-PEF) [5], and their prognosis did not improve over the last years [6]. Currently, adequate treatment of hypertension and other comorbidities, control of heart rate in those with concurrent atrial fibrillation, and diuretics to control sodium and water retention are considered important in HF-PEF [4].

The majority of the elderly patients with HF is diagnosed and managed in primary care [7]. Unfortunately however, recognizing HF in the early stage is challenging, and echocardiography is not readily available in primary care. A diagnosis based on the signs and symptoms only, without echocardiography, results in both false-positive [8,9] and false-negative diagnoses [10]. Moreover, uncertainty about HF diagnosis and fear of side effects have led to underutilization of ACE-inhibitors and beta-blockers in patients with HF in primary care [11,12].

We suspect that especially in older persons presenting with shortness of breath to the general practitioner (GP), the prevalence of undetected HF is high. Therefore, we developed a selective screening strategy, including an open-access outpatient echocardiography facility. In addition we developed an easy to apply up-titration scheme for those newly diagnosed with HF-REF and HF-PEF. Our main objective is to assess whether such a targeted diagnostic-therapeutic approach improves current underdiagnosis and undertreatment.

### Key objectives

- To determine the prevalence of unrecognized heart failure (HF-REF, HF-PEF, and isolated right sided heart failure) in elderly who present themselves with shortness of breath on exertion to the general practitioner.
- To examine the effect of treatment guided by a structured up-titration scheme on functionality, health-related quality of life, and uptake of heart failure medication in patients with newly, screen-detected HF.
- To assess the cost-effectiveness of such an intervention.

## Methods/Design

### Study design

Our design consists of two parts. The first part is a selective screening study (case finding) of HF in elderly with shortness of breath on exertion. The second part is a single-blind, cluster randomized controlled trial comparing an intervention at the level of the GP to improve treatment uptake with care as usual in those with screen-detected HF. The intervention consists of a half-day training in the management of HF, and the practical application of an up-titration scheme for HF-REF and HF-PEF separately. See Figure 1 for the study flowchart.

### Study population and recruitment

Thirty primary care practices in the Zeist region, located in the vicinity of the Diakonessenhuis hospital Zeist, the Netherlands, participate in this study. In this sample of primary care practices, urban, suburban and rural communities are represented.

The study population consists of persons aged 65 years or over who in the previous 12 months presented themselves to one of the participating GPs with shortness of breath on exertion (including those known with a pulmonary disease), irrespective of whether they were suspected of HF or not. Shortness of breath was not necessarily the main reason for contact. Eligible subjects are identified from the electronic medical files of the participating GPs by a single physician (EvR).

Patients already known with an established diagnosis of HF confirmed by a cardiologist with help of an echocardiography are excluded, as are patients with a life expectancy shorter than 6 months, and those unable to give informed consent.

We consider our study sample representative for elderly aged 65 years or over in the community, since in the Netherlands all citizens, except those living in a nursing home or hospice, are registered with a GP, irrespective of (co)treatment by a specialist.

### Randomization and blinding

Random allocation to either management guided by a structured up-titration scheme (intervention group) or care as usual (control group) will be executed at the level of the GP. As a result, patients with HF of one and the same GP (a cluster) will all be managed according to the same arm. This approach was taken to reduce the risk of contamination between patient groups.

Since it is not deemed feasible to keep the GPs in the care as usual group unaware of the existence of an intervention arm, blinding of the participants is considered necessary to minimize bias in assessing the outcome parameters. In addition, the researcher performing the six minutes walking test is blinded to the patient's allocation arm. The risk of observer bias for the other endpoints is

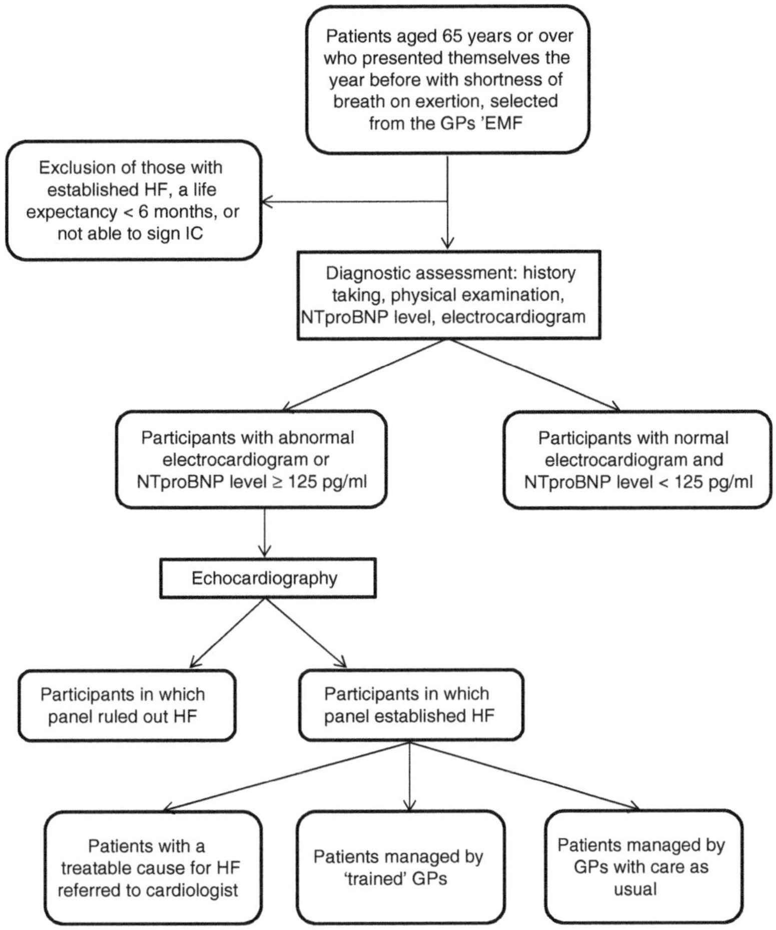


**Figure 1 Flowchart STRETCH – study.** GP = general practitioner, EMF = electronic medical file, HF = heart failure, IC = informed consent, NTproBNP = N-terminal pro B-type natriuretic peptide.

minimized, because questionnaires on quality of life are filled out at home by the participants themselves, and retrieving information on HF medication and HF related doctor appointments from the electronic medical files is not subject to interpretation.

### Sample size

The difference in mean distance walked during the six-minute walking test (6MWT) between the two groups after six months follow-up will be taken as the primary outcome. The average distance walked by HF patients ranges from 242 m (standard deviation 71 m) up to 427 m (standard deviation 100 m), depending on the severity of HF [13]. Since it was shown that an increase of 50 m in walking distance indicated a clinically relevant change [14,15], we consider a mean difference of 50 meters between groups as the minimal important difference to show an effect of the intervention.

We used the two-sample t-test power analysis to examine how many HF patients are needed per group to demonstrate an effect. With an effect size of 0.6, alpha of 0.05, and beta of 0.2, group sample sizes of two times 45 will be sufficient.

We assume that in a standard general practice with 2400 patients, at least 50 patients aged 65 years or over will experience shortness of breath during a one-year period. The prevalence of previously unrecognized HF in such patients is expected to be around 14% (10.4-17.5%) [16]. With a participation rate of 50%, a mean number of 3.5 patients per GP are expected to have newly detected HF (50% HF-REF and 50% HF-PEF). Twenty-six general practitioners are needed to reach the targeted number of HF patients. We will include 4 extra practices to allow for taking clustering into account.

### Diagnostic procedures

Participants will be send two health-related quality of life (HRQoL) questionnaires. They will fill out these questionnaires before the initial baseline assessment that will be performed by a trained physician and research nurse at the outpatient clinic of the Julius Center. If unable to travel to the study center, participants will be visited at home by the physician. Informed consent will be obtained from all participants.

After signing informed consent, participants receive a diagnostic work-up scheme. Diagnostic investigations include history taking, physical examination, an electrocardiogram (ECG), and a blood test for N-terminal pro B-type natriuretic peptide (NTproBNP) levels. For the assessment of medical history, comorbidities, symptoms, and current drug use, a standardised digital questionnaire will be used. Physical examination includes height and weight, blood pressure (two readings), pulse, respiratory rate, pulmonary percussion and auscultation, heart auscultation, palpation of the apex beat, measurement of the jugular venous pressure, palpation of the liver and inspection for signs of venous insufficiency.

Blood serum concentrations of NTproBNP will be analysed with a non-competitive immunoradiometric assay (Roche, Mannheim, Germany). NTproBNP is considered elevated if the value exceeds the exclusionary cut point 15 pmol/L (~125 pg/ml), in line with the ESC guidelines on HF [17].

A standard 12-lead ECGs will be recorded in supine position. All ECGs will be analysed by a trained GP with special expertise in heart failure (FR), according to the Minnesota coding criteria [18], without knowledge of the patients' clinical status.

The ECG is considered abnormal when one of the following is present; atrial fibrillation, sinus tachycardia (heart rate > 100 beats per minute), left and right bundle branch block (complete and incomplete), left anterior and posterior block, left ventricular hypertrophy, pathological Q-waves suspected for previous myocardial infarction, P-wave abnormalities compatible with left atrial enlargement, ST-segment/T-wave abnormalities, or second or third degree AV block.

Only participants with an abnormal ECG or an elevated blood NTproBNP level will undergo additional echocardiography in the outpatient clinic of the Diakonessenhuis Hospital Zeist. Echocardiography is performed by a single trained and experienced cardiac sonographer (HvdH) using a Philips iE33 imaging system, Andover MA, blinded to the patients' test results of the diagnostic work-up. Guidelines of the American Society of Echocardiography [19,20] will be followed to assess structural and functional cardiac properties. The left ventricular ejection fraction (LVEF) will be assessed quantitatively, or semi-quantitatively when necessary. Multiple diastolic parameters will be measured, including pulsed-wave Doppler of the mitral and pulmonary venous inflow and tissue Doppler imaging of the mitral annulus motion. The ratio of peak early (E) diastolic filling velocity to peak of atrial (A) contraction (E/A ratio) will be calculated. The early diastolic mitral annular velocity (e') will be determined at the septal and lateral wall, and the average of both velocities will be used to calculate the E/e' ratio.

Participants will register the experienced burden of the aforementioned investigations on a visual analogue scale (VAS) (0 = not burdening at all, 10 = extremely burdening).

The participating GPs will receive a first preliminary conclusion about the presence or absence of HF, based on all available information from the diagnostic work up. GPs will be asked to initiate treatment in patients with HF according to their allocation (intervention or care as usual). An expert panel consisting of two cardiologists and a GP will finally establish or exclude HF.

Participants with a newly established diagnosis of HF will be asked to perform a 6MWT [21], and again after six months of follow-up. All participants will be asked to fill out the HRQoL questionnaires again six months after the diagnostic assessment.

In addition, information about medication, HF related appointments with the GP, HF related referrals to the cardiologist, and HF related hospitalization rates will be extracted from the electronic medical files at the GP's office during 12 months of follow-up.

#### Intervention

Patients with newly diagnosed HF will participate in the cluster randomize trial, except for those having a potentially treatable cause of their HF; they will immediately be referred to a cardiologist. All other HF patients will receive either care as usual or management guided by a structured up-titration scheme (intervention) by their own GP.

The GPs randomly allocated to the intervention group will receive a half-day training in the management of HF and the practical application of an up-titration scheme for HF-REF and HF-PEF separately, based on the Dutch GPs' heart failure guideline (NHG-standaard Hartfalen 2005) [22], a Dutch equivalent of the recent ESC Guideline on heart failure [4].

In patients with newly established HF-REF, the up-titration scheme will start with a combination of a diuretic and an ACE-inhibitor, or in case of intolerance to an ACE-inhibitor an ARB. In case of acceptable blood pressures, ACE-inhibitors will be further up-titrated until half of the recommended dose. When patients are in euvolemic state and there are no contra-indications, GPs will then start with up-titration of a beta-blocker. The dosage of the beta-blocker will be increased to either the maximal recommended dose or the maximal tolerated dose. After the up-titration period of the beta-blocker, the GP will try to further increase the dosage of the ACE-inhibitor up to either the maximal recommended dose or maximal tolerated dose.

Patients with newly established HF-PEF will receive optimal blood pressure treatment. An ACE-inhibitor (or

ARB) or low dosages of diuretics will be prescribed. In case of tachycardia such as in atrial fibrillation, the GP will aim to regulate the heart rate, preferably with a beta-blocker. A diuretic will also be prescribed if signs or symptoms of fluid or salt retention are present. See Figure 2 for a simplified version of the initiation- and up-titration scheme for HF patients, and Additional file 1 for the full content of the scheme.

The GPs randomly allocated to the control group will manage patients with a newly screen-detected diagnosis of HF as they are used to (care as usual). They are expected to follow the same Dutch heart failure guideline, however, they will lack the guided up-titration scheme and will not receive a special training.

Referral to a cardiologist is possible at any stage in this pragmatic trial. GPs in both groups will receive instructions about when it is advisable to refer patients for specialist consultation in line with the guidelines on HF, e.g. if patients remain symptomatic after the up-titration phase, in case of complications or adverse effects, and when a novel treatable cause of HF is suspected.

### Outcome measures

#### *Heart failure*

An expert panel, consisting of two cardiologists (AL and ML) and one GP with special expertise in heart failure (FR) will determine the presence or absence of HF based on all diagnostic test results. Consensus diagnosis by an

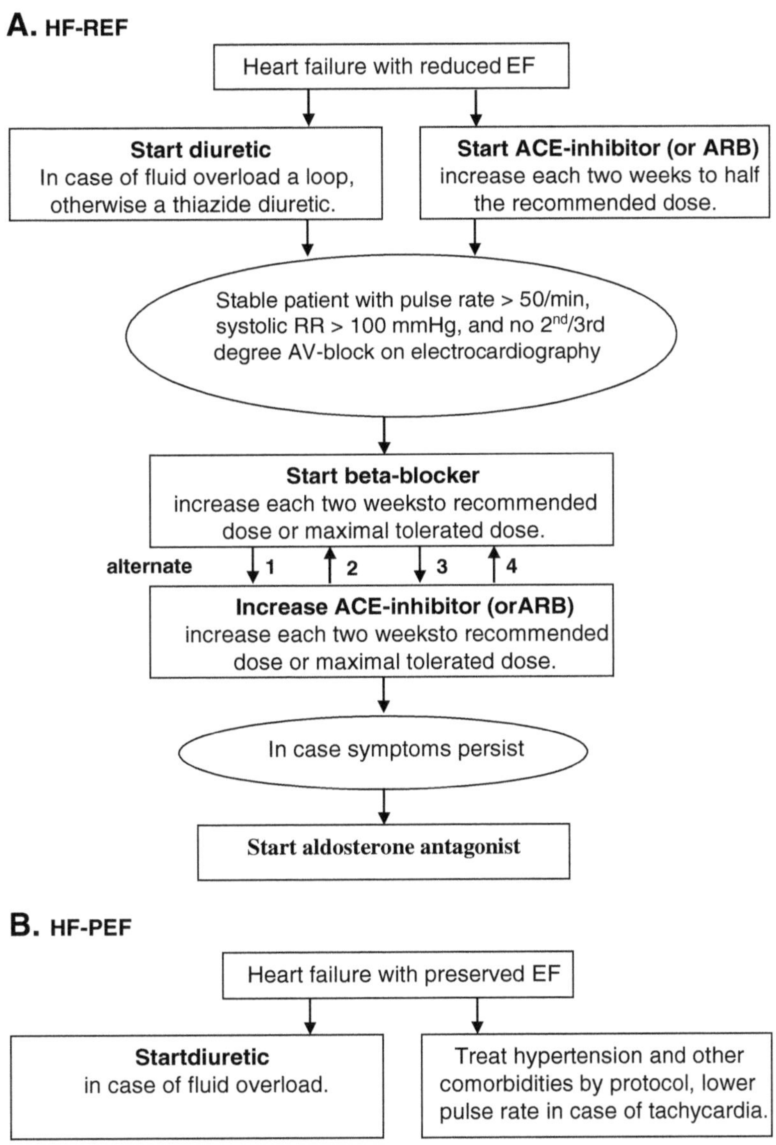


**Figure 2 Simplified version of the treatment scheme for heart failure.** HF-REF = heart failure with reduced ejection fraction, HF-PEF = heart failure with preserved ejection fraction, EF = ejection fraction, ACE = angiotensin converting enzyme, ARB = angiotensin receptor blocker, min = minute, RR = blood pressure, ECG = electrocardiogram, AV-block = atrioventricular block.

outcome panel is the preferred method in case a sufficiently reliable reference standard is lacking, as is the case for HF [7].

The panel moves along three phases in their decision making process; part 1 history taking and physical examination, part 2 adding NTproBNP and ECG, and part 3 adding echocardiography. After part 1 and 2, the panel expresses their suspicion for the presence of HF in a percentage (0-100%). With this approach, we can evaluate which investigations add most in reaching the final decision (set in part 3).

To classify participants as (not) having HF, the panel will follow the latest criteria of the European Society for Cardiology [17]. HF is considered present when participants have suggestive symptoms (typically breathlessness at rest or on exercise, fatigue, tiredness, ankle swelling) and signs (typically tachycardia, tachypnea, pulmonary rales, raised jugular venous pressure, peripheral oedema, laterally displaced apical beat) in combination with objective echocardiographic evidence of cardiac dysfunction at rest. Signs of volume overload could be masked when diuretics are used for hypertension, and therefore in participants on diuretics signs of fluid overload are not mandatory.

Heart failure is further classified in HF-REF, HF-PEF, or isolated right sided HF. Patients in whom signs and symptoms of HF are present in combination with a LVEF ≤ 45%, are classified as having HF-REF. Patients in whom signs and symptoms of HF are present in combination with a LVEF > 45% and echocardiographic evidence of diastolic dysfunction, are classified as having HF-PEF.

The E/e' ratio is regarded as a key parameter for assessing diastolic dysfunction; an E/e' greater than or equal to 15 is considered abnormal, an E/e' value between 9 and 14 indeterminate, and an E/e' less than 9 as normal. In case the E/e' is indeterminate, at least two additional abnormal parameters are needed to establish diastolic dysfunction [20,23]; an E/A ratio below 0.75 or above 1.5, an E-deceleration time >280 ms, a time difference between the duration of the atrial reversal velocity and the late diastolic mitral inflow duration (Ar - A) of more than 30 ms, a left atrial volume index > 34 ml/$m^2$, a left ventricular mass indexed by body surface area > 95 g/$m^2$ in women, and > 115 g/$m^2$ in men (according to the formula of Devereux [24].

A complete assessment of diastolic dysfunction is not possible in participants with atrial fibrillation. In such participants an elevated indexed left atrial volume (≥34 ml/$m^2$) in combination with AF will be considered sufficient to establish diastolic dysfunction.

To diagnose isolated right-sided HF, patients need to have signs and symptoms of HF in combination with a LVEF > 45%, and an increased pulmonary artery pressure (calculated systolic pulmonary artery pressure >40 mmHg), in the absence of (overt) diastolic dysfunction.

By re-assessment of a random sample of 10% by the same outcome panel, blinded to the original decision, the reproducibility of the panel diagnoses will be evaluated.

#### *Functional capacity*

For the elderly HF patient exercise intolerance can be very limiting and of major clinical importance. We chose the 6MWT for the objective evaluation of submaximal functional capacity in patients with newly established HF, because the exercise level is consistent with daily physical activities [21]. The 6MWT is considered a valid, easy, well-tolerated, and inexpensive test [25] that measures the distance that a patient can walk on a flat, hard surface during 6 minutes. The test will be executed according to the guidelines of the American Thoracic Society [21].

#### *Health-related quality of life*

The SF-36 [26,27] and EQ-5D [28,29] were chosen as instruments to measure general health status of all participants. In addition, the scores of the EQ-5D will be converted to a time trade-off utility score to calculate quality-adjusted life years for the cost-effectiveness analysis.

The MLHF questionnaire was added as a condition-specific measurement for HF patients to evaluate the patients' perception of the effects of HF on the physical, socioeconomic and psychological aspects of their life. All questionnaires are well validated and widely used.

#### *Costs*

Relevant cost parameters within and outside the healthcare system will be collected prospectively during a follow-up period of 12 months. Direct costs within the health care system will be monitored through the electronic medical patients files of the GPs, including the costs of further diagnostic testing, time consumption of health care workers (i.e. GP contacts, referrals to medical specialists, hospital admissions), and treatment expenses. Costs outside the healthcare system include the estimation of time-investment and travelling expenses patients make. As the population under study is older than 65 years of age, costs of productivity loss will not be studied. Regarding the standardization of costs, we will use a uniform costing methodology [30].

### Statistical analyses

Prevalence rates of newly established HF-REF, HF-PEF and isolated right sided HF in our population with shortness of breath on exertion will be calculated as proportions with 95% confidence intervals.

Differences in functionality and quality of life after 6 months of follow-up, and uptake of HF medication between both groups after 6 and 12 months of follow-up will be compared taking into account potential difference of relevant parameters at baseline (ANCOVA), although such differences are expected to be minimal because of the randomization procedure. This will be done separately for patients with HF-REF and HF-PEF. A multilevel approach is used in the analyses to correct for the fact that we randomized at the level of the GP and not at the patient level.

The cost-effectiveness of training GPs in the management of HF and the practical application of an up-titration scheme will be evaluated and compared with care as usual. Cost-effectiveness will be expressed in terms of costs per quality-adjusted life year gained (cost-

**Table 1 Baseline characteristics of the 585 participants, divided in the intervention and care as usual group**

| Characteristics | All | Care as usual | Intervention* | |
|---|---|---|---|---|
| | n = 585 | n = 351 (60%) | n = 234 (40%) | p-value |
| General | | | | |
| Mean age in years ± sd | 74.1 ± 6.3 | 73.8 ± 6.1 | 74.4 ± 6.5 | 0.25 |
| Female sex | 319 (54.5) | 181 (51.6) | 138 (59.0) | 0.08 |
| MRC dyspnea score ≥ 3 | 157 (26.8) | 97 (27.6) | 60 (25.6) | 0.59 |
| Cardiovascular comorbidities | | | | |
| Ischemic heart disease | 116 (19.8) | 70 (19.9) | 46 (19.7) | 0.93 |
| Prior myocardial infarction | 43 (7.4) | 27 (7.7) | 16 (6.8) | 0.70 |
| Prior PCI/CABG | 47 (8.0) | 29 (8.3) | 18 (7.7) | 0.80 |
| Vascular comorbidity | 351 (60.0) | 217 (61.8) | 134 (57.3) | 0.27 |
| Hypertension | 310 (53.0) | 196 (55.8) | 114 (48.7) | 0.09 |
| Hypercholesterolemia | 187 (32) | 115 (32.8) | 72 (30.8) | 0.61 |
| Diabetes Mellitus | 79 (13.5) | 47 (13.4) | 32 (13.7) | 0.92 |
| Prior stroke or TIA | 51 (8.7) | 27 (7.7) | 24 (10.3) | 0.28 |
| Peripheral arterial disease | 35 (6.0) | 22 (6.3) | 13 (5.6) | 0.72 |
| Atrial fibrillation | 42 (7.2) | 33 (9.4) | 9 (3.8) | 0.01 |
| Non-cardiovascular comorbidities | | | | |
| Cognitive disorders | 110 (18.8) | 50 (14.2) | 60 (25.6) | 0.001 |
| Asthma/COPD | 323 (55.2) | 200 (57.0) | 123 (52.6) | 0.29 |
| Depression | 72 (12.3) | 39 (11.1) | 33 (14.1) | 0.28 |
| Medication | | | | |
| Loop diuretics | 55 (9.4) | 36 (10.3) | 19 (8.1) | 0.39 |
| Thiazide diuretics | 147 (25.1) | 89 (25.4) | 58 (24.8) | 0.88 |
| ACE-inhibitors | 120 (20.5) | 70 (19.9) | 50 (21.4) | 0.68 |
| ARBs | 128 (21.9) | 83 (23.6) | 45 (19.2) | 0.21 |
| Beta-blockers | 128 (21.9) | 79 (22.5) | 49 (20.9) | 0.65 |
| Digitalis | 5 (0.9) | 4 (1.1) | 1 (0.4) | 0.36 |
| Aldosterone antagonists | 7 (1.2) | 7 (2.0) | 0 (0.0) | 0.03 |
| Oral anticoagulants | 51 (8.7) | 37 (10.5) | 14 (6.0) | 0.06 |
| Antiplatelets | 147 (25.1) | 84 (23.9) | 63 (26.9) | 0.41 |
| Statins | 179 (30.6) | 110 (31.3) | 69 (29.5) | 0.63 |
| Nitrates | 41 (7.0) | 26 (7.4) | 15 (6.4) | 0.64 |
| Calcium channel blockers | 76 (13.0) | 54 (15.4) | 22 (9.4) | 0.04 |

Values are numbers (percentages).
*Intervention = a half-day training in the management of HF and the practical application of an up-titration scheme for HF-REF and HF-PEF.
Sd = standard deviation, MRC = medical research council, PCI = percutaneous coronary intervention, CABG = coronary artery bypass grafting, TIA = transient ischemic attack, COPD = chronic obstructive pulmonary disease, ACE = angiotensin converting enzyme, ARB = angiotensin receptor blocker, HF = heart failure, HF-REF = heart failure with reduced ejection fraction, HF-PEF = heart failure with preserved ejection fraction.

utility analysis). Estimates have to be made in the calculation of the costs and the definition of effects, and these are subjected to different margins of uncertainty. To assess to what extent the results of the analysis depend on prior assumptions and choices made, a sensitivity analysis will be performed conform current Dutch standards for pharmacoeconomic research [31].

### Results of inclusion

Thirty GPs are included in the study, 14 were randomized to the care as usual arm and 16 to the intervention arm. We invited 1,527 elderly patients with shortness of breath on exertion to participate in the study. Of the invited patients, 77% responded, and eventually 38% was willing to participate. Reasons named for non-participation were; expected burden too high (40%), already known to a cardiologist (24%), other demanding health problems (15%), not experiencing shortness of breath anymore (12%), and severe immobility (5%).

Finally, 585 patients signed informed consent and were included in our study. The mean age of the participants was 74.1 (SD ±6.3) years. Stratified by age, 57% was aged between 65 and 74 years, 37% between 75 and 84 years, and 6% was aged 85 years or over. The percentage females was 54.5%. Important comorbidities were pulmonary disease (55.2%), hypertension (53%), hypercholesterolemia (32%), and ischemic heart disease (20%). The 14 GPs in the care as usual arm yielded 351 participants, and the 16 GPs of the up-titration arm 234 participants. Baseline characteristics of included patients divided between both groups are described in Table 1.

## Discussion

The diagnostic part of our study will provide information on the prevalence rate of previously unrecognized HF in older community-dwelling persons with shortness of breath on exertion. The cluster randomized comparison will reveal whether a single half-day training of GPs in the management of HF and the practical appliance of an up-titration scheme results in subsequent improvements in functionality, HRQoL, and uptake of HF medication compared to care as usual. In addition, cost-effectiveness will be examined. We expect that our diagnostic-therapeutic strategy is easy applicable and implementable, and above all, is able to detect a large number of patients with previously unrecognized HF in primary care and optimize their treatment, resulting in increased functional capacity and HRQoL.

### Regulation statement

This study is conducted according to the principles of the current version of the declaration of Helsinki and in accordance with the Dutch law on Medical Research Involving Human Subjects Act (WMO).

### Ethics committee approval

The study was approved by the medical ethical committee (METC) of the University Medical Center Utrecht, the Netherlands.

#### Abbreviations

HF: Heart failure; HF-REF: Heart failure with reduced ejection fraction; ACE: Angiotensin converting enzyme; ARB: Angiotensin receptor blocker; HFPEF: Heart failure with preserved ejection fraction; GP: General practitioner; 6MWT: Six-minute walking test; HRQoL: Health-related quality of life; ECG: Electrocardiogram; NTproBNP: Amino-terminal pro-B-type natriuretic peptide; LVEF: Left ventricular ejection fraction; VAS: Visual analog scale; SF-36: Medical outcomes study 36-item short form health survey; EQ-5D: EuroQol; ANCOVA: Analysis of covariance.

#### Competing interests

All authors declare no competing interests.

#### Authors' contributions

AW and FH designed the study. FH coordinated the study. EvR managed the study and data collection. HvdH performed all echocardiographies. AL, ML and FH were members of the expert panel. EvR conducted the data analyses and wrote the first draft of the manuscript. All authors read and approved the final draft of the manuscript.

#### Acknowledgements

We thank all participating GPs, the personnel of the outpatient clinic of the Julius center (Utrecht, The Netherlands), and the personnel of nursing home Bovenwegen (Zeist, The Netherlands).

The study is conducted with a research grant from the Dutch Heart Foundation ("Nederlandse Hartstichting" project number 2009B048).

#### Author details

[1]Julius Center for Health Sciences and Primary care, University Medical Center Utrecht, PO Box 85500, 3508 AB, Utrecht, The Netherlands.
[2]Diakonessenhuis Zeist, Zeist, The Netherlands.

#### References

1. Schocken DD, Benjamin EJ, Fonarow GC, Krumholz HM, Levy D, Mensah GA, *et al*: **Prevention of heart failure: a scientific statement from the American heart association councils on epidemiology and prevention, clinical cardiology, cardiovascular nursing, and high blood pressure research; quality of care and outcomes research interdisciplinary working group; and functional genomics and translational biology interdisciplinary working group.** *Circulation* 2008, **117:**2544–2565.
2. Levy D, Kenchaiah S, Larson MG, Benjamin EJ, Kupka MJ, Ho KK, *et al*: **Long-term trends in the incidence of and survival with heart failure.** *N Engl J Med* 2002, **347:**1397–1402.
3. Roger VL, Weston SA, Redfield MM, Hellermann-Homan JP, Killian J, Yawn BP, *et al*: **Trends in heart failure incidence and survival in a community-based population.** *JAMA* 2004, **292:**344–350.
4. Dickstein K, Cohen-Solal A, Filippatos G, McMurray JJ, Ponikowski P, Poole-Wilson PA, Strömberg A, *et al*: **ESC guidelines for the diagnosis and treatment of acute and chronic heart failure 2008: the task force for the diagnosis and treatment of acute and chronic heart failure 2008 of the European society of cardiology; developed in collaboration with the**

heart failure association of the ESC (HFA) and endorsed by the European society of intensive care medicine (ESICM). *Eur J Heart Fail* 2008, **10**:933–989.
5. Paulus WJ: **Novel strategies in diastolic heart failure.** *Heart* 2010, **96**:1147–1153.
6. Owan TE, Hodge DO, Herges RM, Jacobsen SJ, Roger VL, Redfield MM: **Trends in prevalence and outcome of heart failure with preserved ejection fraction.** *N Engl J Med* 2006, **355**:251–259.
7. Mosterd A, Hoes AW: **Clinical epidemiology of heart failure.** *Heart* 2007, **93**:1137–1146.
8. Remes J, Miettinen H, Reunanen A, Pyorala K: **Validity of clinical diagnosis of heart failure in primary health care.** *Eur Heart J* 1991, **12**:315–321.
9. Wheeldon NM, MacDonald TM, Flucker CJ, McKendrick AD, McDevitt DG, Struthers AD: **Echocardiography in chronic heart failure in the community.** *Q J Med* 1993, **86**:17–23.
10. Rutten FH, Cramer MJ, Grobbee DE, Sachs AP, Kirkels JH, Lammers JW, *et al*: **Unrecognized heart failure in elderly patients with stable chronic obstructive pulmonary disease.** *Eur Heart J* 2005, **26**:1887–1894.
11. Cleland JG, Cohen-Solal A, Aguilar JC, Dietz R, Eastaugh J, Follath F, *et al*: **Management of heart failure in primary care (the IMPROVEMENT of heart failure programme): an international survey.** *Lancet* 2002, **360**:1631–1639.
12. Rutten FH, Grobbee DE, Hoes AW: **Differences between general practitioners and cardiologists in diagnosis and management of heart failure: a survey in every-day practice.** *Eur J Heart Fail* 2003, **5**:337–344.
13. Rostagno C, Olivo G, Comeglio M, Boddi V, Banchelli M, Galanti G, *et al*: **Prognostic value of 6-minute walk corridor test in patients with mild to moderate heart failure: comparison with other methods of functional evaluation.** *Eur J Heart Fail* 2003, **5**:247–252.
14. Rasekaba T, Lee AL, Naughton MT, Williams TJ, Holland AE: **The six-minute walk test: a useful metric for the cardiopulmonary patient.** *Intern Med J* 2009, **39**:495–501.
15. Spertus J, Peterson E, Conard MW, Heidenreich PA, Krumholz HM, Jones P, *et al*: **Monitoring clinical changes in patients with heart failure: a comparison of methods.** *Am Heart J* 2005, **150**:707–715.
16. Lamberts H, Oskam SK, Okkes IM: **the clinical relationship between symptoms and the final diagnosis in general practice, determined by means of posterior probabilities calculated on the basis of the transition project.** *Ned Tijdschr Geneeskd* 2005, **149**:2566–2572.
17. McMurray JJ, Adamopoulos S, Anker SD, Auricchio A, Bohm M, Dickstein K, *et al*: **ESC guidelines for the diagnosis and treatment of acute and chronic heart failure 2012: the task force for the diagnosis and treatment of acute and chronic heart failure 2012 of the European society of cardiology: developed in collaboration with the heart failure association (HFA) of the ESC.** *Eur J Heart Fail* 2012, **14**:803–869.
18. Rose GA, Blackburn H: *Cardiovascular survey methods.* Geneva: World Health Organisation; 1982.
19. Lang RM, Bierig M, Devereux RB, Flachskampf FA, Foster E, Pellikka PA, *et al*: **Recommendations for chamber quantification: a report from the American society of Echocardiography's guidelines and standards committee and the chamber quantification writing group, developed in conjunction with the European association of echocardiography, a branch of the European society of cardiology.** *J Am Soc Echocardiogr* 2005, **18**:1440–1463.
20. Nagueh SF, Appleton CP, Gillebert TC, Marino PN, Oh JK, Smiseth OA, *et al*: **Recommendations for the evaluation of left ventricular diastolic function by echocardiography.** *J Am Soc Echocardiogr* 2009, **22**:107–133.
21. ATS Committee on Proficiency Standards for Clinical Pulmonary Function Laboratories: **ATS statement: guidelines for the six-minute walk test.** *Am J Respir Crit Care Med* 2002, **166**:111–117.
22. Rutten FH, Walma EP, Kruizinga GI, Bakx HCA, Van Lieshout J: **NHG-standaard hartfalen.** *Huisarts Wet* 2005, **48**(2):64–76.
23. Paulus WJ, Tschope C, Sanderson JE, Rusconi C, Flachskampf FA, Rademakers FE, *et al*: **How to diagnose diastolic heart failure: a consensus statement on the diagnosis of heart failure with normal left ventricular ejection fraction by the heart failure and echocardiography associations of the European society of cardiology.** *Eur Heart J* 2007, **28**:2539–2550.
24. Devereux RB, Reichek N: **Echocardiographic determination of left ventricular mass in man: anatomic validation of the method.** *Circulation* 1977, **55**:613–618.
25. Pollentier B, Irons SL, Benedetto CM, Dibenedetto AM, Loton D, Seyler RD, *et al*: **Examination of the six minute walk test to determine functional capacity in people with chronic heart failure: a systematic review.** *Cardiopulm Phys Ther J* 2010, **21**:13–21.
26. Aaronson NK, Muller M, Cohen PD, Essink-Bot ML, Fekkes M, Sanderman R, *et al*: **Translation, validation, and norming of the dutch language version of the SF-36 health survey in community and chronic disease populations.** *J Clin Epidemiol* 1998, **51**:1055–1068.
27. McHorney CA, Ware JE Jr, Raczek AE: **The MOS 36-item short-form health survey (SF-36): II psychometric and clinical tests of validity in measuring physical and mental health constructs.** *Med Care* 1993, **31**:247–263.
28. EuroQol Group: **EuroQol–a new facility for the measurement of health-related quality of life.** *Health Policy* 1990, **16**:199–208.
29. Brooks R: **EuroQol: the current state of play.** *Health Policy* 1996, **37**:53–72.
30. Oostenbrink JB, Koopmanschap MA, Rutten FF: **Standardisation of costs: the dutch manual for costing in economic evaluations.** *Pharmacoeconomics* 2002, **20**:443–454.
31. Health Insurance Council: *Dutch guidelines for pharmacoeconomic research.* Amstelveen: Ziekenfondsraad; 1999.

# 2

# Prevalence of heart failure in Australia

Berhe W. Sahle[1,2], Alice J. Owen[1], Mutsa P. Mutowo[3], Henry Krum[1] and Christopher M. Reid[1,4*]

**Abstract**

**Background:** In the absence of a systematic collection of data pertaining to heart failure, summarizing the data available from individual studies provides an opportunity to estimate the burden of heart failure. The present study systematically reviewed the literature to estimate the incidence and prevalence rates of heart failure in Australia.

**Methods:** Studies reporting on prevalence or incidence of heart failure published between 1990 and 2015 were identified through a systematic search of Embase, PubMed, Ovid Medline, MeSH, Scopus and websites of the Australian Institute of Health, and Welfare and Australian Bureau of Statistics.

**Results:** The search yielded a total of 4978 records, of which thirteen met the inclusion criteria. There were no studies reporting on the incidence of heart failure. The prevalence of heart failure in the Australian population ranged between 1.0 % and 2.0 %, with a significant proportion of cases being previously undiagnosed. The burden of heart failure was higher among Indigenous than non-Indigenous Australians (age-standardized prevalence rate ratio of 1.7). Heart failure was prevalent in women than men, and in rural and remote regions than in the metropolitan and capital territories.

**Conclusion:** This systematic review highlights the limited available data on the epidemiology of heart failure in Australia. Population level studies, using standardized approaches, are needed in order to precisely describe the burden of HF in the population.

**Keywords:** Heart failure, Incidence, Prevalence, Indigenous, Australia

## Background

Heart failure (HF) causes a significant burden for patients and healthcare systems in developed countries [1, 2]. Approximately 50–75 % of patients with HF die within five years of diagnosis [3, 4]. Evidence shows that HF accounts for 1–3 % of overall healthcare spending, mainly due to repeated hospital admissions and prolonged in-patient length of stay [1]. In developed countries, prevalence of HF ranges from 1–3 %, rising to 10 % or more in those aged 75 years or older [1, 2], while estimates in developing countries are not routinely reported.

The relationship between obesity, hypertension, smoking and cholesterol with cardiovascular morbidity is undisputed. Australia has made significant attempts to address risk factors contributing to the onset of chronic diseases [5]. Public health policy on tobacco control, improvements in surgical treatment and the widespread use of lipid and blood pressure-lowering drugs have resulted in a significant decline in the burden of major cardiovascular diseases [5–8]. Despite these improvements, the burden of diabetes and obesity in the population has steadily increased over time [7].

Data on the incidence of HF is not reported in the Australian Institute of Health and Welfare (AIHW) periodic statistics [9], while the Australian National Health Surveys (NHS) report prevalence rates based on self-report [10]. However, self-reported data may underestimate the true burden of HF because the early stages of HF may be only mildly symptomatic; therefore many people may be unaware that they have the condition [7]. Similarly, estimation based on mortality data may under-report the actual burden of HF, as the international classification of diseases (ICD) recommends coding underlying causes of death such as ischemic heart diseases rather than HF, which is often the

* Correspondence: chris.reid@monash.edu
[1]Centre of Cardiovascular Research and Education in Therapeutics, Department of Epidemiology and Preventive Medicine, Monash University, 99 Commercial Road, Melbourne, Vic 3004, Australia
[4]School of Public Health, Curtin University, Perth, Australia
Full list of author information is available at the end of the article

terminal illness of other cardiovascular diseases [10, 11]. Variation in the definition of HF and process of estimation therefore limit the validity and utility of data from these sources [9, 10].

Despite the morbidity and economic burden to the community and poor patient outcomes, there is a deficiency in the systematic collection of data pertaining the incidence and prevalence of HF. Therefore, summarizing the data available from individual studies provides an opportunity to estimate the burden of HF. The present study systematically reviewed the literature to estimate the incidence and prevalence rates of heart failure in Australia.

## Methods

### Literature search

The process of the review was designed and undertaken according to the Preferred Reporting Items for Systematic Reviews and Meta-Analyses (Additional file 1) guidelines [12]. We searched Embase, PubMed, Ovid Medline, MeSH, and Scopus for articles published under subject terms: heart failure, cardiac failure, congestive heart failure, chronic heart failure, left ventricular dysfunction, systolic heart failure, diastolic heart failure combined with epidemiology, incidence, prevalence, burden and morbidity. The search was limited to articles published in the Australian population in English, between September 1990 and 20 July 2015 (Additional file 2: Table S1). Relevant studies on the prevalence and incidence of HF in Australia were included. We further searched the AIHW and Australian Bureau of Statistics (ABS) websites to identify relevant datasets and reports.

### Study selection

Figure 1 summarises the selection process for the studies. Publications retrieved from all databases were organized in Endnote and duplicate publications were removed (by BW). Two reviewers (BWS and MPM) independently reviewed abstracts and full text citations to screen

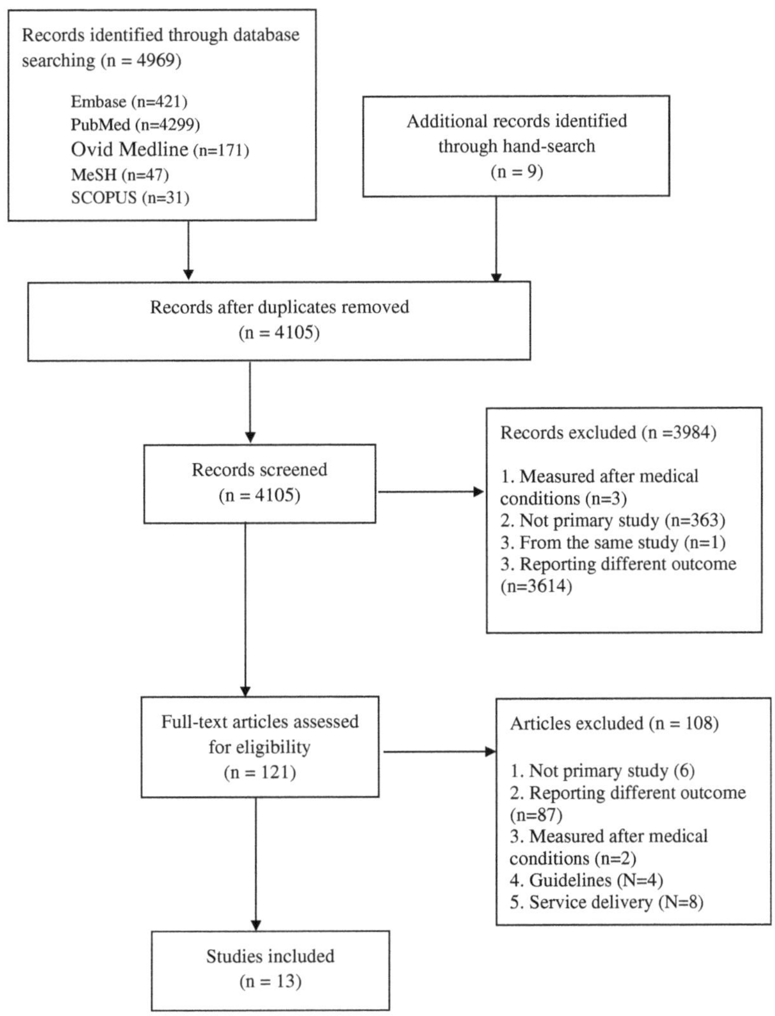


**Fig. 1** PRISMA flow diagram of selection process

for eligibility. The reviewers had no difference regarding to the selection of eligible publications. Studies were eligible if: (1) reported on prevalence or incidence of HF in Australia; (2) not clinical trials or therapeutic studies; (3) and conducted on patients with pre-existing medical conditions such as hypertension and coronary heart disease.

### Data extraction and summarisation

A summary table was prepared to ensure that all relevant data including type of study, sample size, sampling methods, age and sex of the participants, year of study, scope of the study (national or single center), method of diagnosis, and the primary outcomes (incidence and prevalence rates) were extracted. Tables 1 and 2 provides a summary of the studies included in the review. Due to heterogeneity in data sources and design of the individual studies, data were summarised narratively.

### Quality assessment

Quality of the studies selected for the review were assessed using a checklist comprising the items recommended by Sanderson et al. [13]. The items in the checklist include: appropriate source population; measurement methods; methods outlined to deal with any design-specific issues such as recall bias, interviewer bias, biased loss to follow or blinding; design and/or analytical methods; and appropriate use of statistics for primary analysis of effect. Each criterion was given a score of zero or one, which was then summed in to summary score (0 to 5). The score for each article was an average value of the score assigned by two independent reviewers (BWS and DM Emdadul Hoque). The studies selected for the review had an overall quality score of three or more out of five. This study used publicly available data which does not require ethical approval.

## Results

### Description of studies

The search yielded 4978 citations. After screening the titles and abstracts and removing duplicates, 121 studies remained for the full text review. Thirteen studies which met the inclusion criteria were selected (Tables 1 and 2). Ten were cross-sectional studies [14–23], and three studies extrapolated data from other countries to the Australian population [24–26].

### Participants and method of diagnosis

Six studies recruited participants from the community [14–16, 19, 21, 22] three from clinical settings [17, 18, 20] and the remainder used administrative data [14, 23, 25, 26]. Five studies were conducted in adults (≥18 years) [14–16, 22], two in those 60 years or over [19, 20], two in all age groups [17, 18], with participant's age not specified in the reminder [23–26]. Heart failure was defined based self-report [14–16, 22], echocardiography (and physical assessment) [19, 21], using modified World Health Organization criteria [20] while the rest used administrative data [17, 18, 23, 25, 26] (Tables 1 and 2).

**Table 1** Studies reporting prevalence of heart failure

| Author | Participants | Type of study | Method of diagnosis | Prevalence (%) | | | Quality rating |
|---|---|---|---|---|---|---|---|
| | | | | Male | Female | Total | |
| Abhayaratna 2006 [19] | 1275 random sample, aged 60–86 years | Cross sectional | physical examination, and Echo | 8.2 | 4.4 | 6.3 | 4 |
| Knox 2008 [17] | 9156 of all ages, selected from 305 GP centers | Multi-center Cross sectional | Medical record | - | - | 1.8 | 4.1 |
| Harrison 2013 [18] | 8707 of all ages selected from 290 GP centers | Multi-center, Cross sectional | Medical record | - | - | 1.5 | 4 |
| NHS 2004/5 [14] | National survey on ≥18 y | National survey | Self-report | 0.9 | 1.8 | 1.4 | 3 |
| NHS 2007/8 [15] | National survey on ≥18 y | National survey | Self-report | 1.0 | 1.7 | 1.3 | 3 |
| NHS 2011/12 [16] | National survey on ≥18 y | National survey | Self-report | 1.0 | 1.5 | 1.2 | 3 |
| NATSIHS 2008 [22] | National survey on ≥18 y aboriginals | Survey | Self-report | 1.74 | 2.88 | 1.0 | |
| McGrady 2012 [21] | 436 random sample >18 yrs | Cross sectional | Echo | 7 | 4 | 5.3 | 4.3 |
| Clark 2004 [26] | No mentioned | Cross sectional | administrative data | - | - | 2.0 | 3.0 |
| Clark 2005 [23] | No mentioned | Cross sectional | administrative data | - | - | 1.8 | 3.3 |
| Clark 2007 [20] | 23845, ≥60 yrs selected from 341 general practice | Cross sectional | WHO criteria | - | - | 13.1 | 3.5 |

*CHF* congestive heart failure, *GP* general practice, *NHS* national health survey, *WHO* World Health Organization, *NATSIHS* national aboriginal and torres strait islander health survey, *Echo* echocardiography

**Table 2** Studies reporting prevalence of heart failure by geographic locations

| Author | Sample size | Geographic stratum (%) | Quality rating |
|---|---|---|---|
| Clark 2004 [26] | Not mentioned | Central and west Australia (28.8–79.9 per 1000) | 3.2 |
| | | Queensland, New South Wales, Western Australia (20.3–28.7 per 1000) | |
| Clark 2005 [23] | Not mentioned | Australian Capital Territory (14 per 1000) | 3.3 |
| | | Northern Territory (29.5 per 1000) | |
| McGrady 2012 | 436 random sample >18 yrs | Urban (6 %) Remote (4 %) | 4.3 |
| Clark 2007 [20] | 23845, ≥60 yrs selected from 341 GP center | Capital cities and metropolitan (12.4 %) | 3.5 |
| | | Large and small rural towns (16.1 %) | |
| | | Other rural and remote areas (13.9 %) | |

#### Incidence of heart failure

There were no studies reporting the incidence of HF in Australia. According to the AHIW (based up on extrapolation of incidence rates from large scale international cohorts to the Australian population characteristics) an estimated 30,000 new cases of HF are diagnosed each year in Australia [24], which translates in to a crude incidence rate of 2.1 per 1000 population.

#### Prevalence of heart failure

Prevalence of HF was reported in twelve studies [14–23, 25, 26]. Based on self-report, the prevalence of HF and oedema in adults was estimated to be 1.4 % in the 2004/5, 1.3 % in the 2007/8, and 1.2 % in the 2011/12 National Health Surveyes [14–16].

The national population prevalence of HF was reported in four studies, ranging from 1.5–2.0 % [17, 18, 20, 26]. Two studies reported the prevalence of chronic conditions among a sample of 9156 [17] and 8707 [18] general practice patients adjusted for the Australian population. In these studies the prevalence of HF in the population was estimated to be 1.8 % [17] and 1.5 % [18], respectively. In the third study, HF data were derived by applying international HF prevalence data to the Australian population [25]. The study reported a national prevalence of 17.9 per 1000 [25]. Slightly higher prevalence rate (2.0 %) was also reported in a similar study, which extrapolated HF data from Scotland and United Kingdom to the Australian popaultion [26].

In the Canberra Heart Study, which screened 1275 people aged 60–86 years old, 6.7 % (95 % CI: 4.4 %-7.1 %) of them had HF and 0.6 % (95 % CI: 0.3 %-1.2 %) of these were previously undiagnosed [19]. In the same study, the prevalence of HF ranged between 3.1 % in those 60–64 years old to 13.6 % in those 80–86 years old [19]. In another study on a sample of 23845 general practice patients aged 60 years and over, HF was reported in 13.1 % of them comprising previously diagnosed cases (prevalence, 11.2 %) and newly diagnosed cases (prevalence, 1.9 %) [20] However, this rate was not adjusted for the general population.

In a study that screened 436 indigenous adults (18 years or over), HF was diagnosed in 5.3 % of them, of which 65 % were previously undiagnosed [21]. In the 2004/5 National Aboriginal and Torres Strait Islander Health Survey (NATSIHS) [22] the prevalence of HF among Indigenous Australians was 1.0 %. However, following age-standardization the prevalence of HF was 1.7 times higher among Indigenous than non-Indigenous Australians [22].

#### Heart failure by gender

In the NHS [14–16, 22] HF was almost twice common in women than in men. Prevalence rates were 0.89 % vs 1.8 % in the 2004/5 NHS, 1.0 % vs 1.7 % in the NHS 2007/8 and 1.0 % vs 1.5 % in the NHS 2011/12 in men and women, respectively [14–16]. Similarly, in the 2004/5 NATSIHS, the age-standardized prevalence of HF was 17.4 per 1000 in men and 28.8 per 1000 in women [22]. On the other hand, In the Canberra Heart Study, HF was twice as common in men (8.2 %) than in women (4.4 %) [19]. Similarly, the prevalence of HF was 7.0 % in male and 4.0 % in female adult Indigenous Australians [21].

#### Heart failure by geographic location

Four studies reported on HF by geographic location [20, 21, 23, 25]. Clark and colleagues reported a higher prevalence of HF in large and small rural towns (16.1 %) than in the capital city and metropolitan areas (12.4 %) [20]. In the second study, prevalence rates ranged between 2.9 % and 7.8 % in Central and Western Australia and between 2.0 % and 2.9 % in parts of Queensland, New South Wales, and Western Australia [23]. The prevalence of HF also varied from 14 per 1000 in the Australian Capital Territory compared to 29 per 1000 in rural Northern Territory [25]. McGrady and colleagues also reported higher in prevalence of HF in urban Aboriginals (6.0 %) than those in remote communities (4.0 %) [21].

## Discussion

Our findings indicate that the prevalence of HF in the Australian population ranges from 1.0–2.0 %, and varies by Indigenous status, gender, age, and geographic location. The burden of HF was higher among Indigenous than non-Indigenous Australians, and in rural and remote than in capital city and metropolitan areas. In most of the studies reviewed, HF was more prevalent in women than in men.

As indicated in the AIHW reports, there are no studies reporting on the incidence of HF. [7] The only data available was the number of new cases of HF diagnosed each year, estimated based on overseas data, which may not be generalizable to the population due to limitations inherent to the process of extrapolation [24].

Our findings of the prevalence of HF in Australia (1.0–2.0 %) is congruent with data from Europe and North America where prevalence of HF range between 1.3 % and 2.2 % [1, 27–29]. Consistent with existing knowledge [30, 31] HF was three or more times higher in the elderly than in the population. In general, the NHS [14–16] reported a lower prevalence of HF compared with the individual studies [17, 18, 20, 26] which may be related to the use of self-reported diagnosis in the NHS [7]. The significant proportion of previously undiagnosed HF patients [19, 21] also reveal a chance of underestimation when HF is defined based on self-reported diagnosis.

In most of the studies [14–16, 22] HF was twice more prevalent in women than men, although men were more affected than women in two other studies [19, 21]. The inconsistency in the prevalence of HF by gender has been reported in several studies [3, 32, 33]. In Australia, major risk factors of HF including coronary heart diseases, diabetes, and high blood pressure are higher in men than in women [7, 34]. However, risk factors of HF such as diabetes, hypertension, and left ventricular dysfunction have stronger risk of progression to HF in women than men, which may explain the higher prevalence of HF among women [30, 35]. The higher burden of HF among women could be also be attributed to the longer life expectancy and higher incidence of HF in later years of life in women than men [36].

The higher prevalence of HF among Indigenous Australians is consistent with the existing literature. The latest Australian statistics shows that cardiovascular diseases are 1.3 times more common among Indigenous than their non-Indigenous counterparts [8]. The excess burden of HF, cardiovascular diseases in general, in Indigenous population is related to the overall disparity in the social and economic status that impact on their health status [22]. The risk factors of HF are also reported to be more prevalent among Indigenous population than the nationally reported data [21].

According to previous studies [22, 25] the disproportionately higher burden of HF in rural and remote towns is related to the concentration of older age inhabitants and higher prevalence of socio-demographic risk factors in these regions. Indigenous Australians, who have higher prevalence of HF also concentrate in rural and remote towns [25]. The comparatively lower access to healthcare services in rural and remote regions, which may affect early identification and management of the risk factors predisposing to HF, could also contribute to the geographic disparity [20, 23, 25].

The syndrome of HF has different causes and diverse clinical presentations, and long-term clinical evolution that makes its diagnosis challenging [1, 37]. Studies based on self-reported diagnosis are likely to underestimate the burden of HF because participants may not know their HF status [37, 38]. Limitations inherent to use of administrative data such misclassification may also compromise the validity of HF data from such studies. Therefore the overall estimate of the burden of HF is likely to be affected by the use of different definitions and measurement methods for HF.

This systematic review has some limitations. There were limited studies on epidemiology of HF in Australia and therefore studies that used varying HF definition (such as heart failure and oedema) were included in the review. Due to the limited number of studies, further description of the pattern of HF over time was not possible. Moreover, the search was restricted to PubMed indexed journals, and unpublished reports. As a result, articles published non-PubMed indexed journals may have been missed. Despite these limitations, the current review still provides valuable information on the prevalence of HF in the Australian population. Extensive and systematic literature search using pre-defined quality assessment and inclusion criteria were employed.

## Conclusions

This review shows that the prevalence heart failure in Australia is similar to other developed countries, however it has a significant burden in specific demographic profiles in the country, namely Indigenous groups, females and those who reside in rural and remote areas. Further population-level studies, with clearly defined method of diagnosis, are needed for a more accurate description of the burden of HF in Australia.

**Competing interests**

The authors declare that they have no competing interests.

**Authors' contribution**

BWS, AJO, MPM, HK, and CMR contributed to the conception of the study, participated in writing the manuscript. BWS: performed the literature search.

BWS and MMP: screened publications and selected eligible studies. All authors read and approved the final manuscript.

**Acknowledgements**
We are grateful to DM Emdadul Hoque Department of Epidemiology and Preventive Medicine, Monash University, for his assistance in assessing the quality of the publications included in the review. This work was supported by a NHMRC Program Grant (1092642) awarded to HK and CMR. CMR is supported by a Research Fellowship from the National Health and Medical Research Council of Australia (NHMRC). The funding bodies had no role in the design and conduct of the study, the collection, management, analysis and interpretation of the data, or the preparation, review, or approval of the manuscript.

**Author details**
[1]Centre of Cardiovascular Research and Education in Therapeutics, Department of Epidemiology and Preventive Medicine, Monash University, 99 Commercial Road, Melbourne, Vic 3004, Australia. [2]School of Public Health, Mekelle University, Mekelle, Ethiopia. [3]School of Public Health, Department of Epidemiology and Preventive Medicine, Monash University, Melbourne, Australia. [4]School of Public Health, Curtin University, Perth, Australia.

**References**

1. Ponikowski P, Anker SD, AlHabib KF, Cowie MR, Force TL, Hu S, et al. Heart failure: preventing disease and death worldwide. ESC Heart Failure. 2014;1:425.
2. McMurray JJV, Stewart S. The burden of heart failure. Eur Heart J Supplements. 2002;4:D50–8.
3. Bleumink GS, Knetsch AM, Sturkenboom MC, Straus SM, Hofman A, Deckers JW, et al. Quantifying the heart failure epidemic: prevalence, incidence rate, lifetime risk and prognosis of heart failure. The Rotterdam Study. Eur Heart J. 2004;25: 1614–9.
4. Hobbs FD, Roalfe AK, Davis RC, Davies MK, Hare R. Midlands Research Practices Consortium (MidReC). Prognosis of all-cause heart failure and borderline left ventricular systolic dysfunction: 5 year mortality follow-up of the Echocardiographic Heart of England Screening Study (ECHOES). Eur Heart J. 2007;28:1128–34.
5. Willcox S. Chronic diseases in Australia: the case for changing course. Background and policy paper No. 02/2014. Melbourne, Mitchell Institute. Available at: http://www.mitchellinstitute.org.au/reports/chronic-diseases-in-australia-the-case-for-changing-course/ [Cited 28 September 2015].
6. Reid CM. Cardiovascular diseases in Australia: calm before a new storm? Clin Exp Pharmacol Physiol. 2013;40(6):345–6.
7. Australian Institute of Health and Welfare. Cardiovascular disease, diabetes and chronic kidney disease— Australian facts: Prevalence and incidence. In: Cardiovascular, diabetes and chronic kidney disease series no. 2. Cat. no. CDK 2. Canberra: AIHW; 2014.
8. Waters A-M, Trinh L, Chau T, Bourchier M, Moon L. Latest statistics on cardiovascular disease in Australia. Clin Exp Pharmacol Physiol. 2013;40:347–56.
9. Woods JA, Katzenellenbogen JM, Davidson PM, Thompson SC. Heart failure among indigenous Australians: a systematic review. BMC Cardiovasc Disord. 2012;12:99.
10. Snyder ML, Love SA, Sorlie PD, Rosamond WD, Antini C, Metcalf PA, et al. Redistribution of heart failure as the cause of death: the Atherosclerosis Risk in Communities Study. Popul Health Metr. 2014;12:10.
11. Inglis SC, Clark RA, Shakib S, Wong DT, Molaee P, Wilkinson D, et al. Hot summers and heart failure: seasonal variations in morbidity and mortality in Australian heart failure patients (1994–2005). Eur J Heart Fail. 2008;10:540–9.
12. Moher D, Liberati A, Tetzlaff J, Altman D, The PRISMA Group. Preferred Reporting Items for Systematic Reviews and Meta-Analyses: the PRISMA statement. PLoS Med. 2009;6(6):e1000097.
13. Sanderson S, Tatt ID, Higgins JP. Tools for assessing quality and susceptibility to bias in observational studies in epidemiology: a systematic review and annotated bibliography. Int J Epidemiol. 2007;36:666–76.
14. Australian Bureau of Statistics, National Health Survey: Summary of results 2004–05. Cat. no. 4364.0.Canberra:ABS;2006.
15. Australian Bureau of Statistics, National Health Survey: Summary of Results, 2007–2008 (Reissue). Cat. no. 43640DO020_20072008. Canberra: ABS;2009.
16. Australian Bureau of Statistics, National Health Survey: First Results, 2011–12. Cat. no. 43640DO003_20112012. Canberra: ABS; 2012.
17. Knox SA, Harrison CM, Britt HC, Henderson J. Estimating prevalence of common chronic morbidities in Australia. Med J Aust. 2008;189:66–70.
18. Harrison C, Britt H, Miller G, Henderson J. Prevalence of chronic conditions in Australia. PloS One. 2013;8:e67494.
19. Abhayaratna WP, Smith WT, Becker NG, Marwick TH, Jeffery IM, McGill DA. Prevalence of heart failure and systolic ventricular dysfunction in older Australians: the Canberra Heart Study. Med J Aust. 2006;184:151–4.
20. Clark RA, Eckert KA, Stewart S, Phillips SM, Yallop JJ, Tonkin AM, et al. Rural and urban differentials in primary care management of chronic heart failure: new data from the CASE study. Med J Aust. 2007;186:441–5.
21. McGrady M, Krum H, Carrington MJ, Stewart S, Zeitz C, Lee GA, et al. Heart failure, ventricular dysfunction and risk factor prevalence in Australian aboriginal peoples: the Heart of the Heart Study. Heart. 2012;98(21):1562–7.
22. AIHW, Penm E. Cardiovascular disease and its associated risk factors in Aboriginal and Torres Strait Islander peoples 2004–05. In: Cardiovascular disease series no. 29. Cat. no. CVD 41. Canberra: Australian Institute of Health and Welfare; 2008.
23. Clark RA, Driscoll A, Nottage J, McLenan S, Coombie DM, Bamford EJ, et al. Inequitable provision of optimal services for patients with chronic heart failure: a national geo-mapping study. Med J Aust. 2007;186:169e73.
24. AIHW: Field B. Heart failure…what of the future? Bulletin no. 6. AIHW Cat. No. AUS 34. Canberra: AIHW; 2003.
25. Clark RA, McLennan S, Eckert K, Dawson A, Wilkinson D, Stewart S. Chronic heart failure beyond city limits. Rural Remote Health. 2005;5:443.
26. Clark RA, McLennan S, Dawson A, Wilkinson D, Stewart S. Uncovering a hidden epidemic: a study of the current burden of heart failure in Australia. Heart Lung Circ. 2004;13:266–73.
27. Quach S, Blais C, Quan H. Administrative data have high variation in validity for recording heart failure. Can J Cardiol. 2010;26(8):306–12.
28. Zarrinkoub R, Wettermark B, Wändell P, Mejhert M, Szulkin R, Ljunggren G, et al. The epidemiology of heart failure, based on data for 2.1 million inhabitants in Sweden. Eur J Heart Fail. 2013;15(9):995–1002.
29. Valle R, Baccichetto R, Barro S, Calderan A, Carbonieri E, Chinellato M, et al. Heart failure in Eastern Veneto: prevalence, hospitalization rate, adherence to guidelines and social costs. Monaldi Arch Chest Dis. 2006;66(1):63–74.
30. Bui AL, Horwich TB, Fonarow GC. Epidemiology and risk profile of heart failure. Nat Rev Cardiol. 2011;8:30–41.
31. Bhatnagar P, Williams J, Townsend N. The epidemiology of cardiovascular disease in the United Kingdom 2014. Heart 2015 doi:10.1136/heartjnl- 2015–307516
32. Mehta PA, Cowie MR. Gender and heart failure: a population perspective. Heart. 2006;92 suppl 3:iii14–8.
33. Patten RD. Models of gender differences in cardiovascular disease. Drug Discov Today Dis Models. 2007;4(4):227–32.
34. Nichols M, Peterson K, Herbert J, Allender S. Australian heart disease statistics. Overweight, obesity and cardiovascular disease – past, present and future. Melbourne: National Heart Foundation of Australia;2015.
35. Meredith PA, Ostergren J. From hypertension to heart failure – are there better primary prevention strategies? J Renin Angiotensin Aldosterone Syst. 2006;7:64–73.
36. Lenzen MJ, Rosengren A, OP Reimer WJMS, Follath F, Boersma E, Simoons ML, et al. Management of patients with heart failure in clinical practice: differences between men and women. Heart. 2008;94:e10.
37. Adams Jr KF, Zannad F, France N. Clinical definition and epidemiology of advanced heart failure. Am Heart J. 1998;135:S-204–15.
38. Krum H, Abraham WT. Heart failure. Lancet. 2009;373:941–55.

3

# A comparison of risk factors for mortality from heart failure in Asian and non-Asian populations: An overview of individual participant data from 32 prospective cohorts from the Asia-Pacific Region

Rachel R Huxley[1*], Federica Barzi[2], Jean Woo[3], Graham Giles[4], Tai Hing Lam[5], Kazem Rahimi[6,7], Suma Konety[8], Takayoshi Ohkubo[9], Sun Ha Jee[10], Xianghua Fang[11], Mark Woodward[2,12] and Asia Pacific Cohort Studies Collaboration

## Abstract

**Background:** Most of what is known regarding the epidemiology of mortality from heart failure (HF) comes from studies within Western populations with few data available from the Asia-Pacific region where the burden of heart failure is increasing.

**Methods:** Individual level data from 543694 (85% Asian; 36% female) participants from 32 cohorts in the Asia Pacific Cohort Studies Collaboration were included in the analysis. Adjusted hazard ratios (HR) and 95% confidence intervals (CI) for mortality from HF were estimated separately for Asians and non-Asians for a quintet of cardiovascular risk factors: systolic blood pressure, diabetes, body mass index, cigarette smoking and total cholesterol. All analyses were stratified by sex and study.

**Results:** During 3,793,229 person years of follow-up there were 614 HF deaths (80% Asian). The positive associations between elevated blood pressure, obesity, and cigarette smoking were consistent for Asians and non-Asians. There was evidence to indicate that diabetes was a weaker risk factor for death from HF for Asians compared with non-Asians: HR 1.26 (95% CI: 0.74-2.13) versus 3.04 (95% CI 1.76-5.25) respectively; p for interaction = 0.022. Additional adjustment for covariates did not materially change the overall associations. There was no good evidence to indicate that total cholesterol was a risk factor for HF mortality in either population.

**Conclusions:** Most traditional cardiovascular risk factors including elevated blood pressure, obesity and cigarette smoking appear to operate similarly to increase the risk of death from HF in Asians and non-Asians populations alike.

**Keywords:** Meta-analysis, Heart failure, Epidemiology

* Correspondence: r.huxley@uq.edu.au
[1]Epidemiology & Biostatistics Division, School of Population Health, University of Queensland, Brisbane, Australia
Full list of author information is available at the end of the article

## Background

Heart failure (HF) is a complex syndrome with a multifactorial aetiology and is a major cause of death and disability in higher-income countries where it is estimated that 2% of adults are affected [1]. The incidence of HF is strongly age-related so that the prevalence of the condition rises to 6-10% in those over 65 years of age [1]. In the United States (US) alone, an estimated 550,000 new cases occur annually [2] and in 2008, 1 in 9 death certificates mentioned heart failure [3]. Globally, it has been estimated that 23 million individuals worldwide have HF [4] although this may be an underestimate given the lack of reliable population-based studies of the prevalence and incidence of HF for Asia and elsewhere [5,6]. What data there are from Asia suggest that hospitalization for HF is increasing in the region [7,8].

Our knowledge regarding the causes of HF has chiefly been derived from studies from the US [9] and Europe [10] with relatively few data from less developed parts of the world including Asia [11]. As with other forms of cardiovascular disease, the major lifestyle risk factors for HF are reported to include elevated blood pressure, obesity, smoking, and diabetes [12]. Whether these risk factors exert the same effect on Asian populations that tend to have markedly different risk factor profiles compared with non-Asians [13] remains to be determined. In this paper we report on the associations between traditional cardiovascular risk factors and mortality from HF in the Asia-Pacific region and contextualize these findings with respect to the current literature using data from the Asia Pacific Cohort Studies Collaboration (APCSC) [14,15].

## Methods

### Ethics approval

All of the individual studies that participated in APCSC obtained ethics approval from their own ethics approval boards. All participants were aged 18 or over and provided informed consent in accordance with the principles of the Declaration of Helsinki.

Details of the APCSC have been described elsewhere [14,15]. In brief, a study was eligible for inclusion if the population was drawn from the Asia Pacific region; it had a prospective cohort study design without selection being consequent to pre-existing disease; it had accumulated at least 5000 person-years of follow-up; date of birth (or age), sex and blood pressure were recorded at baseline; and date or age at death was recorded during follow-up. Cohorts were excluded if they were based on a positive disease history or diagnosis. Cohorts were classified as Asian if the participants were recruited from mainland China, Hong Kong, South Korea, Japan or Taiwan, and Australian if the cohorts were recruited within Australia. The majority of cohorts were population-based but several of the cohorts were sourced from occupational settings (e.g. KMIC, Guangzhou Occupational, Beijing Steelworkers, and Civil Service Workers).

In most studies, blood pressure was measured at rest in the seated position using a standard mercury sphygmomanometer [16]. TC was obtained using previously described methods [17]. Body mass index (BMI) was calculated as weight (kg) divided by squared height ($m^2$) [18]. The diabetes status of individual participants was determined on the basis of a self-reported history of diabetes at baseline or by applying the World Health Organization (WHO) criteria to baseline blood glucose levels [19]. Cigarette smoking was classified based on self-report at baseline as 'ever' versus 'never' smoking [20].

### End-point

Most studies used database linkage to identify deaths, while others also included scheduled follow-up visits or examined hospital records Information on fatal events was classified according to the Ninth Revision of the International Classification of Diseases (ICD-9). The end point considered in this analysis was fatal HF (ICD-9 428). Data quality of the individual cohorts was centrally checked and, if needed, data were recoded for comparability across studies. Where necessary, further details were sought from the principal investigators of each individual study.

### Statistical analyses

All analyses used individual participant data, restricted to participants aged ≥20 years at the time of the baseline survey. Cox proportional hazards regression was used to estimate hazard ratios (HRs) and 95% confidence intervals (95% CI) for HF for each risk factor, after adjustment for age. All analyses were stratified by sex and study. For linear associations HRs for a unit increase were derived. BMI and HF exhibited a non-linear relationship so the HRs across quarters were reported. In addition, the HR's across five sequential categories of BMI were reported: <18.5, 18.5–21.9, 22–24.9, 25–29.9 and ≥30 kg/$m^2$ [21]. The 95% CI for categories of BMI were obtained by the method of floating absolute risks [22]. The associations for continuous variables were adjusted for regression dilution bias using repeated measurement data [23]. The analyses were repeated within subgroups according to sex, age (≤75 v > 75 years), and region (Asia v Australia) and a p-value less than 0.05 was considered evidence of an interaction. In a sensitivity analysis, the impact of adjustment for SBP, smoking, BMI and diabetes was explored using a restricted sample that had information on these variables. In a further sensitivity analysis, the data were left-censored to exclude events that occurred during the first two years of follow-up. We also examined whether there was an interaction with history of cardiovascular disease at study baseline (CVD) by including an interaction term in the model. Data provided to the Secretariat were checked for completeness and consistency and recoded, when necessary, to maximize comparability across cohorts. Summary reports were referred back to principal investigators of each collaborating study for review and confirmation. Analyses were performed using SAS, version 9.2 and Stata version 11.

## Results

A total of 543694 (85% Asian; 36% female) participants from 32 cohorts were included in this analysis (Table 1). Due to missing values for some variables, the number of subjects available for analysis varied according each to risk factor.

### Systolic blood pressure

Overall, 3,793,229 person years of follow-up data contributed to the analysis of SBP with HF during which time 614 deaths (80% Asian) from HF were recorded. In the Asian cohorts, 56% of HF deaths were from Japan, 42% from China and the remainder from Hong Kong, Taiwan, Japan and Korea. There was a significant and linear positive association between SBP and the risk of mortality from HF ($p = 0.0003$). Every 10 mmHg increment in SBP increased the risk by 13% (95% CI: 6-21%) with no evidence that the effect varied by sex ($p = 0.28$) or region ($p = 0.93$, Figure 1). There was a highly significant interaction with age ($p < 0.0001$), such that the association was only observed for younger compared with older individuals: HR 1.27 (1.15-1.39) and HR 1.00 (0.92-1.09) in individuals ≤75 years and >75 years, respectively. Adjusting for smoking, BMI and diabetes did not materially change the associations (Additional file 1: WebFigure 1). There was some evidence that the association differed by whether or not the individual had a history of cardiovascular disease (CVD) at study baseline (Additional file 1: WebTable 1); In those individuals with no CVD history, there was a positive association whereas there was no apparent association between SBP and heart failure mortality in those with a history of CVD ($p_{\text{interaction with history of CVD}} = 0.024$). This may have been a chance finding due to the small number (<100) of events that occurred in those with a history of CVD.

### Body mass index

The age-adjusted analysis between BMI and HF mortality was based on a total of 2,430,378 person-years and 494 events. There was a U-shaped relationship across quarters of BMI (Figure 2), with the second and third quarters having the lowest risk of mortality compared with the first quarter. There was no indication that the association differed by region ($p = 0.86$), sex ($p = 0.65$), or age ($p = 0.95$). When the relationship was examined using the pre-specified categories for weight with normal weight (18.5–21.9 kg/m$^2$) as the reference group the U-shaped relation was more evident (Table 2). Compared with the reference group, both underweight and obese individuals had more than a 60% increased risk of dying from HF compared with normal weight individuals: HR 1.68 (95% CI: 1.34-2.11) and 1.69 (1.17-2.43) for underweight and obese individuals, respectively which remained unchanged after adjustment for cigarette smoking or after two years left censoring (Table 2). The relationship was consistent in those with and without a history of CVD at study baseline ($p_{\text{interaction with history of CVD}} = 0.92$; Additional file 1: WebTable 1).

### Lifetime cigarette smoking

A total of 3,443,811 person years and 579 events contributed to this analysis. Compared with never smokers ever smoking was significantly associated with 30% increased risk of mortality (95% CI: 6-60%; Figure 3). There was no evidence that the association differed by region ($p = 0.073$), sex ($p = 0.60$) or age ($p = 0.064$). The results remained largely unchanged after adjusting for SBP and BMI (Additional file 1: WebFigure 2). The relationship was consistent in those with and without a history of CVD at study baseline ($p_{\text{interaction with history of CVD}} = 0.10$; Additional file 1: WebTable 1).

### Diabetes

Based on 1,996,642 person years of data and 496 events, individuals with diabetes had 80% (95% CI: 1.24-2.63) greater risk of death from HF compared with those without the condition, with no evidence to suggest that the relationship differed significantly by sex ($p = 0.59$) or by age ($p = 0.21$) (Figure 4). There was suggestive evidence of a stronger effect in cohorts from Australia compared with Asia: HR 3.04 (1.76-5.25) versus 1.26 (0.74-2.13) ($p = 0.022$). There was no material change in these associations once the effect of other covariates was considered (Additional file 1: WebFigure 3). The relationship was consistent in those with and without a history of CVD at study baseline ($p_{\text{interaction with history of CVD}} = 0.15$; Additional file 1: WebTable 1).

### Total cholesterol

Information on the association between TC and HF was based on 2,145,819 person years and 365 events. Test for linearity indicated that there was a weak inverse association between TC and HF ($p = 0.01$). A 1 mmol/L increment in TC was associated with a non-significant reduction in HF mortality with no significant evidence of a regional interaction: HR 0.90 (95% CI: 0.77-1.07); $p = 0.059$; Figure 5. The HR remained largely unchanged after additional adjustment for cigarette smoking, SBP and BMI: HR 0.93 (0.77-1.11) per 1 mmol/L increase in TC

**Table 1 Baseline characteristics of participating studies in Australia and Asia in the Asia Pacific Cohort Studies Collaboration**

| Study name (Country) | N | Baseline years | Female (%) | Age (yrs) | HF deaths | FU (yrs) | SBP (mmHg) | BMI (kg/m2) | TC (mmol/L) | Diab (%) | Smoke (%) |
|---|---|---|---|---|---|---|---|---|---|---|---|
| ALSA (Aus) | 1613 | 1992-93 | 48 | 78 | 20 | 5 | 148 | 26.0 | 5.8 | 8.3 | 7.7 |
| ANHF (Aus) | 9277 | 1989-90 | 51 | 43 | 3 | 8 | 126 | 25.4 | 5.5 | 1.9 | 24.1 |
| Busselton (Aus) | 7866 | 1966-81 | 52 | 45 | 50 | 27 | 138 | 24.6 | 5.9 | 3.5 | 33.8 |
| Canberra (Aus) | 833 | 1990-91 | 46 | 77 | 16 | 9 | 145 | - | - | 6.8 | 11.3 |
| Melbourne (Aus) | 41286 | 1990-94 | 59 | 55 | 18 | 9 | 138 | 26.9 | 5.5 | 5.4 | 11.3 |
| Perth (Aus) | 10230 | 1978-94 | 48 | 45 | 5 | 14 | 130 | 25.2 | 5.8 | 2.1 | 25.5 |
| WAAAA Screenees (Aus) | 12203 | 1996-99 | 0 | 72 | 10 | 3 | 157 | 26.9 | - | 11.6 | 10.9 |
| *Total Australia* | *83308* | | *47* | *55* | *122* | *8* | *139* | *26.3* | *5.6* | *5.4* | *16.4* |
| Aito Town (Japan) | 1717 | 1980-83 | 57 | 51 | 9 | 15 | 136 | 22.6 | 4.6 | 2.7 | 28.6 |
| Akabane (Japan) | 1836 | 1985-86 | 56 | 54 | 16 | 11 | 125 | 22.5 | 5.0 | 2.5 | 28.0 |
| Anzhen (China) | 8378 | 1991 | 55 | 54 | 3 | 4 | 129 | 23.9 | - | 0.0 | 28.5 |
| Beijing Steelworkers (China) | 8957 | 1970 | 12 | 36 | 15 | 28 | 123 | - | - | - | - |
| Civil Service Workers (Japan) | 9319 | 1990-92 | 33 | 47 | 1 | 7 | 126 | 22.5 | 5.2 | 1.8 | 37.9 |
| CVDFACTS (Taiwan) | 5730 | 1988-96 | 55 | 47 | 4 | 6 | 118 | 23.5 | 5.0 | 2.7 | 22.2 |
| East Beijing (China) | 1128 | 1977-94 | 51 | 44 | 3 | 17 | 125 | 23.6 | - | 5.6 | 28.6 |
| Fangshan (China) | 2625 | 1991-92 | 67 | 47 | 1 | 4 | 136 | 24.4 | 4.6 | 7.1 | 39.3 |
| Guangzhou Occupational (China) | 167377 | 1985-97 | 22 | 42 | 11 | 7 | 115 | 22.6 | 5.3 | 10.5 | 47.6 |
| Hisayama (Japan) | 1616 | 1961 | 56 | 56 | 24 | 25 | 135 | 21.6 | 4.1 | 0.0 | 42.7 |
| Hong Kong | 3006 | 1985-91 | 58 | 79 | 4 | 3 | 150 | 21.9 | 5.3 | 8.6 | 18.6 |
| Huashan (China) | 1868 | 1990-92 | 52 | 53 | 2 | 3 | 126 | 23.3 | 4.6 | 13.7 | 24.9 |
| Kinmen (Taiwan) | 2793 | 1993-96 | 48 | 63 | 90 | 3 | 137 | 23.4 | - | 8.6 | 8.3 |
| KMIC (Korea) | 183600 | 1992 | 37 | 44 | 7 | 4 | 122 | 23.0 | 5.0 | 7.7 | 38.5 |
| Konan (Japan) | 1226 | 1987-95 | 55 | 52 | 9 | 6 | 130 | 21.9 | 4.9 | 12.6 | 30.1 |
| Miyama (Japan) | 1078 | 1988-90 | 56 | 61 | 11 | 7 | 132 | 22.1 | 5.1 | 0.0 | 29.5 |
| Ohasama (Japan) | 2240 | 1992-93 | 64 | 60 | 4 | 4 | 128 | 23.3 | 5.0 | 10.9 | 20.0 |
| Saitama (Japan) | 3624 | 1986-90 | 62 | 55 | 28 | 11 | 135 | 22.4 | 5.0 | 1.7 | 28.4 |
| Seven Cities Cohorts (China) | 10811 | 1987 | 55 | 54 | 139 | 3 | 130 | 22.6 | 5.0 | 1.2 | 35.1 |
| Shibata (Japan) | 2350 | 1977 | 58 | 57 | 34 | 20 | 131 | 22.4 | 4.6 | 1.1 | 33.1 |
| Shigaraki Town (Japan) | 3758 | 1991-97 | 60 | 57 | 7 | 4 | 132 | 22.5 | 5.0 | 7.2 | 28.8 |
| Shirakawa (Japan) | 4643 | 1974-79 | 54 | 48 | 27 | 18 | 127 | 21.5 | 4.6 | 0.9 | 34.9 |
| Six Cohorts (China) | 19387 | 1982-86 | 47 | 45 | 6 | 9 | 119 | 21.2 | 4.2 | 0.0 | 46.0 |
| Tanno/Soubetsu (Japan) | 1984 | 1977 | 53 | 51 | 16 | 16 | 133 | 23.6 | 4.9 | 7.2 | 38.6 |
| Tianjin (China) | 9335 | 1984 | 51 | 55 | 21 | 6 | 136 | 23.5 | - | 0.0 | 50.9 |
| *Total Asia* | *460386* | | *34* | *45* | *492* | *6* | *121* | *22.8* | *4.9* | *6.9* | *41.4* |
| Total | 543694 | | 36 | 46 | 614 | 7 | 124 | 23.6 | 5.1 | 6.5 | 37.3 |

FU = mean follow-up in years; SBP = systolic blood pressure; TC = total cholesterol; diab = diabetes; HF = death from heart failure; NHS = National Health Survey; ALSA = Australian Longitudinal Study of Aging; ANHF = Australian National Heart Foundation. WAAAA = West Australian Abdominal Aortic Aneurysm; CISCH = Capital Iron and Steel Hospital; KMIC = Korean Medical Insurance Corporation. - = no data available.

(Additional file 1: WebFigure 4). There was also no material effect after excluding the first two years of follow up (HR 0.98 [95% CI 0.81-1.17]). The relationship was consistent in those with and without a history of CVD at study baseline ($p_{\text{interaction with history of CVD}} = 0.45$; Additional file 1: WebTable 1).

## Discussion

This study comprises the largest amount of prospective data to date on the relationship between major cardiovascular risk factors with HF mortality in populations from the Asia-Pacific region. The key findings from this individual participant data meta-analysis indicate positive and

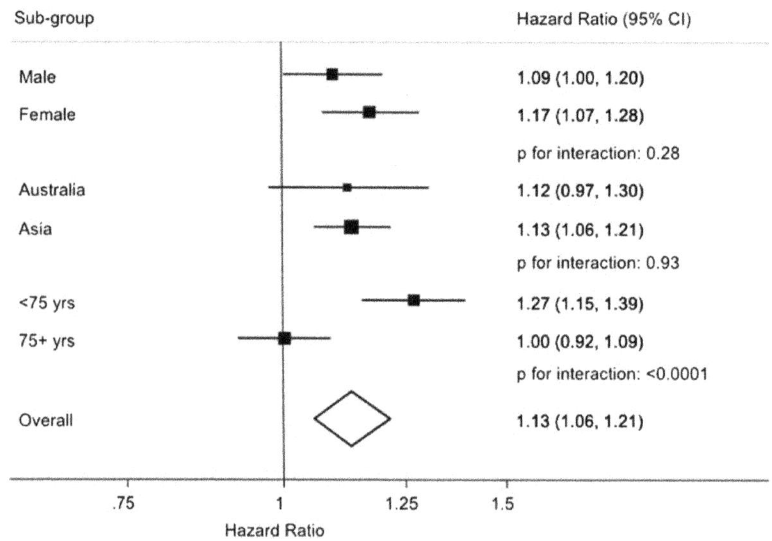


**Figure 1 Hazard ratios for fatal heart failure associated with a 10 mmHg increment in systolic blood pressure, adjusted for age and regression dilution bias and stratified by sex and study in the Asia Pacific Cohort Studies Collaboration, both by subgroup (male versus female; Asia versus Australia; ≤ 75 yrs vs > 75 yrs) and overall.** Bars show 95% confidence intervals. The vertical dimension of the diamond indicates the overall estimate and the horizontal dimension indicates the 95% confidence interval.

independent relationships between elevated blood pressure, obesity, diabetes and cigarette smoking with death from HF in Asians and non-Asians, but no evidence of an association with TC. With the possible exception for blood pressure, the relationships were consistent in those with and without a history of CVD at study baseline. Overall, these current findings are broadly consistent with those reported from Western population-based studies, including Framingham [24,25] and NHANES [12]. Both of these US studies reported hypertension to be a major, if not the leading, modifiable cause of incident HF in addition to diabetes, smoking and obesity [24,25]. Comparative population-based data from Asia are sparse, but those derived from hospital-based studies have also indicated the frequently high co-occurrence of hypertension and diabetes among individuals hospitalized for HF [26].

That diabetes may also be an independent risk factor for incident HF was first shown by the Framingham study where a clinical history of diabetes was associated with a two-fold increased risk in men and a five-fold increased risk for women [25]. Since then, numerous studies have reported higher incidence rates of HF among those with diabetes compared with those without the condition, as well as a relatively higher relative risk of

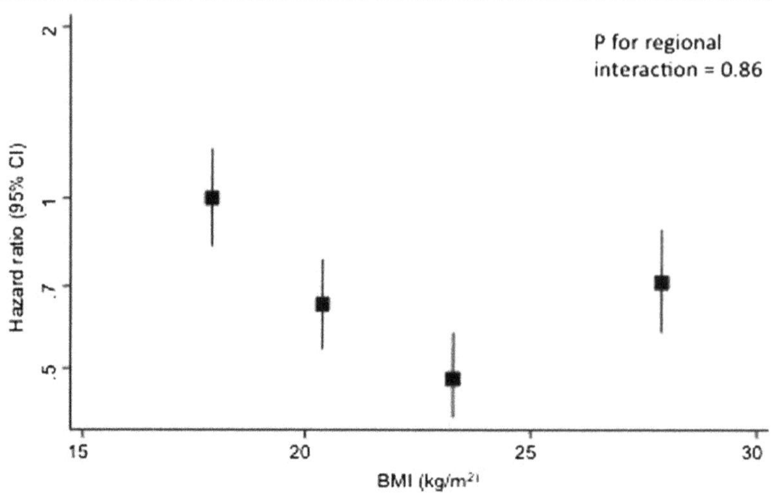


**Figure 2 Hazard ratios for fatal heart failure by fourths of body mass index adjusted for age and regression dilution; stratified by sex and study.** Bars show 95% confidence intervals. Baseline fourths were ≤21.1, 21.2-23.2, 23.3-25.4, ≥25.5 kg/m$^2$.

**Table 2 The categorical association between body mass index (BMI) and mortality from heart failure in the Asia Pacific Cohort Studies Collaboration**

| BMI category (kg/m$^2$) | Age, sex and study adjusted | | Age, sex, study, smoking adjusted | | 2-year left censored | |
|---|---|---|---|---|---|---|
| | HF deaths | HR (95% CI) | HF deaths | HR (95% CI) | HF deaths | HR (95% CI) |
| < 18.5 (underweight) | 100 | 1.68 (1.34-2.11) | 100 | 1.72 (1.37-2.16) | 79 | 1.78 (1.37-2.30) |
| 18.5 – 21.9 (normal, ref) | 157 | 1.00 (0.84-1.18) | 151 | 1.00 (0.84-1.19) | 125 | 1.00 (0.83-1.21) |
| 22 – 24.9 | 103 | 0.81 (0.67-0.98) | 101 | 0.83 (0.68-1.01) | 87 | 0.86 (0.69-1.05) |
| 25 – 29.9 (overweight) | 91 | 0.98 (0.80-1.22) | 90 | 1.02 (0.83-1.27) | 76 | 1.04 (0.82-1.31) |
| > 30 (obese) | 33 | 1.69 (1.17-2.43) | 33 | 1.76 (1.22-2.54) | 27 | 1.75 (1.16-2.63) |

HF in populations of women and young people [27,28]. Data from the current study, confirmed an independent association between diabetes and mortality from HF for non-Asians and (to a lesser extent) Asians. That diabetes may have a slightly weaker association with mortality from HF in Asians than in non-Asians is an intriguing finding that warrants further investigation.

In the current study, a U-shaped association between BMI and mortality from HF was observed such that individuals who were either underweight or obese were at similarly greater risk of dying from HF compared with those of normal weight. This remained unaffected by adjustment for smoking, which may have operated as a confounder of the association given that smokers tend to be relatively leaner than their non-smoking counterparts. Efforts to reduce the impact of reverse causality by excluding the first two years of follow-up also had little impact on the relationship. Our observation that underweight is a risk factor for mortality from HF is tangentially supported by previous hospital-based studies that have shown patients with chronic HF who are underweight have a lower survival than those of normal weight or who are overweight or obese [29]. The increased risk of HF death for underweight individuals may be due to cardiac cachexia, a wasting syndrome observed in patients with advanced HF that has no accepted definition but is characterized by significant weight loss in the absence of peripheral edema [30,31]. Studies have demonstrated that many patients with advanced HF are malnourished, with a calorie and protein intake that is inadequate to meet their energy requirements [32,33]. But, this is unlikely to account for all of the increased risk as even in the absence of cachexia studies have shown that the increased risk of HF for the underweight individual remains [34]. The relationship between low BMI with increased risk of mortality from heart failure may also reflect pre-existing heart failure at study baseline. We did not have information on prevalent HF so could not examine this further but in the sensitivity analysis comparing those with and without a history of CVD at study baseline, the relationship between BMI with mortality from HF was the same. Perhaps of more relevance to Western countries, is the increased risk of mortality from HF for obese compared

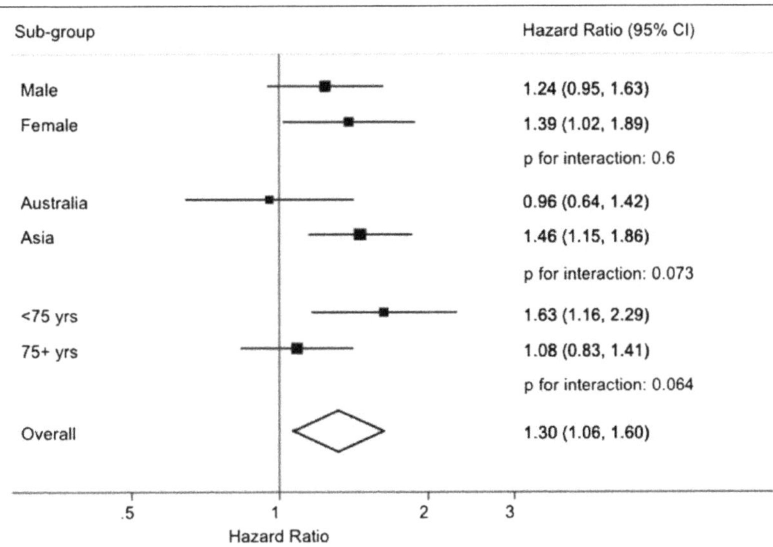


**Figure 3 Hazard ratios for fatal heart failure associated with cigarette smoking (ever versus never) adjusted for age and stratified by sex and study in the Asia Pacific Cohort Studies Collaboration.** Conventions as in Figure 1.

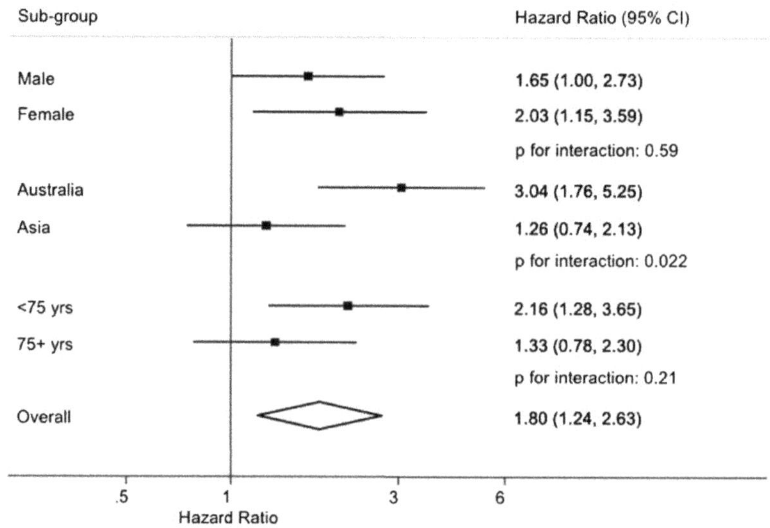


**Figure 4 Hazard ratios for fatal heart failure associated with diabetes (yes versus no) adjusted for age and regression dilution bias and stratified by sex and study in the Asia Pacific Cohort Studies Collaboration.** Conventions as in Figure 1.

with relatively lean individuals that we, and other authors, have shown. In Framingham, for example, there was a continuous association between BMI and risk of new onset HF and each unit increase in BMI was associated with a 5% increase in the risk of HF for men and 7% for women [35].

The epidemiological literature describing the relationship between TC and mortality from HF is inconsistent; some studies have reported a positive [36] or inverse relation [37] between TC and mortality from HF, but others including NHANES have shown no association [12]. In the current study there was no good evidence of an association between TC with mortality from HF –either positive or inverse- as shown by the confidence intervals around the point estimate spanning unity in both the unadjusted and adjusted models. This is consistent with randomized data from two clinical trials –CORONA [38] and GISSI-HF [39]–which demonstrated that in patients with HF the incidence of cardiovascular events, which are greatly driven by non-atherosclerotic events, was not importantly affected with statin therapy. Moreover, the Cholesterol Treatment Trialist's showed that LDL-cholesterol lowering with statin therapy has no benefit on cardiac deaths due to non-occlusive mechanisms, such as HF [40].

There are some important limitations of this analysis. The lack of a universal definition of HF, and between

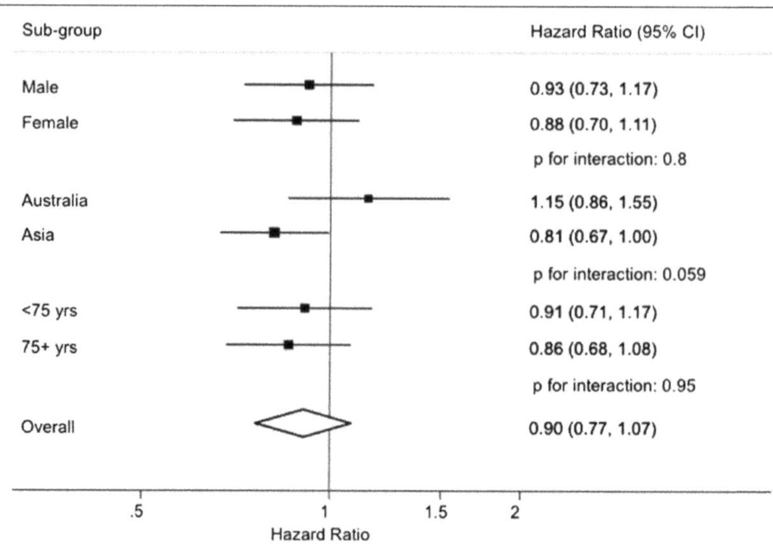


**Figure 5 Hazard ratios for fatal heart failure associated with a 1 mmol/L increment in total cholesterol adjusted for age and regression dilution bias and stratified by sex and study in the Asia Pacific Cohort Studies Collaboration.** Conventions as in Figure 1.

study differences in its diagnosis and reporting, may have introduced bias. For example, misdiagnosis of HF as stroke, myocardial infarction or IHD in the early 1990's has been suggested to account for the observed increase in IHD mortality between 1990–1995 in Japan [41]. In the current analysis, over half of the data from Asia were derived from Japanese cohorts, many of which were initiated in the early 1990's. Therefore, it is conceivable that there was some under-reporting of mortality from HF in these cohorts; such misclassification is likely to draw estimates of association towards the null. We also did not have information on incident heart failure which precludes examination of the possible effects of reverse causality on the results (i.e. whether the association between a particular risk factor with mortality from heart failure is impacted by the development on heart failure at some point during follow-up). Another limitation of our data was the lack of information on rheumatic heart disease, coronary artery disease and Chagas' disease, which are major causes of HF in South Asia and China [8] and which have been reported to be independent predictors of HF risk [42]. Finally, we were unable to examine the relationships between emerging cardiovascular risk factors with HF. In a recent report from the Strong Heart Study, inflammatory markers were shown to be associated with incident HF, although the relationships were substantially attenuated after adjusting for more traditional coronary risk factors [43].

## Conclusions

In summary, findings from this current study indicate that several traditional and modifiable cardiovascular risk factors, namely elevated blood pressure, diabetes, obesity and cigarette smoking, are independently associated with mortality from HF for Asian and non-Asian populations alike in a broadly consistent manner.

## Appendix

### APCSC Executive Committee

M. Woodward (Chair), X. Fang, D.F. Gu, R. Huxley, Y. Imai, H.C. Kim, T.H. Lam, W.H. Pan, A. Rodgers, I. Suh, H. Ueshima

### Participating Studies and Principal Collaborators in APCSC

Aito Town: A. Okayama, H. Ueshima, H. Maegawa; Akabane: M. Nakamura, N. Aoki; Anzhen02: Z.S. Wu; Anzhen: C.H. Yao, Z.S. Wu; Australian Longitudinal Study of Aging: Mary Luszcz; Australian National Heart Foundation: T.A. Welborn; Beijing Aging: Z. Tang; Beijing Steelworkers: L.S. Liu, J.X. Xie; Blood Donors' Health: R. Norton, S. Ameratunga, S. MacMahon, G. Whitlock; Busselton: M.W. Knuiman; Canberra-Queanbeyan: H. Christensen; Capital Iron and Steel Company: X.G. Wu; CISCH: J. Zhou, X.H. Yu; Civil Service Workers: A. Tamakoshi; CVDFACTS: W.H. Pan; East Beijing: Z.L. Wu, L.Q. Chen, G.L. Shan; Electricity Generating Authority of Thailand: P. Sritara; Fangshan: D.F. Gu, X.F. Duan; Fletcher Challenge: S. MacMahon, R. Norton, G. Whitlock, R. Jackson; Guangzhou: Y.H. Li; Guangzhou Occupational: T.H. Lam, C.Q. Jiang; Hisayama: Y. Kiyohara, H. Arima, M. Iida; Hong Kong: J. Woo, S.C. Ho; Huashan: Z. Hong, M.S. Huang, B. Zhou; Kinmen: J.L. Fuh; Konan: H. Ueshima, Y. Kita, S.R. Choudhury; KMIC: I. Suh, S.H. Jee, I.S. Kim; Melbourne: G.G. Giles; Miyama: T. Hashimoto, K. Sakata; Newcastle: A. Dobson; Ohasama: Y. Imai, T. Ohkubo, A. Hozawa; Perth: the late K. Jamrozik, M. Hobbs, R. Broadhurst; Saitama: K. Nakachi; Seven Cities: X.H. Fang, S.C. Li, Q.D. Yang; Shanghai Factory Workers: Z.M. Chen; Shibata: H. Tanaka; Shigaraki Town: Y. Kita, A. Nozaki, H. Ueshima; Shirakawa: H. Horibe, Y. Matsutani, M. Kagaya; Singapore Heart: K. Hughes, J. Lee; Singapore NHS92: D. Heng, S.K. Chew; Six Cohorts: B.F. Zhou, H.Y. Zhang; Tanno/Soubetsu: K. Shimamoto, S. Saitoh; Tianjin: Z.Z. Li, H.Y. Zhang; Western Australia AAA Screenees: P. Norman, the late K. Jamrozik; Xi'an: Y. He, T.H. Lam; Yunnan: S.X. Yao.

## Additional file

**Additional file 1: WebFigure 1.** Hazard ratios for fatal heart failure associated with a 10 mmHg increment in systolic blood pressure, adjusted for age, smoking, body mass index, diabetes, and regression dilution bias and stratified by sex and study in the Asia Pacific Cohort Studies Collaboration, both by subgroup (male versus female; Asia versus Australia; < 75 yrs vs> 75 yrs) and overall. Bars show 95% confidence intervals. The vertical dimension of the diamond indicates the overall estimate and the horizontal dimension indicates the 95% confidence interval. **WebFigure 2.** Hazard ratios for fatal heart failure associated with cigarette smoking (ever versus never) adjusted for age, systolic blood pressure, body mass index and stratified by sex and study in the Asia Pacific Cohort Studies Collaboration. Conventions as in **WebFigure 1. WebFigure 3.** Hazard ratios for fatal heart failure associated with diabetes (yes versus no) adjusted for age, systolic blood pressure, body mass index, cigarette smoking, regression dilution bias and stratified by sex and study in the Asia Pacific Cohort Studies Collaboration. Conventions as in **WebFigure 1. WebFigure 4.** Hazard ratios for fatal heart failure associated with 1 mmol/L increment in total cholesterol (multiply by 38.7 to obtain mg/dL) adjusted for age, systolic blood pressure, body mass index, cigarette smoking, regression dilution bias and stratified by sex and study in the Asia Pacific Cohort Studies Collaboration. Conventions as in **WebFigure 1. WebTable 1.** Associations between risk factors and mortality from heart failure in those with and without a history of cardiovascular disease at study baseline.

#### Competing interests

The authors declare that they have no competing interests.

#### Authors' contributions

RH conceived the manuscript, interpreted the data and wrote the manuscript; FB analyzed the data; JW, GG, THL, TO, SHJ, XF acquired the data and provided critical revision of the manuscript; KZ, SK provided critical revision of the manuscript and MW oversaw the statistical analysis and provided critical revision of the manuscript. All authors read and approved the final manuscript.

#### Acknowledgements

We are grateful to Karice Hyun for preparing the forest plots and to Hirotsugu Ueshima for comments on an earlier draft.

**Funding**
This work was supported by Australian National Health and Medical Research Council (NHMRC) grant 571281; MW is supported by NHMRC fellowship 1020812.

**Author details**
[1]Epidemiology & Biostatistics Division, School of Population Health, University of Queensland, Brisbane, Australia. [2]The George Institute for Global Health, University of Sydney, Sydney, Australia. [3]Department of Medicine and Therapeutics, Faculty of Medicine, The Chinese University of Hong Kong, Hong Kong, China. [4]Cancer Epidemiology Centre, The Cancer Council Victoria, Melbourne, Australia. [5]School of Public Health/Department of Community Medicine, The University of Hong Kong, Hong Kong, China. [6]George Centre for Healthcare Innovation, University of Oxford, Oxford, UK. [7]Department of Cardiovascular Medicine, University of Oxford, Oxford, UK. [8]Division of Epidemiology and Community Health, School of Public Health, University of Minnesota, Minneapolis, Minnesota, USA. [9]Department of Health Science, Shiga University of Medical Science, Shiga, Japan. [10]Institute for Health Promotion, Graduate School of Public Health, Yonsei University, Seoul, Korea. [11]Department of Epidemiology and Social Medicine, Xuanwu Hospital, Capital Medical University, Beijing, China. [12]Division of Epidemiology, Johns Hopkins University, Baltimore, USA.

**References**

1. McMurray JJ, Pfeffer MA: **Heart failure.** *Lancet* 2005, **365:**1877–1889.
2. Rosamond W, Flegal K, Friday G, Furie K, Go A, Greenlund K, Haase N, Ho M, Howard V, Kissela B, Kittner S, Lloyd-Jones D, McDermott M, Meigs J, Moy C, Nichol G, O'Donnell CJ, Roger V, Rumsfeld J, Sorlie P, Steinberger J, Thom T, Wasserthiel-Smoller S, Hong Y, American Heart Association Statistics Committee and Stroke Statistics Subcommittee: **Heart disease and stroke statistics–2007 update: a report from the American Heart Association Statistics Committee and Stroke Statistics Subcommittee.** *Circulation* 2007, **115:**e69–e171. doi:10.1161/CIRCULATIONAHA.106.179918. Accessed September 10, 2013.
3. Roger VL, Go AS, Lloyd-Jones DM, Benjamin EJ, Berry JD, Borden WB, Bravata DM, Dai S, Ford ES, Fox CS, Fullerton HJ, Gillespie C, Hailpern SM, Heit JA, Howard VJ, Kissela BM, Kittner SJ, Lackland DT, Lichtman JH, Lisabeth LD, Makuc DM, Marcus GM, Marelli A, Matchar DB, Moy CS, Mozaffarian D, Mussolino ME, Nichol G, Paynter NP, Soliman EZ, *et al*: **Heart disease and stroke statistics–2012 update: a report from the American Heart Association.** *Circulation* 2012, **125:**e2–e220. doi:10.1161/CIR.0b013e31823ac046. Accessed September 10, 2013.
4. McMurray JJ, Petrie MC, Murdoch DR, Davie AP: **Clinical epidemiology of heart failure: public and private health burden.** *Eur Heart J* 1998, **19**(Suppl P):P9.
5. Cowie MR, Mosterd A, Wood DA, Deckers JW, Poole-Wilson PA, Sutton GC, Grobbee DE: **The epidemiology of heart failure.** *Eur Heart J* 1997, **18:**208–225.
6. Hoes AW, Mosterd A, Grobbee DE: **An epidemic of heart failure? Recent evidence from Europe.** *Eur Heart J* 1998, **19**(Suppl L):L2.
7. Ng TP, Niti M: **Trends and ethnic differences in hospital admissions and mortality for congestive heart failure in the elderly in Singapore, 1991 to 1998.** *Heart* 2003, **89:**865–870.
8. Sanderson JE: **Heart failure; a growing epidemic in Asia.** *Hong Kong Med J* 2004, **10:**76.
9. Lloyd-Jones DM, Larson MG, Leip EP, Beiser A, D'Agostino RB, Kannel WB, Wang TJ, Larson MG, Levy D, Vasan RS, Massaro JM, Beiser A, Wolf PA, Benjamin EJ, Framingham Heart Study: **Lifetime risks for developing congestive heart failure: the Framingham Heart Study.** *Circulation* 2002, **106:**3068–3072.
10. Bleumink GS, Knetsch AM, Sturkenboom MC, Straus SM, Hofman A, Deckers JW, Witteman JC, Stricker BH: **Quantifying the heart failure epidemic: prevalence, incidence rate, lifetime risk and prognosis of heart failure The Rotterdam Study.** *Eur Heart J* 2004, **25:**1614–1619.
11. Schocken DD, Benjamin EJ, Fonarow GC, Krumholz HM, Levy D, Mensah GA, Narula J, Shor ES, Young JB, Hong Y, American Heart Association Council on Epidemiology and Prevention; American Heart Association Council on Clinical Cardiology; American Heart Association Council on Cardiovascular Nursing; American Heart Association Council on High Blood Pressure Research; Quality of Care and Outcomes Research Interdisciplinary Working Group; Functional Genomics and Translational Biology Interdisciplinary Working Group: **Prevention of heart failure: a scientific statement from the American Heart Association Councils on Epidemiology and Prevention, Clinical Cardiology, Cardiovascular Nursing, and High Blood Pressure Research; Quality of Care and Outcomes Research Interdisciplinary Working Group; and Functional Genomics and Translational Biology Interdisciplinary Working Group.** *Circulation* 2008, **117:**2544–2565.
12. He J, Ogden LG, Bazzano LA, Vupputuri S, Loria C, Whelton PK: **Risk factors for congestive heart failure in US men and women: NHANES I epidemiologic follow-up study.** *Arch Intern Med* 2001, **161:**996–1002.
13. Huxley RR, Barzi F, Lam TH, Czernichow S, Fang X, Welborn T, Shaw J, Ueshima H, Zimmet P, Jee SH, Patel JV, Caterson I, Perkovic V, Woodward M, Asia Pacific Cohort Studies Collaboration and the Obesity in Asia Collaboration: **Isolated low levels of high-density lipoprotein cholesterol are associated with an increased risk of coronary heart disease: an individual participant data meta-analysis of 23 studies in the Asia-Pacific region.** *Circulation* 2011, **124:**2056–2064.
14. Asia Pacific Cohort Studies Collaboration: **Determinants of Cardiovascular Disease in the Asian Pacific Region: Protocol for a Collaborative Overview of Cohort Studies.** *CVD Prev* 1999, **2:**281–289.
15. Woodward M, Barzi F, Martiniuk A, Fang X, Gu DF, Imai Y, Lam TH, Pan WH, Rodgers A, Suh I, Jee SH, Ueshima H, Huxley R, Asia Pacific Cohort Studies Collaboration: **Cohort profile: the Asia Pacific Cohort Studies Collaboration.** *Int J Epidemiol* 2006, **35:**1412–1416.
16. Asia Pacific Cohort Studies Collaboration: **Blood pressure and cardiovascular disease in the Asia Pacific Region.** *J Hypertens* 2003, **21:**707–716.
17. Asia Pacific Cohort Studies Collaboration: **Cholesterol, coronary heart disease and stroke in the Asia Pacific region.** *Int J Epidemiol* 2003, **32:**563–572.
18. Asia Pacific Cohort Studies Collaboration: **Body mass index and cardiovascular disease in the Asia Pacific Region: An overview of 33 cohorts involving 310,000 participants.** *Int J Epidemiol* 2004, **31:**1025–1033.
19. Asia Pacific Cohort Studies Collaboration: **The effects of diabetes on the risks of major cardiovascular diseases and death in the Asia-Pacific Region.** *Diabetes Care* 2003, **26:**360–366.
20. Asia Pacific Cohort Studies Collaboration: **Smoking, quitting and the risk of cardiovascular disease among women and men in the Asia-Pacific region.** *Int J Epidemiol* 2005, **34:**1036–1045.
21. WHO Expert Consultation: **Appropriate body-mass index for Asian populations and its implications for policy and intervention strategies.** *Lancet* 2004, **363:**157–163.
22. Woodward M: *Epidemiology: Study design and data analysis.* 2nd edition. Boca Raton: Chapman and Hall/CRC Press; 2005.
23. MacMahon S, Peto R, Cutler J, Collins R, Sorlie P, Neaton J, Abbott R, Godwin J, Dyer A, Stamler J: **Blood pressure, stroke, and coronary heart disease. Part 1. Prolonged differences in blood pressure: prospective observational studies corrected for the regression dilution bias.** *Lancet* 1990, **335:**765–774.
24. Levy D, Larson MG, Vasan RS, Kannel WB, Ho KK: **The progression from hypertension to congestive heart failure.** *JAMA* 1996, **275:**1557–1562.
25. Kannel WB, Hjortland M, Castelli WP: **Role of diabetes in congestive heart failure: the Framingham study.** *Am J Cardiol* 1974, **34:**29–34.
26. Yip GWK, Ho PPY, Woo KS, Sanderson JE: **Comparison of frequencies of left ventricular systolic and diastolic heart failure in Chinese living in Hong Kong.** *Am J Cardiol* 1999, **84:**563–567.
27. Nichols GA, Gullion CM, Koro CE, Ephross SA, Brown JB: **The incidence of congestive heart failure in type 2 diabetes: an update.** *Diabetes Care* 2004, **27:**1879–1884.
28. Bibbins-Domingo K, Lin F, Vittinghoff E, Barrett-Connor E, Hulley SB, Grady D, Shlipak MG: **Predictors of Heart Failure Among Women With Coronary Disease.** *Circulation* 2004, **110:**1424–1430.
29. Curtis JP, Selter JG, Wang Y, Rathore SS, Jovin IS, Jadbabaie F, Kosiborod M, Portnay EL, Sokol SI, Bader F, Krumholz HM: **The obesity paradox: body mass index and outcomes in patients with heart failure.** *Arch Intern Med* 2005, **165:**55–61.
30. Anker SD, Sharma R: **The syndrome of cardiac cachexia.** *Int J Cardiol* 2002, **85:**51–66.

31. Deswal A, Petersen NJ, Feldman AM, Young JB, White BG, Mann DL: **Cytokines and cytokine receptors in advanced heart failure: an analysis of the cytokine database from the Vesnarinone trial (VEST).** *Circulation* 2001, **103:**2055–2059.
32. Aquilani R, Opasich C, Verri M, Boschi F, Febo O, Pasini E, Pastoris O: **Is nutritional intake adequate in chronic heart failure patients?** *J Am Coll Cardiol* 2003, **42:**1218–1223.
33. Freeman LM, Roubenoff R: **The nutrition implications of cardiac cachexia.** *Nutr Rev* 1994, **52:**340–347.
34. Davos CH, Doehner W, Rauchhaus M, Cicoira M, Francis DP, Coats AJ, Clark AL, Anker SD: **Body mass and survival in patients with chronic heart failure without cachexia: the importance of obesity.** *J Card Fail* 2003, **9:**29–35.
35. Kenchaiah S, Evans JC, Levy D, Wilson PW, Benjamin EJ, Larson MG, Kannel WB, Vasan RS: **Obesity and the Risk of Heart Failure.** *N Engl J Med* 2002, **347:**305–313.
36. Velagaleti RS, Massaro J, Vasan RS, Robins SJ, Kannel WB, Levy D: **Relations of lipid concentrations to heart failure incidence: the Framingham Heart Study.** *Circulation* 2009, **120:**2345–2351.
37. Nago N, Ishikawa S, Goto T, Kayaba K: **Low cholesterol is associated with mortality from stroke, heart disease and cancer: The Jichi Medical School Cohort Study.** *J Epidemiol* 2011, **21:**67–74.
38. Kjekshus J, Apetrei E, Barrios V, Böhm M, Cleland JG, Cornel JH, Dunselman P, Fonseca C, Goudev A, Grande P, Gullestad L, Hjalmarson A, Hradec J, Jánosi A, Kamenský G, Komajda M, Korewicki J, Kuusi T, Mach F, Mareev V, McMurray JJ, Ranjith N, Schaufelberger M, Vanhaecke J, van Veldhuisen DJ, Waagstein F, Wedel H, Wikstrand J, CORONA Group: **Rosuvastatin in older patients with systolic heart failure.** *N Engl J Med* 2007, **357:**2248–2261.
39. Gissi-HF Investigators, Tavazzi L, Maggioni AP, Marchioli R, Barlera S, Franzosi MG, Latini R, Lucci D, Nicolosi GL, Porcu M, Tognoni G: **Effect of rosuvastatin in patients with chronic heart failure (the GISSI-HF trial): a randomised, double-blind, placebo-controlled trial.** *Lancet* 2008, **372:**1231–1239.
40. Cholesterol Treatment Trialists' (CTT) Collaboration: **Efficacy and safety of more intensive lowering of LDL cholesterol: a meta-analysis of data from 170 000 participants in 26 randomised trials.** *Lancet* 2010, **376:**1670–1681.
41. Ma E, Iso H, Takahashi H, Yamagishi K, Tanigawa T: **Age-Period-Cohort analysis of mortality due to ischemic heart disease in Japan, 1955 to 2000.** *Circ J* 2008, **72:**966–972.
42. Barac A, Wang H, Shara NM, de Simone G, Carter EA, Umans JG, Best LG, Yeh J, Dixon DB, Devereux RB, Howard BV, Panza JA: **Markers of inflammation, metabolic risk factors, and incident heart failure in American Indians: the Strong Heart Study.** *J Clin Hypertens* 2012, **14:**13–19.
43. Butler J, Kalogeropoulos A, Georgiopoulou V, Belue R, Rodondi N, Garcia M, Bauer DC, Satterfield S, Smith AL, Vaccarino V, Newman AB, Harris TB, Wilson PW, Kritchevsky SB, Health ABC Study: **Incident heart failure prediction in the elderly: the health ABC heart failure score.** *Circ Heart Fail* 2008, **1:**125–133.

# 4

# The role of urine neutrophil gelatinase – associated lipocalin (NGAL) in acute heart failure in patients with ST – elevation myocardial infarction

Simona Kirbiš[1*], Maksimiljan Gorenjak[2] and Andreja Sinkovič[1]

**Abstract**

**Background:** Neutrophil gelatinase-associated lipocalin (NGAL) is a novel early marker of acute kidney injury for which has been shown that it can also be released from the injured myocardium. Our aim was to correlate urine NGAL with markers of in-hospital heart failure in patients with acute ST-elevation myocardial infarction (STEMI).

**Methods:** We prospectively included 61 consecutive STEMI patients after primary percutaneous coronary intervention and estimated admission and in-hospital urine NGAL, serum creatinine, troponin I, leucocytes, CRP, N-terminal pro brain natriuretic peptide (NT-proBNP) levels and ejection fraction by echocardiography. Urine NGAL levels were compared between patients with and without HF defined as serum NT-proBNP > 400 pmol/l and were correlated to markers of heart failure, inflammations and of kidney function.

**Results:** Urine NGAL levels and CRP was significantly higher in participants with heart failure compared to those with NT-proBNP below 400 pmol/l. Urine NGAL level of 50 ng/ml had 90 % specificity for HF, the sensitivity was low at 25 %. Comparison of participants with NGAL levels < 50 ng/ml and ≥ 50 ng/ml at admission and after 12 h revealed a significant difference in NT-proBNP levels, left ventricle ejection fraction, markers of inflammation and of kidney function. Urine NGAL level was independently associated with NT-proBNP level.

**Conclusions:** The level of urine NGAL early after myocardial infarction is associated with NT-proBNP concentration and even NGAL levels below 137 ng/ml, the usually reported normal cut-off value, had high specificity for HF in our sample.

**Keywords:** Neutrophil gelatinase-associated lipocalin - NGAL, Heart failure, Myocardial infarction, Acute kidney injury

## Background

In spite of early contemporary reperfusion therapy by primary percutaneous coronary intervention (PPCI), ST-elevation myocardial infarction (STEMI) can lead to systolic and/or diastolic dysfunction with decreased cardiac output, leading to further decrease in systemic and coronary perfusion and activation of inflammation. It has been shown that inflammation plays an important role in acute heart failure (HF) after acute myocardial infarction (MI) and there is evidence for profound neutrophil activation during acute MI with release of proinflammatory markers [1, 2]. Inflammation is also important in the process of remodeling by influencing matrix degeneration and fibrosis, promoting apoptosis etc. [3–5].

Neutrophil gelatinase-associated lipocalin (NGAL) is a 25 kDa glycoprotein of the lipocalin superfamily, synthesized in granulocyte precursors in bone marrow during a narrow window of their maturation. It is stored in specific granules of mature neutrophils in complex with gelatinase [6, 7]. In recent years, NGAL has been considered mainly a predictor of acute kidney injury (AKI), because its plasma and urine levels rise before any increase in creatinine level is encountered [8]. In addition, NGAL has been associated with cell death, inflammation and matrix degradation and there is increasing evidence for enhanced systemic and myocardial expression of NGAL after acute MI, supporting the role of inflammation in this entity [9–12].

* Correspondence: simona.kirbis@gmail.com
[1]Department of intensive care unit, University Clinical Center Maribor, Ljubljanska 5, Maribor, SI 2000, Slovenia
Full list of author information is available at the end of the article

The aim of our present study was to evaluate the association of urine NGAL early after acute STEMI with markers of myocardial dysfunction and test its predictive value for acute HF.

## Methods

### Study design and participants

We performed an observational prospective monocentric study with patients admitted with acute STEMI to the Department of Medical Intensive Care (ICU), University Medical Centre Maribor. The study was approved by the Republic of Slovenia National Medical Ethics committee (77/01/11) and written informed consent was obtained from all patients. The study protocol conformed to the ethical guidelines of the Declaration of Helsinki.

Consecutive patients admitted with STEMI between April 2010 and July 2011 who had PPCI performed and stayed at the ICU for at least 24 h were included in the study. Criteria for STEMI were ischemic chest pain lasting up to 12 h plus persistent ST-elevation or new bundle-branch block on ECG [13]; PPCI is the primary reperfusion strategy for acute STEMI at our institution. Exclusion criteria were prior malignancy, infectious disease, sepsis and death or discharge from the ICU in less than 24 h.

### Treatment protocol

On admission, blood samples were drawn to estimate complete blood cell count, serum troponin I, creatinine and lipid profile and a urine sample was collected for estimation of urine-NGAL. Immediately after PPCI, patients were transferred from the catheterization laboratory to the medical ICU for continuous ECG-monitoring and pulse oximetry. On admission to the ICU, a clinical examination and standard ECG were performed and the patency of peripheral intravenous catheter, inserted before the PPCI, was checked. In case of hemodynamic compromise, the treating physician assessed the need for invasive monitoring. Combined antiplatelet therapy (acetylsalicylic acid and clopidogrel), initiated either in the emergency department or by outpatient emergency units, was continued, statins and angiotensin-converting enzyme inhibitors were administered to all patients unless contraindicated. After admission to the ICU, all patients were started on intravenous saline infusions 0.5 to 1.0 ml/kg/hour, the total amount of fluid administered depended on clinical signs of acute pulmonary congestion [14].

Complete blood cell count, troponin I, serum creatinine, N-terminal pro brain natriuretic peptide (NT-proBNP) and CRP levels were estimated daily from blood samples collected between 8.00 and 10.00 a.m. in the first two days, later these tests were performed at the discretion of the treating physician. For the study purposes, a urine sample was taken for estimation of NGAL 12 h after admission and serum creatinine level was estimated every 6 h during the first 24 h. Two dimensional transthoracic echocardiography was performed within the first 24–48 h. The biplane method of disks (modified Simpson's rule) was used to calculate left ventricular ejection fraction (EF); values higher than 55 % are considered normal [15]. Other investigations and treatment modalities were indicated by the ICU team individually for each patient. During treatment, we obtained data on prior known arterial hypertension, diabetes, dyslipidemia, prior stroke, prior MI, smoking and physical activity.

For the purpose of this study, HF was defined as NT-proBNP ≥ 400 pmol/l, in accordance with the European guidelines [16]. Other estimates of heart failure were the Kilip-Kimbal classification and ejection fraction of the left ventricle.

### Laboratory methods

The lipid profile - total serum cholesterol, HDL-cholesterol and triglycerides were estimated by the colorimetric method (Ektachem 250 Analyzer, Eastman Kodak Company, Rochester, USA). Urine NGAL by the chemiluminiscent microparticle immunoassay (CMIA) for the quantitative determination of neutrophil gelatinase-associated lipocalin in human urine (Abbott ARCHITECTAnalyzer, Abbott Ireland Diagnostics Division, Lisnamuck, Ireland; normal levels up to 131.7 ng/ml – coefficient of variability 4.6 %). Troponin I was estimated by colorimetric-immune method (Siemens Healthcare Diagnostics Inc., Newark, USA, normal levels up to 0.045 μg/l). Plasma NT-proBNP levels was estimated by the electrochemiluminescence immunoassay on an Elecsys 2010 analyzer (Roche Diagnostics, normal levels up to 20 pmol/L). Complete blood cell count was performed by automatic counter Sysmex XE - 2100, Kobe Japan; normal levels for leukocytes were 4 – $10 \times 10^9$/l, erythrocytes 4.2 – $6.3 \times 10^{12}$/l and platelets 140 – $340 \times 10^9$/l.

### Statistical analysis

Demographic characteristic and laboratory data were analysed using descriptive methods – frequencies, mean with standard deviation or median with interquartile range. Subgroup comparisons were done using $\chi^2$ test for categorical and Student's $t$-test or the nonparametric Mann–Whitney test for numeric variables. Bivariate correlations were tested by Spearmann's coefficient (rho). P value of 0.05 was set as the limit of statistical significance. SPSS Statistics 18.0 (IBM ®) was used for statistical analysis.

Sensitivity and specificity of NGAL concentration for heart failure defined by elevated NT-proBNP level was calculated [16]. A receiver operating characteristic (ROC) diagram was constructed with urine NGAL level as the test variable and NT-proBNP level as the state variable (Fig. 3). Area under the curve of the constructed ROC diagram was 0.67 (95 % CI 0.52, 0.83; $p = 0.02$). Although the area under the curve was relatively low, it still was considered relevant. The cut-off of urine NGAL with 90 % specificity for heart failure was 46.95 ng/ml, the sensitivity of this cut-off was 25 %; the value 50 ng/ml was used in addition to the previously established normal value of 137 ng/ml. This 50 ng/ml cut-off was thus derived from the same dataset as used in all other statistical analyses.

Urine NGAL levels, markers of kidney injury and markers of inflammation were compared between predefined subgroups of patients with NT-proBNP < 400 pmol/l and patients with NT-proBNP ≥ 400 pmol/l. Conversely, markers of heart failure, inflammation and kidney injury were compared in subgroups based on values of urine NGAL. A linear regression model was constructed with NT-proBNP as the dependent and age, gender, NGAL level, CRP, peak creatinine and left ventricular ejection fraction as independent variables.

## Results

In total, 61 patients were included in the study, among them 44 (72 %) men. The mean age was 63.8 years (SD 12.8 years) As shown in Fig. 1, the most prevalent risk factor for vascular disease was arterial hypertension, followed by dyslipidemia and diabetes.

Among the studied patients, 39 were in Kilip class I, 11 in Kilip class II, 5 in Kilip class III and 6 in Kilip class IV as the higher class during their stay in the ICU. The average values of analysed laboratory variables in the whole sample are presented in Table 1 and the distribution of NGAL levels stratified by heart failure is presented in Fig. 2. There was no significant difference between NGAL levels at admission and after 12 h and, overall, the levels were well below the 137 ng/ml as the usual normal cut-off value. Only two patients had urine NGAL above 137 ng/ml both at admission and after 12 h.

We compared markers of inflammation and of cardiac function in patients with NT-proBNP levels above and below 400 pmol/l which was the definition for heart failure in or study ([16]; Table 2). There was a significant difference between subgroups in urine NGAL levels and in markers of inflammation. The subgroups did not differ in the amount of radiologic contrast material infused.

As explained in the methods section, urine NGAL 50 ng/ml was established as the level with 90 % specificity for acute heart failure defined by NT-proBNP (Fig. 3). Comparison of the two subgroups with NGAL levels < 50 ng/ml and ≥ 50 ng/ml at admission and after 12 h revealed a significant difference in NT-proBNP levels and in ejection fraction as well as in markers of inflammation and of kidney function between subgroups (Table 3). When we used 137 ng/ml as the cut-off value, subgroups did not differ in any of the analyzed variables.

Because NGAL has high specificity for heart failure after STEMI in our sample, we attempted to establish correlations between NGAL levels and markers of inflammation and of heart failure. There was a positive

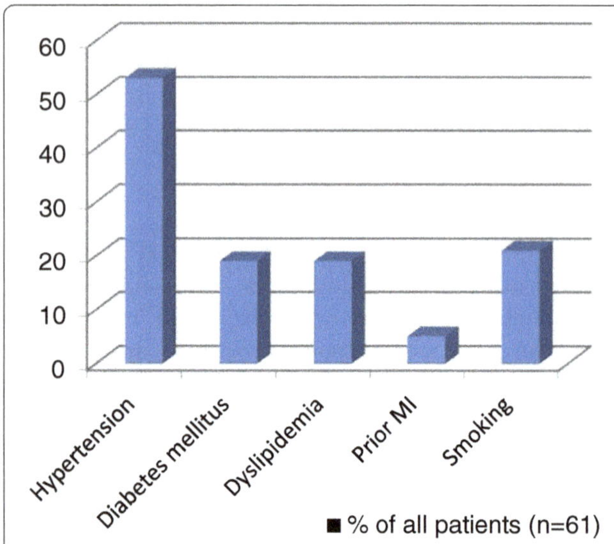


**Fig. 1** Risk factors for vascular diseases in study participants. Legend: MI = myocardial infarction

**Table 1** Admission and in-hospital laboratory data of the included STEMI patients

| Laboratory data (mean ± SD) | *N = 61* |
|---|---|
| Urine NGAL at admission (ng/ml) | 24.5 ± 42.1 |
| Urine NGAL at 12 h (ng/ml) | 27.7 ± 42.7 |
| In-hospital NT-proBNP (pmol/l) | 565.0 ± 882.2 |
| EF (%) | 42.2 ± 12.5 |
| Troponin I at admission (μg/l) | 12.1 ± 20.5 |
| Troponin I after 12 h (μg/l) | 55.7 ± 37.0 |
| CRP at 24 h (mg/l) | 99.0 ± 54.7 |
| Creatinine at admission (μmol/l) | 102.5 ± 45.0 |
| Creatinine at 24 h (μmol/l) | 99.0 ± 54.7 |
| Leucocyte count at 24 h ($1 \times 10^{12}$/l) | 10.9 ± 3.9 |
| Contrast material infused (ml) | 147.2 ± 67.6 |

Data are presented as mean ± standard deviation
*MI* myocardial infarction, *NGAL* neutrophil gelatinase-associated lipocalin, *CRP* C reactive protein, *EF* left ventricular ejection fraction, *NT – proBNP* N-terminal pro brain natriuretic peptide

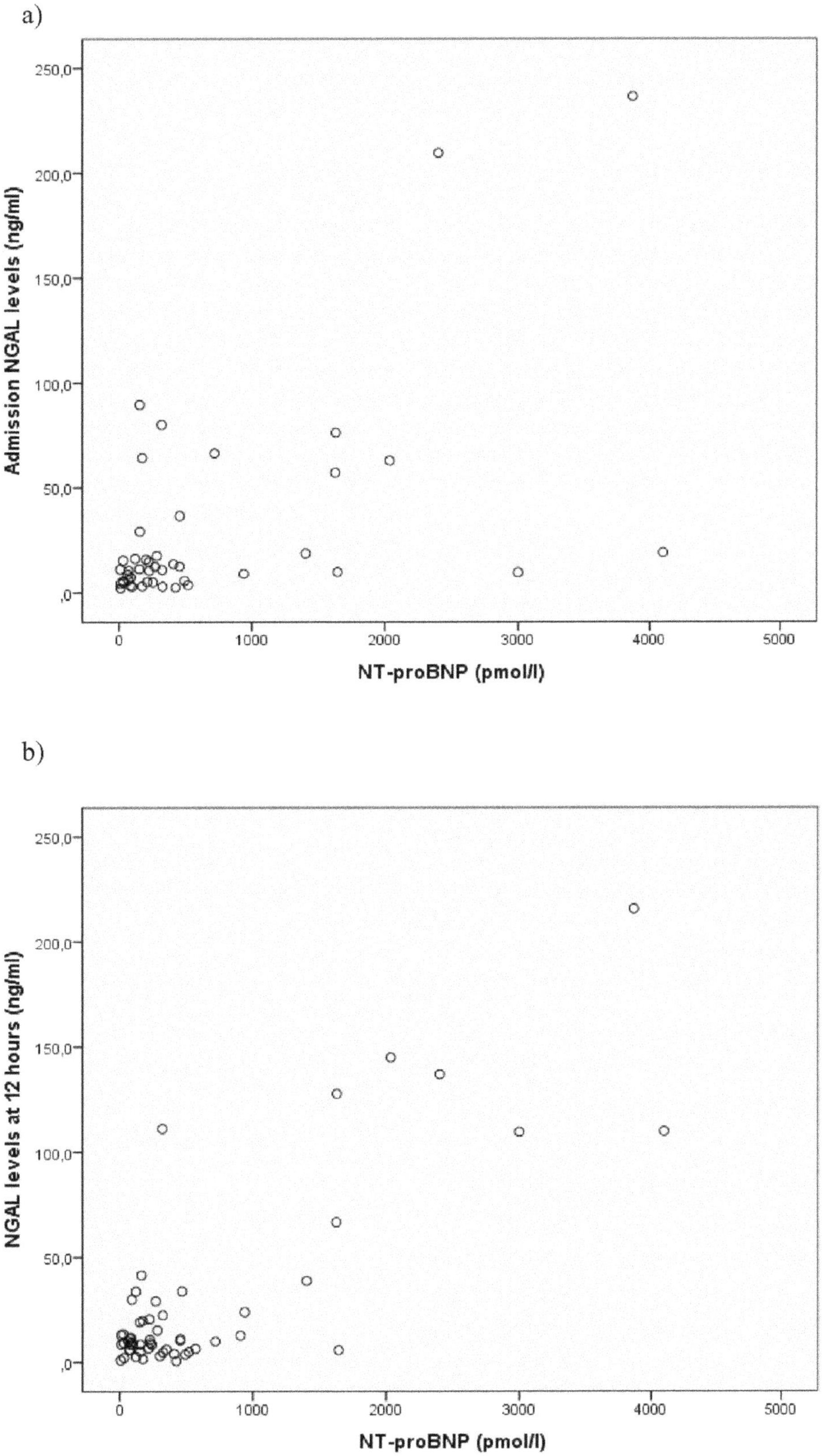


**Fig. 2** (See legend on next page.)

(See figure on previous page.)
**Fig. 2** The distribution of urine neutrophil gelatinase-associated lipocalin (NGAL) concentration at admission (**a**) and 12 h after admission (**b**) and its relation to serum N-terminal pro brain natriuretic peptide (NT-proBNP) concentration. **a** Urine NGAL levels at admission. **b** Urine NGAL levels 12 h after admission. Legend: NGAL = neutrophil gelatinase-associated lipocalin; NT – proBNP = N-terminal pro brain natriuretic peptide

association between admission urine NGAL and in-hospital NT-proBNP (rho$_s$ 0.34, $p = 0.003$) and between admission urine NGAL and in-hospital CRP (rho$_s$ 0.22, $p = 0.04$). Results were similar for urine NGAL estimated 12 h after admission (rho$_s$ 0.34 for NT-proBNP, $p = 0.003$ and rho$_s$ 0.353 for CRP, $p = 0.03$). There was a negative association between NGAL on admission and EF (rhos – 0.122, $p = 0.19$). In a multiple linear regression model, urine NGAL levels ($\beta = 8.91$) and female gender ($\beta = 464.1$) were independently associated with NT-proBNP concentration, while age, peak troponin, creatinine and CRP were not; adjusted $r^2$ for model 0.716.

## Discussion

In our sample of patients with acute STEMI we observed NGAL levels below the usual normal limit 137 ng/ml in the great majority of participants. However, higher levels of NGAL – even though below the above stated limit – had high specificity for development of heart failure and urine NGAL concentration was positively correlated with serum concentration of NT-proBNP. These results suggest that elevated urine NGAL very early after STEMI could be a marker of high risk for acute heart failure in an individual patient and that with regard to MI much lower concentrations of NGAL are of significance compared to when evaluating patients with kidney failure [17].

Urine NGAL was individually correlated with NT-proBNP as well as with CRP and creatinine. In a multiple linear regression model, NGAL was an independent predictor of NT-proBNP concentration, even though in clinical terms the association was weak. This association and the correlation between NGAL and CRP can be viewed as evidence for the importance of early inflammation in acute heart failure after MI. But we must state that NGAL has several possible sources – most commonly is has been associated with inflammation and with kidney dysfunction – and that our study design does not allow deductions about causality.

Damman et al. have shown that increased urine NGAL is highly prevalent in patients with chronic HF and, similarly to our results, positively associated with increased levels of NT-proBNP [18]. Other authors have demonstrated that in patients with chronic HF of ischemic origin with normal renal function, serum NGAL levels were markedly increased in comparison to controls and this increase independently correlated with New York heart Association (NYHA) class and the estimated glomerular filtration rate [19]. It has also been demonstrated that plasma NGAL strongly predicted mortality in patients with chronic heart failure with and without chronic kidney disease [20]. Our results suggest

**Table 2** Comparison of subgroups with heart failure and with no heart failure as defined by N-terminal pro brain natriuretic peptide level (NT-proBNP)

| Variables (mean ± SD) | NT-proBNP < 400 pmol/l ($n = 41$) | NT-proBNP ≥ 400 pmol/l ($n = 20$) | P value |
|---|---|---|---|
| EF at 24–48 h (%) | 48.1 ± 7.8 | 31.3 ± 11.9 | <0.01 |
| Urine NGAL at admission (ng/ml) | 14.8 ± 19.2 | 45.0 ± 65.2 | <0.01 |
| Urine NGAL at 12 h (ng/ml) | 15.5 ± 18.3 | 53.8 ± 63.6 | <0.01 |
| Troponin I at admission (μg/l) | 7.2 ± 13.0 | 22.5 ± 28.7 | <0.01 |
| Creatinine at 24 h (μmol/l) | 83.7 ± 28.9 | 134.0 ± 79.9 | <0.01 |
| CRP at 24 h (mg/l) | 21.3 ± 23.3 | 59.5 ± 74.9 | <0.01 |
| Leucocytes at 24 h (1 × $10^{12}$/l) | 10.1 ± 3.0 | 12.6 ± 5.1 | <0.01 |
| Amount of contrast material (ml) | 142.0 ± 67.3 | 160.3 ± 69.6 | NS |

Data are presented as mean ± standard deviation
*MI* myocardial infarction, *NGAL* neutrophil gelatinase-associated lipocalin, *CRP* C reactive protein, *EF* left ventricular ejection fraction, *NT-proBNP* N-terminal pro brain natriuretic peptide

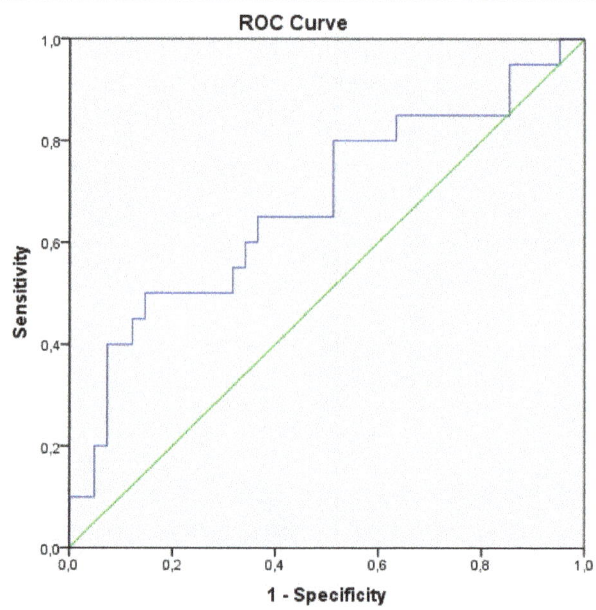


**Fig. 3** The receiver operating characteristic (ROC) curve for determination of cut-off value and predictive values of neutrophil gelatinase-associated lipocalin (NGAL) in urine for heart failure in patients after myocardial infarction

**Table 3** Admission and in-hospital laboratory findings by urine NGAL

| Variables | Admission urine NGAL < 50 ng/ml (*n* = 52) | Admission urine NGAL ≥50 ng/ml (*n* = 9) | *p* | Urine NGAL after 12 h < 50 ng/ml (*n* = 52) | Urine NGAL after 12 h ≥ 50 ng/ml (*n* = 9) | *p* |
|---|---|---|---|---|---|---|
| NT-proBNP after 24 h (pmol/l) | 218.0 (82.5–420.0) | 1627.0 (245.50–2221.5) | $p < 0.05$ | 214.0 (84.0–424.0) | 2221.5 (1628.0–3654.0) | $p < 0.05$ |
| EF (%) | 47 (35–50) | 25 (20–40) | $p < 0.05$ | 45 (35–50) | 20 (20–36.2) | $p < 0.05$ |
| Kilip ≥ 2 (%) | 22 | 78 | $p < 0.05$ | 22 | 78 | $p < 0.05$ |
| Leucocytes after 24 h (1 × 1012/l) | 9.2 (7.8–12.1) | 14.3 (8.5–16.3) | NS | 9.2 (7.8–11.6) | 14.3 (8.9–16.5) | NS |
| CRP after 24 h (mg/l) | 16.0 (10.0–30.0) | 32.0 (6.5–140.5) | NS | 15.0 (7–28.5) | 80.0 (36.0–177.8) | $p < 0.05$ |
| Creatinine admission (μmol/l) | 91.0 (69.8–114.0) | 140.0 (100.0–216.0) | $p < 0.05$ | 92.0 (74.0–114.0) | 153.0 (111.0–217.0) | $p < 0.05$ |
| Creatinine after 24 h (μmol/l) | 78.5 (63.0–94.5) | 142.0 (94.5–273.0) | $p < 0.05$ | 78.0 (63.5–93.5) | 198.5 (133.8–275) | $p < 0.05$ |
| Contrast material (ml) | 140.0 (110.0–178.6) | 90.0 (61.5–198.8) | NS | 135.0 (100.0–168.0) | 174.2 (110.0–240.0) | NS |

Data are presented as median (interquartile range) for numeric and as proportions for categorical variables
*NGAL* neutrophil gelatinase-associated lipocalin, *CRP* C reactive protein, *EF* left ventricular ejection fraction, *NT – proBNP* N-terminal pro brain natriuretic peptide

that NGAL is also associated with markers of acute HF also in the setting of STEMI and this in probably independent of kidney function. Previous (chronic) heart failure is a possible confounding factor, but unfortunately, we did not have reliable enough data about past cardiac function in our participants.

Kidney damage is another possible cause of elevated NGAL. After STEMI, kidney injury may be the consequence of different mechanisms including systolic dysfunction, nephrotoxicity of contrast material used during PPCI, other nephrotoxic drugs, activation of sympathetic and renin-angiotensin-aldosterone system, inflammation and oxidative stress. NGAL can be released by activated neutrophil, epithelial and endothelial cells, smooth muscle cells and cells in in atherosclerotic plaques [19, 21]. Aghel et al. revealed that patients who developed worsening renal function during hospitalization had significantly higher median admission serum NGAL levels (admission NGAL levels ≥ 140 ng/ml) [22]. In our patients, the mean creatinine level was near normal and no one required renal replacement therapy. The amount of contrast material did not differ between patients with and without heart failure nor between patients with NGAL levels above and below 50 ng/ml and we therefore assume that kidney failure is unlikely the sole explanation for elevated NGAL in patients with heart failure in our sample. Palazzuoli et al. showed that NGAL levels above 130 ng/ml predicted not only renal injury, but also an overall risk for cardiac events [17]. According to our data, the NGAL levels predicting heart failure are even lower.

### Study limitations

Several limitations may influence our results. We studied urine NGAL concentrations, which may follow a different timeline than serum concentration and have a different relationship with kidney damage compared to serum concentration. We also had no data on prior heart failure, which has been shown to influence NGAL levels [18]. Importantly, the cut-off value of urine NGAL with high specificity for HF (50 ng/ml) was derived from the analyzed sample itself and this will have to be verified in other, larger samples. Patients who were discharged from the ICU within 24 h were excluded from the study and this diminished the number of participants with a possible bias towards more severe cases.

## Conclusions

The level of urine NGAL early after myocardial infarction is associated with NT-proBNP concentration and even NGAL levels below 137 ng/ml, the usually reported normal cut-off value, had high specificity for HF in our sample. The mechanism of urine NGAL increase after STEMI and its potential value as a predicting factor for acute HF should be investigated in further studies.

**Competing interests**
The authors declare that they have no competing interests.

**Authors' contributions**
SK: concept/design, data collection and analysis/interpretation/drafting article/approval of the submitted and final versions. AS: concept/design, data analysis/statistics, revising article critically/ approval of the submitted and final versions. MG: laboratory analysis/approval of the submitted and final version. All authors read and approved the final manuscript.

**Author details**
[1]Department of intensive care unit, University Clinical Center Maribor, Ljubljanska 5, Maribor, SI 2000, Slovenia. [2]Department of laboratory diagnostics, University Clinical Center Maribor, Maribor, Slovenia.

### References

1. Elneihoum AM, Falke P, Hedblad B, Lindgarde F, Ohlsson K. Leukocyte activation in atherosclerosis: correlation with risk factors. Atherosclerosis. 1997;131:79–84.
2. Falke P, Elneihoum AM, Ohlsson K. Leukocyte activation: relation to cardiovascular mortality after cerebrovascular ischemia. Cerebrovasc Dis. 2000;10:97–101.
3. Hochman JS. Cardiogenic shock complicating acute myocardial infarction: expanding the paradigm. Circulation. 2003;107:2998–3002.

4. Reynolds HR, Hochman JS. Cardiogenic shock: current concepts and improving outcomes. Circulation. 2008;117:686–97.
5. Kirbis S, Breskvar UD, Sabovic M, Zupan I, Sinkovic A. Inflammation markers in patients with coronary artery disease – comparison of intracoronary and systemic levels. Wien Klin Wochenschr. 2010;122:31–4.
6. Kjeldsen L, Bainton DF, Sengelov H, Borregaard N. Identification of neutrophil gelatinase-associated lipocalin as a novel matrix protein of specific granules in human neutrophils. Blood. 1994;83:799–807.
7. Kjeldsen L, Johnsen AH, Sengelov H, Borregaard N. Isolation and primary structure of NGAL, a novel protein associated with human neutrophil gelatinase. J Biol Chem. 1993;268:10425–32.
8. Ronco C. N-GAL: diagnosing AKI as soon as possible. Crit Care. 2007;11:173.
9. Malyszko J, Bachorzewska G, Malyszko JS, Pawlak K, Dobrzycki S. Serum neutrophil gelatinase-associated lipocalin as a marker of renal function in hypertensive and normotensive patients with coronary artery disease. Nephrology. 2008;13:153–6.
10. Vinten-Johansen J. Involvement of neutrophils in the pathogenesis of lethal myocardial reperfusion injury. Cardiovasc Res. 2004;61:481–97.
11. Tang WH, Brennan ML, Philip K, Tong W, Mann S, Van Lente F, et al. Plasma myeloperoxidase levels in patients with chronic heart failure. Am J Cardiol. 2006;98:796–9.
12. Tang WH, Tong W, Troughton RW, Martin MG, Shrestha K, Borowski A, et al. Prognostic value and echocardiographic determinants of plasma myeloperoxidase levels in chronic heart failure. J Am Coll Cardiol. 2007;49:2364–70.
13. Van de Werf F, Blomstrom-Lundqvist CB, Crea F, Falk V, Filippatos G, Fox K, et al. Management of acute myocardial infarction in patients presenting with persistent ST-segment elevation-ESC guidelines. Eur Heart J. 2008;29:2909–45.
14. Wijns W, Kolh P, Danchin N, Di Mario C, Falk V, Folliguet T, et al. Guidelines on myocardial revascularization. The task force on myocardial revascularization of the European society of cardiology (ESC) and the European association for cardio-thoracic surgery. Eur Heart J. 2010;31(20):2501–55.
15. Lang RM, Bierig M, Devereux RB, Flachskampf FA, Pelikka PA, Picard MH, et al. Recommendations for chamber quantification: a report from the American society of echocardiography's guidelines and standards committee and the chamber quantification writing group, developed in conjunction with the European association of echocardiography, a branch of the European society of cardiology. J Am Soc Echocardiogr. 2005;18:1440–63.
16. Dickstein K, Cohen-Solal A, Filippatos G, McMurray JJV, Ponikowski P, Poole-Wilson PA, et al. ESC guidelines for the diagnosis and treatment of acute and chronic heart failure 2008. The task force for the diagnosis and treatment of acute and chronic heart failure 2008 of the European society of cardiology. Developed in collaboration with the Heart failure Association of the ESC (HFA) and endorsed by the European society of intensive care medicine (ESCIM). Eur J Heart Fail. 2008;10:933–89.
17. Palazzuoli A, Ruocco G, Beltrami M, Franci B, Pellegrini M, Lucani B, et al. Admission plasma neutrophil gelatinase-associated lipocalin (NGAL) predicts worsening renal function during hospitalization and post discharge outcome in patients with acute heart failure. Acute Card Care. 2014, (early Online).
18. Damman K, van Veldhuisen DJ, Navis G, Voors AA, Hillege HL. Urinary neutrophil gelatinase associated lipocalin (NGAL), a marker of tubular damage, is increased in patients with chronic heart failure. Eur J Heart Fail. 2008;10:997–1000.
19. Bolignano D, Basile G, Parisi P, Coppolino G, Nicocia G, Buemi M. Increased plasma neutrophil gelatinase-associated lipocalin levels predict mortality in elderly patients with chronic heart failure. Rejuvenation Res. 2009;12:7–14.
20. Van Deursen VM, Damman K, Voors AA, Van der Wal MH, Jaarsma T, Van Veldhuisen DJ, et al. Prognostic value of plasma neutrophil gelatinase-associated lipocalin for mortality in patients with heart failure. Circ Heart Fail. 2014;7(1):35–42.
21. Yndestad A, Landro L, Ueland T, Dahl CP, Flo TH, Vinge LE, et al. Increased systemic and myocardial expression of neutrophil gelatinase-associated lipocalin in clinical and experimental heart failure. Eur Heart J. 2009;30:1229–36.
22. Aghel A, Shrestha K, Mullens W, Borowski A, Tang WH. Serum neutrophil gelatinase-associater lipocalin (NGAL) in predicting worsening renal function in acute decompensated heart failure. J Card Fail. 2010;16:49–54.

# 5

# Association between left ventricular global longitudinal strain and natriuretic peptides in outpatients with chronic systolic heart failure

F Gaborit[1*], H Bosselmann[2], N Tønder[2], K Iversen[1], T Kümler[1], C Kistorp[3], G Sölétormos[4], J P. Goetze[5] and M Schou[1]

**Abstract**

**Background:** Both impaired left ventricular (LV) global longitudinal strain (GLS) and increased plasma concentrations of natriuretic peptides(NP) are associated with a poor outcome in heart failure (HF). Increased levels of NP reflect increased wall stress of the LV. However, little is known about the relationship between LV GLS and NP. This aim of this study was to evaluate the relationship between the echocardiographic measure LV GLS and plasma levels of NP.

**Methods:** We prospectively included 149 patients with verified systolic HF at the baseline visit in an outpatient HF clinic. LV GLS was assessed by two dimension speckle tracking and plasma concentrations of N-terminal-pro-brain-natriuretic-peptide (NT-proBNP) and pro-atrial-natriuretic-peptide (proANP) were analysed.

**Results:** The patients had a median age of 70 years, 28.2 % were females, 26.5 % were in functional class III-IV, median left ventricular ejection fraction (LVEF) was 33 % and median LV GLS was −11 %. LV GLS was associated with increased plasma concentrations of NT-proBNP and proANP in multivariate logistic regression (NT-proBNP: Odds $Ratio_{GLS}$: 7.25, 95 %-CI: 2.48-21.1, $P < 0.001$ and proANP: Odds $Ratio_{GLS}$: 3.26, 95-%-CI: 1.28-8.30, $P = 0.013$) and linear regression (NT-proBNP: $\beta_{GLS}$: 1.19, 95 %-CI: 0.62-1.76, $P < 0.001$ and proANP: $\beta_{GLS}$: 0.42, 95-%-CI: 0.11-0.72, $P = 0.007$) models after adjustment for traditional confounders (age, gender, body-mass-index, atrial fibrillation, renal function) and left atrial volume index.

**Conclusion:** Impaired LV GLS is associated with increased plasma concentrations of NP and our data suggest that left ventricular myocardial mechanics estimated by LV GLS reflects myocardial wall stress in chronic systolic HF.

**Keywords:** Left ventricular global longitudinal strain, Systolic heart failure, Natriuretic peptides

## Background

Left ventricular (LV) global longitudinal strain (GLS) is a novel echocardiographic method to evaluate LV function. It is more sensitive to LV dysfunction than conventional methods, and strain analysis allows for both regional and global assessment of the LV [1, 2]. GLS is reported as a negative value in percentages. A value closer to cero is a sign of impaired function of the LV. The normal range has been explored in some studies and it is reported to be in the region from −15.9 % to −22.1 %. The variation may be due to age, blood pressure and technical circumstances [3, 4]. It has been observed that LV GLS is associated with an increased risk of mortality and cardiovascular events in patients with established cardiac disease [5].

Among patients presenting with acute myocardial infarction, LV GLS is associated with development of heart failure (HF) and an increased mortality risk [6] as well as increased plasma concentrations of aminoterminal pro-brain natriuretic peptide(NT-proBNP) [7]. In chronic HF it has been shown that LV GLS has additional prognostic value and it can predict hospitalization for HF and an increased mortality risk [8–10]. However it remains unknown whether LV GLS reflects e.g., myocardial

* Correspondence: freja.stoltze.gaborit@regionh.dk
[1]Department of Cardiology, Herlev University Hospital, DK-2730 Herlev, Denmark
Full list of author information is available at the end of the article

wall stress [11], fibrosis [12] or subclinical ischemia [13] in chronic HF patients. NT-proBNP is released from the myocardium when it is exposed to stretch and increased wall stress [14]. Only few data exist on the relationship between LV GLS and NT-proBNP in patients with HF, suggesting association between impaired LV GLS and increased NT-proBNP [15]. Among patients suspected of HF LV GLS has been reported to be a strong predictor of NT-proBNP [16]. In asymptomatic patients with echocardiographic verified diastolic dysfunction GLS rate showed the strongest correlation to increased NT-proBNP [17].

In the present study we, therefore, tested the hypothesis that impaired LV GLS is associated with increased plasma concentrations of NT-proBNP and pro-atrial natriuretic peptide (proANP) in chronic systolic HF patients.

## Methods

### Patient selection

Patients were enrolled prospectively at their first visit when referred to the outpatient HF clinic at North Zealand Hospital, University of Copenhagen, Denmark. From January 2011 to November 2012, $N = 230$ patients were referred to the HF clinic with LVEF < 45 %. Patients had to be clinically stable (60 days out of hospital) and have steady state plasma-creatinine concentration for 60 days (+/−10 μg). A total of $N = 149$ patients agreed to participate in an echocardiography study (Cardio-Ren) [18]. All patients provide written informed consent according to the Declaration of Helsinki and the study was approved by the Scientific Ethic Committee (H-1-2010-074).

At baseline all patients were examined by a physician and the following information were obtained: medical history, present symptoms, functional class, medication, height, weight, non-invasive blood pressure, heart rate, 12-lead electrocardiogram. Venous blood samples were taken and advanced echocardiography was preformed according to standard recommendations of the European Society of Cardiology [19, 20].

### Echocardiography

Echocardiography was performed on Vivid 9E (GE Vingmed Ultrasound, Horten, Norway) and analysed offline (Echopac BT 12, 1.0, General Electric, Horten, Norway). All analysis was performed by a single operator blinded to plasma concentrations of NT-proBNP and proANP.

LVEF were determined using the Simpson biplane model. Two dimensional parasternal view were used to measure LV dimension and wall thickness. LV mass were calculated automatically by Echopac software from the linear dimensions and reported indexed to body surface area. Maximal left atrial volume were determined from the biplane area method and indexed to body surface area. Mitral inflow was evaluated by doppler recordings and peak velocity of early (E) and atrial filling (A) and mitral valve deceleration time were measured. Pulsed wave velocity was measured at both lateral and septal mitral annulus for myocardial peak early velocity (e') and peak systolic velocity (s'). Mean e' was calculated from the lateral and septal e', and used for calculating E/e'. In case of atrial fibrillation the mean value of e' from three consecutive cycles was used.

GLS analysis were performed by two-dimensional speckle tracking in the three standard apical projections (long axis, four chambers, two chambers). In the echocardiographic examination we aimed for a frame rate 40–80 frames/sec in all images for strain analysis. The region of interest was set to cover the thickness of the myocardium. Appropriate tracking were verified visually and adjusted if necessary. Aortic valve closure were automated in the analyse and then confirmed visually, when uncertain it was identified with continuous wave doppler in the aortic annulus. LV GLS were analysed for 17 standardised segments, based on these values a mean value were calculated for each of the three apical projections and then a total LV GLS were calculated as the average of the value from the three apical projections. The Echopac software allows up to one missing segment in each projection. If two segment values were missing in one projection we calculated the missing score as the average of neighbouring segments and then calculated LV GLS manually. LV GLS analysis could not be performed when three or more segments were missing over all or two segments were missing in more projections. Reproducibility were tested in 25 random selected patients for both inter- or intra observer variation. No significant bias were found (intra observational: mean diff: −0.08 % +/− 1.16 %, $P = 0.703$; inter observational: mean diff: 0.19 % +/−1.9 %, $P = 0.422$).

### Plasma analyses

Venous blood were obtained after >8 hours overnight fast and 15 min rest. At the time of sampling P-hemoglobin, P-creatinine, P-sodium and P-potassium were measured. For later analyses plasma were collected in ethylenediamine tetracetic (EDTA) vial and centrifuged at 4° (3000 rpm in 10 min) and stored at −80° Celsius. Plasma concentrations of NT-proBNP were measured on the Dimension Vista® 1500 from Siemens Medical Solutions Diagnostics using the LOCI®-technology (Luminescent Oxygen Channeling Assay) according to the manufacturer procedure [21]. Total proANP was measured with a processing-independent radioimmunoassay, which quantitates the total sum of unprocessed and processed N-terminal proANP fragments [22].

### Statistics

Baseline clinical data, biochemical data (Table 1) and echocardiographic measures (Table 2) are presented as percentages for dichotomous variables and interquartile range (25 %-75 %) for continuous variables. Groups were compared with Pearson Chi square-test for discrete variables and t-tests (parametric) and Mann Whitney U-tests (nonparametric) for continuous variables, as appropriate. Multivariate and univariate regression analyses were made test the relationship between LV GLS and NT-proBNP or proANP. Both linear and logistic regression analyses were tested (Tables 3 and 4). Adjustments were made for established confounders: gender, age, body mass index (BMI), atrial fibrillation, left atrial size and plasma eGFR. Additional univariate regression analyses were used to crosscheck the relationship between the ability to obtain sufficient image quality for LV GLS analysis and the co-existing of obesity (BMI >35 kg/m2) or chronic obstructive pulmonary disease (no significant relationship were observed). Statistic results was considered significant when $P < 0.05$ (two-sided).

## Results

We were able to perform LV GLS analysis in 117 of 149 patients, corresponding to 80 %, and median LV GLS was −11 %. Ischemic heart disease determined by coronary angiography was present in 58 % of the patients, and 38 % of all patients had atrial fibrillation. Baseline characteristic are presented in Table 1 according to LV GLS below (more negative) or above (more positive = impaired) median LV GLS. There were no significant differences between baseline characteristics in the two groups.

In Table 2 echocardiographic variables are presented. Patients with a LV GLS above the median had lower LVEF ($P < 0.001$), mildly enlarged LV internal dimension in diastole ($P < 0.001$) and lower s' both laterally ($P < 0.001$) and medially ($P < 0.001$). Diastolic function estimated by mitral valve deceleration time ($P = 0.027$) was reduced in patients with LV GLS above the median, but left atria size and E/e' were not significantly affected by LV GLS. Right ventricular systolic function estimated by TAPSE ($P = 0.012$) was also reduced in patients with LV GLS above the median. LV mass index was significantly

**Table 1** Baseline characteristics according to values below median (more negative) ($n = 65$) or above median (more positive) ($n = 52$), median GLS (median = −11 %)

| Variable | Below median GLS ($n = 65$) | Above median GLS ($n = 52$) | p-value |
|---|---|---|---|
| Age, years | 69 (63–76) | 71 (67–76) | 0.761 |
| Female gender, % | 33.8 | 21.2 | 0.130 |
| BMI[a], kg/m2 | 26.0 (22.6-30.2) | 26.3 (24.5-30.3) | 0.214 |
| NYHA[b] class III-IV, % | 23.1 | 30.8 | 0.349 |
| Systolic BP[c], mmHg | 132 (120–147) | 120 (110–140) | 0.178 |
| Diastolic BP[c], mmHg | 77 (70–82) | 77 (69–84) | 0.889 |
| Heart rate, beats/min | 64 (56–76) | 70 (62–78) | 0.188 |
| HF[d] duration, months | 9 (6–12) | 12 (6–24) | 0.216 |
| Pervious MI[e], % | 33.8 | 44.2 | 0.251 |
| Hypertension, % | 67.7 | 59.6 | 0.395 |
| Atrial fibrillation, % | 24.6 | 40.4 | 0.068 |
| ICD[f], % | 9.5 | 13.5 | 0.507 |
| Diabetes, % | 20 | 25 | 0.518 |
| ApoplexiaCerebri/TCI[g], % | 12.3 | 23.1 | 0.124 |
| ACE-I[h], % | 73.8 | 59.6 | 0.140 |
| ARB[i], % | 21.5 | 32.7 | 0.174 |
| Beta-blocker, % | 87.7 | 86.5 | 0.853 |
| MRA[j], % | 14.1 | 28.8 | 0.051 |
| Diuretics, % | 69.2 | 76.9 | 0.354 |
| Hemoglobine, mmol/l | 8.5 (7.0-9.0) | 8.8 (8.0-9.3) | 0.215 |
| Creatinine, umol/l | 80 (68–97) | 95 (73–119) | 0.254 |
| eGFR[k], ml/min/1,73 m2 | 82 (66–98) | 70 (51–95) | 0.244 |

[a]Body mass index, [b]New York Heart Association, [c]Blood pressure, [d]Heart failure, [e]Myocardial infarction, [f]Implantable cardiac defibrillator, [g]Transitory cerebral ischemia, [h]Angiotensin converting enzyme inhibitor, [i]Aldosterone receptor blocker, [j]Mineralocorticoid receptor antagonist, [k]Estimated glomerular filtration rate

**Table 2** Echocardiographic variable according to values below or above median GLS, with 75 % interquartile range

| Variable | Below median GLS ($n = 65$) | Above median GLS ($n = 52$) | p-value |
|---|---|---|---|
| LVEF biplane[a], % | 38 (32–42) | 27 (20–34) | <0.001 |
| LVIDd[b], cm | 5.00 (4.55-5.55) | 5.70 (5.20-6.30) | <0.001 |
| Peak GLS[c] | −13 (−15 - -12) | −8 (−10 - -6) | <0.001 |
| TAPSE[d], mm | 19.0 (15.0-23.0) | 16.0 (14.0-20.8) | 0.012 |
| TRmax[e],mmHG | 22.52 (8.48-27.25) | 16.98 (4.28-26.70) | 0.474 |
| s' medial[f], cm/s | 5.00 (4.00-6.00) | 4.00 (3.00-5.00) | <0.001 |
| s' lateral[f], cm/s | 6.00 (5.00-7.00) | 5.00 (4.00-5.00) | 0.001 |
| LAVI[g], ml/m2 | 27.09 (21.18-33.00) | 31.57 (23.17-39.10) | 0.093 |
| MV deceleration time[h], ms | 222 (178–277) | 182 (152–223) | 0.027 |
| E[i]/A[j] ratio | 0.89 (0.67-1.36) | 0.86 (0.62-1.65) | 0.937 |
| E[f]/e'[k] | 9.68 (7.53-12.20) | 10.47 (7.75-15.27) | 0.130 |
| LV mass Index, g/m2 | 123.60 (90.85-153.18) | 145 (117.85-194.90) | 0.019 |

[a]Left ventricle ejection fraction, [b]Left ventricle internal dimension diastole, [c]Peak left ventricle global longitudinal strain, [d]Tricuspid annular plane systolic excursion, [e]Maximal pressure gradient of tricuspid regurgitation, [f]Myocardial peak systolic velocity, [g]Left atrial end systolic volume index, [h]Mitral valve, [i]Mitral inflow early filling, [j]Mitral inflow atrial filling, [k]Myocardial early velocity

higher in patients with a GLS above the median ($P = 0.019$).

Plasma concentrations of NT-proBNP and proANP were significantly higher in patients with LV GLS above the median (Fig. 1). The overall linear relationship between LV GLS and log(NT-proBNP) and LV GLS and log(proANP) are shown in Fig. 2. In multivariate linear regression models with log(NT-proBNP) and log(proANP) as response variables and LV GLS as explanatory variable the associations were significant between LV GLS and log(NT-proBNP) ($\beta_{(NT\text{-}proBNP)} = 1.19$ (95 %-CI: 0.62-1.76, $p < 0.001$) and LV GLS and log(proANP) ($\beta_{(proANP)} = 0.42$, (95 %-CI: 0.11-0.72, $P = 0.007$). The associations between impaired LV GLS and log(NT-proBNP), and LV GLS and log(proANP), respectively, were also significant in multivariate logistic regression models (Odds Ratio $GLS_{NT\text{-}proBNP}$ 7.25 (95 %-CI: 2.48-21.18, $P < 0.001$) and (Odds Ratio $GLS_{proANP}$ 3.26 (95 %-CI: 1.28-8.29, $P = 0.013$).

## Discussion

The main finding of this study is that impaired LV GLS is associated with increased cardiac wall stress expressed by elevated plasma concentrations of NT-proBNP and proANP in chronic systolic HF patients.

### Echocardiographic findings and GLS

In the present study of patients with chronic systolic HF the majority of patients had impaired LV GLS. Patients with more impaired LV GLS had lower LVEF, and moreover, LV GLS showed stronger correlation to echocardiographic variables related to systolic function than to diastolic function. Previous studies have observed same association between LV GLS and systolic function [5, 8, 10]. LV GLS has also been evaluated in patients with HF and preserved LVEF and these studies have also identified LV GLS to be associated with systolic function and not conventional echocardiographic measures of diastolic dysfunction [23, 24]. These previous findings, including our result, therefor suggest that LV GLS reflects systolic function of the LV in both HF with reduced and normal LVEF.

### Cardiovascular Biomarkers and GLS

Few studies have examined LV GLS and NP in chronic systolic HF. In a study of 137 patients with suspected HF Yoneyama et al. [16] observed that plasma concentrations of brain-natriuretic-peptide (BNP) were correlated to functional class, decreased LVEF and an impaired GLS in patients with both systolic and diastolic dysfunction. This is supported by Nahum et al. who examined 125 patients with chronic systolic heart failure and found not only prognostic value of LV GLS, but also association between both GLS and NT-proBNP and strain rate and NT-proBNP [15]. In patients with acute myocardial infarction Ersbøll et al. observed that impaired LV GLS was correlated to plasma concentrations of NT-proBNP [7] and risk of HF during the admission [25]. The previous and the present studies, therefore, suggest that LV GLS reflects wall stress in HF patients since plasma concentration of BNP and NT-proBNP reflect myocardial wall stress [10]. It should be noted that both LV GLS and natriuretic peptides may be indirect measures of myocardial wall stress and future studies should evaluate the relationship between wall stress based on invasive measures and LV GLS and plasma concentrations of NP's before any

**Table 3** Univariate and multivariate logistic regression models

| Variable | Univariate | | Multivariate | |
|---|---|---|---|---|
| | Odds ratio (95 % CI[a]) P-value | Beta (95 % CI) P-value | Odds ratio (95 % CI) P-value | Beta (95 % CI) P-value |
| $\text{GLS}^{b\ c}_{\text{NT-proBNP}}$ | 5.92 | 0.47 | 7.25 | 1.19 |
| | (2.59-13.60) | (0.15-0.32) | (2.48-21.18) | (0.62-1.76) |
| | <0.001 | <0.001 | <0.001 | <0.001 |
| $\text{GLS}_{\text{Age}}$ | - | - | 1.03 | 0.03 |
| | | | (0.97-1.09) | (0.00-0.06) |
| | | | 0.310 | 0.025 |
| $\text{GLS}_{\text{GenderFemale}}$ | - | - | 2.29 | 0.07 |
| | | | (0.62-8.47) | (−0.55-0.69) |
| | | | 0.214 | 0.822 |
| $\text{GLS}^{d}_{\text{BMI}}$ | - | - | 0.89 | −0.05 |
| | | | (0.80-1.00) | (−0.10-0.00) |
| | | | 0.047 | 0.063 |
| $\text{GLS}^{e}_{\text{AF}}$ | - | - | 3.05 | 0.52 |
| | | | (0.94-0.85) | (−0.10-1.14) |
| | | | 0.063 | 0.099 |
| $\text{GLS}_{\text{Creatinine}}$ | - | - | 1.03 | 0.01 |
| | | | (1.00-1.05) | (0.00-0.01) |
| | | | 0.010 | <0.001 |
| $\text{GLS}^{f}_{\text{LAVI}}$ | - | - | 1.00 | 0.00 |
| | | | (0.99-1.02) | (−0.01-0.01) |
| | | | 0.647 | 0.569 |

[a]Confidence interval, [b]Global longitudinal strain, [c]Amino-terminal-pro-brain-natriuretic-peptide, [d]Body mass index, [e]Atrial fibrillation, [f]Left atrial volume index
Confounders included in the multivariate logistic regression models: Age, gender, atrial fibrillation, body-mass-index, creatinine, LAVI
A: Univariate and Multivariate logistic regression models (response: NT-proBNP) (confounders: age, gender, body mass index, atrial fibrillation, creatinine, left atrial volume index)

**Table 4** Univariate and multivariate logistic regression models

| Variable | Univariate | | Multivariate | |
|---|---|---|---|---|
| | Odds ratio (95 % CI[a]) P-value | Beta (95 % CI) P-value | Odds ratio (95 % CI) P-value | Beta (95 % CI) P-value |
| $\text{GLS}^{b\ c}_{\text{proANP}}$ | 3.37 | 0.34 | 3.26 | 0.42 |
| | (1.53-7.40) | (0.05-0.16) | (1.28-8.30) | (0.11-0.72) |
| | 0.003 | <0.001 | 0.013 | 0.007 |
| $\text{GLS}_{\text{Age}}$ | - | - | 1.05 | 0.05 |
| | | | (1,00-1.11) | (0.03-0.06) |
| | | | 0.075 | <0.001 |
| $\text{GLS}_{\text{GenderFemale}}$ | - | - | 1.18 | -.023 |
| | | | (0.39-3.58) | (−0.55-0.10) |
| | | | 0.773 | 0.172 |
| $\text{GLS}^{d}_{\text{BMI}}$ | - | - | 0.96 | −0.02 |
| | | | (0.88-1.05) | (−0.05-0.00) |
| | | | 0.402 | 0.097 |
| $\text{GLS}^{e}_{\text{AF}}$ | - | - | 0.80 | −0.05 |
| | | | (0.28-2.29) | (−0.38-0.28) |
| | | | 0.671 | 0.746 |
| $\text{GLS}_{\text{Creatinine}}$ | - | - | 1.02 | 0.00 |
| | | | (1.00-1.04) | (0.00-0.01) |
| | | | 0.030 | <0.001 |
| $\text{GLS}^{f}_{\text{LAVI}}$ | - | - | 1.00 | 0.00 |
| | | | (0.99-1.01) | (0.00-0.01) |
| | | | 0.960 | 0.245 |

[a]Confidence interval, [b]Global longitudinal strain, [c]pro-atrial-natriuretic-peptide, [d]Body mass index, [e]Atrial fibrillation, [f]Left atrial volume index
Confounders included in the multivariate logistic regression models: Age, gender, atrial fibrillation, body-mass-index, creatinine, Left atrial volume index
B: Univariate and Multivariate logistic regression models (response: proANP)(Confounders: age, gender, body mass index, atrial fibrillation, creatinine, left atrial volume index)B: Univariate and Multivariate logistic regression models (response: proANP)(Confounders: age, gender, body mass index, atrial fibrillation, creatinine, left atrial volume index)

firm conclusions can be made. Whether impaired LV GLS also reflects other aspects than increased wall stress in chronic systolic HF needs to be investigated in future biomarker studies including e.g., Galectin 3.

### Methodological considerations and perspectives

Some methodological limitations of this study should be addressed. It is a single center study and consists of a relatively small cohort. Patients in this study have a short history of chronic systolic HF, are in stable clinical condition over past tree month and may not be fully up-titrated in the recommended HF treatment. Therefore the results cannot be extrapolated to other groups of patients or other stages of heart failure.

All patients had performed an echocardiography by a trained physician. Due to poor acoustic conditions or atrial fibrillation we were not able to perform LV GLS analyses in 21.5 % of the patients. Atrial fibrillation is a challenge when LV GLS is analysed, because of variation in the electrocardiographic loop duration, but if cycles of same length are selected, corresponding to a normal heart rate. LV GLS can be calculated in patients with atrial fibrillation [26]. It may be speculated that patients with atrial fibrillation more often have an impaired LV GLS since atrial fibrillation is associated with increased plasma concentrations of NP's [27], but why NP's are increased in atrial fibrillation is unknown, and exclusion of some patients with atrial fibrillation will probably not result in selection bias. In the present study the prevalence of atrial fibrillation did not differ significantly between the two groups of LV GLS above and below the

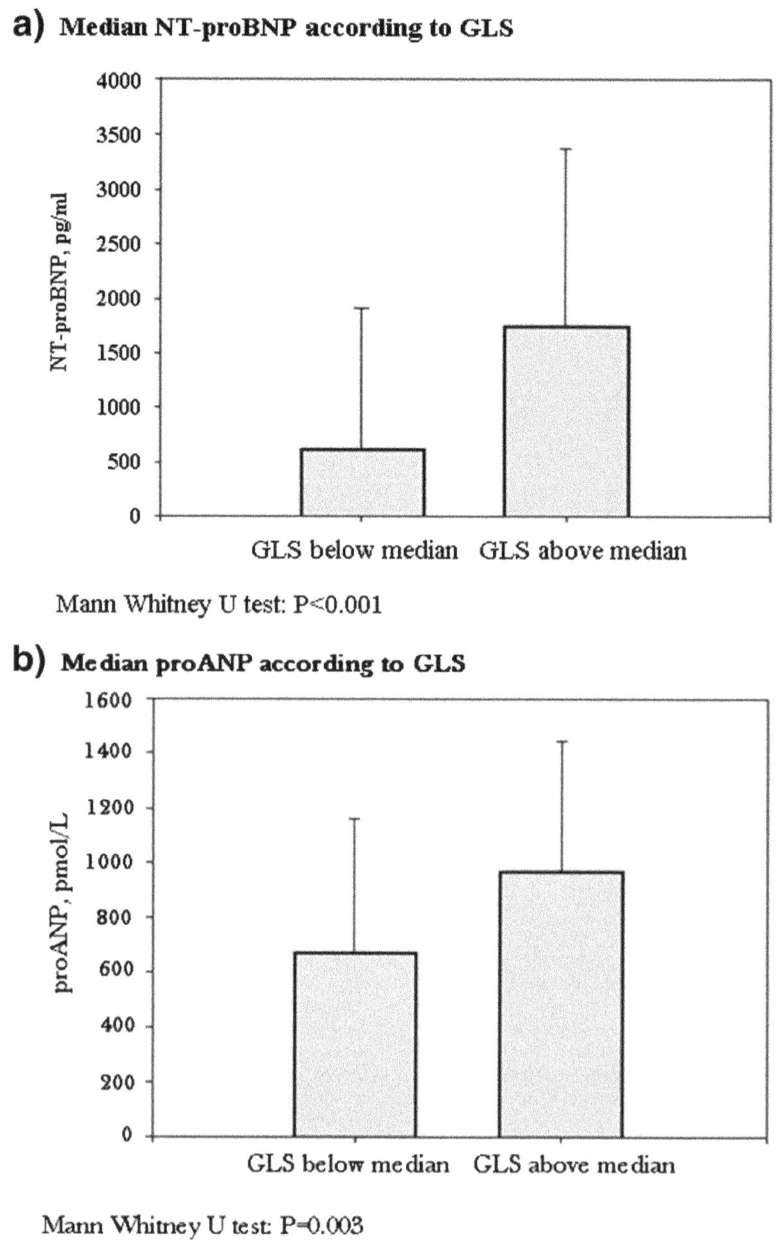


**Fig. 1** **a** Median NT-proBNP according to GLS above or below median, with 75 % interquartile range. **b** Median proANP according to global longitudinal strain above or below median, with 75 % interquartile range. GLS: global longitudinal strain; NT-proBNP: amino-terminal-pro-brain-natriuretic-peptide; proANP: pro-atrial-natriuretic-peptide

median (Table 3). A BMI > 35 kg/m2 and chronic obstructive lung disease (prevalent conditions in HF) did neither influence the echocardiographic image quality and it was possible to analyse LV GLS in these subgroups. Selection bias due poor echocardiographic quality in certain subgroups seems, therefore, not to be the case.

Calculation of LV GLS is not yet a standard procedure in the echocardiographic examination. The challenge of LV GLS is that it requires good imaging quality of all three apical standard projections and sinus rhythm is preferable. LV GLS is only slightly angle dependent [28]. The calculation of LV GLS is automatic after setting the region of interest and intra- and interobserver variation is low. Theoretically, if LV GLS is going to be analysed in clinical practice it may be possible to find patients at high risk of developing decompensating and worsening of HF, and an hospitalization might be prevented if a

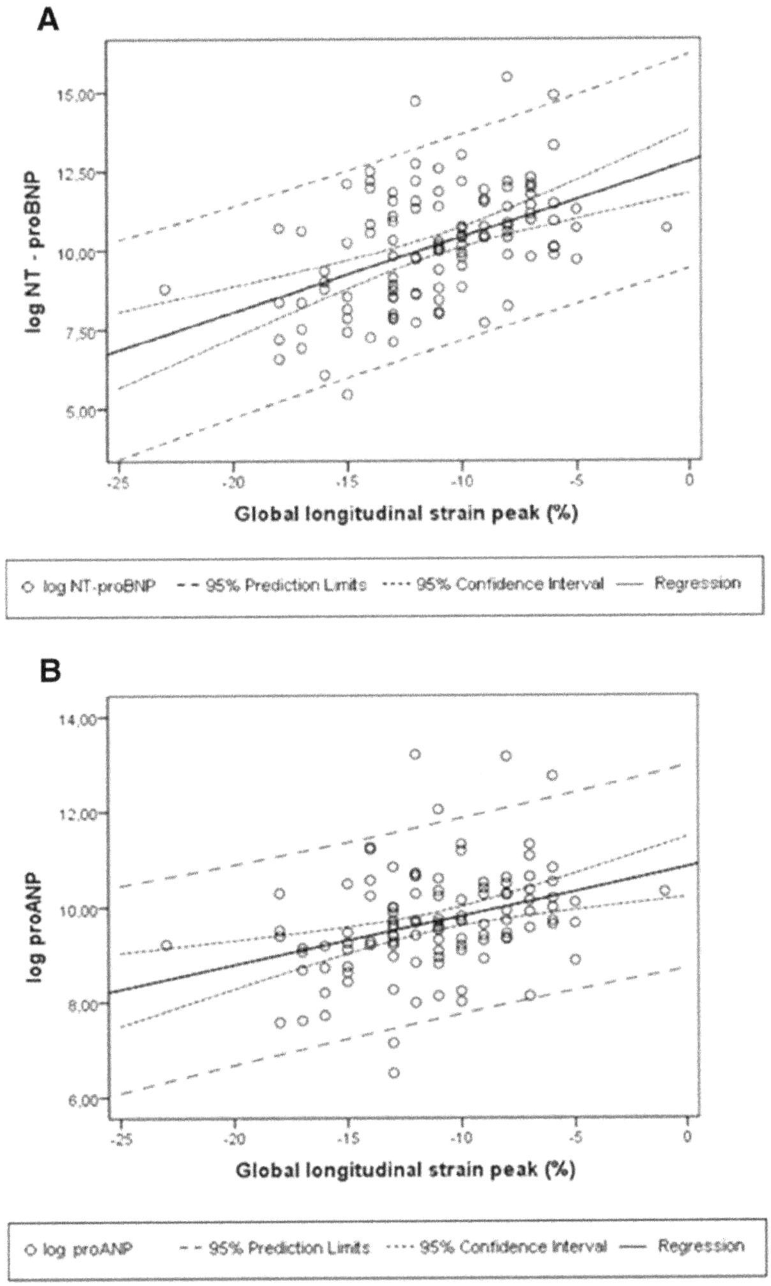


**Fig. 2 a** Correlation between NT-proBNP and GLS. **b** Correlation between MR-proANP and global longitudinal strain. GLS: global longitudinal strain; NT-proBNP: amino-terminal-pro-brain-natriuretic-peptide; proANP: pro-atrial-natriuretic-peptide

relevant intervention is applied, but this hypothesis needs to be validated in a prospective setting.

## Conclusion

Impaired LV GLS is associated with increased plasma concentrations of NP's and patients with impaired LV GLS have more frequent other cardiac abnormalities and diastolic and systolic dysfunction. GLS of the LV is, therefore, both associated with other structural abnormalities of the heart and neurohormonal activity. LV GLS is an accessible echocardiographic meassure and should be used in future studies for risk stratification and to identify clinical or scientific scenarios where GLS might be more useful than NP's.

### Abbreviations

LV: Left ventricle; GLS: Global longitudinal strain; NP: Natriuretic peptide; HF: Heart failure; NT-proBNP: Aminoterminal pro-brain natriuretic peptide; ProANP: Pro-atrial natriuretic peptide; LVEF: Left ventricle ejection fraction;

EDTA: Ethylenediamine tetracetic; NYHA: New York Heart Association; BMI: Body mass index; eGFR: Estimated glomerular filtration rate.

**Competing interests**
The authors declare that they have no competing interest.

**Authors' contributions**
FG: acquisition of data, interpretation of data, drafting the manuscript, final approval of the version. HB: acquisition of data, analysis of data, final approval of the version. NT: analysis of data, interpretation of data (especially regarding echocardiography), final approval of the version. KI: interpretation of data, revising manuscript critically for important intellectual content, final approval of the version. TK: interpretation of data (especially regarding echocardiography), final approval of the version. CK: interpretation of data, final approval of the version. GS: interpretation of data (especially regarding biomarkers), final approval of the version. JPG: interpretation of data (especially regarding biomarkers), final approval of the version. MS: hypothesis generating, revising manuscript critically for important intellectual content, final approval of the version.

**Acknowledgements**
The technical assistance of the nurses Mette Welløv Petersen and Ellen Mouritsen is gratefully acknowledged.
The study was funded by Research Grants from North Zealand Hospital, University of Copenhagen.

**Author details**
[1]Department of Cardiology, Herlev University Hospital, DK-2730 Herlev, Denmark. [2]Department of Internal Medicine KNEA, North Zealand University Hospital, DK-3400 Hillerod, Denmark. [3]Department of Internal Medicine O, Herlev University Hospital, DK-2730 Herlev, Denmark. [4]Department of Clinical Biochemistry, North Zealand University Hospital, DK-3400 Hillerod, Denmark. [5]Department of Clinical Biochemistry, Rigshospitalet, DK-2100 Copenhagen, Denmark.

**References**

1. Feigenbaum H, Mastouri R, Sawada S. A practical approach to using strain echocardiography to evaluate the left ventricle. Circ J. 2012;76:1550–5.
2. Brown J, Jenkins C, Marwick TH. Use of myocardial strain to assess global left ventricular function: a comparison with cardiac magnetic resonance and 3-dimensional echocardiography. Am Heart J. 2009;157:102.e1–5.
3. Tee M, Noble JA, Bluemke DA. Imaging techniques for cardiac strain and deformation: comparison of echocardiography, cardiac magnetic resonance and cardiac computed tomography. Expert Rev Cardiovasc Ther. 2013;11:221–31.
4. Yingchoncharoen T, Agarwal S, Popović ZB, Marwick TH. Normal ranges of left ventricular strain: a meta-analysis. J Am Soc Echocardiogr. 2013;26:185–91.
5. Cho GY, Marwick TH, Kim HS, Kim MK, Hong KS, Oh DJ. Global 2-dimensional strain as a New prognosticator in patients with heart failure. J Am Coll Cardiol. 2009;54:618–24.
6. Ersbøll M, Valeur N, Andersen MJ, Mogensen UM, Vinther M, Svendsen JH, et al. Early echocardiographic deformation analysis for the prediction of sudden cardiac death and life-threatening arrhythmias after myocardial infarction. JACC Cardiovasc Imaging. 2013;6:851–60.
7. Ersbøll M, Valeur N, Mogensen UM, Andersen M, Greibe R, Møller JE, et al. Global left ventricular longitudinal strain is closely associated with increased neurohormonal activation after acute myocardial infarction in patients with both reduced and preserved ejection fraction: a two-dimensional speckle tracking study. Eur J Heart Fail. 2012;14:1121–9.
8. Iacoviello M, Puzzovivo A, Guida P, Forleo C, Monitillo F, Catanzaro R, et al. Independent role of left ventricular global longitudinal strain in predicting prognosis of chronic heart failure patients. Echocardiography. 2013;30:803–11.
9. Stanton T, Leano R, Marwick TH. Prediction of all-cause mortality from global longitudinal speckle strain: comparison with ejection fraction and wall motion scoring. Circ Cardiovasc Imaging. 2009;2:356–64.
10. Motoki H, Borowski AG, Shrestha K, Troughton RW, Tang WHW, Thomas JD, et al. Incremental prognostic value of assessing left ventricular myocardial mechanics in patients with chronic systolic heart failure. J Am Coll Cardiol. 2012;60:2074–81.
11. Iwanaga Y, Nishi I, Furuichi S, Noguchi T, Sase K, Kihara Y, et al. B-type natriuretic peptide strongly reflects diastolic wall stress in patients with chronic heart failure: comparison between systolic and diastolic heart failure. J Am Coll Cardiol. 2006;47:742–8.
12. Saito M, Okayama H, Yoshii T, Higashi H, Morioka H, Hiasa G, et al. Clinical significance of global two-dimensional strain as a surrogate parameter of myocardial fibrosis and cardiac events in patients with hypertrophic cardiomyopathy. Eur Heart J Cardiovasc Imaging. 2012;13:617–23.
13. Eek C, Grenne B, Brunvand H, Aakhus S, Endresen K, Hol PK, et al. Strain echocardiography and wall motion score index predicts final infarct size in patients with non-ST-segment-elevation myocardial infarction. Circ Cardiovasc Imaging. 2010;3:187–94.
14. Hall C. NT-ProBNP: The Mechanism Behind the Marker. J Card Fail. 2005;11:S81–3.
15. Nahum J, Bensaid A, Dussault C, Macron L, Clémence D, Bouhemad B, et al. Impact of longitudinal myocardial deformation on the prognosis of chronic heart failure patients. Circ Cardiovasc Imaging. 2010;3:249–56.
16. Yoneyama A, Koyama J, Tomita T, Kumazaki S, Tsutsui H, Watanabe N, et al. Relationship of plasma brain-type natriuretic peptide levels to left ventricular longitudinal function in patients with congestive heart failure assessed by strain Doppler imaging. Int J Cardiol. 2008;130:56–63.
17. Uraizee I, Cheng S, Hung C-L, Verma A, Thomas JD, Zile MR, et al. Relation of N-terminal pro-B-type natriuretic peptide with diastolic function in hypertensive heart disease. Am J Hypertens. 2013;26:1234–41.
18. Bosselmann H, Tonder N, Sölétormos G, Rossing K, Iversen K, Goetze JP, et al. Influence of renal impairment on myocardial function in outpatients with systolic heart failure: An echocardiographic and cardiac biomarker study. Int J Cardiol. 2014;177:942–8.
19. Lang RM, Bierig M, Devereux RB, Flachskampf FA, Foster E, Pellikka PA, et al. Recommendations for chamber quantification. Eur J Echocardiogr. 2006;7:79–108.
20. Nagueh SF, Appleton CP, Gillebert TC, Marino PN, Oh JK, Smiseth OA, et al. Recommendations for the evaluation of left ventricular diastolic function by echocardiography. Eur J Echocardiogr. 2009;10:165–93.
21. Bruneel A, Dehoux M, Barnier A, Boutten A. External evaluation of the Dimension Vista 1500® intelligent lab system. J Clin Lab Anal. 2012;26:384–97.
22. Hunter I, Rehfeld JF, Goetze JP. Measurement of the total proANP product in mammals by processing independent analysis. J Immunol Methods. 2011;370:104–10.
23. Kraigher-Krainer E, Shah AM, Gupta DK, Santos A, Claggett B, Pieske B, et al. Impaired systolic function by strain imaging in heart failure with preserved ejection fraction. J Am Coll Cardiol. 2014;63:447–56.
24. Carluccio E, Biagioli P, Alunni G, Murrone A, Leonelli V, Pantano P, et al. Advantages of deformation indices over systolic velocities in assessment of longitudinal systolic function in patients with heart failure and normal ejection fraction. Eur J Heart Fail. 2011;13:292–302.
25. Ersbøll M, Valeur N, Mogensen UM, Andersen MJ, Møller JE, Hassager C, et al. Relationship between left ventricular longitudinal deformation and clinical heart failure during admission for acute myocardial infarction: a two-dimensional speckle-tracking study. J Am Soc Echocardiogr. 2012;25:1280–9.
26. Kusunose K, Yamada H, Nishio S, Tomita N, Hotchi J, Bando M, et al. Index-beat assessment of left ventricular systolic and diastolic function during atrial fibrillation using myocardial strain and strain rate. J Am Soc Echocardiogr. 2012;25:953–9.
27. Freestone B, Gustafsson F, Chong AY, Corell P, Kistorp C, Hildebrandt P, et al. Influence of atrial fibrillation on plasma von willebrand factor, soluble E-selectin, and N-terminal pro B-type natriuretic peptide levels in systolic heart failure. Chest. 2008;133:1203–8.
28. Forsha D, Risum N, Rajagopal S, Dolgner S, Hornik C, Barnhart H, et al. The influence of angle of insonation and target depth on speckle-tracking strain. J Am Soc Echocardiogr. 2015;28:580–6.

# 6

# Comparative effects of recombinant human brain natriuretic peptide and dobutamine on acute decompensated heart failure patients with differsent blood BNP levels

Hai-Yan Pan[1], Jian-Hua Zhu[1*], Yong Gu[1], Xiao-Hong Yu[1], Min Pan[1] and Hong-Yin Niu[2]

**Abstract**

**Background:** Recombinant human B-type natriuretic peptide (rhBNP) has been indicated for the treatment of acute decompensated heart failure (ADHF). However, the therapeutic efficacy of intravenous rhBNP is not always satisfactory in patients with extremely high blood BNP levels. In this study, we evaluated the effects of rhBNP on patients with different BNP levels.

**Methods:** One hundred and five patients with ADHF whose left ventricular ejection fraction (LVEF) was <40%, were assigned to a high BNP group (BNP ≤ 3000 pg/mL) or an extra-high BNP group (BNP > 3000 pg/mL) , depending on their admission plasma BNP levels. Each group was then subdivided into rhBNP or dobutamine subgroups according to intravenous administration with either rhBNP or dobutamine for 24-72h. In the high BNP group, 58 patients were randomized to subgroup rhBNP (n = 28) and subgroup dobutamine (n = 30). In the extra-high BNP group, 47 patients were randomized to subgroup rhBNP (n = 24) and subgroup dobutamine (n = 23). The effects of rhBNP and dobutamine on patients in the high and extra-high BNP groups were compared.

**Results:** In the high BNP group, rhBNP was more efficient than dobutamine at improving NYHA classification ($P < 0.05$), decreasing plasma BNP levels ($P < 0.05$), increasing LVEF ($P < 0.05$), and reducing hospital length of stay ($P < 0.05$). However, rhBNP displayed no superior therapeutic efficacy to dobutamine in the extra-high BNP group. Adverse cardiovascular events in patients treated with rhBNP were similar to adverse events in patients treated with dobutamine in both the high and extra-high BNP groups.

**Conclusions:** rhBNP was more efficient than dobutamine at improving heart function in patients with ADHF when plasma BNP was ≤3000 pg/mL. However, rhBNP treatment showed no advantages over dobutamine when plasma BNP reached extremely high levels (>3000 pg/mL).

**Keywords:** Acute decompensated heart failure, Recombinant human brain natriuretic peptide, Dobutamine

## Background

Acute decompensated heart failure (ADHF) is associated with significant morbidity and mortality and remains a common cause of hospitalization worldwide. As a result, therapies targeting both symptoms and cardiovascular outcomes are greatly needed. Two such treatments are dobutamine and recombinant human brain natriuretic peptide (rhBNP).

Dobutamine is a synthetic catecholamine that acts mainly through stimulation of β1-receptors and partly through β2-receptors to produce dose-dependent positive inotropic and chronotropic effects [1]. It has long been used as a potent positive inotrope for the management of severe heart failure. rhBNP is a recombinant formulation of BNP that is identical to the endogenous hormone released from the cardiac ventricle in response

* Correspondence: dr.zhujianhua@gmail.com
[1]Department of Cardiology, Affiliated Hospital of Nantong University, and Institute of Cardiovascular Research, Nantong University, Jiangsu 226001, China
Full list of author information is available at the end of the article

to increases in wall stress, hypertrophy, and volume overload [2]. It is a potent vasodilator that is proven to rapidly reduce cardiac filling pressures and improve dyspnea in patients with ADHF [3]. In 2005, rhBNP was recommended in the ADHF treatment guidelines by the European Society of Cardiology [4].

Some evidence suggests that rhBNP is more effective than dobutamine in the treatment of heart failure [5-7]. However, in our clinical work, we have found that the effects of rhBNP are not always satisfactory in patients with extremely high blood BNP levels, with the heart function of some patients not improved until rhBNP is replaced by dobutamine. Although comparison of rhBNP and dobutamine in ADHF patients has been reported in several studies [5-7], no comparative study has been performed on ADHF patients with different plasma BNP levels. Thus, the purpose of this study was to determine the therapeutic efficacy of rhBNP in ADHF patients with different plasma BNP levels in comparison to that of dobutamine in order to provide valuable information for the treatment of heart failure.

## Methods

### Patient selection

Between January 2011 and June 2012, patients with ADHF who required hospitalization were enrolled in the study. The mean age was 66 ± 13 years (range = 29–88). The ADHF etiology included idiopathic dilated cardiomyopathy (IDC), coronary heart disease (CHD), fulminant viral myocarditis (FVM), hyperthyroid heart disease (HHD), and valvulopathy. All patients were classified as New York Heart Association (NYHA) class III–IV and had an ejection fraction of <40%. Exclusion criteria included intravenous administration with rhBNP or dobutamine in the 2 weeks before study entry, acute myocardial infarction, significant valvular stenosis, serious ventricular arrhythmia (frequent ventricular premature beat of >5 bpm, nonsustained and sustained ventricular tachycardia), blood pressure <95/60 mmHg or >140/90 mmHg, shock, hypovolemia, and hepatic or renal impairment [alanine aminotransferase or aspartate aminotransferase >2 times the upper limit of the normal value, serum creatinine >177 μmol/L (2.0 mg/dl) for man or >146 μmol/L (1.7 mg/dl) for women]. In addition, pregnant and lactating women, those who had to change medication due to adverse events during the study were also excluded. All patients provided informed consent, and the Ethics Committee of Affiliated Hospital of Nantong University approved the protocol.

### Study design

Previous studies evaluating the correlation between BNP level and heart failure severity used 3000 pg/mL as the cut-off for extremely high BNP elevation [8,9]. In this open-label prospective cohort study we also used value of 3000 pg/mL (30 times the upper normal range) as the cut-off for stratifying patients into high and extra BNP groups. Enrolled patients were stratified into a high BNP group (BNP ≤ 3000 pg/mL) or extra-high BNP group (BNP > 3000 pg/mL) depending on their admission plasma BNP levels. Each group was then subdivided into two subgroups (rhBNP or dobutamine) according to the intravenous administration of either rhBNP or dobutamine. Patients in the high and extra-high BNP groups were randomly assigned to rhBNP or dobutamine subgroups using a computer-generated random number table. In total, 58 patients were enrolled in the high BNP group, of which 28 were randomized to the rhBNP subgroup and 30 were randomized to the dobutamine subgroup. In addition, 47 patients were enrolled in the extra-high BNP group, of which 24 were randomized to the rhBNP subgroup and 23 were randomized to the dobutamine subgroup.

### Procedure

In addition to conventional heart failure therapy, patients in the rhBNP and dobutamine subgroups received rhBNP (marketed as Xinhuosu, Chengdu Rhodiola Bio-Pharmacy, Chengdu, China) and dobutamine (Shanghai No. 1 Biochemical & Pharmaceutical, Shanghai, China) infusion, respectively, for a period of 24–72 h. rhBNP was administered as an intravenous bolus of 1.5 μg/kg followed by continuous infusion in doses of 0.0075–0.01 μg/kg/min according to each patient's clinical status. Patients in the dobutamine subgroup initially received 2.5 μg/kg/min dobutamine and were up-titrated to 10 μg/kg/min if hemodynamic goals were not achieved.

Plasma creatinine and BNP levels were measured at baseline and 5 days after the start of the study. Creatinine was detected by a creatinine assay kit (Abcam, MA, USA). BNP levels were determined with the ARCHITECT BNP Reagent Kit (Abbott Laboratories, IL, USA). Left ventricle end diastolic dimension (LVEDD) and left ventricular ejection fraction (LVEF) were measured by one observer blinded to the clinical data with a GE Vivid E9 ultrasound scanner (GE Healthcare, Horten, Norway) at the time of blood sample drawing.

### Assessment of efficacy

The drug therapeutic efficacy was assessed as improvement of functional class; changes in BNP levels, LVEDD, and LVEF from baseline to fifth day after the beginning of treatment. According to the assessed dyspnea and systemic symptoms, the functional improvement was graded as "excellent" (NYHA class was improved ≥2 functional classes), "improved" (NYHA class was improved 1 functional class) or "failed" (NYHA class remained the same or deteriorated). The overall effective rate was calculated as (patients with "excellent" + patients with "improved"/all patients) × 100%.

In addition, the length of hospitalization and the effects of the study drugs on blood pressure, heart rate (HR), blood creatinine, and cardiovascular adverse events during infusion were also analyzed.

### Statistical analysis

Statistical analysis was performed with SigmaStat 3.5 (Systat Software, Point Richmond, CA, USA) statistical software. Quantitative data are presented as mean ± standard deviation (SD), while categorical data are presented as numbers. Comparisons between the two groups were made using a two-sample *t*-test for continuous variables and chi-squared test or Fishe exact test for categorical data. Differences between baseline and treatment values were assessed using a paired *t*-test. $P < 0.05$ was considered significant.

## Results

### Baseline characteristics

In the extra-high BNP group, one patient who was assigned to the rhBNP subgroup had to withdraw from the study because of symptomatic hypotension 3 h after rhBNP administration; thus, 23 patients in the rhBNP subgroup finished this study. Basal blood pressure and plasma creatinine and baseline demographics and medical history information for patients in the high and extra-high BNP groups are summarized. Basal SBP level tended to be lower in the extra-high BNP group than in the high BNP group (P = 0.079), while plasma creatinine was significantly higher in the extra-high BNP group (P < 0.01) (Table 1). However, the baseline characteristics of the patients and heart failure medications in patients randomized to the rhBNP subgroup or the dobutamine subgroup were well balanced in both the high and extra-high BNP groups (Table 2).

### Changes in NYHA class

Functional improvements, as assessed by NYHA class, were observed so as to evaluate the therapeutic efficacy of the treatments. Both rhBNP and dobutamine could effectively improve patient cardiac function. In the high BNP group, rhBNP was significantly more efficacious than dobutamine in improving NYHA class. The proportion of patients showing a functional improvement of at least 1 grade in NYHA class was significantly greater in the rhBNP subgroup (92.86%, 26/28) than in the dobutamine subgroup (70%, 21/30) ($P < 0.05$). However, in the extra-high BNP group, the overall effective rates of the two subgroups did not differ significantly [56.52% (13/23) vs. 65.22 (15/23) ($P > 0.05$)] (Table 3).

**Table 1 Baseline blood pressure and plasma creatinine in the high and Extra-high BNP groups**

| Parameters | High-BNP group (n = 58) | Extra-high BNP group (n = 46) | P value* |
|---|---|---|---|
| SBP (mmHg) | 121.0 ± 12.3 | 116.7 ± 12.5 | 0.079 |
| DBP (mmHg) | 72.9 ± 7.2 | 71.3 ± 6.5 | 0.229 |
| Cr (μmol/L) | 81.6 ± 30.7 | 97.0 ± 27.1 | 0.009 |

*Unpaired *t* test.
*Abbreviations*: *BNP* brain natriuretic peptide, *Cr* creatinine, *DBP* diastolic blood pressure, *SBP* systolic blood pressure.

### Changes in blood BNP, LVEDD and LVEF in the high BNP group

Changes in blood BNP, LVEDD, and LVEF were analyzed to assess the therapeutic efficacy. In the high BNP group, both rhBNP and dobutamine were able to significantly reduce the plasma BNP levels ($P < 0.01$), decrease LVEDD ($P < 0.01$), and increase LVEF ($P < 0.01$). Compared to dobutamine, rhBNP was significantly more efficacious in reducing plasma BNP ($P < 0.05$) and increasing LVEF ($P < 0.05$), but the decrease of LVEDD in the rhBNP subgroup was similar to that of the dobutamine subgroup ($P > 0.05$) (Table 4).

### Changes in blood BNP, LVEDD and LVEF in the extra-high BNP group

The measurement range for the ARCHITECT BNP assay is 10–5000 pg/mL. In the extra-high BNP group, there were 10 patients (6 from the dobutamine subgroup and 4 from the rhBNP subgroup) whose plasma BNP levels were >5000 pg/mL before the study; therefore, as we only selected patients with plasma BNP levels ≤5000 pg/mL for statistical analyses of BNP changes, their BNP levels could not be used for calculating the mean BNP values. Nonetheless, the changes in LVEDD and LVEF were still analyzed in all enrolled patients. Of the 10 patients with plasma BNP >5000 pg/mL, there were 5 and 3 patients in the dobutamine and rhBNP subgroups, respectively, whose plasma BNP levels were reduced to <5000 pg/mL. The average plasma BNP level in the rhBNP subgroup was slightly, but not significantly, higher than that of the dobutamine subgroup (4020 ± 710 pg/mL vs. 3508 ± 654 pg/mL; $P > 0.05$) at day 5 after treatment. Similarly, the BNP levels in patients with plasma BNP ≤ 5000 pg/mL was effectively reduced by rhBNP and dobutamine ($P < 0.01$) (Table 5). In addition, both rhBNP and dobutamine slightly, but significantly decreased the LVEDD ($P < 0.05$), and significantly increased the LVEF ($P < 0.05$) of all enrolled patients. The therapeutic efficacy of dobutamine in improving these parameters tended to be better than that of rhBNP, although the difference was not statistically significant ($P > 0.05$) (Table 5).

**Table 2 Baseline characteristics and treatment information**

| Characteristics | High BNP group | | | Extra-high BNP group | | |
|---|---|---|---|---|---|---|
| | Dobutamine (n = 30) | rhBNP (n = 28) | P value | Dobutamine (n = 23) | rhBNP (n = 23) | P value |
| Age (y) | 63 ± 13 | 65 ± 13 | 0.495† | 68 ± 14 | 67 ± 12 | 0.709† |
| Male/female | 19/11 | 18/10 | 0.843‡ | 15/8 | 16/7 | 0.935‡ |
| HF etiology | | | | | | |
| IDC | 13 | 11 | 0.963‡ | 10 | 12 | 0.768‡ |
| CHD | 8 | 10 | 0.645‡ | 10 | 8 | 0.763‡ |
| FVM | 2 | 1 | 1.000§ | 0 | 1 | 1.000§ |
| HHD | 1 | 2 | 0.605§ | 0 | 1 | 1.000§ |
| Valvulopathy | 6 | 4 | 0.732§ | 3 | 1 | 0.608§ |
| NHYA | | | 0.645‡ | | | 0.489§ |
| III | 8 | 10 | | 0 | 2 | |
| IV | 22 | 18 | | 23 | 21 | |
| Concomitant medications | | | | | | |
| ACEI | 14 | 16 | 0.593‡ | 14 | 12 | 0.766‡ |
| ARB | 12 | 7 | 0.349‡ | 5 | 8 | 0.513‡ |
| Digitalis | 24 | 23 | 0.899‡ | 18 | 20 | 0.699§ |
| β-blockers | 11 | 14 | 0.448‡ | 4 | 6 | 0.722§ |
| Spironolactone | | | | | | |
| 20 (mg/d) | 15 | 18 | 0.405‡ | 11 | 6 | 0.324‡ |
| 40 (mg/d) | 10 | 8 | 0.914‡ | 10 | 12 | 0.768‡ |
| Average dosage | 28.0 ± 10.0 | 26.2 ± 9.4 | 0.500† | 29.5 ± 10.2 | 33.3 ± 9.7 | 0.243† |
| Furosemide (mg/d) | | | | | | |
| 20 (mg/d) | 12 | 15 | 0.440‡ | 7 | 4 | 0.328§ |
| 40 (mg/d) | 11 | 8 | 0.707‡ | 11 | 9 | 0.766‡ |
| 80 (mg/d) | 2 | 3 | 0.665§ | 3 | 5 | 0.699§ |
| Average dosage | 33.6 ± 17.0 | 33.1 ± 19.5 | 0.919† | 39.0 ± 19.5 | 46.7 ± 22.8 | 0.267† |

†Unpaired *t*-test; ‡Chi-square test; §Fisher exact test.
*Abbreviations*: *ACEI* angiotensin-converting enzyme inhibitor, *ARB* angiotensin II receptor blocker, *BNP* brain natriuretic peptide, *CHD* coronary heart disease, *HF* heart failure, *HHD* hyperthyroid heart disease, *IDC* idiopathic dilated cardiomyopathy, *NHYA* New York Heart Association, *rhBNP* recombinant human brain natriuretic peptide. Values are expressed as number or mean ± SD.

### Length of hospitalization and All cause mortality

No patients died during administration of dobutamine or rhBNP. One patient with dilated cardiomyopathy in the extra-high BNP group whose symptoms were much improved by dobutamine suffered sudden death due to ventricular fibrillation at 8 days after withdrawal of dobutamine infusion during hospitalization; we excluded this patient from analysis of hospitalization length. In the high BNP group, length of hospitalization for rhBNP-treated patients was significantly shorter than for patients treated with dobutamine (8.0 ± 1.9 versus 9.3 ± 2.2 days, $P < 0.05$). However, in the extra-high BNP group, the length of hospitalization was not significantly different between the two subgroups (13.0 ± 3.1 versus 12.2 ± 2.7 days, $P > 0.05$). All-cause mortality during hospitalization was similar between the dobutamine and rhBNP

**Table 3 Changes in NYHA class from baseline to day 5 after treatment**

| Groups | Dobutamine | | | | | rhBNP | | | | |
|---|---|---|---|---|---|---|---|---|---|---|
| | Total | Ex | Im | Fa | OER (%) | Total | Ex | Im | Fa | OER (%) |
| High BNP | 30 | 12 | 9 | 9 | 21 (70.00) | 28 | 9 | 17* | 2 | 26 (92.86)* |
| Extra-high BNP | 23 | 6 | 9 | 8 | 15 (65.22) | 23 | 5 | 8 | 10 | 13 (56.52) |

*Abbreviations*: *Ex* Excellent, *Fa* failed, *Im* improved, *OER* overall effective rate. Other abbreviations are same as in Table 2. *P < 0.05 versus (Fisher exact test) dobutamine.

**Table 4 Changes in blood BNP, LVEDD, and LVEF in the high BNP group**

| Parameters | Dobutamine (n = 30) | | | rhBNP (n = 28) | | |
|---|---|---|---|---|---|---|
| | Baseline | 5 Days | Changes | Baseline | 5 Days | Changes |
| BNP (pg/mL) | 1890 ± 742 | 1261 ± 560** | 629 ± 715 | 1819 ± 665 | 843 ± 450**ΔΔ | 976 ± 566Δ |
| LVEDD (mm) | 63.8 ± 4.6 | 61.2 ± 6.5** | 2.6 ± 4.3 | 64.3 ± 4.9 | 60.9 ± 5.7** | 3.3 ± 3.2 |
| LVEF (%) | 32.1 ± 6.1 | 39.6 ± 10.9** | 7.5 ± 8.1 | 31.3 ± 6.8 | 43.7 ± 11.2** | 12.4 ± 7.5Δ |

*Abbreviations: LVEDD* left ventricle end diastolic dimension, *LVEF* left ventricular ejection fraction, Other abbreviations are same as in Table 2. Values are mean ± SD. **P < 0.01 (paired *t*- test) versus baseline; ΔP < 0.05, ΔΔP < 0.01 (unpaired *t*- test) versus dobutamine.

subgroups in the high and extra-high BNP groups (both P = 1.000).

### Effects of the study drugs on blood pressure, HR and plasma creatinine

Ambulatory changes in systolic blood pressure (SBP), diastolic blood pressure (DBP), and HR were monitored during infusion. The SBP, DBP, and HR values at the end of infusion and the levels of plasma creatinine at day 5 after treatment were measured. Both rhBNP and dobutamine did not significantly affect HR and plasma creatinine ($P > 0.05$). The systolic and diastolic pressure were significantly decreased by rhBNP ($P < 0.01$), while no significant changes were observed in dobutamine-treated patients ($P > 0.05$) (Table 6).

### Cardiovascular adverse events

The incidence of selected cardiovascular adverse events during administration was similar between the rhBNP- and dobutamine-treated patients. However, symptomatic hypotension tended to be more common in the rhBNP-treated patients than the dobutamine-treated patients, although the difference was not statistically significant (Table 7). In the extra-high BNP group, one patient who was initially enrolled to the rhBNP subgroup had to withdraw from this study due to symptomatic hypotension. We still included this patient in the statistical analysis of adverse events.

## Discussion

Our study is the first to compare the effects of rhBNP and dobutamine on ADHF patients with different plasma BNP levels. The results revealed that rhBNP was not superior to the traditional inotropic agent dobutamine at improving cardiac function in patients with extra-high BNP levels (>3000 pg/mL). On the contrary, rhBNP-treated patients tended to be more likely to experience hypotension than dobutamine-treated patients.

Dobutamine, a dopamine derivative, produces positive inotropic and chronotropic effects on myocardium mainly through stimulation of β1-receptors and by causing a reflex decrease in sympathetic tone [1,10,11]. At low doses, dobutamine induces mild arterial vasodilatation, which augments stroke volume by reductions in afterload [4], and has little influence on HR, blood pressure, and cardiovascular adverse events.

BNP, a natriuretic peptide, is produced and released from the ventricles in response to increased wall stretch and tension [2]. It binds to the A-type natriuretic peptide receptor that is present on the surface of vascular smooth muscle and endothelial cells [2], resulting in activation of guanylate cyclase and the subsequent accumulation of intracellular cyclic GMP in target tissues [12]. Cyclic GMP, as a second messenger, mediates natriuretic, diuretic and smooth muscle relaxant effects, which lead to the therapeutic benefits of venous and arterial vasodilation and decreases in preload and afterload, resulting in increased cardiac output with improved dyspnea and systemic symptoms [12].

In addition, BNP also serves as a physiological antagonist of the renin-angiotensin-aldosterone system and the sympathetic nervous system [13]. It inhibits renin-aldosterone secretion, suppresses the sympathetic nervous system, and antagonizes the action of antidiuretic hormone in inducing antidiuresis, antinatriuresis, and vasoconstriction, leading to a decrease in systemic vascular resistance and cardiac pre- and afterload [4,14,15]. Thus, as a compensatory mechanism for heart failure, circulating BNP levels strongly correlate with the severity of heart failure [16,17].

**Table 5 Changes in blood BNP, LVEDD, and LVEF in the extra-high BNP group**

| Parameters | Dobutamine (n = 23) | | | rhBNP (n = 23) | | |
|---|---|---|---|---|---|---|
| | Baseline | 5 Days | Changes | Baseline | 5 Days | Changes |
| BNP (pg/mL) | 3790 ± 740 | 2806 ± 859** | 985 ± 931§ | 3912 ± 726 | 3207 ± 900** | 705 ± 884× |
| LVEDD (mm) | 66.6 ± 5.1 | 64.2 ± 5.1* | 2.4 ± 4.6 | 67.7 ± 5.4 | 65.6 ± 6.3* | 2.1 ± 4.2 |
| LVEF (%) | 24.4 ± 5.7 | 31.6 ± 6.9** | 7.2 ± 6.1 | 23.8 ± 5.6 | 29.0 ± 6.5** | 5.2 ± 7.1 |

Abbreviations are same as in Table 2 and Table 4. Values are mean ± SD. §n = 17, ×n = 19. *P < 0.05, **P < 0.01 (paired *t*- test) versus baseline.

**Table 6 Effects of the study drugs on blood pressure (mmHg), HR (bpm) and plasma creatinine (μmol/L)**

| Parameters | High BNP group | | | | Extra-high BNP group | | | |
|---|---|---|---|---|---|---|---|---|
| | Dobutamine (n = 30) | | rhBNP (n = 28) | | Dobutamine (n = 23) | | rhBNP (n = 23) | |
| | Baseline | 5 Days | Baseline | 5 Days | Baseline | 5 Days | Baseline | 5 Days |
| SBP | 119.3 ± 12.7 | 121.3 ± 12.0 | 122.9 ± 11.9 | 115.4 ± 12.4** | 114.8 ± 11.9 | 116.0 ± 12.5 | 118.6 ± 13.0 | 113.2 ± 13.2** |
| DBP | 72.4 ± 6.8 | 74.3 ± 5.3 | 73.5 ± 7.7 | 69.6 ± 7.9** | 70.7 ± 6.7 | 71.8 ± 6.6 | 71.9 ± 6.5 | 68.7 ± 6.6** |
| HR | 77.6 ± 12.5 | 80.3 ± 13.1 | 81.8 ± 11.1 | 83.9 ± 11.5 | 83.2 ± 13.9 | 85.7 ± 13.0 | 82.3 ± 12.4 | 84.6 ± 9.3 |
| Cr | 84.4 ± 29.8 | 79.3 ± 20.4 | 78.5 ± 31.9 | 80.9 ± 26.3 | 95.4 ± 24.4 | 90.3 ± 23.3 | 98.6 ± 30.1 | 105.5 ± 32.9 |

*Abbreviations: HR* heart rate. Other abbreviations are same as in Table 1 and Table 2. Values are mean ± SD. **P < 0.01 (paired *t*- test) versus baseline.

rhBNP has the same 32 amino acid sequence and biological activity as endogenous BNP, with a mean terminal elimination half-life of 18–20 min [18,19], which means that it is almost completely cleared at 3 h post infusion withdrawal (approximately 9–10 elimination half-lives). Several studies indicated that BNP changes during the first 5 days of hospitalization had a very high prognostic value in patients with heart failure [20,21]. Accordingly, we assayed the plasma BNP levels at day 5 after treatment to evaluate the efficacy of rhBNP and dobutamine. At this time, the exogenous rhBNP had been completely eliminated and did not interfere with the measurement of the endogenous BNP level, allowing accurate assessment of the therapeutic efficacy of the study drugs.

Numerous studies reported that BNP levels reflect heart failure severity [16,17,22]. However, Law et al. found that extremely high BNP level ( > 3000pg/mL) did not correlate with heart failure severity when patients had complications such as neurological disorder, sepsis, or subarachnoid hemorrhage. The possible reasons might be that in these patients, an increase in sympathetic stimulation causes the hypothalamus to secrete excess vasopressin and BNP [9,23]. In our study, all patients with these confounders were excluded. Thus, BNP level might well reflect the status of heart function.

We found that rhBNP was more efficient than dobutamine at improving heart function in patients with BNP levels ≤3000 pg/mL. However, their efficacies were similar in patients with extra-high BNP levels. The difference might be explained by the following reasons. First, BNP exerts its biological activities through binding to the A-type natriuretic peptide receptor, which is present on the surface of vascular smooth muscle and endothelial cells [2]. When the compensatorily increased endogenous BNP is not sufficient to bind to all the free receptors, the introduced exogenous BNP (rhBNP) can fully activate the remaining free receptors, resulting in a marked improvement in heart function. However, when the circulating BNP increases to even greater levels, with subsequent full activation of their receptors, an insufficient number of free BNP receptors can be bound by exogenous BNP, meaning that the additional effects of exogenous BNP on decreasing cardiac pre- and afterload are inhibited. Second, patients with extremely high BNP levels might be resistant to the biological action of BNP. This phenomenon is characterized by extremely high circulating BNP levels in patients with congestive heart failure who have physical signs of fluid retention and vasoconstriction from poor biological activity of the BNP system [14]. A deficient response to BNP is attributed to inactivation of BNP by plasma and tissue proteases

**Table 7 Selected cardiovascular adverse events during drug administration**

| Adverse events | High BNP group | | | Extra-high BNP group | | |
|---|---|---|---|---|---|---|
| | Dobutamine (n = 30) | rhBNP (n = 28) | P value | Dobutamine (n = 23) | rhBNP (n = 24) | P value |
| Symptomatic hypotension | 0 | 0 | 1.000 | 0 | 1 | 1.000 |
| Asymptomatic hypotension | 0 | 2 | 0.229 | 0 | 3 | 0.234 |
| Sustained VT | 0 | 0 | 1.000 | 0 | 0 | 1.000 |
| Nonsustained VT | 2 | 0 | 0.492 | 2 | 1 | 0.609 |
| VF | 0 | 0 | 1.000 | 0 | 0 | 1.000 |
| Sudden death | 0 | 0 | 1.000 | 0 | 0 | 1.000 |
| Cardiac arrest | 0 | 0 | 1.000 | 0 | 0 | 1.000 |

*Abbrevations: VF* ventricular fibrillation, *VT* ventricular tachycardia, Other abbreviations are same as in Table 2. Fisher exact text was used.

before they bind to their receptors, downregulation or desensitization of BNP-specific receptors, and mechanisms that counteract the biological effects of BNP at postreceptor level [14]. Third, patients with extremely high BNP levels usually suffer from more severe heart failure, accompanied by serious renal congestion and low renal blood flow [24], which could inhibit the effects of rhBNP on renal vessel dilation, natriuresis, and diuresis, but would not affect the positive inotropic effects of dobutamine on myocardium. In this study, basal plasma creatinine was significantly higher in the extra-high BNP group, suggesting deterioration of renal function might be responsible for the low efficiency of rhBNP in patients with extremely high BNP. In addition, patients with more severe heart failure usually also have lower arterial pressure. The SBP level in the extra-high BNP group tended to be lower than in the high BNP group, although the difference was not significant (P = 0.079). Vasodilator drugs such as rhBNP might lead to more satisfactory clinical improvements in heart failure patients with high-normal blood pressure.

The blood pressure in the rhBNP subgroup was decreased after treatment (Table 6). One patient in the extra-high BNP group with low baseline blood pressure (96/64 mmHg) experienced symptomatic hypotension (84/50 mmHg) at 3 h after rhBNP infusion and had to withdraw from the study. Plasma creatinine remained unchanged in patients with plasma BNP ≤3000 pg/mL after treatment, but it tended to increase in patients with extra-high BNP levels after rhBNP treatment (Table 6). One male patient in the extra-high BNP group who received rhBNP had an increase in plasma creatinine from 165 μmol/L (1.9 mg/dl, baseline) to 243 μmol/L (2.7 mg/dl). These results indicate that rhBNP, as an antagonist of the renin-angiotensin-aldosterone system (RAAS), might impair renal function and induce azotemia in patients with severe heart failure whose renal function depends on RAAS. Dobutamine had no obvious effect on plasma creatinine.

### Study limitations

The results of this study are limited by its open-label design and the relatively small number of patients in each subgroup. Moreover, the effects of rhBNP and dobutamine on hospital readmissions and long-term survival were not assessed. More information from a larger blinded study will be required to confirm the results of this study.

## Conclusions

We found that rhBNP was more efficient than dobutamine in ADHF patients who had plasma BNP ≤3000 pg/mL. However, rhBNP therapy was not superior to dobutamine when BNP reached extremely high level (>3000 pg/mL).

### Abbreviations

ADHF: Acute decompensated heart failure; CHD: Coronary heart disease; DBP: Diastolic blood pressure; FVM: Fulminant viral myocarditis; HHD: Hyperthyroid heart disease; HR: Heart rate; IDC: Idiopathic dilated cardiomyopathy; LVEDD: Left ventricular end diastolic diameter; LVEF: Left ventricular ejection fraction; NYHA: New York Heart Association; RAAS: Renin-angiotensin-aldosterone system; rhBNP: Recombinant human B-type natriuretic peptide; SBP: Systolic blood pressure.

### Competing interests

The authors declare that they have no competing interests.

### Authors' contributions

PHY conceived and designed the study, analyzed and interpreted the data, drafted the manuscript and critically revised the manuscript for intellectual content. ZJH was responsible for acquisition, analysis and interpretation of data, drafting of the manuscript, and final approval of the published version. GY was responsible for analysis and interpretation of data and critical revision of the manuscript. YXH and PM inspected and approved the final version of the manuscript. NHY was responsible for analysis and interpretation of data. All authors read and approved the final manuscript.

### Acknowledgement

This work was supported by the Special Coordination Funds for 226 Project of Nantong City.

### Author details

[1]Department of Cardiology, Affiliated Hospital of Nantong University, and Institute of Cardiovascular Research, Nantong University, Jiangsu 226001, China. [2]Department of Echocardiography, Affiliated Hospital of Nantong University, Jiangsu, China.

### References

1. Leier CV, Unverferth DV: **Drugs five years later: dobutamine.** *Ann Intern Med* 1983, **99**:490–496.
2. Arora S, Clarke K, Srinivasan V, Gradman A: **Effect of nesiritide on renal function in patients admitted for decompensated heart failure.** *QJM* 2007, **100**:699–706.
3. Colucci WS: **Nesiritide for the treatment of decompensated heart failure.** *J Card Fail* 2001, **7**:92–100.
4. Nieminen MS, Böhm M, Cowie MR, Drexler H, Filippatos GS, Jondeau G, Hasin Y, Lopez-Sendon J, Mebazaa A, Metra M, Rhodes A, Swedberg K, Priori SG, Garcia MA, Blanc JJ, Budaj A, Cowie MR, Dean V, Deckers J, Burgos EF, Lekakis J, Lindahl B, Mazzotta G, Morais J, Oto A, Smiseth OA, Garcia MA, Dickstein K, Albuquerque A, Conthe P, *et al*: **Executive summary of the guidelines on the diagnosis and treatment of acute heart failure: the Task Force on Acute Heart Failure of the European Society of Cardiology.** *Eur Heart J* 2005, **26**:384–416.
5. Silver MA, Horton DP, Ghali JK, Elkayam U: **Effect of nesiritide versus dobutamine on short-term outcomes in the treatment of patients with acutely decompensated heart failure.** *J Am Coll Cardiol* 2002, **39**:798–803.
6. Burger AJ, Elkayam U, Neibaur MT, Haught H, Ghali J, Horton DP, Aronson D: **Comparison of the occurrence of ventricular arrhythmias in patients with acutely decompensated congestive heart failure receiving dobutamine versus nesiritide therapy.** *Am J Cardiol* 2001, **88**:35–39.
7. Burger AJ, Horton DP, LeJemtel T, Ghali JK, Torre G, Dennish G, Koren M, Dinerman J, Silver M, Cheng ML, Elkayam U: **Effect of nesiritide (B-type natriuretic peptide) and dobutamine on ventricular arrhythmias in the treatment of patients with acutely decompensated congestive heart failure: the PRECEDENT study.** *Am Heart J* 2002, **144**:1102–1108.
8. Guglin M, Hourani R, Pitta S: **Factors determining extreme brain natriuretic peptide elevation.** *Congest Heart Fail* 2007, **13**:136–141.
9. Law C, Glover C, Benson K, Guglin M: **Extremely high brain natriuretic peptide does not reflect the severity of heart failure.** *Congest Heart Fail* 2010, **16**:221–225.
10. Nakajima-Takenaka C, Sakata S, Kato S, Ohga Y, Murata KY, Taniguchi S: **Detrimental effects after dobutamine infusion on rat left ventricular function: mechanical work and energetics.** *Exp Physiol* 2005, **90**:635–644.

11. Ruffolo RR Jr: **The pharmacology of dobutamine.** *Am J Med Sci* 1987, **294**:244–248.
12. Michaels AD, Klein A, Madden JA, Chatterjee K: **Effects of intravenous nesiritide on human coronary vasomotor regulation and myocardial oxygen uptake.** *Circulation* 2003, **107**:2697–2701.
13. Omland T, Hagve TA: **Natriuretic peptides: physiologic and analytic considerations.** *Heart Fail Clin* 2009, **5**:471–487.
14. Clerico A, Recchia FA, Passino C, Emdin M: **Cardiac endocrine function is an essential component of the homeostatic regulation network: physiological and clinical implications.** *Am J Physiol Heart Circ Physiol* 2006, **290**:H17–H29.
15. Fermepín MR, Vatta MS, Bianciotti LG, Wolovich TJ, Fernández BE: **B-Type and C-type natriuretic peptides modify norepinephrine uptake in discrete encephalic nuclei of the rat.** *Cell Mol Neurobiol* 2000, **20**:763–771.
16. Maisel A: **B-type natriuretic peptide levels: diagnostic and prognostic in congestive heart failure: what's next?** *Circulation* 2002, **105**:2328–2331.
17. Cowie MR, Jourdain P, Maisel A, Dahlstrom U, Follath F, Isnard R, Luchner A, McDonagh T, Mair J, Nieminen M, Francis G: **Clinical applications of B-type natriuretic peptide (BNP) testing.** *Eur Heart J* 2003, **24**:1710–1718.
18. Reichert S, Ignaszewski A: **Molecular and physiological effects of nesiritide.** *Can J Cardiol* 2008, **24**(Suppl B):15B–18B.
19. DeWald TA, Hernandez AF: **Efficacy and safety of nesiritide in patients with acute decompensated heart failure.** *Expert Rev Cardiovasc Ther* 2010, **8**:159–169.
20. Cohen-Solal A, Logeart D, Huang B, Cai D, Nieminen MS, Mebazaa A: **Lowered B-type natriuretic peptide in response to levosimendan or dobutamine treatment is associated with improved survival in patients with severe acutely decompensated heart failure.** *J Am Coll Cardiol* 2009, **53**:2343–2348.
21. Valle R, Aspromonte N, Giovinazzo P, Carbonieri E, Chiatto M, di Tano G, Feola M, Milli M, Fontebasso A, Barro S, Bardellotto S, Milani L: **B-type natriuretic Peptide-guided treatment for predicting outcome in patients hospitalized in sub-intensive care unit with acute heart failure.** *J Card Fail* 2008, **14**:219–224.
22. Cheng V, Kazanagra R, Garcia A, Lenert L, Krishnaswamy P, Gardetto N, Clopton P, Maisel A: **A rapid bedside test for B-type peptide predicts treatment outcomes in patients admitted for decompensated heart failure: a pilot study.** *J Am Coll Cardiol* 2001, **37**:386–391.
23. Benvenga S: **What is the pathogenesis of hyponatremia after subarachnoid hemorrhage?** *Nat Clin Pract Endocrinol Metab* 2006, **2**:608–609.
24. Clerico A: **Pathophysiological and clinical relevance of circulating levels of cardiac natriuretic hormones: is their assay merely a marker of cardiac disease?** *Clin Chem Lab Med* 2002, **40**:752–760.

7

# Can BNP-guided therapy improve health-related quality of life, and do responders to BNP-guided heart failure treatment have improved health-related quality of life? Results from the UPSTEP study

Patric Karlström[1*], Peter Johansson[2], Ulf Dahlström[2], Kurt Boman[3] and Urban Alehagen[2]

**Abstract**

**Background:** To investigate whether B-type natriuretic peptide (NP)-guided treatment of heart failure (HF) patients improved their health related quality of life (Hr-QoL) compared to routine HF treatment, and whether changes in Hr-QoL differed depending on whether the patient was a responder to NP-guided therapy or not.

**Methods:** A secondary analysis of the UPSTEP-study, a Scandinavian multicentre study using a prospective, randomized, open, blinded evaluation design on patients with HF with New York Heart Association (NYHA) class II-IV. NP-guiding was aimed to reduce BNP <150 ng/L if < 75 years or BNP < 300 ng/L if > 75 years. A responder was defined as a patient with a BNP < 300 ng/L and/or a decrease in BNP of at least 40 % in week 16 compared to study start. Short form-36 (SF-36) was used to measure Hr-QoL. At the study start, 258 patients presented evaluable SF-36 questionnaires, 131 in the BNP group and 127 in the control group. At the study end 100 patients in the NP-guided group and 98 in the control group, presenting data from both the study start and the study end.

**Results:** There were no significant differences in Hr-QoL between NP-guided HF treatment and control group; however significant improvements could be seen in four of the eight domains in the NP-guided group, whereas in the control group improvements could be seen in six of the domains.
Among the responders improvements could be noted in four domains whereas in the non-responders improvements could be seen in only one domain evaluating within group changes.

**Conclusions:** Improved Hr-QoL could be demonstrated in several of the domains in both the NP-guided and the control group. In the responder group within group analyses showed more increased Hr-QoL compared to the non-responder group. However, all groups demonstrated increase in Hr-QoL.

**Keywords:** Heart failure, Treatment guided by natriuretic peptides, Health related quality of life, Responders, BNP, SF-36

* Correspondence: patric.karlstrom@rjl.se
[1]Department of Medicine, Division of Cardiology, County Hospital Ryhov, Jönköping, Sweden
Full list of author information is available at the end of the article

## Background

In developed countries, approximately 1-2 % of the adult population has heart failure (HF) and the prevalence is over 10 % among persons older than 70 years of age [1]. There was an increase in the absolute numbers of patients hospitalized because of HF in Sweden between 1990 until 2007, but the age-adjusted prevalence in Sweden has shown a decreasing trend since 2002 [2]. Improved diagnostics, pharmacological therapies and interventions on patients with cardiovascular (CV) diseases have resulted in a decrease in the incidence of HF after acute myocardial infarction in Sweden [3]. However, despite recent improvements in pharmacological treatment, the prognosis is poor, with an estimated five-year survival of approximately 50 % [4]. Moreover, HF patients' perceived health-related quality of life (HR-QoL) is poorer compared to patients with other chronic diseases [5].

There have been several attempts to improve and individualize HF treatment through guiding with natriuretic peptides (NP). Troughton et al. showed that NP-guided HF therapy reduced all-cause mortality as well as HF and CV hospitalization in patients younger than 75 years [6]. However, only mortality and hospitalization were evaluated, and in a review article by Anker et al. the importance of patient-reported outcomes such as Hr-QoL was emphasized, and it was recommended that these outcomes should be reported in all clinical CV trials, in addition to mortality and morbidity [7]. There are only a limited number of NP-guided studies that have evaluated the impact of NP-guiding on Hr-QoL [8–13]. Bhardwaj et al. showed that NT-proBNP-guided care was associated with greater and more sustained improvement in Hr-QoL compared to standard of care [11]. However, an association between NP-guiding and improvement in Hr-QoL was not reported in five other NP-guiding studies [8–10, 12, 13]. One reason for the differences in study findings may be that not all HF patients seem to benefit from NP-guided therapy, i.e. their NP levels do not decrease despite increased doses of angiotensin-converting enzyme inhibitors, angiotensin II receptor blockers, beta-blockers and mineralocorticoid receptor antagonists. Thus, these patients, defined as non-responders to HF pharmacological treatment, may have obscured the effects of NP-guided therapy on Hr-QoL. Gaggin et al. [14] and the UPSTEP study [15, 16] have previously shown that the responders had significantly reduced risk of CV- and HF hospitalization and CV- and HF mortality compared to non-responders. However, to our knowledge no studies have reported whether responders to NP-guided HF treatment also show beneficial effects of their treatment on Hr-QoL.

### Aim

The primary aim was to investigate whether B-type natriuretic peptide-guided treatment of HF patients compared to routine HF treatment improves the perceived Hr-QoL. The secondary aim was to evaluate whether changes in HR-QoL differed depending on whether the patient was a responder to NP-guided therapy or not.

## Methods

### Population

This study is based on data from the UPSTEP-study and has been described elsewhere [15]. In brief, the UPSTEP study was a Scandinavian multicentre study (15 centres in Sweden and four centres in Norway), on patients with HF with New York Heart Association (NYHA) class II-IV, using a PROBE design (prospective, randomized, open, blinded evaluation) [15]. The patients were randomized into a BNP-guided treatment group (BNP group) and a control group (conventionally treated), (CTR group). In the CTR group, medical treatment was adjusted at the discretion of the investigator based on changes in signs and/or symptoms of worsening HF, in accordance with the guidelines [15].The patients were recruited after an episode of worsening HF and a verified left ventricular ejection fraction (LVEF) < 40 %, NYHA class II–IV and a BNP > 150 ng/L if < 75 years, and >300 ng/L if >75 years, were required to be included. Most patients were in NYHA functional class III (55 %) and 14 % were in NYHA class IV. The mean values of BNP were 808 ng/L in the BNP group and 899 ng/L in the CTR group at the study start (Table 1). Both groups were well treated at baseline regarding HF medication. In the BNP group 146 out of 147 patients (99 %) were receiving treatment with renin-angiotensin system (RAS)-blockers versus 129 of 132 patients (98 %) in the CTR group. Approximately 50 percent of those in both groups had impaired renal function defined as an estimated Glomerular Filtration Rate (eGFR) < 60 mL/min/1.73 $m^2$ [15].

### Definition of a responder

The definition of a responder was carefully evaluated with different percentage changes in different weeks, and the best definition to a responder was a patient with a decrease in BNP concentration of at least 40 percent in week 16 of follow-up, compared to study start and/or a BNP < 300 ng/L in week 16 [16]. According to that definition, 78 responders (60 %) and 53 non-responders could be identified (Fig. 1). In the conventionally treated group, it was not allowed to control BNP, so responders and non responders are derived from the BNP-group, (Fig. 1). The non-responders had a greater degree of impaired renal function compared to the responders (eGFR 56.1 vs. 66.5; $p = 0.005$) and the non-responders were older (74.0 years vs. 69.6 years; $p = 0.009$) (Table 1). There were no differences in medication, blood pressure, heart rate, serum-potassium or BNP levels between the responders and non-responders at study start [16].

**Table 1** Baseline characteristics for conventionally treated (CTR group) and patients whose treatment was guided by BNP (BNP group) and for non-responders and responders (defined as a patient with a BNP < 300 ng/l and/or a decrease in BNP of at least 40 % in week 16 compared to BNP at study start) (ref art 2)

| Characteristics | BNP group | CTR group | p-value | Responders | Non-responders | p-value |
|---|---|---|---|---|---|---|
| | *n* = 147 | *n* = 132 | | *n* = 78 | *n* = 53 | |
| Background | | | | | | |
| Age years (SD) | 71.6 (±9.7) | 70.1 (±10) | 0.19 | 69.6 (±10.2) | 74.0 (±8.1) | 0.009 |
| Gender male, n (%) | 107 (73 %) | 96 (73 %) | 0.99 | 63 (81 %) | 34 (64 %) | 0.33 |
| IHD n (%) | 81 (55 %) | 76 (58 %) | 0.68 | 43 (55 %) | 30 (57 %) | 0.87 |
| Hypertension n (%) | 39 (27 %) | 30 (23 %) | 0.46 | 35 (45 %) | 25 (47 %) | 0.80 |
| Diabetes Mellitus n (%) | 39 (27 %) | 48 (36 %) | 0.08 | 19 (24 %) | 13 (25 %) | 0.98 |
| Physical examination | | | | | | |
| Heart rate beats/min (SD) | 74 (±18) | 73 (±19) | 0.89 | 78 (±20) | 71 (±15) | 0.93 |
| Systolic blood pressure, mm Hg (SD) | 126 (±22) | 122 (±22) | 0.12 | 126 (±23) | 125 (±21) | 0.77 |
| Diastolic blood pressure, mm Hg (SD) | 75 (±13) | 74 (±13) | 0.42 | 75 (±13) | 74 (±12) | 0.71 |
| NYHA functional classes | | | | | | |
| II n (%) | 47 (32 %) | 36 (27 %) | 0.39 | 28 | 18 | 0.09 |
| III n (%) | 76 (52 %) | 78 (59 %) | 0.22 | 42 | 27 | 0.74 |
| IV n (%) | 22 (15 %) | 18 (14 %) | 0.75 | 8 | 8 | 0.41 |
| Medication | | | | | | |
| ACEi n (%) | 113 (77) | 92 (70) | 0.17 | 65 (83) | 37 (70) | 0.67 |
| ARB n (%) | 51 (35) | 46 (35) | 0.98 | 23 (29) | 23 (43) | 0.10 |
| BB n (%) | 137 (93) | 125 (95) | 0.60 | 75 (96) | 48 (91) | 0.19 |
| MRA n (%) | 81 (55) | 78 (59) | 0.50 | 43 (55) | 28 (55) | 0.80 |
| Echocardiography (LVEF) | | | | | | |
| <30 % n | 84 (57 %) | 76 (58 %) | 0.94 | 50 (64 %) | 27 (51 %) | 0.13 |
| 30-40 % n | 63 (43 %) | 56 (42 %) | 0.94 | 28 (36 %) | 26 (49 %) | 0.13 |
| Laboratory results | | | | | | |
| BNP ng/l mean (SD) | 808 (±676) | 899 (±915) | 0.34 | 805 (±704) | 778 (±651) | 0.82 |
| eGFR mL/min/1.73 m$^2$ mean (SD) | 61.4 (±20.9) | 60.1 (±20.9) | 0.59 | 66.5 (±21.1) | 56.1 (±19.2) | 0.005 |
| Potassium mmol/l mean (SD) | 4.3 (±0.5) | 4.2 (±0.5) | 0.38 | 4.3 (±0.50) | 4.3 (±0.52) | 0.80 |

Notes: *ACEi* Angiotensin Converting Enzyme inhibitor, *ARB* Angiotensin receptor blockers, *BB* Beta blocker, *BNP* B-type natriuretic peptide, *CTR* Conventionally treated, *eGFR* estimated glomerular filtration rate (MDRD formula), *IHD* Ischemic Heart Disease, *LVEF* Left Ventricular Ejection Fraction, *MRA* mineralocorticoid receptor antagonist, *NYHA* New York Heart Association functional class, *SD* standard deviation

#### Health-related Quality of life

The patients' self-assessed Hr- QoL was measured using the Swedish and Norwegian version of the SF-36 [17, 18]. SF-36 is a well-established Hr-QoL instrument and is frequently used in studies of patients with HF and other diseases [19, 20]. The 36-item instrument includes eight domains of Hr-QoL: physical functioning (PF), role limitations due to physical health problems (RP), bodily pain (BP), general health (GH), vitality (VT), social functioning (SF), role limitations due to emotional health problems (RE) and mental health (MH). The scores were transformed into values between 0-100, with a higher score indicating a better Hr-QoL [21]. The physical component score (PCS) and mental component score (MCS), are two higher order components [17]. All patients filled out the inventory at the study start and at the study end. We used a normative Swedish population evaluated with SF-36 to illustrate the effect ageing has on Hr-QoL. The population 65-74 years consisted of 460 males and 481 females and the population over 75 years of 108 males and 125 females [22].

#### BNP analyses

BNP analyses were analysed on site by means of an immunoassay technique (Triage, Biosite Inc., San Diego, CA, USA) as described in a previous publication [15].

### Statistics

Continuous variables were presented as means and standard deviation (SD) values and categorical variables were

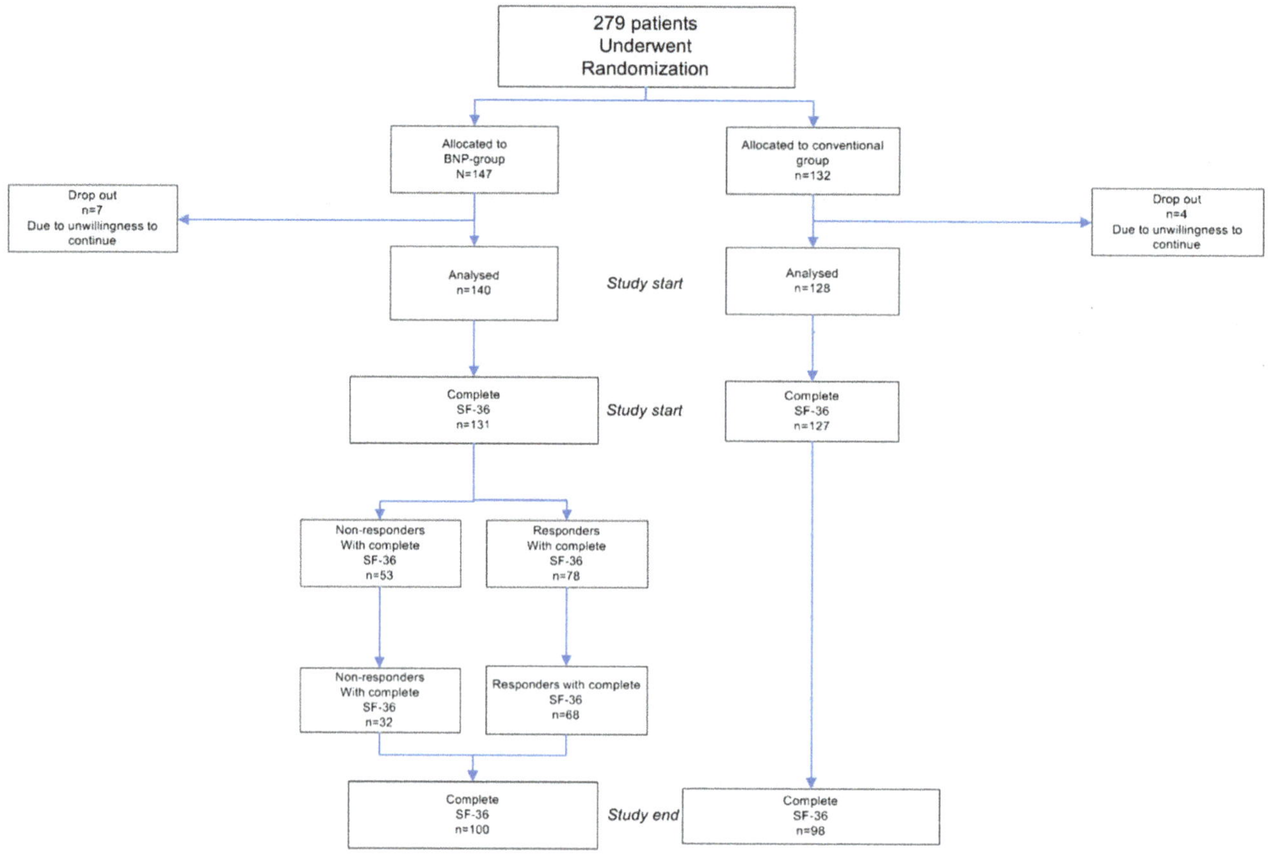


**Fig. 1** Flow chart of the patients in the UPSTEP-study. Conventionally treated (CTR group) and BNP group, BNP group divided into responders and non-responders. Responder defined as a patient with a BNP under 300 ng/l and/or a decrease in BNP of at least 40 percent in week 16 of follow-up, compared to study start

presented using percentages. Differences in mean values between groups were analysed using the Student's two-tailed *T*-test for normal distributed data. For non-normal distributed variables, the non-parametric Mann–Whitney U-test was used. Continuous variables were analysed with the student unpaired two-sided *T*-test, whereas the $\chi^2$-test was used for discrete variables. Within group differences were analysed with a Wilcoxon paired test. Spearman Rank Order correlations was used to analyse possible correlations between background characteristics and changes in Hr-QoL as indicated by the composite scores PCS and MCS. A p-value <0.05 was considered statistically significant. All calculations were performed on commercial statistical software packages (Statistica v.10,Statsoft Inc, Tulsa, OK, USA).

### Ethical considerations

The study protocol of UPSTEP was approved by the Regional Ethical Committee (Diary nr: M180-04) in Linkoping, Sweden. Every patient signed an informed consent before entering the trial. The study conforms to the Helsinki Declaration.

## Results

### Study sample

The total study population consisted of 279 patients, of whom 147 were randomized to the BNP-guided group and 132 patients to the CTR group. The mean follow-up time of the 198 patients who completed the study was 712 (SD ± 279) days. Eleven patients, seven in the BNP group and four in the control group, discontinued the study for various reasons (Fig. 1), mainly because of unwillingness to continue [15]. At the study start, 258 patients presented evaluable SF-36 questionnaires, 131 in the BNP group and 127 in the control group. As seen in Table 1, no significant differences between the groups regarding baseline characteristics were found. At the study end there were 100 patients in the BNP-guided group and 98 in the control group, presenting evaluable questionnaires from both the study start and the study end.

Of the 147 patients who were randomized to the BNP group in the UPSTEP study, there were 78 responders and 53 non-responders who had answered the Hr-QoL questionnaire at the study start (Fig. 1). The responders had a mean follow-up time of 649 days (SD ± 268) and non-responders 640 (SD ± 365) days ($p = 0.86$). The cohort of patients with SF-36 questionnaires available at both the study start and at the final visit consisted of 68 responders with 675 days (SD ± 266) of follow-up and 32 non-responders with 794 days (SD ± 286) of follow up, $p = 0.04$. The total numbers of worsening HF was 57 in the CTR-group versus 41 in BNP-group, and the amount of serious adverse events was 301 events versus 252 events in BNP group.

### Health-related Quality of life BNP-guided and CTR group

Figure 2 presents the change in perceived Hr-QoL during the study. No significant differences between the groups at baseline regarding scores in the eight dimensions could be noted (Appendix 1).

Within-group analyses of changes from the study start showed that significant improvements could be found in four of the eight domains in the NP-guided group (PF, $p < 0.01$, RP, $p < 0.01$, VT, $p < 0.001$ and MH, $p < 0.01$). In the CTR group, significant improvements could be seen in six of the eight domains (RP, $p < 0.001$, BP, $p < 0.001$, VT, $p = 0.03$, SF, $p < 0.0001$, RE, $p < 0.01$, MH, $p < 0.01$) (Appendix 2). For the composite dimension scores PCS and MCS, the NP-guided group improved significantly in PCS, ($p < 0.001$) whereas those with conventional treatment improved in the PCS ($p < 0.001$), and MCS ($p < 0.002$) (Appendix 2).

### Health-related Quality of life responders and non-responders

Figure 3 shows the mean changes of the scores between the study start and the study end in the eight different SF-36 domains including the PCS and MCS. Compared to non-responders, the responders at the study start already had significantly better scores in three of the eight SF-36 domains (PF ($p = 0.001$), GH ($p = 0.01$), SF ($p = 0.006$) and in the summary score PCS ($p = 0.007$) (Appendix 1). Within group analyses of changes from the study start showed significant improvements for responders in four domains; RP ($p < 0.004$), VT ($p < 0.002$), SF ($p = 0.03$), MH ($p = 0.02$) and for PCS ($p < 0.004$). For the non-responders the within group analysis was significantly improved in one domain; PF ($p = 0.03$) and for the summary score, PCS ($p < 0.03$) (Appendix 2).

### Correlates of patient characteristics to changes in Health-related Quality of life

Few background characteristics correlated significantly to changes in PCS and MCS. Instead of presenting data on eight dimensions we presented the two summary scores PCS and MCS. In the total study group (i.e. NP-guided and CRT group), a higher heart rate correlated weakly with improvements in PCS ($r = 0.23$) and MCS ($r = 0.25$) whereas a previous myocardial infarct correlated weakly to a worse MCS ($r = -0.23$), In the 100 patients defined as responders or non-responders, no significant correlations were found.

## Discussion

The main finding is that BNP guided HF therapy did not improve the perceived Hr-QoL compared to the conventionally guided HF therapy. However, the BNP group improved in four out of the eight domains, whereas the CTR groups improved in six of the eight domains. We could also demonstrate that the responders improved in four of the eight domains, whereas among the non-responders improvement could only be seen in one single domain. It could also be demonstrated

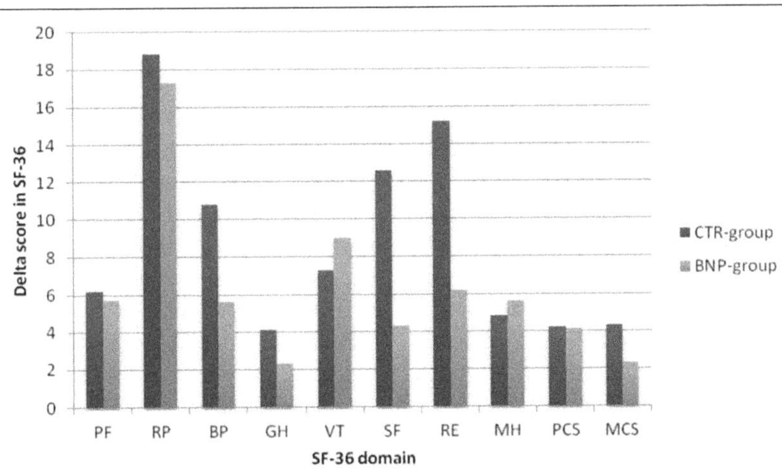


**Fig. 2** Change in Health-related Quality-of-Life between the NP-guided group (BNP group, $n = 100$) and conventionally treated (CTR group, $n = 98$) group at the study start and the study end regarding different dimensions of the SF-36 questionnaire

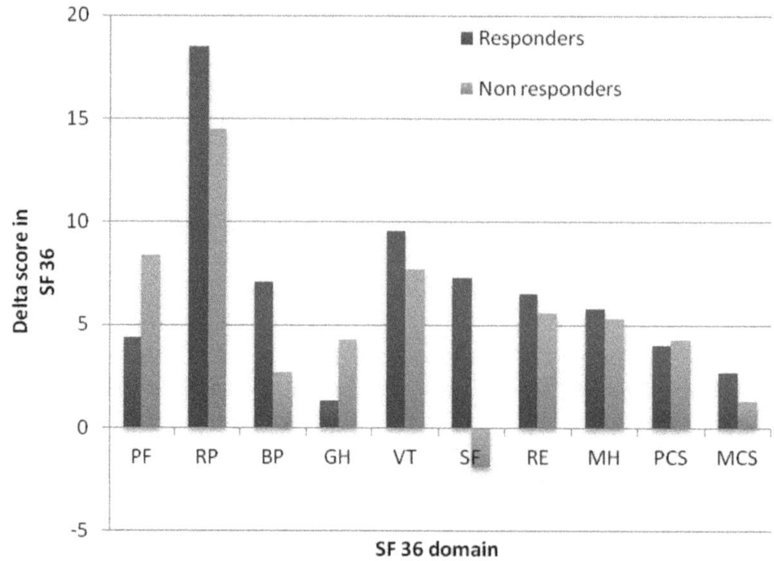


**Fig. 3** Change in Health-related Quality-of-Life between the responders ($n = 68$) and non-responders ($n = 32$) at the study start and the study end regarding different dimensions of the SF-36 questionnaire

that improvements could be seen irrespective if BNP guided therapy were applied, or if randomized to conventional therapy. Even if a difference could be seen in the size of improvement between responders compared to non-responders, all groups did improve in Hr-QoL. The mechanism behind this could only be speculated on, but it is independent of the use of BNP-guided therapy.

The fact that NP-guided therapy group did not improve in the perceived Hr-QoL compared to the conventionally guided therapy group concurs with studies that have addressed Hr-QoL and NP-guiding [8–10, 12, 13]. However, the Pro-B Type Natriuretic Peptide Outpatient Tailored Chronic Heart Failure (PROTECT) study did present improved HR-QoL [11]. That study showed that those receiving NP-guided medical treatment had a greater and more sustained improvement in HR-QoL compared to those who received conventional handling of their HF. However, our study and the PROTECT study differed in populations and in study design, which may partly explain the differences regarding the perceived Hr-QoL. The patients in the PROTECT study were around 64 years of age, whereas the mean age of our patients was 71 years, thus ours was an older population. As it is documented that with increased age, a decrease in Hr-QoL is to be expected, the margin to influence this variable diminishes as the population is getting older.

We converted our BNP levels to an estimated NT-proBNP level. We found that the UPSTEP population had higher levels of NT-proBNP compared to the population in PROTECT study. Thus, the present study population was older and had higher NT-proBNP concentrations, indicating a more severe HF compared to the PROTECT population. It is therefore possible that our study population was less likely to benefit from the BNP-guided therapy, and thus lesser differences were reported between the two groups in the perceived Hr-QoL. In the evaluation, the score differences between the different groups are small, however as the patients evaluated are elderly and the progress of Hr-QoL can be expected to decrease even small difference can therefore be of importance. In our study we have demonstrated that the responders survive in a higher percentage compared to non-responders [16]. Therefore the demonstration of small differences in domains could be adequate in this patient population.

It has been discussed in the literature a potential advantage using a disease-specific Hr-QoL instrument in terms of better sensitivity for small changes in HF symptoms compared to a generic instrument. One of the most well-known disease specific instrument in the area of HF is the Minnesota Living with Heart Failure (MLWHF) [11]. However, there are studies indicating is a better ability to differentiate physical and emotional aspects of HR-QoL by SF-36 compared to MLwHF [23]. In the study Trial of Intensified versus standard Medical therapy in Elderly patients with Congestive Heart Failure (TIME-CHF), MLwHF and SF-12, were used to evaluate HR-QoL [9]. The result were consistent with ours, improvement of Hr-QoL within the two groups during the first 12 months, but after that no significant differences between the NP-guided and the control group. This could be interpreted as perceived improvement in Hr-QoL can be detected with both generic and disease specific Hr-QoL instrument if represented by SF-12 and MLWHF. In our study we used the SF-36, but there is no reason to believe that there are fundamental differences in this perspective between the two instruments. Interestingly, all four groups (i.e. the BNP-guided group, the CTR group, responders and non-responders) investigated had improved Hr-QoL. This is interesting since it might be expected that patients with a severe chronic and disabling disease such as HF over time at best may have shown a maintained or a slowly decreased Hr-QoL level. In the Prospective Comparison of ARNI (Angiotensin Receptor–Neprilysin Inhibitor) with ACEI (Angiotensin-Converting–Enzyme Inhibitor) to Determine Impact on Global Mortality and Morbidity in Heart Failure Trial (PARADIGM-HF) study [24], the control group, despite being on optimal treatment, had a significantly decreased Hr-QoL, indicating that Hr-QoL are to be expected to decrease in patient with HF in spite of continuous pharmacologic treatment. In healthy elderly persons the Hr-QoL also decreases as a result of increased age (Fig. 4 ) [22]. In our study, the study population had an age of 71 years at the study start and the follow-up time was almost two years. Instead of an expected decline in the eight domain scores during the study, we saw an improvement in both groups.

HR-QoL is an important tool to determine whether different treatment actions are of any benefit for the patients. Wyrwich et al. evaluated the smallest amount on the SF-36 scale score that would show that a patient moved up or down one response level of the scale items. [25] The smallest points in a state change which represents the smallest amount that an SF-36 scale would change if a patient moved up or down one response level on only one of the SF-36 scale items are; PF 5 points, RH 6.25 points, BP 10 points, GH 5 points, VT 6.25 points, SF 12.5 points, RE 8.33 points and MH 5 points [25]. According to Wyrwich definition the CTR group moved up one response level in PF, RP, BP, VT, SF, RE and the BNP-guided group moved up in PF, RP, VT and MH. The responders moved up in RP, VT, MH and non responders in PF, RP VT and MH. There was no response down in any of the four groups (Table 2).

The exact mechanisms behind the improvements in Hr-QoL are not easy to explain. However, support from health care professionals has been found to be an important factor influencing HF patients' Hr-QoL [26]. Thus, all patients had scheduled visits at weeks 2, 6, 10, 16, 24, 36, 48 and then every six months until the study end where they met the HF nurse/doctor at the HF clinic. This is more often than clinical routine in the Nordic countries. The mechanism that more use of health resources also influences the perceived Hr-QoL in HF patients has also been reported from primary health care [27, 28]. In the present study NP-guiding has been shown to improve the perceived Hr-QoL in patients with HF. As the perceived Hr-QoL is a complex mechanism other factors also influences the reported result, as seen in this study from the group with conventional HF-treatment where improvement of Hr-QoL was equally reported.

As the design of the present study does not permit the differentiation between effect of the NP-guiding, and the effect of contacts with the HF-professionals, we suggest further research in this important area. From the patient perspective increased Hr-QoL was reported, an important difference compared to what was

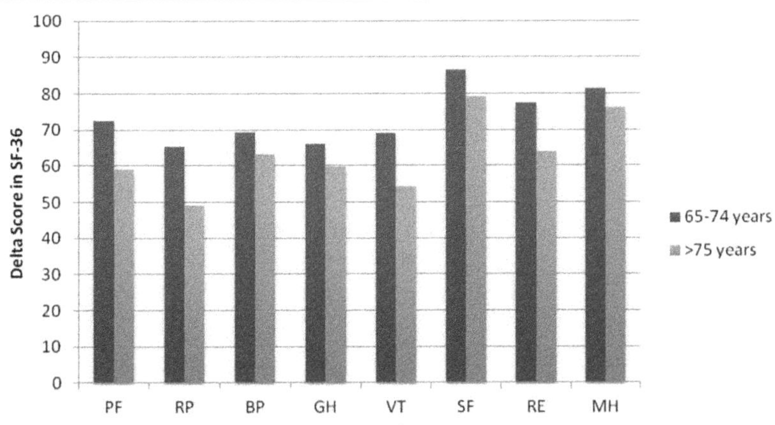


**Fig. 4** SF 36 scores for a normative Swedish population in the eight domains at age 65-74 years and a population older than 75 years [22], showing decreasing scores in all eight domains with increasing age

**Table 2** The clinically important difference for each SF-36 scale to indicate that the patient moved up (+) or down (-) one response level on only one of the scale items [25] in BNP-guided group, CTR group, responders and non responders

| SF-36 scales | Points per state change[a] | CTR group | BNP group | Responders | Non responders |
|---|---|---|---|---|---|
| PF | 5 | + | + | 0 | + |
| RP | 6.25 | + | + | + | + |
| BP | 10 | + | 0 | 0 | 0 |
| GH | 5 | 0 | 0 | 0 | 0 |
| VT | 6.25 | + | + | + | + |
| SF | 12.5 | + | 0 | 0 | 0 |
| RE | 8.33 | + | 0 | 0 | 0 |
| MH | 5 | 0 | + | + | + |

Abbreviations: *PF* Physical functioning, *RP* Role limitations due to physical health problems, *BP* Bodily pain, *GH* General health, *VT* Vitality, *SF* Social functioning, *RE* Role limitations due to emotional health problems, *MH* Mental health, *BNP* B-type natriuretic peptide, *CTR* conventionally treated group, *SF-36* Short Form 36

Note: [a]A state change represents the smallest amount that an SF-36 scale score would change if a patient moved up (+) or down (-) one response level on only one of the scales items according to Wyrwich et al.

expected. Therefore more research in this important area is suggested.

### Study limitations

There are limitations to this study that need to be discussed; the relatively small size of the study population restricts the possibilities for drawing conclusions. The population consisted of a homogenous Caucasian population. Therefore it is not possible to draw conclusions about other populations; the age of the study population was high, why the obtained results might be difficult to apply to a general population with HF in the society. The Hr-QoL questionnaire was only filled out at study start and at study end this might influence the possibility to detect changes during the study. The use of a non-disease-specific quality-of-life instrument limits the interpretation of small changes in Hr-QoL.

## Conclusion

Hr-QoL improved in several domains in both the NP-guided therapy group and the control group. Comparing the responder group to the non-responder group, the within group analyses showed improvements in four out of eight domains in the responder group compared to one out of eight domains in the non-responder group.

The perceived Hr-QoL is a complex mechanism that is influenced not only by the pharmacological treatment given, but also by the repeated contacts with health professionals. Both components positively influenced the Hr-QoL in the patients in this study. Therefore more research in perceived Hr-QoL and how to influence it is suggested.

## Appendix 1

**Table 3** Short Form-36 (SF-36) for conventionally treated (CTR) and patients whose treatment was guided by BNP and for responders and non-responders at study start and at study end. Responder defined as a patient with a BNP under 300 ng/l and/or a decrease in BNP of at least 40 percent in week 16 of follow-up, compared to study start

| | Study start Mean (SD) | | | Study end Mean (SD) | | | Study start Mean (SD) | | | Study end Mean (SD) | | |
|---|---|---|---|---|---|---|---|---|---|---|---|---|
| | CTR group *n* = 127 | BNP group *n* = 131 | p | CTR group *n* = 98 | BNP group *n* = 100 | p | Responders *n* = 78 | Non-responders *n* = 53 | p | Responders *n* = 68 | Non-responders *n* = 32 | p |
| SF-36 | | | | | | | | | | | | |
| PF | 46.4 (±27) | 45.3 (±26) | 0.80 | 54.8 (±26) | 55.2 (±27) | 0.78 | 51.3 (±25) | 36.5 (±24) | 0.001 | 52.7 (±26) | 42.3 (±23) | 0.055 |
| RP | 19.1 (±33) | 28.4 (±38) | 0.06 | 39.8 (±44) | 46.4 (±44) | 0.21 | 32.4 (±38) | 22.6 (±37) | 0.15 | 33.5 (±44) | 22.7 (±38) | 0.20 |
| BP | 56.4 (±31) | 60.6 (±29) | 0.26 | 65.8 (±29) | 69.6 (±29) | 0.39 | 62.7 (±29) | 57.4 (±29) | 0.32 | 64.6 (±29) | 64.2 (±30) | 0.95 |
| GH | 47.1 (±20) | 48.5 (±18) | 0.45 | 50.9 (±20) | 53.8 (±19) | 0.51 | 51.8 (±18) | 43.8 (±17) | 0.01 | 52.2 (±20) | 45.5 (±17) | 0.07 |
| VT | 43.1 (±22) | 42.0 (±21) | 0.61 | 50.2 (±25) | 51.9 (±22) | 0.63 | 43.3 (±22) | 40.2 (±19) | 0.40 | 42.5 (±25) | 43.0 (±18) | 0.91 |
| SF | 62.4 (±25) | 67.8 (±25) | 0.10 | 75.1 (±24) | 73.8 (±25) | 0.60 | 72.6 (±25) | 60.5 (±23) | 0.006 | 72.6 (±24) | 62.5 (±22) | 0.056 |
| RE | 41.1 (±45) | 49.0 (±45) | 0.19 | 54.5 (±44) | 57.1 (±42) | 0.75 | 52.8 (±44) | 43.4 (±45) | 0.24 | 55.7 (±44) | 44.8 (±45) | 0.26 |
| MH | 70.0 (±20) | 69.6 (±19) | 0.82 | 74.1 (±19) | 76 (±17) | 0.61 | 70.1 (±18) | 68.8 (±20) | 0.69 | 70.1 (±19) | 69.5 (±19) | 0.87 |
| PCS | 31.5 (±11) | 32.7 (±11) | 0.24 | 35.6 (±11) | 37.8 (±12) | 0.18 | 34.9 (±10) | 29.6 (±11) | 0.007 | 35.5 (±11) | 31.6 (±11) | 0.09 |
| MCS | 42.7 (±12) | 43.6 (±11) | 0.60 | 46.0 (±11) | 46.5 (±10) | 0.87 | 44.3 (±11) | 42.7 (±11) | 0.45 | 44.3 (±11) | 43.1 (±11) | 0.63 |

Abbreviations: *PF* Physical functioning, *RP* Role limitations due to physical health problems, *BP* Bodily pain, *GH* General health, VT Vitality, *SF* Social functioning, *RE* Role limitations due to emotional health problems, *MH* Mental health, *PCS* Physical component score, *MCS* Mental component score, *SD* Standard Deviation

## Appendix 2

**Table 4** Changes in Short Form-36 within groups, conventionally treated (CTR) and BNP-guided group and responders versus non-responders. Responder defined as a patient with a BNP under 300 ng/l and/or a decrease in BNP of at least 40 percent in week 16 of follow-up, compared to study start

| | Change in Hr-QoL Mean (SD) | | | Within group analysis | | Change in Hr-QoL Mean (SD) | | | Within group analysis | |
|---|---|---|---|---|---|---|---|---|---|---|
| | CTR group $n = 98$ | BNP group $n = 100$ | p-value | CTR group p-value | BNP group p-value | Responders $n = 68$ | Non-responders $n = 32$ | p-value | Responders p-value | Non-responders p-value |
| SF-36 | | | | | | | | | | |
| PF | 6.2 (±28) | 5.7 (±22) | 0.88 | 0.06 | <0.01 | 4.4 (±22) | 8.4 (±22) | 0.39 | 0.06 | 0.03 |
| RP | 18.8 (±46) | 17.3 (±49) | 0.83 | <0.001 | <0.01 | 18.5 (±49) | 14.5 (±49) | 0.71 | <0.004 | 0.11 |
| BP | 10.8 (±32) | 5.6 (±34) | 0.27 | <0.001 | 0.07 | 7.1 (±35) | 2.7 (±32) | 0.55 | 0.07 | 0.65 |
| GH | 4.1 (±22) | 2.3 (±17) | 0.52 | 0.08 | 0.25 | 1.3 (±17) | 4.3 (±17) | 0.40 | 0.55 | 0.21 |
| VT | 7.3 (±27) | 9.0 (±23) | 0.64 | 0.03 | <0.001 | 9.6 (±25) | 7.7 (±19) | 0.71 | <0.002 | 0.06 |
| SF | 12.6 (±28) | 4.3 (±27) | 0.04 | <0.0001 | 0.13 | 7.3 (±26) | -1.9 (±29) | 0.11 | 0.03 | 0.75 |
| RE | 15.2 (±46) | 6.2 (±47) | 0.18 | <0.01 | 0.23 | 6.5 (±26) | 5.6 (±55) | 0.93 | 0.21 | 0.67 |
| MH | 4.8 (±21) | 5.6 (±19) | 0.77 | 0.04 | <0.01 | 5.8 (±20) | 5.3 (±17) | 0.91 | 0.02 | 0.12 |
| PCS | 4.2 (±11) | 4.1 (±9) | 0.94 | 0.001 | <0.001 | 4.0 (±10) | 4.3 (±9) | 0.87 | <0.004 | <0.03 |
| MCS | 4.3 (±12) | 2.3 (±11) | 0.25 | 0.002 | 0.17 | 2.7 (±11) | 1.3 (±12) | 0.57 | 0.10 | 0.91 |

Abbreviations: *PF* Physical functioning, *RP* Role limitations due to physical health problems, *BP* Bodily pain, *GH* General health, *VT* Vitality, *SF* Social functioning, *RE* Role limitations due to emotional health problems, *MH* Mental health, *PCS* Physical component score, *MCS* Mental component score, *SD* Standard Deviation

**Abbreviations**

ACEI: Angiotensin-Converting–Enzyme Inhibitor; ARNI: Angiotensin Receptor–Neprilysin Inhibitor; BNP: B-type natriuretic peptide; BNP-group: BNP-guided group; BP: bodily pain; CTR-group: conventional treated group; CV: cardiovascular; GH: general health; HF: heart failure; Hr-QoL: health related quality of life; MCS: mental component score; MH: mental health; MLWHF: Minnesota Living with Heart Failure; NP: natriuretic peptide; NYHA: New York Heart Association; PARADIGM-HF: prospective comparison of ARNI with ACEI to determine impact on global mortality and morbidity in heart failure; PCS: physical component score; PF: physical functioning; PROBE: prospective, randomized, open, and blinded evaluation; PROTECT: Pro-B Type Natriuretic Peptide Outpatient Tailored Chronic Heart Failure; RE: role limitations due to emotional health problems; RP: role limitations due to physical health problems; SD: standard deviation; SF: social functioning; SF-36: Short Form 36; TIME-CHF: The Trial of Intensified vs Standard Medical Therapy in Elderly Patients With Congestive Heart Failure; UPSTEP: Use of PeptideS in Tailoring hEart failure Project; VT: vitality.

**Competing interests**

None to report for UA, PJ and PK. UD, consulting honoraria's from Novartis, and research grant from Astra Zeneca. KB, consulting honoraria's from Novartis, and grant from Roche Diagnostics.

**Authors' contributions**

PK had full access to all of the data in the study and takes responsibility for the integrity of the data and the accuracy of the data analysis. Study concept and design: UA, KB, UD, PJ, PK. Acquisition of data: UA, KB, UD, PK. Analysis and interpretation of data: UA, PJ, PK. Drafting of the manuscript: UA, PJ, PK. Critical revision of the manuscript: UA, KB, UD, PJ, PK. Statistical analysis: UA, PJ, PK. Obtained funding: UA, KB, UD, PK. Study supervision: UA, KB, UD, PK. All authors read and approved the final manuscript.

**Acknowledgements**

We thank our patients in the UPSTEP study, the investigators and their staff who all made the UPSTEP study possible.

**Funding**

This work was supported by The Swedish Heart-lung foundation, grant number 20060596. The Regional Research Foundation in south-eastern Sweden (Diary nr: FORSS-3963) and the Regional Research Foundation in northern Sweden funded the study. Biosite international and Infiniti Medical AB gave an unrestricted grant and provided the BNP analysis equipment.

**Author details**

[1]Department of Medicine, Division of Cardiology, County Hospital Ryhov, Jönköping, Sweden. [2]Department of Cardiology and Department of Medical and Health Sciences, Linköping University, Linköping, Sweden. [3]Research unit Skellefteå Department of Medicine, Institution of Public Health and Clinical Medicine, Umeå University, Umeå, Sweden.

**References**

1. Mosterd A, Hoes AW. Clinical epidemiology of heart failure. Heart. 2007;93(9):1137–46.
2. Paren P et al. Trends in prevalence from 1990 to 2007 of patients hospitalized with heart failure in Sweden. Eur J Heart Fail. 2014;16(7):737–42.
3. Shafazand M et al. Decreasing trends in the incidence of heart failure after acute myocardial infarction from 1993-2004: a study of 175,216 patients with a first acute myocardial infarction in Sweden. Eur J Heart Fail. 2011;13(2):135–41.
4. Levy D et al. Long-term trends in the incidence of and survival with heart failure. N Engl J Med. 2002;347(18):1397–402.
5. Hobbs FD et al. Impact of heart failure and left ventricular systolic dysfunction on quality of life: a cross-sectional study comparing common chronic cardiac and medical disorders and a representative adult population. Eur Heart J. 2002;23(23):1867–76.
6. Troughton RW et al. Effect of B-type natriuretic peptide-guided treatment of chronic heart failure on total mortality and hospitalization: an individual patient meta-analysis. Eur Heart J. 2014;35(23):1559–67.

7. Anker SD et al. The importance of patient-reported outcomes: a call for their comprehensive integration in cardiovascular clinical trials. Eur Heart J. 2014;35(30):2001–9.
8. Troughton RW et al. Treatment of heart failure guided by plasma aminoterminal brain natriuretic peptide (N-BNP) concentrations. Lancet. 2000;355(9210):1126–30.
9. Pfisterer M et al. BNP-guided vs symptom-guided heart failure therapy: the Trial of Intensified vs Standard Medical Therapy in Elderly Patients With Congestive Heart Failure (TIME-CHF) randomized trial. JAMA. 2009;301(4):383–92.
10. Eurlings LW et al. Management of chronic heart failure guided by individual N-terminal pro-B-type natriuretic peptide targets: results of the PRIMA (Can PRo-brain-natriuretic peptide guided therapy of chronic heart failure IMprove heart fAilure morbidity and mortality?) study. J Am Coll Cardiol. 2010;56(25):2090–100.
11. Bhardwaj A et al. Quality of life and chronic heart failure therapy guided by natriuretic peptides: results from the ProBNP Outpatient Tailored Chronic Heart Failure Therapy (PROTECT) study. Am Heart J. 2012;164(5):793–9. e1.
12. Persson H et al. Improved pharmacological therapy of chronic heart failure in primary care: a randomized Study of NT-proBNP Guided Management of Heart Failure–SIGNAL-HF (Swedish Intervention study–Guidelines and NT-proBNP AnaLysis in Heart Failure). Eur J Heart Fail. 2010;12(12):1300–8.
13. Lainchbury JG et al. N-terminal pro-B-type natriuretic peptide-guided treatment for chronic heart failure: results from the BATTLESCARRED (NT-proBNP-Assisted Treatment To Lessen Serial Cardiac Readmissions and Death) trial. J Am Coll Cardiol. 2009;55(1):53–60.
14. Gaggin HK et al. Characterization and prediction of natriuretic peptide "nonresponse" during heart failure management: results from the ProBNP Outpatient Tailored Chronic Heart Failure (PROTECT) and the NT-proBNP-Assisted Treatment to Lessen Serial Cardiac Readmissions and Death (BATTLESCARRED) study. Congest Heart Fail. 2013;19(3):135–42.
15. Karlstrom P et al. Brain natriuretic peptide-guided treatment does not improve morbidity and mortality in extensively treated patients with chronic heart failure: responders to treatment have a significantly better outcome. Eur J Heart Fail. 2011;13(10):1096–103.
16. Karlstrom P, et al. Responder to BNP-guided treatment in heart failure. The process of defining a responder. Scand Cardiovasc J. 2015;49:316–324.
17. Sullivan M, Karlsson J, Ware Jr JE. The Swedish SF-36 Health Survey–I. Evaluation of data quality, scaling assumptions, reliability and construct validity across general populations in Sweden. Soc Sci Med. 1995;41(10):1349–58.
18. Loge JH, Kaasa S. Short form 36 (SF-36) health survey: normative data from the general Norwegian population. Scand J Soc Med. 1998;26(4):250–8.
19. Johansson P et al. Measurement of health-related quality of life in chronic heart failure, from a nursing perspective-a review of the literature. Eur J Cardiovasc Nurs. 2004;3(1):7–20.
20. Ware Jr JE. SF-36 health survey update. Spine (Phila Pa 1976). 2000;25(24):3130–9.
21. Ware Jr JE, Sherbourne CD. The MOS 36-item short-form health survey (SF-36). I. Conceptual framework and item selection. Med Care. 1992;30(6):473–83.
22. Sullivan M, Karlsson J. The Swedish SF-36 Health Survey III. Evaluation of criterion-based validity: results from normative population. J Clin Epidemiol. 1998;51(11):1105–13.
23. Sneed NV et al. Evaluation of 3 quality of life measurement tools in patients with chronic heart failure. Heart Lung. 2001;30(5):332–40.
24. McMurray JJ et al. Angiotensin-neprilysin inhibition versus enalapril in heart failure. N Engl J Med. 2014;371(11):993–1004.
25. Wyrwich KW et al. Clinically important differences in health status for patients with heart disease: an expert consensus panel report. Am Heart J. 2004;147(4):615–22.
26. Grady KL et al. Predictors of quality of life in patients with advanced heart failure awaiting transplantation. J Heart Lung Transplant. 1995;14(1 Pt 1):2–10.
27. Agvall B, Alehagen U, Dahlstrom U. The benefits of using a heart failure management programme in Swedish primary healthcare. Eur J Heart Fail. 2013;15(2):228–36.
28. Benatar D et al. Outcomes of chronic heart failure. Arch Intern Med. 2003;163(3):347–52.

# 8

# Characterization of exercise limitations by evaluating individual cardiac output patterns: a prospective cohort study in patients with chronic heart failure

Ruud F. Spee[1*], Victor M. Niemeijer[1], Bart Wessels[2], Jasper P. Jansen[3], Pieter F.F. Wijn[3,4], Pieter A.F.M. Doevendans[5] and Hareld M.C. Kemps[1,6]

**Abstract**

**Background:** Patients with chronic heart failure (CHF) suffer from exercise intolerance due to impaired central hemodynamics and subsequent alterations in peripheral skeletal muscle function and structure. The relative contribution of central versus peripheral factors in the reduced exercise capacity is still subject of debate. The main purpose was to investigate heterogeneity in the nature of exercise intolerance by evaluating individual cardiac output (Q) patterns. The secondary purpose was to evaluate whether patient and disease characteristics were associated with a central hemodynamic exercise limitation.

**Methods:** Sixty-four stable CHF patients performed a symptom limited incremental exercise test with respiratory gas analysis and simultaneous assessment of Q, using a radial artery pulse contour analysis method. A central hemodynamic exercise limitation was defined as a plateau or decline in Q from 90 to 100 % of exercise duration.

**Results:** Data from 61 patients were analyzed. A central hemodynamic exercise limitation was observed in 21 patients (34 %). In these patients, a higher occurrence of a plateau/decrease in oxygen uptake ($VO_2$) (52 % vs 23 %, $p = 0.02$), stroke volume (SV) (100 % vs. 75 %, $p = 0.01$) and chronotropic incompetence (31 % vs. 2.5 %, $p = 0.01$) was observed, while presence of a left bundle branch block (LBBB) occurred significantly less (19 % vs 48 %, $p = 0.03$) There was no difference in disease characteristics such as etiology, duration, NYHA class, mitral regurgitation or ischemia.

**Conclusions:** The study revealed considerable heterogeneity in the nature of exercise limitations between moderately impaired CHF patients. In one third of the study population a plateau or decrease in Q towards peak exercise was demonstrated, which is indicative of a central hemodynamic exercise limitation. A central hemodynamic exercise limitation was associated with an impairment to augment stroke volume and heart rate.

**Keywords:** Cardiac output, Oxygen uptake, Patterns, Chronic heart failure, Exercise intolerance

## Background

Chronic heart failure (CHF) is a clinical syndrome resulting from inadequate tissue oxygenation due to impaired cardiac function. Although it is well established that patients with CHF suffer from exercise intolerance, the underlying pathophysiological mechanisms remain controversial. From a theoretical point of view, reduced exercise capacity may be the consequence of $O_2$ diffusion abnormalities in the lungs, impaired central hemodynamics or peripheral derangements such as a reduced skeletal muscle capillarization or metabolic capacity. Whereas it is generally accepted that pulmonary $O_2$ diffusion does not limit exercise capacity in compensated CHF patients, the role of central and peripheral factors is still under debate [1]. Previous studies showed associations between maximal exercise capacity and central hemodynamics [2, 3], whereas other studies revealed a relation between exercise capacity and skeletal muscle function [4, 5]. A possible explanation

* Correspondence: r.spee@mmc.nl
[1]Department of Cardiology, Máxima Medical Centre, De Run 4600, P.O. Box 7777, Veldhoven 5500 MB, The Netherlands
Full list of author information is available at the end of the article

for these seemingly discrepant findings is that the nature of exercise limitations differs between CHF patients. In fact, results from an animal study demonstrated that the primary response of microvascular oxygen pressure in the muscle was speeded in rats with moderate left ventricular (LV) dysfunction, while in rats with severe LV dysfunction, this response was significantly slowed [6]. These results suggest that the dynamic balance between oxygen delivery and utilization in the muscle is dependent of the severity of cardiac dysfunction, indicating physiological heterogeneity. Although additional physiological insight is needed in humans, some clinical studies suggested heterogeneity in exercise limitations. As such, CHF patients with a severe central hemodynamic limitation did not benefit from exercise training [7], but may benefit most from a heart transplantation [8]. Characterization of exercise limitations in individual CHF patients and more knowledge on disease characteristics associated with the nature of these limitations may lead to a more tailored therapeutic strategy in CHF patients. An approach that can be used to characterize exercise limitations is to examine the pattern of the cardiac output (Q) response to symptom-limited exercise, with a failure to augment or a decrease in cardiac output towards peak exercise being indicative of a central hemodynamic exercise limitation [9]. Although previous studies investigated the cardiac output response to exercise with respect to prognosis [10, 11], no studies used cardiac output patterns during incremental exercise to characterize exercise limitations in CHF patients.

The primary goal of this study was to investigate the nature of the limitation of maximal exercise capacity in CHF patients by evaluation of cardiac output patterns. Furthermore we evaluated whether patient and disease characteristics are associated with a central hemodynamic exercise limitation.

## Methods

The present study was designed as a prospective cohort study. All tests were conducted at the Department of Cardiology of the Máxima Medical Centre, the Netherlands. The research protocol was approved by the medical ethics committee of the Máxima Medical Centre. The study complies with the Declaration of Helsinki. All patients provided written and signed informed consent, prior to the study.

### Population

All consecutive symptomatic CHF patients visiting the outpatient clinic of cardiology were considered for participation in the study. Additional inclusion criteria were: CHF secondary to ischemic or dilated cardiomyopathy, New York Heart Association functional class II-III, left ventricular ejection fraction $\leq 40$ % and optimized medical treatment. Exclusion criteria were: recent myocardial infarction, unstable angina (less than 3 months prior to inclusion), hemodynamically significant aortic valve disease, participation in a training program (≥2/week) in the last year, significant chronic obstructive pulmonary disease (FEV1/FVC $< 60$ %) and orthopedic or neuromuscular conditions limiting the ability to perform exercise.

### Exercise testing

All patients performed a symptom-limited incremental exercise test on an electromagnetically braked cycle ergometer in an upright position (Corrival, Lode, Groningen, The Netherlands), using an individualized ramp protocol with a duration of 8 to 12 min. The test ended when a patient was not able to maintain the required pedaling frequency of 70 per minute. A 12-lead electrocardiogram was registered continuously. Ventilatory parameters were measured breath-by-breath (ZAN 680 USB, ZAN Messgeräte, Oberthulba, Germany). Volume and gas analyzers were calibrated before each test.

### Assessment of central hemodynamics

Assessment of central hemodynamics was performed by a radial artery pulse contour analysis method (LiDCO, LiDCO Ltd, London, UK). This technique provides beat-to-beat changes in central hemodynamics, by calculating nominal stroke volume (SV) from a pressure-volume transform of the radial artery pressure waveform [12]. In order to convert nominal SV to absolute SV, the system has to be calibrated at rest for each subject by an independent method. We used echocardiography or lithium dilution for this purpose [13, 14]. Before the exercise test, a 20-gauge arterial catheter was inserted into the radial artery. The radial artery catheter was connected to the LiDCO *plus* monitor. Subsequently, the calibration procedure to determine resting Q was performed in the supine position. Thereafter patients were positioned upright on the cycle ergometer and the exercise protocol was started. Patients were instructed to keep the measured arm on the handlebar of the ergometer in the same position to keep an optimal arterial waveform. Previous studies showed that LiDCO is a reproducible and accurate method for assessment of cardiac output (Q) under a variety of physiological conditions [15, 16]. Moreover, in a study using the Fick method as a reference, we showed that this technique is highly accurate for continuous assessment of Q during incremental symptom-limited exercise testing in CHF patients [13].

### Data analysis

Breath-to-breath data of oxygen uptake and beat-to-beat data of central hemodynamics were filtered for outliers using Python (Python 2.7, Python Software Foundation). Outliers were defined as values deviating more than three standard deviations from a calculated moving average [17]. All data were time aligned using manual set markers at the start of exercise and filtered using a central moving average filter with a window of 11 data points. In order to compare gas exchange and central hemodynamic variables during exercise between CHF patients, data were expressed as a percentage of total exercise time. Baseline values were calculated as the mean of the first 60 s of the unloaded phase prior to the start of loaded exercise. Peak values were defined as the average values during the final 20 s of the test. We characterized exercise limitations by using the pattern of the cardiac output response to maximal exercise. A failure to increase or a decrease in cardiac output towards the end of exercise was considered to be indicative of a central hemodynamic exercise limitation. A central hemodynamic exercise limitation was defined as a plateau or decline in Q from 90 to 100 % of exercise time. Chronotropic incompetence was defined as a peak HR below 80 % of the age-predicted heart rate, using the Brawner formula [18].

### Statistical analysis

Data were analyzed using SPSS 19.0.0 statistical software (SPSS Inc, Chicago, IL, USA). Continuous variables were tested for normality and presented as mean or mean ± SD. Between-group differences of continuous variables were evaluated by an independent *t*-test. Categorical variables are presented as absolute and relative frequencies. The $\chi2$ test was used to evaluate differences between categorical data. Differences were presented as $\chi2$ value with concomitant degree of freedom (df) Relations between variables were assessed by Pearson's correlation coefficient (*r*). For all statistical comparisons, the level of significance was set at $p < 0.05$.

## Results

All 64 patients completed the combined hemodynamic and cardiopulmonary exercise test, without adverse events. Central hemodynamic data from 3 patients were excluded because of insufficient data quality due to excessive damping of the arterial pressure waveform during exercise. In total, data of 61 patients were analyzed.

The majority of the study population were males (84 %); the mean age was 63 ± 9 years. At the time of inclusion, patients were diagnosed with CHF for a mean duration of 45 ± 51 months. Ninety-eight percent used ACE inhibitors or an angiotensin II receptor blocker, 93 % used beta blockers. Thirty-four patients had an ischemic cardiomyopathy (due to one or more myocardial infarctions > 3 months prior to inclusion), 2 patients showed signs of myocardial ischemia during evaluation by non-invasive stress testing (i.e. positive exercise test or myocardial perfusion scintigraphy) or coronary angiography, which required percutaneous coronary intervention (PCI). Six patients had severe mitral regurgitation at resting echocardiography. Twenty-three patients had Left Bundle Branch Block (LBBB) and seven patients had atrial fibrillation.

### Central hemodynamic and gas exchange variables at rest and maximal exercise

Gas exchange and hemodynamic variables at rest and peak exercise are presented in Table 1. The mean peak workload was 125 ± 49 Watt. The mean peak $VO_2$ was 19.0 ± 5.9 mL $min^{-1}$ $kg^{-1}$ and $VO_2$ at the ventilatory threshold was 11.9 ± 2.9 mL $min^{-1}$ $kg^{-1}$, corresponding to 63 % of peak $VO_2$. Mean peak RER was 1.07 ± 0.1. There was a significant correlation between peak $VO_2$ and peak Q ($r$ =0.64, $p < 0.001$).

### Patterns of central hemodynamic variables during incremental exercise

Fig. 1a and b show respectively, exercise-induced changes of $VO_2$ and Q at a group level. Both $VO_2$ and Q show a continuous increase throughout the exercise test. Looking at patterns of Q in individual patients, 21 patients (34 %) showed a plateau or decrease in Q during the final 10 % of exercise duration (Fig. 2b), while 40 patients (66 %) showed a continuous increase in Q (Fig. 2a).

Table 2 shows a comparison of patient and disease characteristics between patients with a plateau/decrease in Q and patients with a continuous increase in Q. There was no significant between-group difference in beta blocker use ($\chi2$ value 0.17, df = 1, $p$ =0.68). Peak $VO_2$, peak Q and SV did not differ between both groups. In 11 of the 21 patients with a plateau/decrease in Q (52 %), a plateau/decrease in $VO_2$ was also observed. Nine out of 40 patients (23 %) with a continuous increase in Q, showed a plateau/decrease in $VO_2$ ($\chi2$ value 5.58, df = 1, $p = 0.02$ for between group comparison). In patients with a plateau/decrease in Q, all patients showed a plateau/decrease in SV as opposed to 30 patients (75 %) in the group with a continuous increase in Q ($\chi2$ value 6.28, df = 1, $p = 0.01$ for between group comparison) (Table 2). Chronotropic incompetence was observed more often in patients with a plateau or decrease in Q (31 % versus 2.5 %, $\chi2$ value 7.05, df = 1, p < 0.01). There was a higher occurrence of a plateau/decrease in SV in patients with chronotropic incompetence (83 % versus 52 %, $p$ =0.047), but no significant difference

**Table 1** Hemodynamic and gas exchange variables at rest and during exercise ($n$ =61)

| | Baseline | Peak exercise |
|---|---|---|
| $VO_2$ (mL $min^{-1}$ $kg^{-1}$) | 4.3 ± 1.3 | 19.0 ± 5.9 |
| HR (beats $min^{-1}$) | 80 ± 17 | 124 ± 26 |
| SV (mL) | 62 ± 14 | 87 ± 23 |
| Q (L $min^{-1}$) | 4.9 ± 1.5 | 10.9 ± 4.1 |

$VO_2$ oxygen uptake, HR heart rate, SV stroke volume, Q Cardiac Output

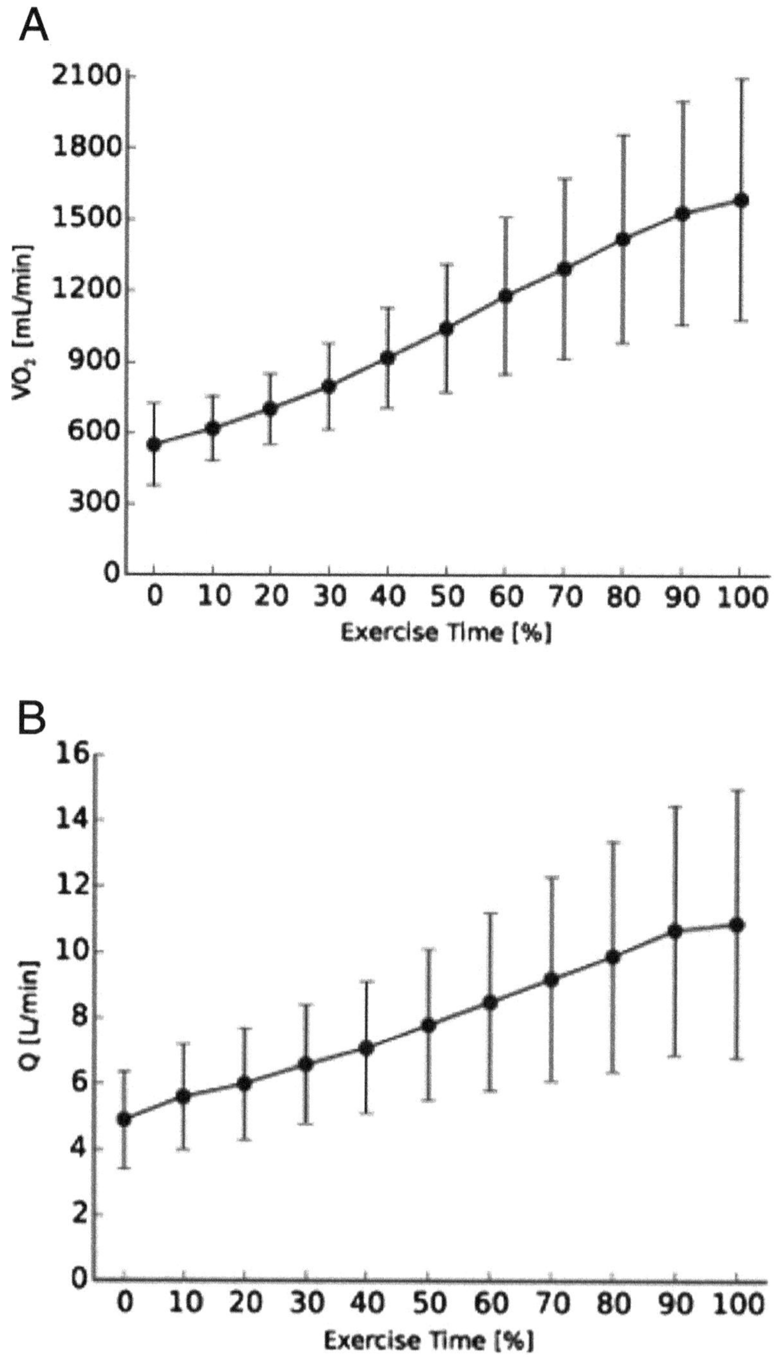


**Fig. 1 a**: Mean oxygen uptake ($VO_2$) and **b**: mean cardiac output (Q) response during a symptom limited exercise test. Error bars represent one standard deviation above and below the mean

in peak SV between patients with and without chronotropic incompetence (74 ± 22 versus 89 ± 22 mL respectively, $p$ =0.29). Left Bundle Branch Block was observed significantly less in patients with a Q plateau/decrease ($\chi 2$ value 4.84, df = 1, p = 0.03). No differences between groups were observed for patients with severe mitral regurgitation at rest or myocardial ischemia.

## Discussion

This is the first study in patients with CHF to characterize physiological limitations at maximal exercise by assessment of the pattern of Q during incremental exercise. In one third of the study population we demonstrated a failure to augment Q towards the end of the exercise test, (Fig. 2b) while a continuous increase was

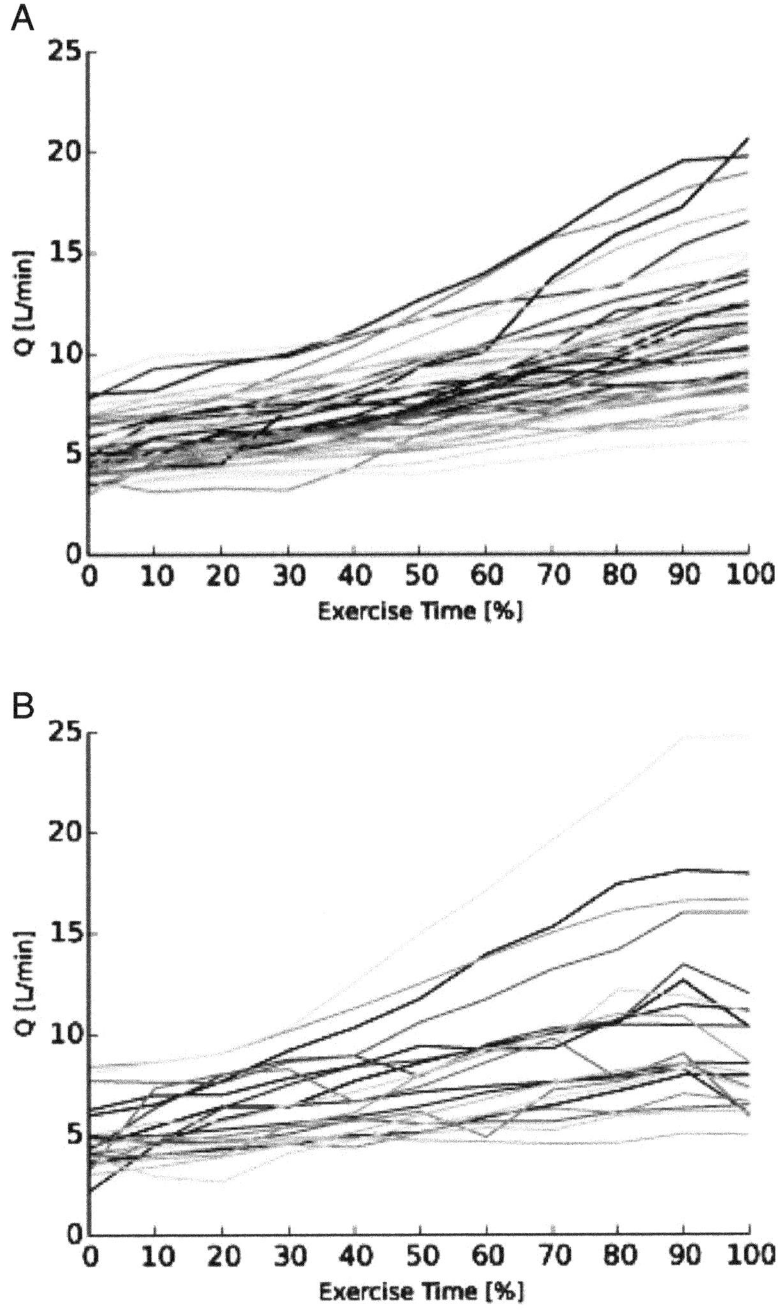


**Fig. 2** **a**: Individual cardiac output (Q) responses with an continuous increase during exercise (*n* =40) and **b**: individual cardiac output (Q) responses with a plateau or decrease during the final 10 % of exercise during a symptom limited exercise test (*n* =21)

observed in the other patients (Fig. 2a). These results indicate that physiological heterogeneity in exercise limitations exists among CHF patients.

As the nature of the exercise limitation may be an important determinant for the selection of patients for specific treatments, (e.g. exercise training, heart transplantation, cardiac resynchronization therapy) these observations may be relevant for clinical practice.

Although we demonstrated a continuous increase in Q throughout the incremental symptom-limited exercise test at group level, we observed a wide inter-individual variation in Q patterns. These observations are different from earlier findings in healthy individuals, showing a continuous increase in Q in all subjects [19]. Whereas individual Q patterns during symptom-limited exercise were not used previously to characterize exercise limitations in

**Table 2** Characteristics comparison between subjects with increase in Q or plateau/decrease in Q (n = 61)

| | Increase in Q (*n* = 40) | Plateau/decrease in Q (*n* = 21) | $\chi 2$ value (df) | *p-value* |
|---|---|---|---|---|
| Age (years) | 63 ± 10 | 64 ± 9 | n.a. | NS |
| Gender male/female (%) | 33 (83)/7 (17) | 18 (86)/3 (14) | 0.10 (1) | NS |
| Etiology ICM/DCM (%) | 21 (53)/19 (47) | 13 (62)/8 (38) | 0.49 (1) | NS |
| Duration CHF (months) | 45 ± 50 | 46 ± 54 | n.a. | NS |
| Beta blocker (%) | 93 | 95 | 0.17 (1) | NS |
| NYHA class II/III (%) | 24 (60)/16 (40) | 11 (52)/10 (48) | 0.33 (2) | NS |
| LVEF (%) | 31 ± 8 | 33 ± 10 | n.a. | NS |
| Peak $VO_2$ (mL $min^{-1}$ $kg^{-1}$) | 19.4 ± 6.0 | 18.2 ± 5.9 | n.a. | NS |
| Peak Q (L $min^{-1}$) | 11.3 ± 3.6 | 10.2 ± 5.0 | n.a. | NS |
| Peak SV (mL) | 90 ± 24 | 83 ± 22 | n.a. | NS |
| Plateau/decrease in $VO_2$ | 9 (23 %) | 11 (52 %) | 5.58 (1) | 0.02 |
| Plateau/decrease in SV | 30 (75 %) | 21 (100 %) | 6.28 (1) | 0.01 |
| Rest HR (beats $min^{-1}$) | 81 ± 16 | 77 ± 18 | n.a. | NS |
| Peak HR (beats $min^{-1}$) | 126 ± 20 | 121 ± 35 | n.a. | NS |
| Chronotropic incompetence | 1 (2.5 %) | 5 (31 %) | 7.05 (1) | 0.01 |
| Rhythm (SR, Afib, paced) (%) | 35 (88)/2 (5)/3 (7) | 15 (71)/5 (24)/1 (5) | 4.85 (2) | NS |
| LBBB | 19 (48 %) | 4 (19 %) | 4.84 (1) | 0.03 |
| Severe mitral regurgitation | 3 (7.5 %) | 3 (14 %) | 0.72 (1) | NS |
| Myocardial ischemia | 2 (5 %) | 0 (0 %) | 1.09 (2) | NS |

$\chi 2$ value, chi-squared value for categorical values, df degree of freedom,n.a. not applicable, ICM ischemic cardiomyopathy, DCM dilated cardiomyopathy, CHF chronic heart failure, NYHA New York Heart Association, LVEF left ventricular ejection fraction, $VO_2$ oxygen uptake, Q cardiac output, SV stroke volume, HR heart rate, SR sinus rhythm, Afib atrial fibrillation, LBBB left bundle branch block, . NS non significant

CHF patients, earlier studies did show heterogeneity in central hemodynamic responses to exercise in CHF populations by relating Q to $VO_2$. In these studies, 32-55 % of CHF patients were classified as having a central hemodynamic limitation of maximal exercise capacity [7, 8], which is in line with our study. Studies using other methods to investigate determinants of maximal exercise capacity in CHF patients demonstrated strong relations between maximal exercise capacity and both skeletal muscle function, e.g. reduced skeletal muscle metabolic capacity or peripheral $O_2$ transport [4, 5, 20], as well as central hemodynamics [2, 3]. However, these results did not allow to draw conclusions on the relative contributions of central and peripheral factors to impaired maximal exercise capacity, nor on the presence of physiological heterogeneity in CHF patients. Studies investigating the influence of peripheral and central factors on exercise capacity simultaneously are scarce and yielded conflicting results. Whereas some of these studies indicate that intrinsic differences in skeletal muscle metabolism are the main determinants of a reduced exercise capacity [21, 22], other studies show that a reduced $O_2$ delivery to exercising muscles is the primary limiting factor [23, 24]. Possible explanations for this discrepancy may be the variety in exercise protocols that were used but also physiological heterogeneity in exercise limitations in these study populations.

One third of our population showed a central hemodynamic limitation of maximal exercise capacity. This limitation was associated with a more frequent occurrence of a plateau/ decrease in $VO_2$. Furthermore a central exercise limitation was associated both with a higher occurrence of a plateau/decrease in SV and a higher occurrence of chronotropic incompetence. From a physiological point of view, the inability to augment forward SV may be caused by impaired global left atrial [25] or ventricular contractile reserve, regional contractility disorders due to ischemia, valvular disorders such as mitral regurgitation and dyssynchrony. As severe mitral regurgitation at rest and ischemia were not identified as determinants of a central exercise limitation, an impaired global contractile reserve is likely to be the most important determinant of impaired SV augmentation in our population. In addition to a failure to augment SV, a central exercise limitation was also associated with a higher occurrence of chronotropic incompetence . In theory, this observation may be caused by neurohormonal dysregulation or the use of beta blockers. Previous studies showed that the lower peak heart rate during long-term administration of beta blockers is associated with a higher peak SV [26, 27]. In contrast, in our study population, patients with chronotropic incompetence, had a higher occurrence of failure to augment SV and a non-statistically significant lower peak SV. A previous study in CHF patients showed a significant correlation between peak oxygen uptake and change in heart rate, with no significant difference for patients with or without beta blockers [28]. As 93 % patients in our study used beta blockers and there was no difference in beta blocker use in both groups, this could not explain the difference in occurrence of chronotropic incompetence. Therefore, we postulate that chronotropic incompetence based on neurohormonal dysregulation (i.e. an imbalance between sympathic and parasympathic nerve activity) can be a contributory factor limiting exercise capacity in patients with a central exercise limitation. Our results showed significantly less patients with LBBB in the centrally limited group. This could be explained by studies that provide evidence that left ventricular (i.e. mechanical) dyssynchrony is irrespective of the QRS duration. Moreover, it is suggested that dyssynchrony is a dynamic condition and may worsen during exercise [29].

Characterization of exercise limitations may be beneficial in clinical practice for a better understanding of the causes of impairments in daily functioning. In addition, this approach may contribute to a more tailored therapeutic strategy in individual CHF patients. As such, Wilson et al. showed that patients with a reduced cardiac output response to exercise benefit less from a moderate intensity exercise training program than patients with a normal cardiac output response [7]. Yet, other studies showed that patients with a more pronounced central exercise limitation may benefit more from interventions aimed at improving central hemodynamics such as heart transplantation [8] and cardiac resynchronization therapy [30]. Whether the approach used in the present study will contribute to a better prediction of treatment results in individual CHF remains to be determined.

Before drawing conclusion from this study, several limitations should be acknowledged. First, we used an arbitrary method to classify exercise limitations. In fact, some patients that were not classified as having a central exercise limitation showed only small increases in Q during the final part of exercise. Second, the limited sample size did not permit to perform additional subgroup analyses. For instance, due to the fact that most patients were moderately impaired, we were unable to test the hypothesis, generated from animal studies that patient with more severe left ventricular dysfunction at rest have a more pronounced peripheral limitation than those with moderate left ventricular dysfunction [6]. Third, assessment of valvular disease and dyssynchrony was performed by resting echocardiography. However, as both may worsen during exercise [31], we cannot fully exclude that this factor played a role in the failure to augment SV and Q towards maximal exercise.

## Conclusion

This study revealed heterogeneity in exercise limitations in CHF patients. In one third of the study population a plateau or decrease in Q towards peak exercise was demonstrated, which is indicative of a central exercise limitation. Factors associated with a central exercise limitation included a higher occurrence of a failure to augment SV and chronotropic incompetence, suggesting that both impaired contractile reserve and neurohormonal dysregulation are determinants of reduced exercise capacity in centrally limited patients. Future research should focus on the clinical utility of characterizing exercise limitations to predict treatment effects in CHF patients.

#### Competing interests

The authors declare that they have no competing interests.

#### Authors' contributions

RS was involved in the study design, acquisition and analysis of data and drafting the manuscript. VN was involved in data collection, drafting and revision of the manuscript. BW and JJ were involved in collection and analysis of the data and revising the manuscript. PW and PD were involved in the study design and revising the manuscript. HK carried out data collection, analysis and was involved in the study design and drafting of the manuscript. All authors read and approved the final manuscript.

#### Acknowledgements

This project was supported by unrestricted research grants from "Friends of the Heart" foundation, Eindhoven, the Netherlands, "scientific foundation Máxima" of Máxima Medical Center and Medtronic.

#### Author details

[1]Department of Cardiology, Máxima Medical Centre, De Run 4600, P.O. Box 7777, Veldhoven 5500 MB, The Netherlands. [2]Department of Biomedical Engineering, Eindhoven University of Technology, Eindhoven, The Netherlands. [3]Department of Clinical Physics and Clinical Informatics, Máxima Medical Centre Veldhoven, Veldhoven, The Netherlands. [4]Department of Applied Physics, Eindhoven University of Technology, Eindhoven, The Netherlands. [5]Department of Cardiology, University Medical Centre Utrecht, Utrecht, The Netherlands. [6]Department of Medical Informatics, Academic Medical Centre, University of Amsterdam, Amsterdam, The Netherlands.

#### References

1. Cohen-Solal A, Logeart D, Guiti C, Dahan M, Gourgon R. Cardiac and peripheral responses to exercise in patients with chronic heart failure. Eur Heart J. 1999;20:931–45.
2. Hummel YM, Bugatti S, Damman K, Willemsen S, Hartog JWL, Metra M, et al. Functional and hemodynamic cardiac determinants of exercise capacity in patients with systolic heart failure. Am J Cardiol. 2012;110:1336–41.
3. Sullivan MJ, Knight JD, Higginbotham MB, Cobb FR. Relation between central and peripheral hemodynamics during exercise in patients with chronic heart failure. Muscle blood flow is reduced with maintenance of arterial perfusion pressure. Circulation. 1989;80:769–81.
4. Okita K, Yonezawa K, Nishijima H, Hanada A, Ohtsubo M, Kohya T, et al. Skeletal Muscle Metabolism Limits Exercise Capacity in Patients With Chronic Heart Failure. Circulation. 1998;98:1886–91.
5. Hopkinson NS, Dayer MJ, Antoine-Jonville S, Swallow EB, Porcher R, Vazir A, et al. Central and peripheral quadriceps fatigue in congestive heart failure. Int J Cardiol. 2013;167:2594–9.
6. Diederich ER, Behnke BJ, McDonough P, Kindig CA, Barstow TJ, Poole DC, et al. Dynamics of microvascular oxygen partial pressure in contracting skeletal muscle of rats with chronic heart failure. Cardiovasc Res. 2002;56:479–86.

7. Wilson JR, Groves J, Rayos G. Circulatory status and response to cardiac rehabilitation in patients with heart failure. Circulation. 1996;94:1567–72.
8. Chomsky DB, Lang CC, Rayos GH, Shyr Y, Yeoh TK, Pierson RN, et al. Hemodynamic exercise testing. A valuable tool in the selection of cardiac transplantation candidates. Circulation. 1996;94:3176–83.
9. Critoph CH, Patel V, Mist B, Elliott PM. Cardiac output response and peripheral oxygen extraction during exercise among symptomatic hypertrophic cardiomyopathy patients with and without left ventricular outflow tract obstruction. Heart. 2014;100:639–46.
10. Myers J, Wong M, Adhikarla C, Boga M, Challa S, Abella J, et al. Cardiopulmonary and noninvasive hemodynamic responses to exercise predict outcomes in heart failure. J Card Fail. 2013;19:101–7.
11. Lang CC, Karlin P, Haythe J, Lim TK, Mancini DM. Peak cardiac power output, measured noninvasively, is a powerful predictor of outcome in chronic heart failure. Circ Heart Fail. 2009;2:33–8.
12. Jonas MM, Tanser SJ. Lithium dilution measurement of cardiac output and arterial pulse waveform analysis: an indicator dilution calibrated beat-by-beat system for continuous estimation of cardiac output. Curr Opin Crit Care. 2002;8:257–61.
13. Kemps HMC, Thijssen EJM, Schep G, Sleutjes BTHM, De Vries WR, Hoogeveen AR, et al. Evaluation of two methods for continuous cardiac output assessment during exercise in chronic heart failure patients. J Appl Physiol. 2008;105:1822–9.
14. Lang RM, Bierig M, Devereux RB, Flachskampf FA, Foster E, Pellikka PA, Picard MH, Roman MJ, Seward J, Shanewise J, Solomon S, Spencer KT, St. John Sutton M, Stewart W: Recommendations for chamber quantification. Eur J Echocardiogr 2006;7:79–108.
15. Hamilton TT, Huber LM, Jessen ME. PulseCO: a less-invasive method to monitor cardiac output from arterial pressure after cardiac surgery. Ann Thorac Surg. 2002;74:S1408–12.
16. Linton NW, Linton RA. Estimation of changes in cardiac output from the arterial blood pressure waveform in the upper limb. Br J Anaesth. 2001;86:486–96.
17. Lamarra N, Whipp B, Ward S, Wasserman K. Effect of interbreath fluctuations on characterizing exercise gas exchange kinetics. J Appl Physiol. 1987;62:2003–12.
18. Brubaker PH, Kitzman DW. Chronotropic incompetence: causes, consequences, and management. Circulation. 2011;123:1010–20.
19. Higginbotham MB, Morris KG, Williams RS, McHale PA, Coleman RE, Cobb FR. Regulation of stroke volume during submaximal and maximal upright exercise in normal man. Circ Res. 1986;58:281–91.
20. Esposito F, Mathieu-Costello O, Shabetai R, Wagner PD, Richardson RS. Limited maximal exercise capacity in patients with chronic heart failure: partitioning the contributors. J Am Coll Cardiol. 2010;55:1945–54.
21. Shoemaker JK, Naylor HL, Hogeman CS, Sinoway LI. Blood Flow Dynamics in Heart Failure. Circulation. 1999;99:3002–8.
22. Wiener DH, Fink LI, Maris J, Jones RA, Chance B, Wilson JR. Abnormal skeletal muscle bioenergetics during exercise in patients with heart failure: role of reduced muscle blood flow. Circulation. 1986;73:1127–36.
23. Toussaint JF, Koelling TM, Schmidt CJ, Kwong KK, LaRaia PJ, Kantor HL. Local relation between oxidative metabolism and perfusion in leg muscles of patients with heart failure studied by magnetic resonance imaging and spectroscopy. J Heart Lung Transplant. 1998;17:892–900.
24. Sperandio PA, Borghi-Silva A, Barroco A, Nery LE, Almeida DR, Neder JA. Microvascular oxygen delivery-to-utilization mismatch at the onset of heavy-intensity exercise in optimally treated patients with CHF. Am J Physiol Heart Circ Physiol. 2009;297:H1720–8.
25. Ceresa M, Capomolla S, Pinna GD, Febo O, Caporotondi A, Guazzotti GP, et al. Left atrial function: bridge to central and hormonal determinants of exercise capacity in patients with chronic heart failure. Monaldi Arch Chest Dis. 2002;58:87–94.
26. Metra M, Nardi M, Giubbini R, Dei Cas L. Effects of short- and long-term carvedilol administration on rest and exercise hemodynamic variables, exercise capacity and clinical conditions in patients with idiopathic dilated cardiomyopathy. J Am Coll Cardiol. 1994;24:1678–87.
27. Eynon N, Sagiv M, Amir O, Ben-Sira D, Goldhammer E, Amir R. The effect of long-term beta-adrenergic receptor blockade on the oxygen delivery and extraction relationship in patients with coronary artery disease. J Cardiopulm Rehabil Prev, 2008;28:189–94.
28. Magrì D, Palermo P, Cauti FM, Contini M, Farina S, Cattadori G, et al. Chronotropic Incompentence and Functional Capacity in Chronic Heart Failure: No Role of β-Blockers and β-Blocker Dose. Cardiovasc Ther. 2012;30:100–8.
29. Lancellotti P, Moonen M. Left ventricular dyssynchrony: a dynamic condition. Heart Fail Rev. 2012;17:747–53.
30. Schlosshan D, Barker D, Pepper C, Williams G, Morley C, Tan LB. CRT improves the exercise capacity and functional reserve of the failing heart through enhancing the cardiac flow- and pressure-generating capacity. Eur J Heart Fail. 2006;8:515–21.
31. Lapu-bula R, Robert A, Craeynest D Van, Dhondt A, Gerber BL, Pasquet A, Melin JA, Kock M De. Contribution of Exercise-Induced Mitral Regurgitation to Exercise Stroke Volume and Exercise Capacity in Patients. Circulation 2002;106(11):1342–8.

# 9

# Inotropic agents use in patients hospitalized with acute decompensated heart failure: a retrospective analysis from a 22-year registry in a Middle-Eastern Country (1991–2013)

Amer H. S. Aljundi[1], Shaban F. K. Mohammed[1], Ashfaq Patel[3], Rajvir Singh[2], Abdulrahman Arabi[3], Hajar A. AlBinali[3] and Jassim Al Suwaidi[1*]

**Abstract**

**Background:** Data about the use of positive inotropic agents in patients hospitalized with acute decompensated heart failure (ADHF) is limited.

**Methods:** The records of 8066 patients with ADHF who were hospitalized at Hamad Medical Corporation, Qatar from 1991 to 2013 were analyzed to explore demographics and clinical characteristics of the patients according to inotropic agents use.

**Results:** Eight hundred fifty eight patients [10.6 %, 95 % CI (10 to 11.3 %)] received intravenous inotropic support. Patients receiving inotropes were more likely to be female and have preserved ejection fraction when compared to those not receiving inotropic agents. Comorbidities associated with higher likelihood of receiving inotropic treatment included acute myocardial infarction, chronic renal impairment, dyslipidemia, hypertension, obesity and hyperglycemia. Patient on inotropes were more likely to undergone percutaneous coronary intervention (PCI), intra-aortic balloon pump support and intubation. There were no differences in the mean plasma BNP and CK-MB levels between the 2 groups. Heart failure patients receiving inotropes also were more likely to have complications including ventricular tachycardia (2.0 % vs. 0.9 %, $p = 0.003$), prolonged hospital stay (8.0 vs. 5.0 days, $p = 0.001$), cardiac arrest (14.6 % vs. 3.2 %, $p = 0.001$) and in-hospital mortality (30.8 % vs. 9.1 %, $p = 0.001$). Over the study period there was an increase use of inotropic agents and decreased mortality rates.

**Conclusion:** Inotropic use increased over the period whereas; female gender and conventional cardiac risk factors were predictors of inotropic agents use in the study.

**Keywords:** Inotropes, Acute decompensated heart failure, Predictors, Length of stay, Mortality

* Correspondence: jalsuwaidi@hotmail.com
[1]Department of Clinical Pharmacology, Heart Hospital, Hamad Medical Corporation, P.O Box 3050, Doha, Qatar
Full list of author information is available at the end of the article

## Background

Acute heart failure refers to a group of clinical syndromes due to either new-onset heart failure (HF) or decompensation of chronic HF with symptoms necessitating hospitalization, emergency department visits, or unscheduled medical attention [1]. Heart failure is a growing problem resulting in significant morbidity and mortality and is the most common cause of hospital admissions in the United States resulting in approximately 1.1 million hospitalizations annually [2–4].

Common causes of ADHF are coronary artery disease (CAD) or valvular abnormalities. However, most patients hospitalized with ADHF have a worsening of preexisting HF, while up to 20 % of patients have no prior diagnosis of HF [5].

Patients with ADHF typically present with symptoms that range in severity from mild volume overload to life-threatening cardiogenic shock and multi-organ failure [6]. A general goal in the management includes improved symptoms with hemodynamic stabilization and increased use of evidence-based therapies to reduce recurrent hospitalization and mortality.

Based on the recent American College of Cardiology/American Heart Association guidelines for the diagnosis and management of heart failure, patients who are refractory to diuretics should be managed with vasodilators as first-line therapy in the absence of symptomatic hypotension or systolic blood pressure of less than 90 mmHg. These guidelines also state that the use of intravenous positive inotropic agents is a valid option to improve contractility for hospitalized patients with heart failure who have evidence of low ejection fraction, hemodynamic compromise, cardiogenic shock, or decreased organ perfusion [7]. Of note, the clinical practice guidelines of the Heart Failure Society of America [8] and the European Society of Cardiology [9] have similar recommendations to that of the American College Cardiology/American Heart Association. Positive inotropic agents, on the other hand, have not been shown to reduce length of hospital stay or mortality when added to standard care [10]. Additionally, milrinone and dobutamine have also been shown to be proarrhythmic and cause more symptomatic hypotension in randomized controlled trials compared to standard care [11]. Several observational studies including that of the Acute Decompensated Heart Failure National Registry (ADHERE) have also shown increases in mortality with inotropes when compared with vasodilator therapy [12]. However, data about trends of inotropic agents use in ADHF patients over a period of time is lacking.

We analyzed predictors of overall use of positive inotropic agents and associated outcomes in patients hospitalized with acute decompensated heart failure over 22-years period.

## Methods

a. Study setting
   This study was conducted in Heart hospital, Doha, Qatar. Heart Hospital is committed to deliver safe, high quality care in cardiology and cardiothoracic surgery for the residents of Qatar, nationals and expatriates where more than 95 % of cardiac patients are being treated in the Hospital, making it an ideal center for observational-based studies. The state of Qatar is located in the Arabian Peninsula having approximately 1.7 million population in 2010 most of them being Arab (40 %) followed by Indians (18 %), Pakistani (18 %), Iranian (10 %) and others (14 %). In the past decade, cardiovascular diseases were the leading cause of morbidity and mortality in the country. Database for patients admitted to the hospital are maintained electronically and registered at the cardiology department since January 1991. Based on these records, patients hospitalized due to ADHF between 1991 and 2013 were retrospectively evaluated. Study (#11355) was exempted for review from Institutional Review Board (IRB), MRC, Hamad Medical Corporation (HMC) due to its retrospective nature and study did not contain identifiable private information and were not collected by investigators through intervention or interaction with individuals. The Framingham criteria were used for the diagnosis of heart failure. The concurrent presence of either 2 major criteria or 1 major and 2 minor criterion was required to establish a diagnosis of HF [13]. Major criteria included paroxysmal nocturnal dyspnea, neck vein distention, weight loss of 4.5 kg in 5 days in response to treatment, acute pulmonary edema, rales, hepatojugular reflux, S3 gallop, central venous pressure greater than 16 cm water, circulation time of 25 s, radiographic cardiomegaly, pulmonary edema, visceral congestion, or cardiomegaly at autopsy. Minor criteria on the other hand included nocturnal cough, dyspnea on ordinary exertion, a decrease in vital capacity by one third the maximal value recorded, pleural effusion, tachycardia (heart rate of at least 120 beats per minute), or bilateral ankle edema that are not attributed to any other medical condition (e.g., cirrhosis, ascites, nephrotic syndrome) [14–17]. Inotropic support is defined as the use of adrenergic agonists and phosphodiesterase III (PDE) inhibitors. Doses of inotropic support were defined as the use of dopamine $\geq 5$ µg/kg/min; any dose of epinephrine, norepinephrine, dobutamine, or milrinone. On the

other hand, definition of acute myocardial infarction (MI) in this study was consistent to the World Heart Organization criteria. Bedside transthoracic echocardiography (TTE) was used to measure EF at admission to coronary intensive care unit. The presence of diabetes mellitus was based on documentation in the patient's previous or current medical record. The diagnosis of hyperlipidemia was made by a fasting cholesterol >5.2 mmol/L in the patient's medical record or any history of treatment of hyperlipidemia by the patient's physician. Chronic renal impairment was defined as creatinine >1.5 upper normal range. Presence of hypertension was determined by any documentation in the medical record or treatment by the patient's physician.

b. Statistical analysis

Descriptive statistics were calculated for all variables of interest. Patient characteristics were in the form of mean ± standard deviation (SD) and frequency with percentages for interval and categorical variables respectively. The frequencies of categorical variables were compared using chi-square test while comparisons were based on independent student *t*-test for interval data. To determine the patient characteristics that were associated with the use of inotropic agents, variables including age, sex, diabetes mellitus, hypertension, obesity, dyslipidemia, chronic renal impairment, ejection fraction, and prior MI were considered for multivariate logistic regression analysis using enter method. Adjusted odds ratios (ORs) and corresponding 95 % confidence intervals (CIs) for each factor were reported. All tests were 2-tailed and statistical difference was defined as a $p$ value < =0.05. All data analyses were carried out using the Statistical Package for Social Sciences version 19.0 (SPSS, IBM, Armonk, NY).

## Results

The study included 8066 patients, of whom 858 patients received inotropic agents. Baseline characteristics of the study population hospitalized with ADHF are displayed in Tables 1 and 2. The study patients were racially diverse; fewer patients in the inotropic group were Asians but more Middle-Eastern Arabs. Patients receiving inotropes were more likely to be female (38.9 % vs. 33.1 %, $p = 0.001$), older age (63 vs. 62 years, $p = 0.004$), with chronic renal impairment (18.4 % vs. 8.5 %, $p = 0.001$), on dialysis (1.9 % vs. 0.3 %, $p = 0.001$), dyslipidemic (11.2 % vs. 5.5 %, $p = 0.001$), hypertensive (69.3 % vs. 56.9 %, $p = 0.001$), obese (8.7 % vs. 6.1 %, $p = 0.003$) and have diabetes mellitus (66.3 % vs. 57.1 %, $p = 0.001$) at the time of admission. The inotropes group was also more likely to have elevated troponin levels (40.8 % vs. 25.9 %, $p = 0.001$) and to present with both STsegment

**Table 1** Heart Failure Patient Characteristics and Comorbidities

| Variable | Inotropes | No Inotropes | *p* Value |
|---|---|---|---|
| Demographics | | | |
| Total number, n (%) | 858 (10.6) | 7208 (89.4) | |
| Age, mean (SD) | 63 ± 12 | 62 ± 12 | 0.04 |
| Male, n (%) | 419 (61.1) | 4270 (66.9) | 0.001 |
| Middle-Eastern Arabs | 674 (78.6) | 5472 (73.7) | |
| South Asians | 164 (19.1) | 1562 (21.7) | |
| Others | 20 (2.3) | 174 (2.4) | 0.001 |
| Patient Characteristics, n (%) | | | |
| Smoker | 141 (16.4) | 1043 (14.5) | 0.12 |
| Chronic renal impairment | 158 (18.4) | 612 (8.5) | 0.001 |
| Dyslipidemia | 96 (11.2) | 394 (5.5) | 0.001 |
| Hypertension | 595 (69.3) | 4100 (56.9) | 0.001 |
| Diabetes Mellitus | 569 (66.3) | 4115 (57.1) | 0.001 |
| Obesity | 75 (8.7) | 443 (6.1) | 0.003 |
| Menopause | 34 (4) | 206 (2.9) | 0.07 |
| Labs, mean (SD) | | | |
| Hemoglobin (g/dl) | 11.8 ± 5 | 12 ± 4.9 | 0.04 |
| Fasting blood sugar, mmol/L | 11 ± 16 | 12 ± 48 | 0.81 |
| Serum creatinine, mmol/L | 164 ± 127 | 131 ± 265 | 0.01 |
| BNP, (pg/ml) | 4195 ± 7450 | 3090 ± 7650 | 0.22 |
| Cholesterol, mmol/L | 4.3 ± 1.5 | 4.4 ± 6 | 0.57 |
| Low density lipoprotein (LDL), mmol/L | 2.46 ± 1.0 | 2.9 ± 9.8 | 0.42 |
| High density lipoprotein (HDL), mmol/L | 1.2 ± 1.6 | 1.6 ± 1.9 | 0.63 |
| Triglycerides, mmol/L | 1.6 ± 1.3 | 1.6 ± 7.8 | 0.98 |
| Creatinine kinase -MB, μ/L | 61 ± 192 | 74 ± 559 | 0.6 |
| Labs, n (%) | | | |
| Troponin positive | 350 (40.8) | 1866 (25.9) | 0.001 |
| Cardiac History, n (%) | | | |
| Admission ejection fraction ≤ 40 % | 200 (59.2) | 1305 (69.6) | 0.001 |
| Rheumatic heart disease | 3 (0.3) | 43 (0.6) | 0.36 |
| ST-elevation myocardial infarction (STEMI) | 74 (8.6) | 309 (4.3) | 0.001 |
| Non-STEMI (NSTEMI) | 53 (6.2) | 256 (3.6) | 0.001 |
| Unstable angina | 64 (7.5) | 421 (5.8) | 0.06 |
| Cardiomyopathy | 125 (14.6) | 860 (11.9) | 0.03 |
| Pulmonary hypertension | 12 (1.4) | 80 (1.1) | 0.45 |
| Valvular Heart Disease, n (%) | | | |
| Mitral regurgitation | 44 (5.1) | 373 (5.2) | 0.95 |
| Aortic regurgitation | 11 (1.3) | 106 (1.5) | 0.66 |

**Table 2** In-hospital Procedures and Complications

| Variable | Inotropes | No Inotropes | p Value |
|---|---|---|---|
| Procedures, n (%) | | | |
| Intraaortic balloon pump (IABP) | 22 (2.6) | 28 (0.4) | 0.001 |
| Swan-Ganz catheterization | 47 (5.5) | 82 (1.1) | 0.001 |
| Percutaneous coronary intervention (PCI) | 17 (2) | 54 (0.7) | 0.001 |
| Coronary artery bypass grafting (CABG) | 61 (7.1) | 652 (9) | 0.06 |
| Intubation | 58 (6.8) | 76 (1.1) | 0.001 |
| Dialysis | 16 (1.9) | 22 (0.3) | 0.001 |
| Complications, n (%) | | | |
| Cerebrovascular accident (CVA) | 4 (0.5) | 39 (0.5) | 0.78 |
| Left bundle branch block (LBBB) | 29 (3.4) | 223 (3.1) | 0.65 |
| Supraventricular tachycardia (SVT) | 3 (0.3) | 13 (0.2) | 0.3 |
| Ventricular tachycardia | 17 (2) | 65 (0.9) | 0.003 |
| Atrial fibrillation | 53 (6.2) | 726 (10.1) | 0.001 |
| Ventricular fibrillation | 5 (0.6) | 10 (0.1) | 0.004 |
| Cardiac arrest | 125 (14.6) | 232 (3.2) | 0.001 |
| In-hospital mortality | 193 (30.8) | 407 (9.1) | 0.001 |
| Complications, mean (SD) | | | |
| Length of CCU stay | 5 ± 7 | 4 ± 5 | 0.02 |
| Total days hospitalized | 8 ± 34 | 5 ± 103 | 0.001 |

elevation (8.6 % vs. 4.3 %, $p = 0.001$) and non-ST-segment elevation (6.2 % VS. 3.6 %, $P = 0.001$) myocardial infarction when compared to the non-intropes group. The inotrope group was also more likely to undergo percutaneous coronary revascularization (2.0 % vs. 0.7 %, $p = 0.001$), and have intra-aortic balloon pump support (2.6 % vs. 0.4 %, $p = 0.001$). Interestingly, patients in the no inotropic support group were more likely to have lower LV ejection fraction (LVEF ≤ 40 %; 69.6 % vs. 59.2 %, $p = 0.001$) and more likely to develop atrial fibrillation (10.1 % vs. 6.2 %, $p = 0.001$) when compared to those who received inotropic agents. There were no significant differences between the 2 groups in regards to the mean plasma BNP levels (4195 ± 7450 vs. 3090 ± 7650) and CKMB levels (61 ± 192 vs. 74 ± 559) ($p$ = 0.22 and 0.60 respectively).

### Outcome

Patients on inotropes group had more cardiovascular complications including; ventricular tachycardia (2.0 % vs. 0.9 %, $p = 0.003$), prolonged hospital stay (8.0 vs. 5.0 days, $p = 0.001$), cardiac arrest (14.6 % vs. 3.2 %, $p = 0.001$) and in-hospital mortality (30.8 % vs. 9.1 %, $p = 0.001$) (Table 2).

### Trends

Inotropes use over the study period significantly increased; 4.6, 9.0, 9.9 14.2 and 17.6 % ($p = 0.001$) in 1991–95, 1996–2000, 2001–05, 2006–2010 and after 2010 years respectively (Table 3).

The average mortality rates in patients with ADHF receiving inotropic agents over 22 years was variable but decreased recently; 17.7, 27.1, 29.2, 18.8, and 7.3 % ($p = 0.001$) in 1991–95, 1996–2000, 2001–05, 2006–2010 and after 2010 years respectively (Table 4).

### Multivariate analysis

Table 5 shows multivariate logistic regression analysis; the adjusted odds of being treated with any positive inotropic agent were highest in patients who were a history of hypertension (OR: 1.66, 95 % CI: 1.10 to 2.5) or having chronic renal impairment (OR: 1.76, 95 % CI: 1.19 to 2.6) or preserved ejection fraction (OR: 1.92, 95 % CI: 1.27 to 2.9) after adjusting age, gender, hyperglycemia, obesity, ethnicity and old myocardial infraction.

In terms of evidence-based discharge medications, more patients in the inotropic support received beta-blockers at discharge and but ACE inhibitors when compared to patients who did not receive inotropes agents (Table 6).

## Discussion

This 22-year observational study of patients hospitalized with HF demonstrates 10.6 % need to use inotropic agents. Patients who received inotropic agents were older, more likely to be female, local Arabs rather than Asians with worse cardiovascular risk profile. Inotropic agents group were more likely to present with acute coronary syndrome when compared to the non-inotropic agents group. Interestingly, low left ventricular ejection fraction and BNP were not predictors of its use.

The current observation of inotropic agents use is consistent with that reported from the ADHERE Registry, which reported ≈ 10 % use of inotropic agents in patients hospitalized for ADHF in the United States. It is also consistent with other reports in the literature, which varied from 3 to 12 % [4, 12, 18]. Interestingly we report significant increase of inotropic support over the 22 years period, which may suggest hospitalization of "sicker" patients, while patients with less severe heart failure are increasingly managed in the outpatient setting.

### Predictors of inotropic agents use

Our study found that the strongest predictors of inotrope use were hypertension and chronic renal impairment. Based on data from ADHERE Registry, about 9.6 % of patients hospitalized for ADHF in the United States received an intravenous inotrope (either milrinone or dobutamine). Such patients tended to have more

**Table 3** Trend of inotropic support in Heart Failure patients

| Trend in years | 1991–95 | 1996–2000 | 2001–05 | 2006–10 | >2010 | *P* value |
|---|---|---|---|---|---|---|
| Inotropic Support | 65(4.6 %) | 159(9.0 %) | 201(9.9 %) | 277(14.2 %) | 154(17.6 %) | 0.001 |

severe disease, including lower blood pressure, lower ejection fraction, and higher blood urea nitrogen. The use of inotropes in the context of normal ejection fraction in our study is also striking because this signifies an overuse of inotropic medications, a fact that is consistently discouraged. Based on (ADHERE) Registry, out of more than 150,000 patients, fewer than 3 % had a systolic BP of <90 mmHg while approximately 50 % had a preserved systolic function. [19] However, about 14 % of the patients in ADHERE were treated with an intravenous inotropic agent indicating an overuse of such agents. Many studies have revealed that the use of inotropic agents may be associated with increased mortality, especially in patients with preserved left ventricular function. Therefore, it is recommended that positive inotropes only be used in patients who require inotropic support for low cardiac output.

However, better LVEF observed in inotropic group in our study may be explained by the susceptibility of these patients to a sudden drop in ejection fraction, even though small, compared to patients pre-conditioned to chronic low ejection fraction. Moreover, our study patients were not stratified based on other reversible conditions like sepsis or infection that can lead to an increase in demand and where the use of inotropes is assumed to improve outcomes.

One of the strongest predictors of inotrope use in our study was hypertension. Large multicenter registries revealed that about 70 % of patient hospitalized with ADHF have fluid overload, normal to elevated blood pressure with relatively preserved end-organ function, and no evidence of cardiogenic shock [4, 6, 20]. Therefore, the use of inotropes, with the main goal of improving end-organ perfusion, in such patients is not rational. Of note, for the majority of patients with ADHF with normal or elevated systemic blood pressure, there are no data to support a role for inotropic therapy. In this context, it is worth mentioning that 9 % of patients in the ADHERE Registry received a positive inotrope (dobutamine or milrinone), although only 2 % of patients were hypotensive. This means that more than 75 % of patients had no clinical indication for their use signifying an overuse of such medications.

Based on the European Society of Cardiology guidelines for the diagnosis and treatment of acute HF, patients with ADHF can be classified into one of six groups based on the clinical presentation [9]. The first 3 categories of patients comprise more than 90 % of ADHF presentations. These patients normally have relatively preserved left ventricular function with signs and symptoms of pulmonary edema and hypertension. Regardless, these findings emphasize the need for well-designed prospective trials to further establish the appropriate use of intravenous inotropic therapy in this population of patients.

The presence of renal dysfunction is relatively common in heart failure and can reduce the adequacy of diuresis. Renal dysfunction in our analysis was a strong predictor of inotropic use. This observation can be explained by the fact that when increases in intravenous boluses or infusions of loop diuretics and addition of metolazone does not lead to an adequate diuretic response, facilitation of diuresis may be enhanced by inotropic therapy by presumably improved renal blood flow through modest increases in cardiac output [21]. Moreover, at our institution, low-dose dopamine is used in combination with diuretic therapy, on the supposition that it can increase renal perfusion and subsequent diuresis. In general, patients with clinical evidence for end-organ hypoperfusion are mostly referred to as having a low output state. While hypotension is classically considered a powerful predictor of this hemodynamic profile, clinical exam findings may inaccurately identify such patients who may not even present with hypotension [22] Of note, patients with long standing heart failure, low output states can be associated with more subtle clinical findings, such as nausea, abdominal pain, slowed mentation, and fatigue [23]. An extremely important clinical finding indicating impaired end-organ perfusion is worsening renal function (so- called cardiorenal syndrome), a finding that usually occurs after initiating intravenous loop diuretics [24]. More recent data suggest that many

**Table 4** Trend of mortality in Heart Failure patients

| Trend in years | 1991–95 | 1996–2000 | 2001–05 | 2006–10 | >2010 | *P* value |
|---|---|---|---|---|---|---|
| Mortality | 17.7 % | 27.1 % | 29.2 % | 18.8 % | 7.3 % | 0.001 |

**Table 5** Multivariate predictors of Inotropes in Patients Hospitalized with ADHF

| Variable | Adjusted OR | 95 % CI | *p* value |
|---|---|---|---|
| Age | 0.99 | 0.98–1.01 | 0.33 |
| Male | 0.90 | 0.64–1.27 | 0.55 |
| Diabetes Mellitus | 1.04 | 0.72–1.50 | 0.84 |
| Hypertension | 1.66 | 1.10–2.50 | 0.02 |
| Obesity | 1.06 | 0.66–1.70 | 0.81 |
| Chronic renal failure | 1.76 | 1.19–2.60 | 0.005 |
| Ejection fraction >40 | 1.92 | 1.27–2.90 | 0.002 |
| Middle-Eastern Arabs | 1.10 | 0.76–1.58 | 0.62 |
| Old myocardial infarction | 1.19 | 0.82–1.71 | 0.36 |

patients with cardiorenal syndrome have a relatively preserved cardiac output and hypertension making them amenable to treatment with inotropes [25].

### Outcomes

Our analysis provides data that focus on outcomes related to the mortality of patients treated with inotropic medications. This consideration is important when comparing our results to other published studies evaluating mortality. Inotropic therapy in certain studies has been shown to have detrimental effects [5, 10, 26–36], although another meta-analysis was unable to confirm this view [37]. In ADHERE registry; more than 65,000 patients from 263 centers across the United States admitted with heart failure were retrospectively analyzed. Data were utilized to describe the management trends and outcomes of those patients. Based on the registry, use of short-term vasodilator therapy was associated with significantly lower in hospital mortality when compared to positive inotropic treatment. A propensity score matching was used to adjust for confounding factors when comparing patients in both arms. Similarly, the impact of intravenous inotropic therapy on mortality in patients hospitalized with ADHF has been validated in the Outcomes of a Prospective Trial of Intravenous Milrinone for Exacerbation of Chronic Heart Failure (OPTIMECHF) study. In this placebo-controlled, randomized, double-blind clinical trial, the use of intravenous milrinone when compared to placebo was associated with a higher rate of early treatment failure, sustained hypotension (10.7 % vs. 3.2 %, $p < 0.001$), and new onset atrial fibrillation or flutter (4.6 % vs. 1.5 %, $p$=0 .004) [10]. There were no improvements in total days hospitalized, symptomatic relief, or mortality with milrinone compared with placebo. Our analysis revealed that intravenous inotrope use was associated with a significant increase in the risk of mortality. This risk association could not be attributed to the use of inotropic medications. Therefore, controlling for other potential risk factors as possible using a propensity score–adjusted multivariable analysis would be better utilized to conclude a significant worse prognosis with the independent use of inotropes compared with the other group. Of note, in terms of predictors of in-hospital mortality, of the 39 variables examined in ADHERE, the strongest predictor was a blood urea nitrogen (BUN) of 43 mg/dL or higher. This was followed by a systolic blood pressure of less than 115 mmHg and a SCr of 2.75 mg/dL or greater.

**Table 6** Medication Use at Discharge

| Variable | Inotropes | No Inotropes | *P* Value |
|---|---|---|---|
| ß-blocker | 275 (32.1) | 1908 (26.5) | 0.001 |
| ACE/ARB[a] | 321 (37.4) | 4346 (60.3) | 0.001 |
| Calcium channel blockers | 352 (41) | 768 (10.7) | 0.001 |
| Digoxin | 28 (3.3) | 389 (5.4) | 0.008 |
| Amiodarone | 53 (6.2) | 394 (5.5) | 0.39 |
| Frusemide | 545 (63.5) | 6012 (83.4) | 0.001 |
| Spiranolactone | 35 (4.1) | 456 (6.3) | 0.009 |

[a]ACE/ARB: Angiotensin converting enzyme inhibitors/Angiotensin receptor blockers

In-hospital mortality in the inotrope-treated patients in our study was close to 31 %. In ADHERE, patients treated with Inotrops had a high mortality rate (19 %) than all other non-inodilator-treated patients (14 %) or patients with preserved ejection fraction not treated with inotropes (2 %) [12]. Proposed mechanisms of increased mortality with inotropes in our study include in-hospital events such as tachyarrhythmias or subclinical myocardial ischemia and apoptosis through increased sympathetic stimulation and intramyocardial calcium accumulation with the use of inotropes. Additionally, many studies have revealed that the use of inotropic agents may be associated with increased mortality, especially in patients with preserved left ventricular function, which is also consistent with our observations.

The use of intravenous inotropes increased over the last years despite the absence of a reasonable indication with a trend in increasing mortality.

In addition to evaluating the in-hospital mortality rate, our study also considered other relevant end points, such as complications of inotropic support, length of CCU stay, and length of hospital stay. As opposed to the results of (OPTIME-CHF), our analysis revealed lower incidence of atrial fibrillation in patients treated with inotropic support. This fact is interesting as patients in this group had more cardiovascular risk factors for developing atrial fibrillation. However, patients on inotropes had more episodes of ventricular tachycardia and cardiac arrest; associated rhythm was ventricular fibrillation. We infer that to the use of inotropic agents that are known to trigger ventricular tachyarrhythmia as such complications have been confirmed in randomized trials of inotropic agents versus placebo or vasodilator medications used for heart failure [38, 39]. Therefore, the use of such medications warrant close monitoring and correction of any cause that can contribute to development of arrhythmias.

Length of CCU stay and overall hospital stay was longer in patients treated with inotropic medications group. This result is consistent with other registries. For example, patients who received inotropic agents in ADHERE had more than double the length of stay (12.9 vs. 5.8 days; $P <$ 0.0001) compared with those who were not treated with inotropes. Moreover, in a subgroup analysis of ADHERE, patients with preserved systolic function treated with inotropic agents had longer length of hospital stay (12.9 vs. 5.8 days; $P < 0.0001$) and more than nine-fold increase in mortality rate (19 vs. 2 %; $P < 0.0001$) compared with patients who did not receive inotropes [40].

One of the important goals in the management of patients with ADHF is to implement the use of evidence-based therapies to reduce recurrent hospitalization and mortality, which include angiotensin converting enzyme (ACE) inhibitors and beta-blockers [41]. According to our analysis, more patients in the inotropic support received beta-blockers but less ACE inhibitors compared to no inotropes group (Table 6). This can be explained by the fact that patients in the inotropic support had more tachy-arrhythmias that augmented the use of beta-blockers. . Of note, ACE inhibitors provide rapid improvement in hemodynamics and renal function that may facilitate the subsequent initiation of betablockers.

### Limitations of the study

Our study had several limitations. First, it is historical and observational in design with its inherent limitations including missing data or measurement errors. Additionally, patients were not randomly assigned to the treatment groups and, as a result, both groups differed in demographics and disease-associated factors related to the outcomes of interest. Because it is not possible to identify and adjust for all possible factors, the differences between patients in both group and the influences of other nonmeasured factors cannot be totally excluded. However, we controlled for between-group differences through multivariate analysis that took into consideration differences in baseline demographics and disease-associated factors related to the predictors of inotropes use. We also did not categorize patients based on the inotropic medication given. The study design cannot also overcome a bias from the inclusion of a select group of severe patients who may have been channeled to the inotropic support group with subsequent worse outcomes. Additionally, our database did not include clinical data of left ventricular ejection fraction and BNP throughout 22 years, which are important determinants of inotrope use and thus may contribute to improved risk adjustments.

## Conclusion

Conventional cardiac risk factors predict the use of inotropic support in heart failure patients. However, there was some overuse of inotropes in patients with hypertension and preserved ejection fraction. Inotopic agents use increased over the years.

#### Abbreviations

ADHF: acute decompensated heart failure; BNP: brain natriuretic peptide; CK-MB: Creatinine kinase-MB fraction; PCI: Percutaneous coronary intervention; MI: myocardial infarction; ADHERE: Acute Decompensated Heart Failure National Registry.

#### Competing interests

The authors declare that they have no competing interests.

#### Authors' contributions

AJ and SM: Literature search, data extraction and manuscript writing; RS: Data extraction, Statistical analysis and tabulations; LZ: AA, AP & HA; Involved in patients recruitment and critical review of the manuscript. JAL is responsible for the overall content as the guarantor. All authors have read and approved the final manuscript

#### Acknowledgement

We would like to thank the staff of the Department of Cardiology and Cardiovascular Surgery at Heart Hospital for providing data and Institutional Review Board (IRB),Medical Research Centre, Hamad Medical Corporation for permitting to publish the study. There is no financial involvement in writing, data collection, analysis and interpretation of data; and in the decision to submit the manuscript for publication.

#### Author details

[1]Department of Clinical Pharmacology, Heart Hospital, Hamad Medical Corporation, P.O Box 3050, Doha, Qatar. [2]Cardiovascular Research, Heart Hospital, Hamad Medical Corporation, Doha, Qatar. [3]Cardiology and Cardiovascular Surgery, Heart Hospital, Hamad Medical Corporation, Doha, Qatar.

#### References

1. Felker GM, Adams KF, Konstam MA, O'Connor CM, Gheorghiade M. The problem of decompensated heart failure: Nomenclature, classification, and risk stratification. Am Heart J. 2003;145:S18–25.
2. Najafi F, Jamrozik K, Dobson AJ. Understanding the 'epidemic of heart failure': a systematic review of trends in determinants of heart failure. Eur J Heart Fail. 2009;11:472–9.
3. Roger VL, Go AS, Lloyd-Jones DM, Adams RJ, Berry JD, Brown TM. Heart disease and stroke statistics-2011 update: a report from the American Heart Association. Circulation. 2011;123:e18–e209.
4. Adams KF, Fonarow GC, Emerman CL, LeJemtel TH, Costanzo MR, Abraham WT. Characteristics and outcomes of patients hospitalized for heart failure in the United States: rationale, design, and preliminary observations from the first 100,000 cases in the Acute Decompensated Heart Failure National Registry (ADHERE). Am Heart J. 2005;149:209–16.
5. Joseph SM, Cedars AM, Ewald GA, et al. Acute decompensated heart failure: contemporary medical management. Tex Heart Inst J. 2009;36:510–20.
6. Gheorghiade M, Zannad F, Sopko G, Klein L, Piña IL, Konstam MA, et al. Acute heart failure syndromes: Current state and framework for future research. Circulation. 2005;112:3958–68.
7. Hunt SA, Abraham WT, Chin MH, Feldman AM, Francis GS, Ganiats TG, et al. 2009 focused update incorporated into the ACC/AHA 2005 guidelines for the diagnosis and management of heart failure in adults. A report of the American College of Cardiology Foundation/American Heart Association Task Force on Practice guidelines developed in

collaboration with the International Society for Heart and Lung Transplantation. J Am Coll Cardiol. 2009;53:e1–e90.

8. Heart Failure Society of America, Lindenfeld J, Albert NM, Boehmer JP, Collins SP, Ezekowitz JA, et al. HFSA 2010 comprehensive heart failure practice guideline. J Card Fail. 2010;16:e1–e194.
9. Dickstein K, Cohen-Solal A, Filippatos G, McMurray JJ, Ponikowski P, PooleWilson PA, et al. ESC guidelines for the diagnosis and treatment of acute and chronic heart failure 2008: the Task Force for the Diagnosis and Treatment of Acute and Chronic Heart Failure 2008 of the European Society of Cardiology. Developed in collaboration with the Heart Failure Association of the ESC (HFA) and endorsed by the European Society of Intensive Care Medicine (ESICM). Eur J Heart Fail. 2008;10:933–89.
10. Cuffe MS, Califf RM, Adams Jr KF, et al. Outcomes of a Prospective Trial of Intravenous Milrinone for Exacerbations of Chronic Heart Failure (OPTIMECHF) Investigators. Short-term intravenous milrinone for acute exacerbation of chronic heart failure: a randomized controlled trial. JAMA. 2002;287(12):1541–7.
11. Burger AJ, Horton DP, LeJemtel T, et al. Effect of nesiritide (B-type natriuretic peptide) and dobutamine on ventricular arrhythmias in the treatment of patients with acutely decompensated congestive heart failure: the PRECEDENT study. Am Heart J. 2002;144:1102–8.
12. Abraham WT, Adams KF, Fonarow GC, et al. In-hospital mortality in patients with acute decompensated heart failure requiring intravenous vasoactive medications: an analysis from the acute decompensated heart failure national registry (ADHERE). J Am Coll Cardiol. 2005;46:57–64.
13. Ho KK, Pinsky JL, Kannel WB, Levy D. The epidemiology of heart failure: the Framingham Study. J Am Coll Cardiol. 1993;22(4 Suppl A):6A–13A.
14. Al Suwaidi J, Bener A, Hajar HA, Numan MT. Does hospitalisation for congestive heart failure occur more frequently in Ramadan: a population- based study (1991–2001). Int J Cardiol. 2004;96:217–21.
15. Al Suwaidi J, Asaad N, Al-Qahtani A, Al-Mulla AW, Singh R, Albinali HA. Prevalence and outcome of Middle-eastern Arab and South Asian patients hospitalized with heart failure: insight from a 20-year registry in a Middle-eastern country (1991–2010). Acute Card Care. 2012;14(2):81–9.
16. Al Suwaidi J, Al-Qahtani A, Asaad N, Al-Mulla AW, Singh R, Albinali HA. Comparison of women versus men hospitalized with heart failure (from a 20-year registry in a middle-eastern country 1991–2010). Am J Cardiol. 2012; 109(3):395–400.
17. McKee PA, Castelli WP, McNamara PM, et al. The natural history of congestive heart failure: the Framingham Study. N Engl J Med. 1971;285:1441–6.
18. Yancy CW, Lopatin M, Stevenson LW, et al. Clinical presentation, management, and in-hospital outcomes of patients admitted with acute decompensated heart failure with preserved systolic function: a report from the Acute Decompensated Heart Failure National Registry (ADHERE) database. J Am Coll Cardiol. 2006;47:76–84.
19. Fonarow GC, for the ADHERE Scientific Advisory Committee. The Acute Decompensated Heart Failure National Registry (ADHERE): opportunities to improve care of patients hospitalized with acute decompensated heart failure. Rev Cardiovasc Med. 2003;4 suppl 7:S21–30.
20. Shah MR, Hasselblad V, Stinnett SS, et al. Hemodynamic profiles of advanced heart failure: Association with clinical characteristics and long-term outcomes. J Card Fail. 2001;7:105–13.
21. Stevenson LW, Massie BM, Francis GS. Optimizing therapy for complex or refractory heart failure: A management algorithm. Am Heart J. 1998;135:S293–309.
22. Forman DE, Butler J, Wang Y, et al. Incidence, predictors at admission, and impact of worsening renal function among patients hospitalized with heart failure. J Am Coll Cardiol. 2004;43:61–7.
23. Stevenson LW, Nohria A, Mielniczuk L. Torrent or torment from the tubules? Challenge of the cardiorenal connections. J Am Coll Cardiol. 2005;45:2004–7.
24. Cleland JGF, Swedberg K, Follath F, et al. The EuroHeart Failure survey programme—A survey on the quality of care among patients with heart failure in Europe: Part 1: Patient characteristics and diagnosis. Eur Heart J. 2003;24:442–63.
25. Goldberg LI. Dopamine: clinical uses of an endogenous catecholamine. N Engl J Med. 1974;291:707–10.
26. Leier CV. Positive inotropic therapy: an update and new agents. Curr Probl Cardiol. 1996;21(8):521–81.
27. Felker GM, Benza RL, Chandler AB, et al. Heart failure etiology and response to milrinone in decompensated heart failure: results from the OPTIME-CHF study. J Am Coll Cardiol. 2003;41:997–1003.
28. Young JB. Evolv ing concepts in the treatment of heart failure: should new inotropic agents carry promise or paranoia? Pharmacotherapy. 1996;16(2 Pt 2):78S–84S.
29. Sasayama S. What do the newer inotropic drugs have to offer? Cardiovasc Drugs Ther Feb. 1992;6(1):15.
30. Packer M, Carver JR, Rodeheffer RJ, et al. Effect of Oral Milrinone on mortality in severe chronic heart failure. N Engl J Med. 1991;325:1468–75.
31. Packer M, Leir CV. Survival in congestive heart failure during treatment with drugs with positive inotropic actions. Circulation. 1987;75(Suppl IV):55–63.
32. Elis A, Bental T, Kimchi O, et al. Intermittent dobutamine treatment in patients with chronic refractory congestive heart failure: a randomized, double-blind, placebo-controlled study. Clin Pharmacol Ther. 1998;63:682–5.
33. Oliva F, Latini R, Politi A, et al. Intermittent 6-month low-dose dobutamine infusion in severe heart failure: DICE multicenter trial. Am Heart J. 1999; 138:247–53.
34. O'Connor CM, Gattis WA, Uretsky BF, et al. Continuous intravenous dobutamine is associated with an increased risk of death in patients with advanced heart failure: insights from the Flolan International Randomized Survival Trial (FIRST). Am Heart J. 1999;138:78–86.
35. Coletta AP, Cleland JG, Freemantle N, et al. Clinical trials update from the European Society of Cardiology Heart Failure meeting: SHAPE, BRING-UP 2 VAS, COLA II, FOSIDIAL, BETACAR, CASINO and meta-analysis of cardiac resynchronisation therapy. Eur J Heart Fail. 2004;6:673–6.
36. Cleland JG, Ghosh J, Freemantle N, et al. Clinical trials update and cumulative meta-analyses from the American College of Cardiology: WATCH, SCD HeFT, DINAMIT, CASINO, INSPIRE, STRATUS-US, RIO-Lipids and cardiac resynchronisation therapy in heart failure. Eur J Heart Fail. 2004;6:501–8.
37. Thackray S, Easthaugh J, Freemantle N, et al. The effectiveness and relative effectiveness of intravenous inotropic drugs acting through the adrenergic pathway in patients with heart failure-a meta-regression analysis. Eur J Heart Fail. 2002;4(4):515–29.
38. Silver MA, Horton DP, Ghali JK, et al. Effect of nesiritide versus dobutamine on short-term outcomes in the treatment of patients with acutely decompensated heart failure. J Am Coll Cardiol. 2002;39:798–803.
39. Pflugfelder PW, O'Neill BJ, Ogilvie RI, et al. A Canadian multicentre study of a 48 h infusion of milrinone in patients with severe heart failure. Can J Cardiol. 1991;7:5–10.
40. Reassessing treatment of acute heart failure syndromes: the ADHERE Registry Mihai Gheorghiade1* and Gerasimos Filippatos2 European Heart Journal Supplements (2005) 7 (Supplement B), B13–B19. doi:10.1093/eurheartj/sui008
41. Johnson D, Jin Y, Quan H, Cujec B. Beta-blockers and angiotensinconverting enzyme inhibitors/receptor blockers prescriptions after hospital discharge for heart failure are associated with decreased mortality in Alberta, Canada. J Am Coll Cardiol. 2003;42(8):1438–45.

# Galectin 3: association to neurohumoral activity, echocardiographic parameters and renal function in outpatients with heart failure

Freja Stoltze Gaborit[1,7*], Helle Bosselmann[2,4], Caroline Kistorp[3,7], Kasper Iversen[1,7], Thomas Kumler[1], Finn Gustafsson[4], Jens P. Goetze[5], György Sölétormos[6], Niels Tønder[2] and Morten Schou[1,7]

**Abstract**

**Background:** Galectin 3 (Gal-3) reflects cardiac fibrosis in heart failure HF, but has also been associated to renal fibrosis and impaired renal function. Previous research has suggested that Gal-3 could be a cardio-renal biomarker, but it has never been tested simultaneous in a single study whether Gal-3 reflects echocardiographic measures, neurohumoral activity and renal function.

The aim of this study was to evaluate the relationship between plasma concentrations of Gal-3 and neurohumoral activity, myocardial and renal function in patients with HF, including advanced echocardiographic measures and 24-h urinary albumin excretion (albuminuria).

**Methods:** We prospectively enrolled 132 patients with reduced left ventricular ejection fraction (LVEF) referred to an outpatient HF clinic. The patients had a median age of 70 years (interquartile rage: 64–75), 26.5 % were female, median LVEF was 33 % (27–39 %) and 30 % were in NYHA class III-IV.

**Results:** Patients with plasma concentrations of Gal-3 above the median had significantly lower estimated glomerular filtration rate (eGFR) and this association remained significant in multivariate regression analysis (β: −0.010; 95 % CI −0.012–-0.008; $P < 0.001$), adjusted for age, gender, medical treatment. Plasma concentrations of Gal-3 were not associated with albuminuria (Beta: 0.008; 95 % CI:-0.028–0.045; $P = 0.652$). There were no association between plasma concentrations of Gal-3 and myocardial function or structure estimated by LVEF, LVmassIndex, LVIDd, E/é or LV global longitudinal strain ($P > 0.05$ for all). In multivariate analyses plasma concentrations of Gal-3 were significantly associated with the cardiac biomarkers: NT-proBNP (β: 0.047; 95 % CI: 0.008–0.086; $P = 0.020$), proANP (β: 0.137; 95 % CI: 0.067–0.207;
$P < 0.001$), chromogranin A (β: 0.123; 95 % CI: 0.052–0.194; $P < 0.001$) and Copeptin (β: 0.080; 95 % CI: 0.000–0.160; $P = 0.049$). Multivariate analysis was adjusted for eGFR, age, gender and medical treatment.

**Conclusions:** Increased plasma concentrations of Gal-3 are associated with reduced eGFR and increased plasma concentrations of NT-proBNP, proANP, chromogranin A and Copeptin, but not with echocardiographic parameters reflecting myocardial function. These results suggest that Gal-3 reflects both increased neurohumoral activity and reduced eGFR, but not myocardial function in patients with systolic HF.

**Keywords:** Heart failure reduced ejection fraction, Galectin 3, Renal function, Echocardiography, Natriuretic peptides

* Correspondence: freja.stoltze.gaborit@regionh.dk
[1]Department of Cardiology, Herlev University Hospital, Herlev, Denmark
[7]Department of Clinical Medicine, University of Copenhagen, Copenhagen, Denmark
Full list of author information is available at the end of the article

## Background

Galectin 3 (Gal-3) is a soluble β-galactoside-binding lectin. It is expressed in epithelial and inflammatory cells in several organs and it is located both intra- and extracellularly [1, 2]. Gal-3 is involved in cellular functions related to cell adhesion, proliferation and differentiation [3]. Gal-3 has been linked to fibrosis in a spectrum of medical conditions including heart failure (HF) [4–7].

Increased plasma concentrations of plasma Gal-3 are inversely associated to renal function evaluated by estimated glomerular filtration rate (eGFR) in both the general population and in HF patients [8, 9]. Increased plasma concentrations of Gal-3 have predictive value of deteriorating renal function and de novo renal disease [10]. It is, however, unknown whether plasma concentrations of Gal-3 are related to 24 h urine albumin excretion (albuminuria), a renal biomarker which also provides prognostic value in HF [11].

Increased plasma concentrations of Gal-3 are observed in both acute and chronic HF and it has been associated to increased risk of mortality and re-hospitalization [12–14]. Previous studies have suggested an association between plasma concentrations of Gal-3 and NT-proBNP [12, 14]. Plasma concentrations of Gal-3 have also been linked to cardiac fibrosis and it seems reasonable to hypothesize that it would also be associated to echocardiographic measures of left ventricular (LV) function [15, 16].

Thus, the clinical potential of Gal-3 and its pathophysiological aspects are not fully investigated in HF. We, therefore, wanted to evaluate whether plasma concentrations of Gal-3 were associated with I) neurohumoral activity (natriuretic peptides), II) myocardial function estimated by echocardiography and III) renal function evaluated by eGFR and albuminuria.

## Methods

### Population

This study was conducted using data from the CardioRen cohort [17]. Patients were enrolled at their first visit at the outpatient HF clinic at the North Zealand University Hospital, in the period from January 2011 to November 2012. Inclusion criteria were LVEF < 45 %, clinical stable (60 days out of hospital) and stable plasma-creatinine (+/– 10 μM the last 60 days). A total of 149 patients fulfilled all inclusion criteria and agreed to participate in the study. A total of 17 patients were excluded from the analyses due to missing venous blood samples or a missing Gal-3 value. As a result 132 patients with complete data were included in this study. All patients provided written informed consent. The study was approved by the Committee on Health Research Ethics for the Capital Region of Denmark (H-1-2010-074) and was conducted according to the Declaration of Helsinki.

Data were collected at the second visit to the HF clinic, including medical history, present symptoms, functional class, medication, height, weight, non-invasive blood pressure, heart rate, 12-lead electrocardiogram. Additionally venous blood samples were taken and patients collected a 24 h urine sample. Advanced echocardiography was preformed according to standard recommendations of the European Society of Cardiology [18].

### Biomarkers

Hemoglobin and creatinine were analyzed successively for each patient. Plasma samples for later analysis were collected in ethylenediamine tetracetic (EDTA) vial, centrifuged at 4 degrees (3,000 rpm in 10 min) and stored in –80 degrees Celsius.

Plasma concentrations of NT-proBNP, Troponin I and high sensitive c-reactive protein (hsCRP) were measured on the Dimension Vista®1500 from Siemens Medical Solutions Diagnostics using the LOCI®-technology (Luminescent Oxygen Channeling Assay) according to the manufacturer's instructions [19]. Plasma concentrations of Copeptin were measured on the Kryptor Compact platform (BRAHMS), assay and validation has been reported previously [20]. Plasma concentrations of proANP were measured using an automated immunoluminometric assay (Thermo-Fisher, Hennigsdorf/Berlin, Germany). Plasma concentrations of Chromogranin A were measured with an immuno assay in two steps to quantify the total amount of Chromogranin A in plasma, as previously described [21]. Gal-3 plasma concentrations were measured with a commercial enzyme-linked immunosorbent assay (BG Medicine, Waltham, MA, USA) [22].

### Renal function

Renal function was calculated as eGFR by the Chronic Kidney Disease Epidemiology Collaboration (CKD-EPI) equation incorporating age, race, gender, and plasma creatinine concentration [23]. Impaired renal function was defined as eGFR <60 mL/min per 1.73 $m^2$. Patients collected a 24 h urine specimen for albumin excretion analysis (albuminuria, mg/24 h).

### Echocardiography

Echocardiography was performed with the Vivid E9 (General Electric, Vingmed, Horten, Norway) and analyzed offline (Echopac BT 12, 1.0, General Electric, Horten, Norway) by a single trained operator blinded to renal function and plasma concentrations of Gal-3.

LVEF was calculated by the Simpson biplane model. LV mass was calculated from the linear dimensions in the parasternal view and indexed to body surface area according to gender (LVmassIndex). Maximal left atrial volume index was determined from the biplane area method and indexed to body surface area LAESVindex).

Mitral inflow was determined by pulse wave Doppler recordings and peak velocity of early (E) and atrial filling (A) and mitral valve deceleration time. Tissue Doppler velocity was measured at both lateral and septal mitral annulus for myocardial peak early velocity (e') and peak systolic velocity (s'). Mean e' was calculated from the lateral and septal e', and used for calculating E/e'. In case of atrial fibrillation mean value of e' was calculated from three consecutive heart cycles. LV global longitudinal strain (GLS) was assessed by two-dimensional speckle tracking in the three apical projections (long axis, four chambers and two chambers). LV GLS was analysed in 17 standardised segments and total LV GLS was calculated automatically by Echopac software.

### Statistics

Baseline clinical and biochemical data were calculated according to median Gal-3. Dichotomous variables as proportion in percentages and continuous variables as median with interquartile range (25–75 %). The two groups were compared with Pearson Chi square-test for discrete variables and t-tests (parametric) and Mann Whitney U-tests (nonparametric) for continuous variables, as appropriate. Univariate and multivariate linear regressions analyses were performed for the relation between plasma concentrations of Gal-3 and each cardiovascular biomarker and echocardiographic variable, with the cardiovascular biomarker or echocardiographic variable as the response variable (+/−median), in separate models. Explanatory variables (covariates) were chosen from available established confounders: eGFR, age and gender. All other potential confounders (diabetes, NYHA class, LVEF, ischemic heart disease, body mass index, atrial fibrillation) were eliminated by backward elimination ($P > 0.10$) to avoid overfitting of the statistical models. Data quality of covariates included in the statistical models was > 90 %. Results were considered statistically significant when $P < 0.05$ (two-sided).

## Results

Baseline characteristic are presented in Table 1. Patients were divided in two groups with plasma concentrations of Gal-3 above or below median (median Gal-3: 16.90 ng/mL). Impaired renal function was present in 28 % of all patients, defined as eGFR < 60 mL/min/1.73 $m^2$. Ischemic heart disease verified by previous coronary angiography was present in 40 %.

Patients with Gal-3 plasma concentrations above the median were older ($P = 0.010$), were more symptomatic ($P < 0.001$) and more often received a mineralocorticoid receptor antagonist ($P = 0.039$) (Additional file 1: Table S1 and Additional file 2). Table 1 also demonstrates that patients with increased Gal-3 plasma concentrations had higher plasma creatinine ($P = 0.001$), lower eGFR ($P < 0.001$), lower plasma hemoglobin ($P = 0.004$) and higher concentrations of NT-proBNP ($P < 0.001$), hsCRP ($P = 0.001$), Copeptin ($P < 0.001$) and Chromogranin A ($P = 0.001$). These findings suggest that patients with Gal-3 plasma concentrations above median suffer from more advanced stages of heart failure. In Fig. 1 echocardiographic variables are presented according to median plasma Gal-3. Patients with Gal-3 plasma concentrations above the median had a decreased TAPSE ($P = 0.031$) and a decreased s' medial ($P = 0.022$). Other echocardiographic variables did not differ significant between the two groups, this included test for LVmassIndex ($P = 0.832$) and s' lateral ($P = 0.473$).

Table 2 illustrates the associations between both Gal-3 and echocardiographic variables and the associations between Gal-3 and cardiovascular biomarkers. In univariate analysis both the echocardiographic variables: TAPSE, E/e', s' medial, LAESVindex and the biomarkers: NT-proBNP, proANP, Chromogranin A, Copeptin, hsCRP and Troponin I were associated with Gal-3. In multivariate analysis, adjusted for age, gender, eGFR, treatment with ACE-inhibitor, Aldosterone Receptor Antagonist, Mineralocorticoid receptor antagonist, beta-blocker, NT-proBNP (β: 0.047; 95 % CI: 0.008–0.086; $P = 0.020$), proANP (β: 0.137; 95 % CI: 0.067–0.207; $P < 0.001$), Chromogranin A (β: 0.123; 95 % CI: 0.052–0.194; $P < 0.001$), Copeptin (β: 0.080; 95 % CI 0.000–0.160; $P = 0.049$) and hsCRP (β: 0.051; 95 % CI: 0.001–0.101; $P = 0.047$) were still associated with Gal-3 (Fig. 2). Patients with Gal-3 plasma concentrations above median had markedly lower eGFR (55 vs. 80 ml/min, $P < 0.001$). This association remained significant in multivariate linear regression with Gal-3 as response variable and eGFR as explanatory variable (β: −0.010; 95 % CI −0.012–-0.008; $P < 0.001$), adjusted for age, gender, treatment with ACE-inhibitor, Aldosterone Receptor Antagonist, Mineralocorticoid receptor antagonist, beta-blocker. There were no significant association between Gal-3 and albuminuria (Beat: 0.012; 95 % CI: −0.041–0.065; $P = 0.652$) (Fig. 3).

## Discussion

The main finding of this present study is threefold. First, plasma concentrations of Gal-3 are associated with neurohumoral activity. Second, plasma concentrations of Gal-3 are associated with renal function evaluated by eGFR, but not with albuminuria. Finally, plasma concentrations of Gal-3 are not associated with myocardial function evaluated by echocardiography in patients with systolic HF.

### Neurohumoral activity and Gal-3

Plasma concentrations of both Gal-3 and NT-proBNP are elevated in HF patients. In the present study we observed significant positive associations between Gal-3 and NT-proBNP and proANP, respectively. These observations are supported by similar findings in other studies [12–14]. Previous studies that also

**Table 1** Baseline characteristics according to Galectin 3 plasma concentration above or below median (median = 16.90 ng/mL). Linear variables presented: median (25–75 % percentiles)

| Variable | Below median Galectin 3 (*n* = 64) | Above median Galectin 3 (*n* = 68) | *P*-value |
|---|---|---|---|
| Age, years | 68 (62–73) | 73 (68–78) | 0.010 |
| Female sex, % | 21.9 | 30.9 | 0.241 |
| BMI, kg/m2 | 26 (24–29) | 27 (23–31) | 0.191 |
| NYHA class III-IV, % | 15.6 | 44.1 | <0.001 |
| Systolic BP, mmHg | 130 (113–143) | 122 (110–137) | 0.225 |
| Diastolic BP, mmHg | 77 (70–84) | 73 (68–81) | 0.174 |
| Heart rate, beats/min | 67 (59–75) | 68 (60–78) | 0.292 |
| HF duration, months | 7.5 (6–12) | 12 (6–24) | 0.257 |
| Medical history: | | | |
| Pervious MI, % | 46.9 | 32.4 | 0.088 |
| Hypertension, % | 57.8 | 64.7 | 0.405 |
| Atrial fibrillation, % | 35.9 | 32.4 | 0.664 |
| ICD, % | 10.9 | 13.4 | 0.663 |
| Diabetes, % | 18.8 | 26.5 | 0.290 |
| Apoplexia Cerebri/ TCI, % | 12.5 | 22.1 | 0.148 |
| Medication: | | | |
| ACE-I, % | 64.1 | 72.1 | 0.333 |
| ARB, % | 31.7 | 22.1 | 0.211 |
| Beta-blocker, % | 85.9 | 85.3 | 0.916 |
| MRA, % | 12.5 | 26.9 | 0.039 |
| Blood sample analysis: | | | |
| Hemoglobin, mmol/L | 8.9 (8.3–9.4) | 8.2 (7.6–8.8) | 0.004 |
| Creatinine, umol/L | 76.0 (66.0–84.0) | 98.0 (81.0–130.5) | 0.001 |
| eGFR, mL/min/1.73 m2 | 81.0 (70.0–88.0) | 55.0 (40.5–70.0) | <0.001 |
| Galectin 3, ng/mL | 13.90 (12.43–14.49) | 21.85 (18.65–27.58) | <0.001 |
| NTproBNP, pg/mL | 920.15 (393.75–1712.30) | 1931.15 (736.20–4059.25) | <0.001 |
| ProANP, pmol/L | 726.89 (470.29–1099.33) | 1205 (658.80–1627.44) | 0.006 |
| Troponin I, % above median | 32,8 | 38,2 | 0.519 |
| hsCRP, mg/L | 1.64 (0.87–3.30) | 3.64 (1.61–8.21) | 0.001 |
| Chromogranin A, pmol/L | 79.0 (49.0–116.0) | 106.5 (72.0–240.0) | 0.001 |
| Copeptin, pmol/L | 7.89 (5.07–12.62) | 10.88 (7.03–32.85) | <0.001 |
| Urine Sample analysis: | | | |
| Albuminuria, mg/24 h | 11.0 (9.0–23.5) | 14.0 (8.0–29.5) | 0.213 |

*Abbreviations*: *BMI* Body mass index, *NYHA* New York Heart Association, *BP* Blood pressure, *HF* Heart failure, *MI* Myocardial infarction, *ICD* Implantable cardiac defibrillator, *TCI* Transitory cerebral ischemia, *ACE-I* Angiotensin converting enzyme inhibitor, *ARB* Aldosterone receptor blocker, *MRA* Mineralocarticoide receptor antagonist, *eGFR* Estimated glomerular filtration rate, *NTproBNP* N-terminal-pro Brain Natriuretic Peptide, *proANP* Pro-atrial-natriuretic-peptide, *hsCRP* high sensitive C-reactive protein

evaluated the long term prognostic value of Gal-3 have demonstrated that the independent prognostic value of Gal-3 disappears after adjusting for NT-proBNP [12, 14, 24–26]. Therefore, although plasma concentrations of Gal-3 are elevated in HF, most likely there are no independently associated with increased mortality risk. This present study is the first to evaluate the relationship of plasma concentrations of Gal-3 and proANP. The positive association is anticipated and confirms the relationship to natriuretic peptides. Natriuretic peptides are part of the neurohumoral activation in HF and markers of increased wall stress in the cardiac cambers. Whether plasma concentrations of Gal-3 are influenced directly by

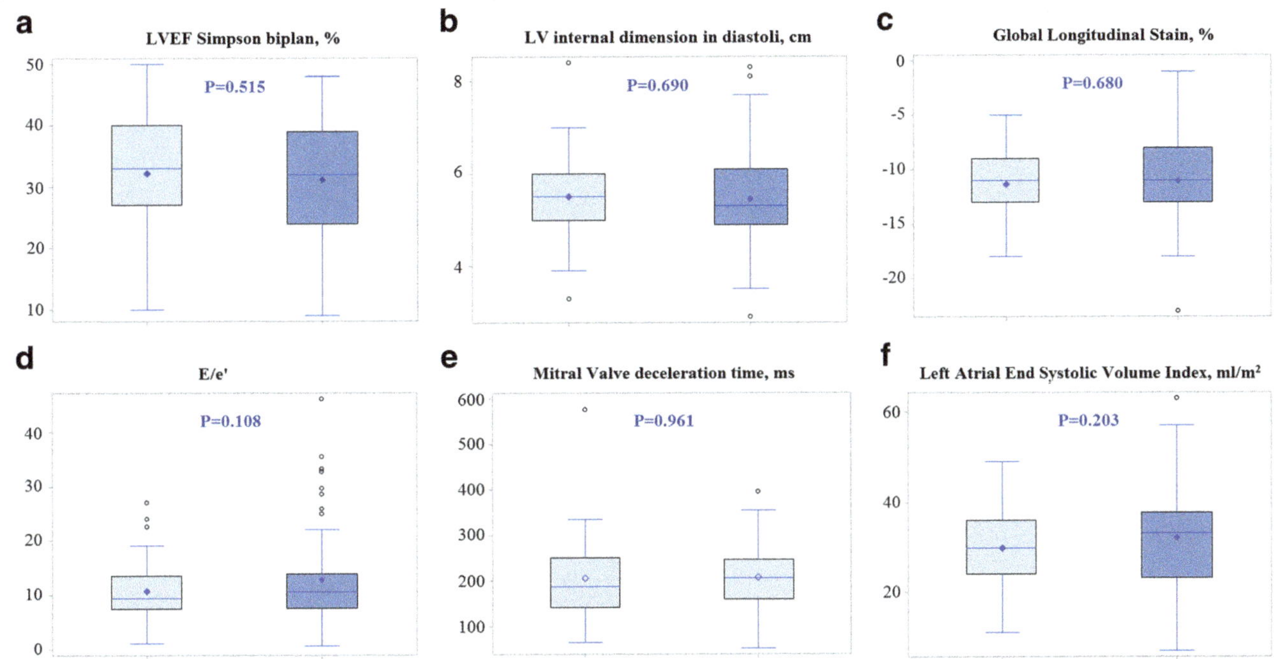


**Fig. 1 a-f** Box plot of medians of echocardiographic variables according to Galectin 3 plasma concentration above median ($n = 68$) (light blue) or Galectin 3 plasma concentration below median ($n = 64$) (dark blue). Patients with plasma concentrations of Galectin 3 above median had a lower TAPSE and lower s' medial, other echocardiographic variables did not show signs of an uneven distribution ($P > 0.05$ for all)

**Table 2** Echocardiographic parameters and biomarkers. Linear regression models (response variable: Galectin 3). Multivariate analyses adjusted for age, gender, eGFR, treatment with beta-blocker, ACE-inhibitor, Aldosterone Receptor Antagonist, Mineralocorticoid receptor antagonist, beta-blocker

| | Univariate: Beta (95 %-CI) | *P*-value | Multivariate: Beta (95 % CI) | *P*-value |
|---|---|---|---|---|
| Echocardiographic parameters: | | | | |
| LVIDd | -0.036 (-0.124--0.510) | 0.410 | -- | -- |
| LVmassIndex | $0.442\times10^{-3}$ ($-0.912\times10^{-3}$–$1.796\times10^{-3}$) | 0.520 | -- | -- |
| EF biplane | -0.002 (-0.011–0.007) | 0.691 | -- | -- |
| GLS | -0.002 (-0.029–0.024) | 0.861 | -- | -- |
| TAPSE | -0.195 (-0.353--0.038) | 0.015 | -0.073 (-0.211–0.065) | 0.298 |
| MV decel time | $-9.655\times10^{-5}$ (-0.001–0.001) | 0.868 | -- | -- |
| E/e' | 0.012 (0.000–0.023) | 0.049 | 0.005 (-0.005–0.014) | 0.338 |
| s' medial | -0.070 (-0.128--0.011) | 0.020 | -0.014 (-0.065–0.036) | −0.575 |
| s' lateral | -0.035 (-0.090–0.019) | 0.199 | -- | -- |
| LAESVi | 0.009 (0.001–0.017) | 0.021 | 0.004 (-0.003–0.011) | 0.222 |
| Biomarkers: | | | | |
| Troponin I | 0.175 (0.008–0.341) | 0.040 | 0.055 (-0.089–0.198) | 0.451 |
| NTproBNP | 0.110 (0.072–0.147) | <0.001 | 0.047 (0.008–0.086) | 0.020 |
| proANP | 0.320 (0.232–0.407) | <0.001 | 0.137 (0.067–0.207) | <0.001 |
| ChromagraninA | 0.203 (0.125–0.280) | <0.001 | 0.123 (0.052–0.194) | <0.001 |
| Copeptin | 0.211 (0.139–0.282) | <0.001 | 0.080 (0.000–0.160) | 0.049 |
| hsCRP | 0.080 (0.021–0.138) | 0.008 | 0.051 (0.001–0.101) | 0.047 |

*Abbreviations*: *LVIDd* Left ventricle internal diameter diastoli, *LVmassIndex* Left ventricle mass index, *EF* Ejection Fraction, *GLS* Global longitudinal strain, *TAPSE* Tricuspid annular plane systolic excursion, *MV decel time* Mitral valve deceleration time, E/e', *s'* Myocardial peak systolic velocity, *LAESVi* Left atrial end systolic volume index, *NTproBNP* N-terminal pro brain natriuretic peptide, *proANP* Pro atrial natriuretic protein, *hsCRP* High sensitive C-reactive protein, *eGFR* Estimated glomerular filtration rate

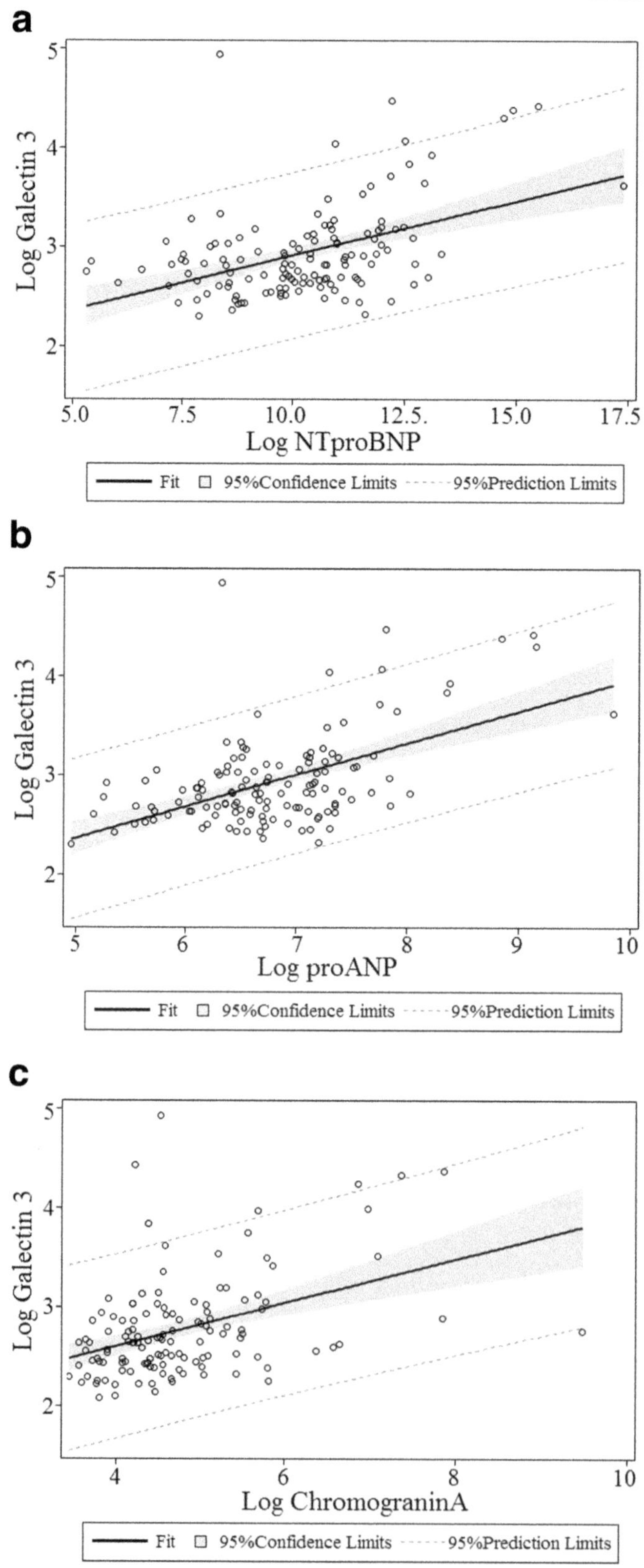


**Fig. 2** Scatterplot of the correlation between (**a**) Galectin 3 plasma concentration and NT-proBNP; (**b**) Galectin 3 plasma concentration and proANP and (**c**) Galectin-3 plasma concentration and Chromogranin A

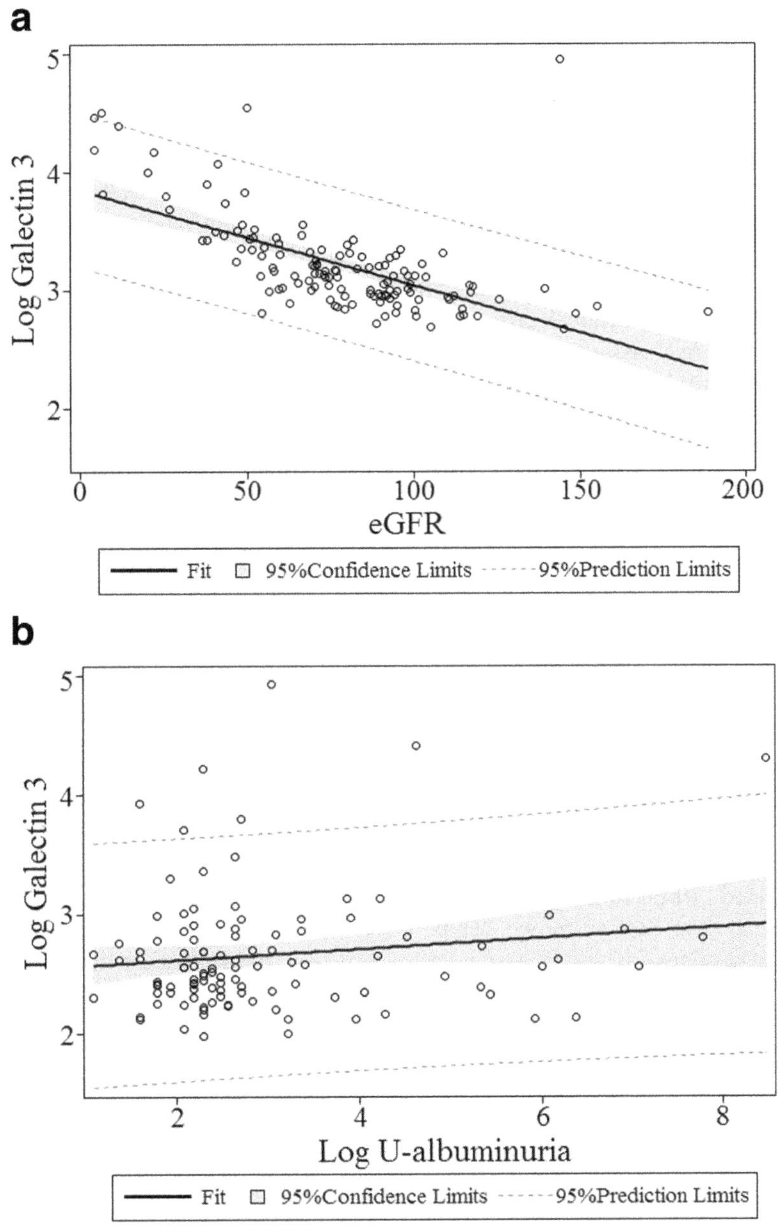


**Fig. 3** Scatterplot of the correlation between (**a**) Galectin 3 plasma concentration and eGFR and (**b**) Galectin 3 plasma concentration and albuminuria. Plasma concentration of Galectin 3 were significantly associated to eGFR in linear univariate (Beta: −0.009; 95%CI: −0.011–−0.007; $P < 0.001$) and multivariate analysis (β -0.010; 95%CI: −0.012–−0.008; $P < 0.001$), adjusted for age and gender, treatment with beta-blocker, ACE-inhibitor, Aldosterone Receptor Antagonist, Mineralocorticoid receptor antagonist, beta-blocker. Plasma concentration of Galectin 3 were not associated to albuminuria in linear univariate analyses (Beta: 0.042; 95%CI: −0.018–0.102; $P = 0.170$)

increased wall stress or through neurohumoral activation needs to be examined.

Another cardiac biomarker reflecting neurohumoral activation is Chromogranin A [21, 27]. No prior study has evaluated the relationship between plasma concentrations of Gal-3 and Chromogranin A. Our findings suggest a significantly association between plasma concentrations of Gal-3 and Chromogranin A, thereby reaffirming the relation with the neurohumoral response.

Copeptin, a surrogate marker for vasopressin, involved in volume regulation and electrolyte homeostasis, is also a cardiac biomarker reflecting neurohumoral activity. Copeptin is elevated in HF and predicts mortality risk and risk of re-hospitalization [28, 29]. In the present study plasma concentrations Gal-3 are significantly associated to copeptin. This finding is new and not observed previously.

Another finding of this study is a positive association between plasma concentrations of Gal-3 and elevated plasma concentrations of hsCRP. This finding is in accordance with other studies including HF patients [30, 31]. Gal-3 is also involved in the inflammatory response, and this could explain a positive association between hsCRP and Gal-3.

### Myocardial function and Gal-3

Gal-3 has been linked to cardiac fibrosis in HF, and it would therefore be reasonable to believe that elevated plasma concentrations of Gal-3 would be linked to echocardiographic findings. In the present study of patients with chronic HF and reduced LVEF none of the conventional echocardiographic measures were statistically associated to plasma concentrations of Gal-3. We evaluated both LV systolic (LVEF, global longitudinal strain, s') and diastolic parameters (E/e', e', E/A, LAESVindex), LVmassIndex, LVIDd and right ventricle systolic function (TAPSE).

Few prior studies have systematically evaluated the relationship between echocardiographic measures and plasma concentrations of Gal-3. The DEAL-HF trial performed serial echocardiographic measures in 240 patients with HF reduced LVEF and found a positive association between increased plasma concentrations of Gal-3 and LV remodeling estimated by change in LV end diastolic volume [32]. In a large study of 1440 patients hospitalized with HF plasma concentrations of Gal-3 did not differ significantly between patients with reduced LVEF compared to patients with preserved LVEF after stratifying by New York Heart Association functional class. However, plasma concentrations of Gal-3 were associated LVEF and LV mass index in univariate analysis [14]. Shah et al. [33] examined 115 patients admitted with acute dyspnea, in whom a standard echocardiography had been performed. It was reported that plasma concentrations of Gal-3 were associated to several echocardiographic parameters reflecting higher LV filling pressure and valvular disease (mitral inflow ratio, right ventricular fractional area, right ventricle systolic pressure, more severe mitral-valve or tricuspid-valve regurgitation) [33]. On the contrary other studies have found no association between plasma concentrations of Gal-3 and myocardial function. In a study of 133 chronic HF patients and 45 decompensated HF patients Tang et al. [9] did not observe any association between plasma concentrations of Gal-3 and echocardiographic findings neither systolic (LVEF, LV end systolic diameter, LV end diastolic diameter, LVmassIndex) nor diastolic (mitral inflow ratio, e', left atrial volume index). Weir et al. [34] examined 100 patients with LV dysfunction after acute myocardial infarction and performed cardiac magnetic resonance imaging at baseline and at 24-week follow-up. Plasma concentrations of Gal-3 were associated to biomarkers reflecting cardiac remodeling, however, there were no association to myocardial function evaluated by cardiac MRI at baseline or change in parameters over time. It is uncertain whether plasma concentrations of Gal-3 reflect myocardial function, and based on previous and the present study plasma concentrations of Gal-3 should likely not play a significantly role in the evaluation of systolic or diastolic function of the LV in HF.

### Renal function and Gal-3

The relationship between plasma concentrations of Gal-3 and eGFR is well established in both HF patients and the general population. Gal-3 has been accepted as a new cardiac biomarker in HF, but also carries potential to be a renal biomarker due to the close association between plasma concentrations of Gal-3 and eGFR.

In the present as in previous studies a negative association between plasma concentrations of Gal-3 and eGFR in HF patients was observed [9, 14]. Moreover, Zamora et al. [24] observed that the prognostic value of plasma concentrations of Gal-3 disappeared after adjusting for renal function. Gopal et al. [35] examined the relationship between plasma concentrations of Gal-3 and renal function in patients with HF and controls. They found plasma concentrations of Gal-3 to be correlated to eGFR in both groups, but Gal-3 were not related to LVEF or clinical congestion.

No previous studies have examined the relationship between albuminuria and plasma concentrations of Gal-3 in HF patients. In patients with impaired renal function O'Seaghdha et al. [10] found no association between albuminuria and plasma concentrations of Gal-3. Meijers et al. [36] have studied the excretion of Gal-3 in both animal models and in HF and dialysis patients. They observed increased plasma concentrations of Gal-3 in HF patients, but they did not observe an increased urinary excretion. They propose that renal clearance of plasma Gal-3 is impaired in HF patients, which explains the elevated plasma concentrations of Gal-3 and the association between renal function and plasma concentrations of Gal-3 [36]. This supports the finding in the present study, where no association was observed between plasma concentrations of Gal-3 and albuminuria. Albuminuria and plasma concentrations of Gal-3 may, therefore, reflect different pathology in the kidneys.

### Methodological considerations and perspectives

Some methodological limitations of this study should be addressed. It is a single center study with a limited sample size. Patients in this study have a short history of HF, they have been in clinically stable through the past 3 months and not all patients have been fully up-titrated in recommended HF treatment. Therefore the results cannot be extrapolated to other groups of patients or other stages of heart failure. This study was conducted as a cross sectional study without follow-up. Therefore, any firm conclusion concerning causal relationship between Gal-3 and NT-proBNP and vice versa has to be interpreted with caution. In this study we measured Troponin I, and no subsequent analyses for high sensitive troponin were made. Due to missing follow-up information we were unable to evaluate the prognostic value of Gal-3.

Plasma concentrations of cardiac biomarkers with renal excretion must be interpreted with caution in patients with renal dysfunction, as increased levels could reflect both decreased clearance and increased cardiac secretion.

While further clinical studies will be necessary to establish the full benefit of Gal-3 as a cardiac biomarker in HF, due to its close relationship with eGFR and NT-proBNP, our studies supports that Gal-3 is elevated in more severe HF and related to other risk markers. The close relationship with eGFR should be evaluated to create a better understanding of this relationship. Future studies could evaluate whether Gal-3 is a cardio-renal marker that e.g. increases before plasma concentrations of creatinine during an acute HF event, a scenario where a new biomarker is needed. And since no clear association has been found between Gal-3 and echocardiographic parameters, future studies should explore the association between plasma concentrations of Gal-3 and myocardial fibrosis e.g. by late gate enhancement with magnetic resonance scanning or by fibrosis identified by myocardial biopsy.

## Conclusion

Increased plasma concentrations of Gal-3 are associated with reduced eGFR and increased neurohumoral activity (NTproBNP, proANP, Copeptin and Chromogranin A), but not with echocardiographic parameters of myocardial function in patients with systolic HF.

### Abbreviations

's, Myocardial peak systolic velocity; A, Peak velocity of atrial filling; Albuminuria, Urine albumin excretion, mg/24 h; CKD-EPI, Chronic Kidney Disease Epidemiology Collaboration; E, Mitral flow peak velocity; É, Myocardial peak early velocity; EDTA, Ethylenediamine tetracetic; eGFR, Estimated Glomerular Filtration Rate; Gal-3, Galectin 3; GLS, Global longitudinal strain; HF, Heart failure; hsCRP, High sensitive C-reactive peptide; LAESVindex, Left atrial end systolic index; LV, Left Ventricular; LVEF, Left ventricle Ejection fraction; LVIDd, Left ventricle inter diameter diastolic; NT-proBNP, Aminoterminal pro-brain natriuretic peptide; ProANP, Pro-atrial natriuretic peptide.

### Acknowledgement

Technical assistance of nurse Mette Welløv Petersen and nurse Ellen Mouritsen is gratefully appreciated.

### Funding

The study was funded by Research Grant from North Zealand Hospital, University of Copenhagen and Research Grant from Herlev University Hospital, University of Copenhagen.

### Authors' contribution

FSG: acquisition of data, interpretation of data, drafting the manuscript, final approval of the version. HB: acquisition of data, analysis of data, final approval of the version. CK: interpretation of data, final approval of the version. KI: interpretation of data, revising manuscript critically, final approval of the version. TK: interpretation of data (especially regarding echocardiography), final approval of the version. FG: interpretation of data, revising manuscript critically, final approval of the version. JPG: interpretation of data (especially regarding biomarkers), final approval of the version. GS: interpretation of data (especially regarding biomarkers), final approval of the version. NT: analysis of data, interpretation of data (especially regarding echocardiography), final approval of the version. MS: hypothesis generating, revising manuscript critically for important intellectual content, final approval of the version.

### Competing interests

The authors declare that they have no competing interests.

### Author details

[1]Department of Cardiology, Herlev University Hospital, Herlev, Denmark. [2]Department of Internal Medicine KNEA, North Zealand University Hospital, Hillerod, Denmark. [3]Department of Internal Medicine, Endocrinology Unit, Herlev University Hospital, Herlev, Denmark. [4]Department of Cardiology, Rigshospitalet, Copenhagen, Denmark. [5]Department of Clinical Biochemistry, Rigshospitalet, Copenhagen, Denmark. [6]Department of Clinical Biochemistry, North Zealand University Hospital, Hillerod, Denmark. [7]Department of Clinical Medicine, University of Copenhagen, Copenhagen, Denmark.

### References

1. Frimodt-Møller M, Nielsen AH, Kamper A-L, Strandgaard S. Reproducibility of pulse-wave analysis and pulse-wave velocity determination in chronic kidney disease. Nephrol Dial Transplant. 2008;23:594–600.
2. Krześlak A, Lipińska A. Galectin-3 as a multifunctional protein. Cell Mol Biol Lett. 2004;9:305–28.
3. Dumic J, Dabelic S, Flögel M. Galectin-3: an open-ended story. Biochim Biophys Acta. 2006;1760:616–35. Available from: http://www.sciencedirect.com/science/article.
4. Henderson NC, Mackinnon AC, Farnworth SL, Kipari T, Haslett C, Iredale JP, et al. Galectin-3 expression and secretion links macrophages to the promotion of renal fibrosis. Am J Pathol. 2008;172:288–98.
5. Henderson NC, Mackinnon AC, Farnworth SL, Poirier F, Russo FP, Iredale JP, et al. Galectin-3 regulates myofibroblast activation and hepatic fibrosis. Proc Natl Acad Sci U S A. 2006;103:5060–5.
6. Sharma UC, Pokharel S, Van Brakel TJ, Van Berlo JH, Cleutjens JPM, Schroen B, et al. Galectin-3 marks activated macrophages in failure-prone hypertrophied hearts and contributes to cardiac dysfunction. Circulation. 2004;110:3121–8.
7. Newlaczyl AU, Yu L-G. Galectin-3–a jack-of-all-trades in cancer. Cancer Lett. 2011;313:123–8.
8. Böhm M, Voors A a., Ketelslegers J-M, Schirmer SH, Turgonyi E, Bramlage P, et al. Biomarkers: optimizing treatment guidance in heart failure. Clin Res Cardiol. 2011;100:973–81.
9. Tang WHW, Shrestha K, Shao Z, Borowski AG, Troughton RW, Thomas JD, et al. Usefulness of plasma galectin-3 levels in systolic heart failure to predict renal insufficiency and survival. Am J Cardiol. 2011;108:385–90.
10. O'Seaghdha C, Hwang S. Elevated galectin-3 precedes the development of CKD. J Am Soc Nephrol. 2013;24(9):1470–7. http://jasn.asnjournals.org/content/early/2013/06/04/ASN.2012090909.short.
11. Damman K, Jaarsma T, Voors A a, Navis G, Hillege HL, Van Veldhuisen DJ. Both in- and out-hospital worsening of renal function predict outcome in patients with heart failure: Results from the Coordinating Study Evaluating Outcome of Advising and Counseling in Heart Failure (COACH). Eur J Heart Fail. 2009;11:847–54.

12. Felker GM, Fiuzat M, Shaw LK, Clare R, Whellan DJ, Bettari L, et al. Galectin-3 in Ambulatory Patients With Heart Failure Results From the HF-ACTION Study. Circ Fail. 2012;5(1):72–8.
13. van der Velde a R, Gullestad L, Ueland T, Aukrust P, Guo Y, Adourian A, et al. Prognostic value of changes in galectin-3 levels over time in patients with heart failure: data from CORONA and COACH. Circ Heart Fail. 2013;6:219–26.
14. Zhang Y, Zhang R, An T, Huang Y, Guo X, Yin S, et al. The utility of galectin-3 for predicting cause-specific death in hospitalized patients with heart failure. J Card Fail. 2015;21(1):51–9.
15. Iwanaga Y, Nishi I, Furuichi S, Noguchi T, Sase K, Kihara Y, et al. B-type natriuretic peptide strongly reflects diastolic wall stress in patients with chronic heart failure: comparison between systolic and diastolic heart failure. J Am Coll Cardiol. 2006;47:742–8.
16. Yoneyama A, Koyama J, Tomita T, Kumazaki S, Tsutsui H, Watanabe N, et al. Relationship of plasma brain-type natriuretic peptide levels to left ventricular longitudinal function in patients with congestive heart failure assessed by strain Doppler imaging. Int J Cardiol. 2008;130:56–63.
17. Bosselmann H, Tonder N, Sölétormos G, Rossing K, Iversen K, Goetze JP, et al. Influence of renal impairment on myocardial function in outpatients with systolic heart failure: An echocardiographic and cardiac biomarker study. Int J Cardiol. 2014;177:942–8.
18. Lang RM, Bierig M, Devereux RB, Flachskampf F a, Foster E, Pellikka P a, et al. Recommendations for chamber quantification. Eur J Echocardiogr. 2006;7: 79–108.
19. Bruneel A, Dehoux M, Barnier A, Boutten A. External evaluation of the Dimension Vista 1500® intelligent lab system. J Clin Lab Anal. 2012;26:384–97.
20. Alehagen U, Dahlström U, Rehfeld JF, Goetze JP. Association of copeptin and N-terminal proBNP concentrations with risk of cardiovascular death in older patients with symptoms of heart failure. JAMA. 2011;305:2088–95.
21. Goetze JP, Hilsted LM, Rehfeld JF, Alehagen U. Plasma chromogranin A is a marker of death in elderly patients presenting with symptoms of heart failure. Endocr Connect. 2014;3:47–56.
22. REF #: 12836 US IVD BGM Galectin-3® Kit: 12836 Enzyme-linked Immunosorbent Assay for the Quantitative Determination of Galectin-3 in Human Serum and Plasma. :1–35.
23. Levey AS, Stevens L a, Schmid CH, Zhang YL, Castro AF, Feldman HI, et al. A new equation to estimate glomerular filtration rate. Ann. Intern. Med. 2009;150:604–12.
24. Zamora E, Lupón J, de Antonio M, Galán A, Domingo M, Urrutia A, et al. Renal function largely influences Galectin-3 prognostic value in heart failure. Int J Cardiol. 2014;177:171–7. Available from: http://www.sciencedirect.com/science/article.
25. Ho JE, Liu C, Lyass A, Courchesne P, Pencina MJ, Vasan RS, et al. Galectin-3, a marker of cardiac fibrosis, predicts incident heart failure in the community. J Am Coll Cardiol. 2012;60:1249–56.
26. Gullestad L, Ueland T, Kjekshus J, Nymo SH, Hulthe J, Muntendam P, et al. The predictive value of galectin-3 for mortality and cardiovascular events in the Controlled Rosuvastatin Multinational Trial in Heart Failure (CORONA). Am Heart J. 2012;164:878–83.
27. Rosjo H, Masson S, Latini R, Flyvbjerg A, Milani V, La Rovere MT, et al. Prognostic value of chromogranin A in chronic heart failure: data from the GISSI-Heart Failure trial. Eur J Heart Fail. 2010;12:549–56.
28. Balling L, Kistorp C, Schou M, Egstrup M, Gustafsson I, Goetze JP, et al. Plasma copeptin levels and prediction of outcome in heart failure outpatients: relation to hyponatremia and loop diuretic doses. J Card Fail. 2012;18:351–8.
29. Masson S, Latini R, Carbonieri E, Moretti L, Rossi MG, Ciricugno S, et al. The predictive value of stable precursor fragments of vasoactive peptides in patients with chronic heart failure: Data from the GISSI-heart failure (GISSI-HF) trial. Eur J Heart Fail. 2010;12:338–47.
30. Celik T, Iyisoy A, Celik M, Yuksel UC, Kardesoglu E. C-reactive protein in chronic heart failure: a new predictor of survival. Int J Cardiol. 2009;135:396–7.
31. Kalogeropoulos A, Georgiopoulou V, Psaty BM, Rodondi N, Smith AL, Harrison DG, et al. Inflammatory Markers and Incident Heart Failure Risk in Older Adults The Health ABC (Health, Aging, and Body Composition) Study. J Am Coll Cardiol. 2010;55:2129–37.
32. Lok DJ, Lok SI, Bruggink-André de la Porte PW, Badings E, Lipsic E, van Wijngaarden J, et al. Galectin-3 is an independent marker for ventricular remodeling and mortality in patients with chronic heart failure. Clin Res Cardiol. 2013;102:103–10.
33. Shah RV, Chen-Tournoux AA, Picard MH, Van Kimmenade RRJ, Januzzi JL. Galectin-3, cardiac structure and function, and long-term mortality in patients with acutely decompensated heart failure. Eur J Heart Fail. 2010;12:826–32.
34. Weir RAP, Petrie CJ, Murphy CA, Clements S, Steedman T, Miller AM, et al. Galectin-3 and Cardiac Function in Survivors of Acute Myocardial Infarction. Circ Hear Fail. 2013;6:492–8.
35. Gopal DM, Kommineni M, Ayalon N, Koelbl C, Ayalon R, Biolo A, et al. Relationship of plasma galectin-3 to renal function in patients with heart failure: effects of clinical status, pathophysiology of heart failure, and presence or absence of heart failure. J Am Heart Assoc. 2012;1:e000760.
36. Meijers WC, van der Velde AR, Ruifrok WP, Schroten NF, Dokter MM, Damman K, et al. Renal handling of galectin-3 in the general population, chronic heart failure, and hemodialysis. J Am Heart Assoc. 2014;3:e000962.

# 11

# Self-reported recall and daily diary-recorded measures of weight monitoring adherence: associations with heart failure-related hospitalization

Christine D Jones[1,2,8*], George M Holmes[2,3], Darren A DeWalt[1,2], Brian Erman[2], Jia-Rong Wu[4], Crystal W Cene[1,2], David W Baker[5], Dean Schillinger[6], Bernice Ruo[5], Kirsten Bibbins-Domingo[6], Aurelia Macabasco-O'Connell[7], Victoria Hawk[2], Kimberly Broucksou[2] and Michael Pignone[1,2]

**Abstract**

**Background:** Weight monitoring is an important element of HF self-care, yet the most clinically meaningful way to evaluate weight monitoring adherence is uncertain. We conducted this study to evaluate the association of (1) self-reported recall and (2) daily diary-recorded weight monitoring adherence with heart failure-related (HF-related) hospitalization.

**Methods:** We conducted a prospective cohort study among 216 patients within a randomized trial of HF self-care training. All patients had an initial self-care training session followed by 15 calls (median) to reinforce educational material; patients were also given digital scales, instructed to weigh daily, record weights in a diary, and mail diaries back monthly. Weight monitoring adherence was assessed with a self-reported recall question administered at 12 months and dichotomized into at least daily versus less frequent weighing. Diary-recorded weight monitoring was evaluated over 12 months and dichotomized into ≥80% and <80% adherence. HF-related hospitalizations were ascertained through patient report and confirmed through record review.

**Results:** Over 12 months in 216 patients, we identified 50 HF-related hospitalizations. Patients self-reporting daily or more frequent weight monitoring had an incidence rate ratio of 1.34 (95% CI 0.24-7.32) for HF-related hospitalizations compared to those reporting less frequent weight monitoring. Patients who completed ≥80% of weight diaries had an IRR of 0.37 (95% CI 0.18-0.75) for HF-related hospitalizations compared to patients who completed <80% of weight diaries.

**Conclusions:** Self-reported recall of weight monitoring adherence was not associated with fewer HF hospitalizations. In contrast, diary-recorded adherence ≥80% of days was associated with fewer HF-related hospitalizations. Incorporating diary-based measures of weight monitoring adherence into HF self-care training programs may help to identify patients at risk for HF-related hospitalizations.

**Keywords:** Heart failure, Patient compliance, Monitoring, Physiologic

* Correspondence: delong.christine@gmail.com
[1]Division of General Medicine and Clinical Epidemiology, University of North Carolina at Chapel Hill, Chapel Hill, NC, USA
[2]The Cecil G. Sheps Center for Health Services Research, University of North Carolina at Chapel Hill, Chapel Hill, NC, USA
Full list of author information is available at the end of the article

## Background

Heart Failure (HF) causes significant morbidity and mortality. Multiple trials have shown that self-care training can reduce HF-related hospitalizations [1]. Weight monitoring is an important element of HF self-care that enables patients to monitor their volume status [2]. Weight gain can often be the first sign of volume overload in patients with HF; if such weight gains are treated promptly, clinically significant HF exacerbations can be avoided. In clinical practice, self-reported measures are frequently used to assess whether patients perform components of HF self-care, including weight monitoring [3-5]. However, the most clinically meaningful way to evaluate adherence to weight monitoring is unclear. Using weight monitoring adherence measures to determine which patients are optimally performing HF self-care could help identify which patients may benefit from more intensive HF self-care training and support.

In a prior case–control analysis, we identified that optimal diary-recorded adherence to weight monitoring (≥80% adherence) measured over seven days was associated with a lower odds of HF-related ED visits or hospitalizations [6]. However, tracking adherence to weight monitoring by diary may be cumbersome for both patients and providers, leading us to speculate how a self-reported measure of weighing frequency that more closely approximates what is commonly used in practice might compare to a diary-recorded measure of weight monitoring adherence. We conducted this study to compare the association of self-reported and diary-recorded measures of weight monitoring adherence with HF-related hospitalizations. Since the optimal frequency to define weight monitoring adherence has not been established, we performed additional analyses to explore thresholds for weight monitoring adherence.

## Methods

### Study design

We performed a prospective cohort study that was nested in the intensive self-care intervention arm of a randomized clinical trial that compared different levels of HF self-care training [7]. Details of this trial have been described previously and will be summarized here. Patients in this study had either diastolic or systolic HF with New York Heart Association (NYHA) class II-IV symptoms within the prior 6 months, adequate cognitive function, were on a loop diuretic, and were fluent in either English or Spanish. Patients were recruited between 2006 and 2009 from Internal Medicine and Cardiology clinics at the University of North Carolina (UNC) at Chapel Hill, Northwestern University, Olive View – UCLA Medical Center, and UCSF – San Francisco General Hospital. Institutional Review Boards (IRB) from UNC, Northwestern University, Olive View-UCLA, and UCSF approved the protocol and all patients provided informed consent. The investigation conformed to the principles outlined in the Declaration of Helsinki.

### Intervention description

All patients in the intensive self-care intervention arm received an in-person 40-minute education session followed by a series of educator calls (median of 15) over 1 year. The education session and calls reinforced the importance of daily weight monitoring, taking proper diuretic doses, medication adherence, salt reduction, and exercise. Most patients (72% of intervention arm patients) were taught how to adjust their diuretic doses based on their daily weights. Among the four educators who delivered the intervention, two were registered dieticians with experience counseling patients in clinical settings; the other two had bachelor's degrees and experience working as health educators. The educators convened for a one-day training prior to enrollment and participated in weekly calls with an investigator to develop the educational protocol and ensure similar education delivery across sites.

All patients were provided a digital bathroom scale and a diary in which they were to record their daily weights. Patients were instructed to mail weight diaries back to their educator on a monthly basis in self-addressed, stamped envelopes. The educator reviewed the diaries to assess how well a patient was following the protocol and incorporated that information in their ongoing interactions with that patient. At the conclusion of the study period (12 months after enrollment), trained study personnel collected the diaries from each site and entered them into a central database for analysis.

The initial number of patients in the intensive self-care training arm was 303. For this analysis, we made exclusions for submitting no diary data during the trial (n = 67) or for a missing response to the self-reported weighing adherence measure from the 12 month survey (n = 20 additional exclusions), leaving a sample of 216 patients.

### Measures and data collection

A trained research assistant (RA) at each site administered baseline questionnaires and collected information about race/ethnicity, income, and insurance status. Socioeconomic status (SES) was measured with the MacArthur Scale of Subjective Social Status; this measure asks individuals to indicate on which ladder rung they feel that they stand relative to other people in the United States with regard to money, education, and jobs (range 0–9) [8]. HF severity was assessed using a single item with a series of structured statements to categorize patients by New York Heart Association (NYHA) class. HF-related quality of life was assessed using the Improving Chronic Illness Care Evaluation (ICICE) HF Symptom Scale (HFSS); [9] HFSS scores were transformed to a 100-point scale with 100 representing the least symptoms/best health. Literacy was measured with a Short Test of Functional health Literacy in Adults (s-TOFHLA) and categorized into adequate literacy (≥ 23 out of 36) or inadequate/marginal literacy (< 23 out of 36) [10]. The RA abstracted medical records to collect additional demographic and clinical data.

### Outcome assessment

The primary end-point for this study was HF-related hospitalization. The University of North Carolina Survey Research Unit conducted telephone surveys at 1, 6, and 12 months during which patients were asked about any hospitalizations or other events that occurred in the previous time period. Upon identification of a hospitalization, admission and discharge summaries were requested from the hospital; these records were reviewed by one of three adjudication committee members masked to intervention status to determine if the hospitalization was HF-related. Adjudication committee members used a study protocol and their clinical judgment to assess whether HF was present at admission and whether HF was an important contributing factor to the hospitalization. If the first assessor concluded that a hospitalization was definitely HF-related or definitely not HF-related, no further assessment was done. For all other hospitalizations, another assessor conducted a second assessment. If the first two assessors disagreed, a third assessor reviewed the hospitalization and the case was discussed by the full committee to resolve differences.

### Weight monitoring adherence: self-reported and diary-recorded

Weight monitoring adherence was measured using two methods: self-reported frequency of weighing and diary-recorded weights. Self-reported weight monitoring adherence was collected at baseline and during telephone interviews using the following question: "How often do you weigh yourself?" Patients who reported weighing at least once a day ("every day" or "twice a day or more") were considered optimally adherent; those who reported weighing less frequently ("several times a week", "once every week or two", or "less frequently than every 1 to 2 weeks") were considered sub-optimally adherent. This threshold was chosen because weighing "every day" indicates a stricter adherence level that is closer to our ≥80% diary threshold than "several days a week", which could represent a wide range of adherence. Our main predictor variable in the self-reported weight monitoring adherence analysis was collected following completion of the full intervention at the 12-month interview. Diary-recorded weight monitoring adherence was determined from weight diaries and dichotomized into ≥80% and <80% days of adherence to weight monitoring over a patient's days in the trial to reflect optimal and sub-optimal adherence, respectively. The ≥80% threshold was chosen because this threshold is commonly used to define optimal medication adherence, [11-13] and because we used this threshold to define weight monitoring adherence in a prior publication [6]. We also performed sensitivity analyses to evaluate how different thresholds of weight monitoring adherence were associated with HF-related hospitalizations.

### Statistical analysis

We compared demographic and clinical data by adherence groups for both self-reported and diary-recorded data for descriptive purposes with a chi-square test for dichotomous variables and Student's t-test for continuous variables. A Fisher's exact test was used to compare dichotomous variables with 5 or fewer individuals in 25% of categories. A Kolmogorov-Smirnov test was used to assess for normal distribution of continuous variables; for continuous variables found to have a non-normal distribution, a Wilcoxon-Mann–Whitney test was used to compare groups.

We compared the incidence rates of HF hospitalizations between (1) self-reported optimal versus sub-optimal adherence groups and (2) diary-recorded optimal versus sub-optimal adherence groups using negative binomial regression. In one negative binomial regression model we adjusted only for site; in the fully adjusted negative binomial regression model, we included demographic and clinical factors that were either statistically significantly different between groups in bivariate analyses (i.e., site, age, race/ethnicity, SES, HF QOL, previous MI/angina, self-reported weighing at baseline, and systolic dysfunction) or have been previously associated with HF-related hospitalizations (i.e., gender) [14]. Standard errors were adjusted for clustering by site. Of note, we did not include total educator calls in the final model because educator calls were likely to have been part of the causal pathway in the association between weight monitoring adherence and HF-related hospitalizations.

We performed sensitivity analyses in which we used different adherence thresholds for diary-recorded weight monitoring adherence (i.e., ≥90%, ≥70%, and ≥60% thresholds). We considered a two-sided p value of <0.05 statistically significant. All data analyses were performed using Stata 12.0 (College Station, TX).

## Results

### Patient characteristics

Among 216 patients the mean age was 62.2 years, about half were male, and 40% were African American (Table 1). Nearly half of patients reported an income < $15,000/year, 34% had inadequate literacy, and approximately half had NYHA Class II HF. Of interest, only 28% of patients

**Table 1 Baseline characteristics of individuals: optimal and Sub-optimal weight monitoring adherence from self-reported and diary-recorded measures**

| Characteristics | Overall sample (N = 216) | Self-reported weighing daily or more (N = 184) | Self-reported weighing less than daily (N = 32) | P value | Diary-recorded ≥80% weighing adherence (N = 107) | Diary-recorded <80% weighing adherence (N = 109) | P value |
|---|---|---|---|---|---|---|---|
| Age (mean, SD) | 62.2 (13.9) | 62.4 (13.9) | 61.1 (13.5) | 0.638 | 64.3 (12.6) | 60.1 (14.8) | 0.024 |
| Men (N, %) | 103 (48) | 83 (45) | 20 (63) | 0.069 | 45 (42) | 58 (53) | 0.101 |
| Race/Ethnicity | | | | | | | |
| White, Non-Hispanic | 80 (37) | 71 (39) | 9 (28) | 0.024 | 47 (44) | 33 (30) | 0.071 |
| Hispanic | 35 (16) | 24 (13) | 11 (34) | | 12 (11) | 23 (21) | |
| African American | 87 (40) | 76 (41) | 11 (34) | | 43 (40) | 44 (40) | |
| Other | 14 (6) | 13 (7) | 1 (3) | | 5 (5) | 9 (8) | |
| NYHA Class (N, %) | | | | | | | |
| I | 45 (21) | 39 (21) | 6 (19) | 0.536 | 23 (21) | 22 (20) | 0.168 |
| II | 111 (51) | 96 (52) | 15 (47) | | 61 (57) | 50 (46) | |
| III | 35 (16) | 27 (15) | 8 (25) | | 15 (14) | 20 (18) | |
| IV | 25 (12) | 22 (12) | 3 (9) | | 8 (7) | 17 (16) | |
| Study site (N, %) | | | | | | | |
| UNC | 87 (40) | 80 (43) | 7 (22) | <0.001[a] | 56 (52) | 31 (28) | <0.001 |
| Northwestern University | 66 (31) | 62 (34) | 4 (13) | | 33 (31) | 33 (30) | |
| UCSF | 39 (18) | 22 (12) | 17 (53) | | 6 (6) | 33 (30) | |
| Olive view, UCLA | 24 (11) | 20 (11) | 4 (13) | | 12 (11) | 12 (11) | |
| Socioeconomic status, median (IQR) | 4 (3, 6) | 5 (3,7) | 4 (1, 5) | 0.026[b] | 4 (2, 6) | 4 (3, 6) | 0.455[b] |
| Inadequate literacy (N, %) | 74 (34) | 59 (32) | 15 (47) | 0.103 | 30 (28) | 44 (40) | 0.06 |
| Heart failure related QOL: Heart failure symptom scale, median (IQR) | 61 (43, 79) | 61(46, 79) | 59 (43, 75) | 0.272[b] | 64 (46, 82) | 57 (43, 71) | 0.014[b] |
| Income level | | | | | | | |
| <$15,000 | 101 (47) | 79 (43) | 22 (69) | 0.052 | 43 (40) | 58 (53) | 0.098 |
| $15,000-$24,999 | 40 (19) | 34 (18) | 6 (19) | | 20 (19) | 20 (18) | |
| >$25,000 | 71 (33) | 67 (36) | 4 (12) | | 41 (38) | 30 (28) | |
| Previous MI/Angina (N, %) | 83 (38) | 76 (41) | 7 (22) | 0.037 | 49 (46) | 34 (31) | 0.027 |
| Systolic dysfunction (N, %) | 123 (57) | 112 (61) | 11 (34) | 0.005 | 65 (61) | 58 (53) | 0.263 |
| ACE-Inhibitor or ARB (N, %) | 178 (82) | 154 (84) | 24 (75) | 0.233 | 86 (80) | 92 (84) | 0.437 |
| Beta-Blocker (N, %) | 176 (81) | 153 (83) | 23 (72) | 0.130 | 90 (84) | 86 (79) | 0.324 |
| Thiazide | 22 (10) | 18 (10) | 4 (13) | 0.750 | 10 (9) | 12 (11) | 0.823 |
| Spironolactone | 50 (23) | 46 (25) | 4 (13) | 0.172 | 22 (21) | 28 (25) | 0.425 |
| Telephone calls with educator, median (IQR) | 16 (14, 18) | 16 (15, 18) | 15 (13, 16) | <0.001[b] | 17 (16, 18) | 15 (13, 17) | <0.001[b] |
| Self-reported weighing daily or more at baseline, (N, %) | 61 (28) | 58 (32) | 3 (9) | 0.005[a] | 35 (33) | 26 (24) | 0.148 |
| Taught weight-based diuretic self-adjustment | 178 (82) | 152 (83) | 26 (81) | 0.852 | 87 (81) | 91 (83) | 0.674 |

[a]Groups compared using Fisher's exact test.
[b]Groups compared using both t-test and Wilcoxon-Mann-Whitney test.
NYHA: New York Heart Association; MI: Myocardial Infarction; ACE: Angiotensin-Converting Enzyme; ARB: Angiotensin Receptor Blocker; IQR: Interquartile Range; QOL: Quality of Life.

reported weighing daily or more frequently at baseline. The 87 patients excluded from this analysis because they either submitted no diary data during the trial (n = 67) or a were missing a 12 month self-reported weighing adherence measure (n = 20) were more likely to be younger (58.4 years), male (63%), have NYHA Class III or IV HF (42%), and were less likely to have a prior MI or angina (25%).

### Weight monitoring adherence: self-reported and diary-recorded

At 12 months, 85% of patients completing a survey (184 of 216) self-reported weighing themselves at least daily (Table 1). Those self-reporting weighing daily or more were more likely to be White, Non-Hispanic (39% versus 28% reporting less than daily, p 0.024), have a higher SES (score of 5 versus 4, p 0.026) , report previous MI or angina (41% versus 22%, p 0.037), systolic dysfunction (61% versus 34%, p 0.005), and on average completed one more telephone call with the clinical educator than patients who reported weighing less than daily (16 calls versus 15 calls, p <0.001, Table 1).

Over 12 months, 50% of patients (107 of 216) recorded and returned ≥80% of daily weights. Those who recorded ≥80% of weights were more likely to be older (64.3 versus 60.1 years for <80% weighing adherence, p 0.024), report a higher HF quality of life (score of 64 versus 57 of 100, p 0.014), report previous MI or angina (46% versus 31%, p 0.027), and on average completed two more telephone calls with the clinical educator than patients who recorded <80% of daily weights (17 versus 15 calls, p <0.001, Table 1). Those who were taught weight-based diuretic self-adjustment were distributed evenly among all groups.

### Weight monitoring adherence and HF hospitalization

Among 216 patients, we identified 50 HF-related hospitalizations over 12 months; 20 patients had 1 hospitalization, 8 patients had 2 hospitalizations, and 4 patients had 3 or more HF-related hospitalizations. Patients with optimal self-reported weight monitoring adherence at 12 months had 0.26 events per person-year (47 events in 184 patients) and those self-reporting sub-optimal adherence had 0.09 events per person-year (3 events in 32 patients). Patients with ≥80% diary-recorded weight monitoring adherence had 0.14 events per person-year (15 events in 107 patients) and those with <80% diary-recorded weight monitoring adherence had 0.32 events per person-year (35 events in 109 patients).

Table 2 shows incidence rate ratios (IRR) for HF hospitalizations both for self-reported and diary-recorded weight monitoring adherence. Ten patients were missing one or more covariate and were excluded from the adjusted models (adjusted model N = 206). In those with optimal self-reported weight monitoring adherence, the IRR for HF hospitalization 1.99 (95% CI 0.69-5.72) adjusted only for study site and 1.34 (95% CI 0.24-7.32) in a fully adjusted model; neither result was statistically significant. In those with diary-recorded weight monitoring adherence of ≥80%, we found a statistically significant lower incidence of HF hospitalization, both in a model adjusted only for study site (IRR 0.32, 95% CI 0.15-0.70) and in a fully adjusted model (IRR 0.37, 95% CI 0.18-0.75).

**Table 2 Association of weight monitoring adherence with HF hospitalizations, self-reported and diary-recorded**

| Models | N | Incidence rate ratios | 95% confidence intervals |
|---|---|---|---|
| **Self-reported daily or more weight monitoring adherence (at 12 months)** | | | |
| Adjusted for site only | 216 | 1.99 | (0.69-5.72) |
| Overall adjusted[a] | 206 | 1.34 | (0.24-7.32) |
| **Diary-recorded weight monitoring adherence (≥ 80% over 12 months)** | | | |
| Adjusted for site only | 216 | 0.32 | (0.15-0.70) |
| Overall adjusted[a] | 206 | 0.37 | (0.18-0.75) |

[a]Model adjusted for age, gender, race, site, subjective SES, HF quality of life, previous MI/angina, systolic dysfunction, and self-reported weight monitoring adherence (daily or more) at baseline.

### Sensitivity analyses

When we changed the diary-recorded optimal adherence threshold to ≥60%, ≥70%, and ≥90%, the magnitude of effect strengthened with each step up in adherence (Table 3). Thresholds for adherence that ranged down to ≥60% were associated with a lower risk for HF-related hospitalization that was statistically significant. Figure 1 demonstrates the association between HF-related hospitalization and diary-recorded adherence as a continuous measure over 12 months; of note, confidence intervals widened considerably with diary-recorded adherence less than 60%, which was related to smaller sample sizes. To address potential selection bias that may have been introduced

**Table 3 Association of weight monitoring adherence with HF hospitalizations, sensitivity analyses**

| Models | Incidence rate ratios | 95% confidence intervals |
|---|---|---|
| **Diary-recorded adherence: varying adherence thresholds** | | |
| ≥ 90%[a] | 0.24 | (0.11-0.54) |
| ≥ 80% (main analysis)[a] | 0.37 | (0.18-0.75) |
| ≥ 70%[a] | 0.41 | (0.25-0.67) |
| ≥ 60%[a] | 0.42 | (0.25-0.70) |

[a]Model adjusted for age, gender, race, site, subjective SES, HF quality of life, previous MI/Angina, systolic dysfunction, and self-reported weight monitoring adherence (daily or more) at baseline.

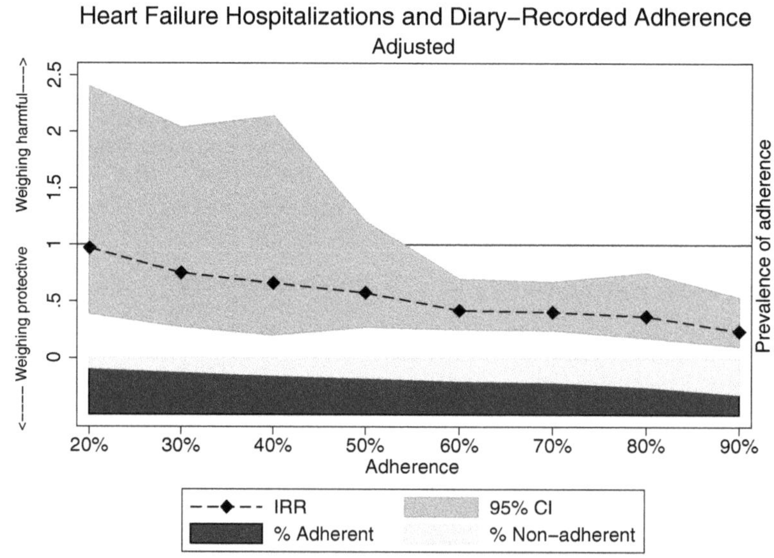


**Figure 1 Association of heart failure-related hospitalization with diary-recorded adherence over 12 months, adjusted incidence rate ratio[a].** [a]Model adjusted for age, gender, race, site, subjective SES, HF quality of life, previous MI/angina, systolic dysfunction, and self-reported weight monitoring adherence (daily or more) at baseline.

by excluding patients who never submitted a diary, we performed sensitivity analyses including this group and found similar IRRs for HF-related hospitalizations when we adjusted only for study site, both for the self-reported recall measure (IRR 1.92, 95% CI 0.80-4.62) and for the diary-recorded measure of adherence (IRR 0.24, 95% CI 0.14-0.41).

## Discussion

In this study, we found that patients self-reporting at least daily weight monitoring adherence did not have reduced rates of HF hospitalization compared to those self-reporting less frequent weighing adherence at 12 months. In contrast, we found that patients with ≥80% diary-recorded weight monitoring adherence had a statistically significantly lower rate of HF hospitalization than those with <80% adherence over 12 months of follow-up. Our findings suggest that diary-recorded measures of adherence may accurately identify optimal self-care that is associated with a reduced risk of HF-related hospitalizations.

HF self-care behaviors are frequently assessed through global self-reported measures, including the Self-Care of HF Index (SCHFI), [3] the revised Heart Failure Self-Care Behavioral Scale [15,16], the European HF Self-Care Behavioral Scale (EHFScB Scale), [4] and the Revised HF Compliance scale, [5,17] all of which contain an item to assess weighing behavior. Better HF care/behavior scores on respective indices/scales have been associated with improved clinical outcomes [17,18]. In studies that have specifically evaluated the association between weight monitoring adherence and clinical outcomes, the association between adherence and clinical outcomes has been variable based on the adherence measure used [17,19,20].

Daily weight monitoring is a mainstay of HF self-care, yet the most clinically meaningful measure to evaluate adherence to this behavior is not clear. Comparisons have been made between measures that are self-reported and measures obtained from repeated sampling of current behaviors or symptoms over a time period, termed "ecological momentary assessment" (EMA), in the work of Shiffman and colleagues [21]. EMA measures have the potential to "minimize recall bias, maximize ecological validity, and allow study of microprocesses that influence behavior in real-world contexts" (pg 1) [21]. EMA can be collected many ways, including diaries, telephone calls, and electronic records. The main objective of EMA is to ascertain multiple samples of symptoms or behaviors experienced at the time the sample is collected. Self-reported and EMA measures have been found to be discrepant in studies from various populations, including patients with alcoholism, [22] tobacco use, [23] urinary incontinence, [24] and headaches [25].

Discrepancies between self-reported and EMA measures of medication adherence [e.g., medication event monitoring systems (MEMS) caps (medication bottle caps that record times/dates that bottles are opened)], have also been noted in patients with HF [19,20]. Such discrepancies between adherence measures can be attributed to a number of characteristics, such as the frequency with which measures are collected, the duration of time over which measures estimate behavior, the types of behaviors being evaluated, and other factors [21]. Overall, self-reported measures are at risk for systematic recall bias when compared to EMA measures [21].

In our study, measures used to assess daily weight monitoring adherence fall into the general categories of self-reported recall and EMA from a daily diary. We found that a self-reported recall of optimal adherence at 12 months was associated with a somewhat higher risk of HF-related hospitalizations that was not statistically significant; the small size of the group self-reporting optimal adherence likely contributed to less precision in this outcome. Yet, we did find an association between diary-recorded weight monitoring adherence and HF-related hospitalizations at multiple thresholds of adherence, with an effect size that strengthened with increasing thresholds. Adherence thresholds ranging down to ≥60% of days were associated with decreased risk for HF-related hospitalization, suggesting benefit even at thresholds lower than our pre-specified cut-point of ≥80%.

One may speculate whether completion of weight diaries in this study is merely a reflection of program engagement and/or more advanced HF self-care skills/knowledge. To evaluate whether program engagement may have explained some of this association, we added the number of educator calls into our adjusted model and found that this did not lead to attenuation of the IRRs from our main analyses (results not shown). We theorize this is because the number of educator calls may have varied based on a range of factors including: a patient's engagement in the program, lack of mastery of educational material that required more calls, or even patient-initiated calls due to concerns about their regimen or symptoms. Of note, the weight diaries in this study were used to teach a majority of patients (72% of intervention arm patients) how to self-adjust their diuretics based on weight. Although the observed association could have been partly related to this aspect of the intervention, the proportion of patients who were taught diuretic self-adjustment did not differ significantly by adherence in either self-reported or diary-recorded groups (Table 1).

### Limitations

With regard to study limitations, our self-reported adherence question did not specify the duration of time for which patients were to report weighing behavior, which likely increased recall bias in responses. In addition, given that 85% of patients self-reported weighing at least daily at 12 months, patient responses to this question may not have accurately reflected behavior, potentially due to social desirability or other factors. It is important to note that the surveys were delivered by masked outcome assessors. The smaller sample size and very low rate of HF-related hospitalization in the group that self-reported sub-optimal adherence contributed to less precision in our results and lack of statistically significant findings.

In addition, our measure of diary-recorded weight monitoring averaged adherence over the entire follow-up period. As such, it is possible that adherence directly preceding HF hospitalizations differed from overall adherence; however, in a prior case–control study nested in this same study population, we found that diary-recorded weight monitoring adherence (≥80%) in the week preceding HF emergency department visits or hospitalizations was similarly protective [6].

Our comparison between self-reported and diary-recorded adherence measures was not a direct comparison between randomized groups of individuals, but instead a comparison of how different measures of adherence were associated with clinical outcomes in the same group of individuals. We noted baseline differences between groups who were optimally adherent and sub-optimally adherent to both self-reported and diary-recorded measures; thus selection bias or unmeasured confounding may have affected our results. However, we attempted to mitigate such differences by adjusting for these variables in our analysis; in addition, we found comparable results to our main analysis when we performed a sensitivity analysis in which we included patients who never submitted a weight diary. The generalizability of our findings may be limited by our younger patients with less advanced HF than in other studies of HF self-care [1,26]. Strengths of this study include a diverse, well-characterized sample drawn from a multi-site trial and rigorous outcome assessment.

## Conclusions

In conclusion, we found that ≥80% adherence to a daily diary-recorded measure was associated with fewer HF hospitalizations, but that a self-reported recall measure of weight monitoring adherence was not associated with fewer HF hospitalizations. Diary-recorded weight monitoring adherence may identify more rigorous adherence to HF self-management skills as well as program engagement and may provide more clinically meaningful information than a self-reported recall measure.

#### Competing interests

The authors declare that they have no competing interests.

#### Authors' contributions

CDJ conceived of the study, participated in design of study and drafted the manuscript; GMH participated in the design of the study and performed the statistical analysis; DAD conceived of the study, participated in design of study, acquisition of data, and provided key revisions to manuscript; BE participated in the design of the study and participated in performing statistical analyses; JRW participated in the design of the study and provided key revisions to the manuscript; CWC participated in the design of the study and provided key revisions to the manuscript; DWB participated in the design of the study, acquisition of data, and provided key revisions to the manuscript; DS participated in the design of the study, acquisition of data, and provided key revisions to the manuscript; BR participated in acquisition of data, and provided key revisions to the manuscript; KBR participated in acquisition of data and provided key revisions to the manuscript; AMO participated in the acquisition of data and provided key revisions to the manuscript; VH participated in the design of the study and acquisition of data; KB participated in the design of the study and acquisition of data; MP conceived of the study, participated in design of study, acquisition of data, and provided key revisions to manuscript. All authors read and approved the final manuscript.

### Authors' information

Work performed at: The University of North Carolina at Chapel Hill, Northwestern University, The University of California at San Francisco, and Olive View-UCLA Medical Center.

### Acknowledgements

The authors would like to thank all of the study patients for their valuable contributions. This work was supported by the National Heart, Lung, and Blood Institute at the National Institutes of Health [grant number R01 HL081257] and the National Institutes of Health American Recovery and Reinvestment Act [grant number A10-0586-001]. Dr. Christine Jones is supported by a NIH/HRSA training grant and is a NRSA Primary Care Research Fellow (T32HP14001-25). The authors would also like to thank the University of North Carolina Health Sciences Library and University Libraries for providing funding to support open access publishing costs.

### Author details

[1]Division of General Medicine and Clinical Epidemiology, University of North Carolina at Chapel Hill, Chapel Hill, NC, USA. [2]The Cecil G. Sheps Center for Health Services Research, University of North Carolina at Chapel Hill, Chapel Hill, NC, USA. [3]Department of Health Policy and Management, University of North Carolina at Chapel Hill, Chapel Hill, NC, USA. [4]School of Nursing, University of North Carolina at Chapel Hill, Chapel Hill, NC, USA. [5]Division of General Internal Medicine, Feinberg School of Medicine, Northwestern University, Chicago, IL, USA. [6]Division of General Internal Medicine and Center for Vulnerable Populations, Department of Medicine at San Francisco General Hospital, University of California San Francisco, San Francisco, CA, USA. [7]Olive View-UCLA Medical Center, UCLA School of Nursing, University of California, Los Angeles, CA, USA. [8]NRSA Primary Care Fellowship, Division of General Medicine and Clinical Epidemiology, University of North Carolina at Chapel Hill, 5034 Old Clinic Building, CB# 7110, Chapel Hill, NC 27599, USA.

### References

1. Inglis SC, Clark RA, McAlister FA, Ball J, Lewinter C, Cullington D, Stewart S, Cleland JG: **Structured telephone support or telemonitoring programmes for patients with chronic heart failure.** *Cochrane Database Syst Rev* 2010, **8**:CD007228.
2. Jessup M, Abraham WT, Casey DE, Feldman AM, Francis GS, Ganiats TG, Konstam MA, Mancini DM, Rahko PS, Silver MA, *et al*: **2009 focused update: ACCF/AHA Guidelines for the Diagnosis and Management of Heart Failure in Adults: a report of the American College of Cardiology Foundation/American Heart Association Task Force on Practice Guidelines: developed in collaboration with the International Society for Heart and Lung Transplantation.** *Circulation* 2009, **119**(14):1977–2016.
3. Riegel B, Lee CS, Dickson W, Carlson B: **An update on the self-care of heart failure index.** *J Cardiovasc Nurs* 2009, **24**(6):485–497.
4. Jaarsma T, Arestedt KF, Martensson J, Dracup K, Stromberg A: **The European Heart Failure Self-care Behaviour scale revised into a nine-item scale (EHFScB-9): a reliable and valid international instrument.** *Eur J Heart Fail* 2009, **11**(1):99–105.
5. Evangelista LS, Berg J, Dracup K: **Relationship between psychosocial variables and compliance in patients with heart failure.** *Heart Lung* 2001, **30**(4):294–301.
6. Jones CD, Holmes GM, DeWalt DA, Erman B, Broucksou K, Hawk V, Cene CW, Wu JR, Pignone M: **Is adherence to weight monitoring or weight-based diuretic self-adjustment associated with fewer heart failure-related emergency department visits or hospitalizations?** *J Card Fail* 2012, **18**(7):576–584.
7. DeWalt DA, Schillinger D, Ruo B, Bibbins-Domingo K, Baker DW, Holmes GM, Weinberger M, Macabasco-O'Connell A, Broucksou K, Hawk V: **A multisite randomized trial of a single- versus multi-session literacy sensitive self-care intervention for patients with heart failure.** *Circulation* 2012, **125**(23):2854–2862.
8. Adler NE, Epel ES, Castellazzo G, Ickovics JR: **Relationship of subjective and objective social status with psychological and physiological functioning: preliminary data in healthy white women.** *Health Psychol* 2000, **19**(6):586–592.
9. Baker DW, Brown J, Chan KS, Dracup KA, Keeler EB: **A telephone survey to measure communication, education, self-management, and health status for patients with heart failure: the improving chronic illness care evaluation (ICICE).** *J Card Fail* 2005, **11**(1):36–42.
10. Baker DW, Williams MV, Parker RM, Gazmararian JA, Nurss J: **Development of a brief test to measure functional health literacy.** *Patient Educ Couns* 1999, **38**(1):33–42.
11. Monane M, Bohn RL, Gurwitz JH, Glynn RJ, Levin R, Avorn J: **The effects of initial drug choice and comorbidity on antihypertensive therapy compliance: results from a population-based study in the elderly.** *Am J Hypertens* 1997, **10**(7 Pt 1):697–704.
12. Rosen MI, Rigsby MO, Salahi JT, Ryan CE, Cramer JA: **Electronic monitoring and counseling to improve medication adherence.** *Behav Res Ther* 2004, **42**(4):409–422.
13. Schedlbauer A, Davies P, Fahey T: **Interventions to improve adherence to lipid lowering medication.** *Cochrane Database Syst Rev* 2010, **3**, CD004371.
14. Krumholz HM, Parent EM, Tu N, Vaccarino V, Wang Y, Radford MJ, Hennen J: **Readmission after hospitalization for congestive heart failure among Medicare beneficiaries.** *Arch Intern Med* 1997, **157**(1):99–104.
15. Artinian NT, Magnan M, Sloan M, Lange MP: **Self-care behaviors among patients with heart failure.** *Heart Lung* 2002, **31**(3):161–172.
16. Artinian NT, Harden JK, Kronenberg MW, Vander Wal JS, Daher E, Stephens Q, Bazzi RI: **Pilot study of a Web-based compliance monitoring device for patients with congestive heart failure.** *Heart Lung* 2003, **32**(4):226–233.
17. van der Wal MH, van Veldhuisen DJ, Veeger NJ, Rutten FH, Jaarsma T: **Compliance with non-pharmacological recommendations and outcome in heart failure patients.** *Eur Heart J* 2010, **31**(12):1486–1493.
18. Lee CS, Moser DK, Lennie TA, Riegel B: **Event-free survival in adults with heart failure who engage in self-care management.** *Heart Lung* 2011, **40**(1):12–20.
19. Lynga P, Persson H, Hagg-Martinell A, Hagglund E, Hagerman I, Langius-Eklof A, Rosenqvist M: **Weight monitoring in patients with severe heart failure (WISH). A randomized controlled trial.** *Eur J Heart Fail* 2012, **14**(4):438–444.
20. Wright SP, Walsh H, Ingley KM, Muncaster SA, Gamble GD, Pearl A, Whalley GA, Sharpe N, Doughty RN: **Uptake of self-management strategies in a heart failure management programme.** *Eur J Heart Fail* 2003, **5**(3):371–380.
21. Shiffman S, Stone AA, Hufford MR: **Ecological momentary assessment.** *Annu Rev Clin Psychol* 2008, **4**:1–32.
22. Litt MD, Cooney NL, Morse P: **Reactivity to alcohol-related stimuli in the laboratory and in the field: predictors of craving in treated alcoholics.** *Addiction* 2000, **95**(6):889–900.
23. Shiffman S, Balabanis MH, Gwaltney CJ, Paty JA, Gnys M, Kassel JD, Hickcox M, Paton SM: **Prediction of lapse from associations between smoking and situational antecedents assessed by ecological momentary assessment.** *Drug Alcohol Depend* 2007, **91**(2–3):159–168.
24. Homma Y, Ando T, Yoshida M, Kageyama S, Takei M, Kimoto K, Ishizuka O, Gotoh M, Hashimoto T: **Voiding and incontinence frequencies: variability of diary data and required diary length.** *Neurourol Urodyn* 2002, **21**(3):204–209.
25. van den Brink M, Bandell-Hoekstra EN, Abu-Saad HH: **The occurrence of recall bias in pediatric headache: a comparison of questionnaire and diary data.** *Headache* 2001, **41**(1):11–20.
26. Koehler F, Winkler S, Schieber M, Sechtem U, Stangl K, Bohm M, Boll H, Baumann G, Honold M, Koehler K, *et al*: **Impact of remote telemedical management on mortality and hospitalizations in ambulatory patients with chronic heart failure: the telemedical interventional monitoring in heart failure study.** *Circulation* 2011, **123**(17):1873–1880.

# 12

# Inverted stress- induced cardiomyopathy as a unusual variant of acute heart failure after cesarean delivery

Anna Ledakowicz-Polak[1*], Jarosław Bartodziej[2], Agata Majos[3] and Marzenna Zielińska[1]

**Abstract**

**Background:** Stress- induced cardiomyopathy is acute, reversible left ventricle mainly apical dysfunction in patients with normal coronary angiography. Rarely it regards basal segments, therefore defined as "inverted stress- induced cardiomyopathy". While classic form mostly affects postmenopausal women, inverted variant occurs essentially in younger females, always triggered by stress. It can also develop after medical procedures and surgery. Herein we report such unique case of 36- year old woman after cesarean delivery.

**Case presentation:** A 36- year- old white woman at 40 week of gestation was admitted to hospital for elective repeated cesarean delivery. During caesarean delivery under spinal anaesthesia a previously healthy woman became hypotensive, requiring ephedrine to maintain her blood pressure. Three hours after delivery the patient presented acute heart failure and pulmonary oedema. Due to low blood pressure she demanded the administration of inotropic agents. Owing to respiratory failure and gradual deterioration of consciousness, mechanical ventilation was applied. Results of additional tests finally excluded pulmonary thromboembolism and acute coronary syndrome. The transthoracic echocardiography revealed severe left ventricular systolic dysfunction, ejection fraction 30 % with hypokinesis of the mid and basal segments of posterior, anterior and lateral wall with preserved contractility of the apical segments. The diagnosis of inverted stress- induced cardiomyopathy was set upon the overall clinical data. Both echocardiography and magnetic resonance imaging performed on the fifth day showed complete recovery of myocardial function. The patient was discharged after 15 days in good overall condition. At 12- month follow- up she remained asymptomatic with no echocardiographic abnormalities.

**Conclusions:** Inverted stress- induced cardiomyopathy may occur in postpartum period, especially in combination with spinal anesthesia and adrenergic stimulants administration. The clinical awareness and multimodality imaging of possible diagnosis and further management of this unexpected variant of acute heart failure after caesarean delivery is required.

**Keywords:** Inverted stress- induced cardiomyopathy, Acute heart failure, Cesarean delivery

## Background

Stress- induced cardiomyopathy (SIC) also known as "takotsubo cardiomyopathy" is characterized by reversible left ventricular dysfunction with chest symptoms (pain or dyspnea), electrocardiogram changes that mimic those of acute coronary syndrome (ACS) and minor elevation in serum levels of cardiac enzymes in patients with normal coronary angiography [1]. While echocardiography revealed apical ballooning in the majority of cases, a small part of patients present with basal dysfunction also defined as "inverted or reverse SIC". Inversely to classic form of SIC, which mainly affects postmenopausal women, the reverse variant of SIC occurs essentially in younger females and is always triggered by emotional or physical stress [2].

We report an extremely rare case of inverted SIC which occurred in young women after cesarean delivery.

* Correspondence: anialedakowicz@wp.pl
[1]Intensive Cardiac Therapy Clinic, Department of Cardiology and Cardiosurgery, Medical University, Pomorska 251, 92-213 Lodz, Poland
Full list of author information is available at the end of the article

## Case presentation

A 36- year- old white woman at 40 week of gestation was admitted to a local obstetric clinic for elective repeated cesarean delivery due to slanting position of the fetus. Both her previous and current pregnancy were uncomplicated. Her past medical history was unremarkable and no family history of cardiac disease was reported. The caesarean delivery was performed following the administration of standard spinal anesthesia. During surgery the patient became hypotensive and ephedrine was injected to maintain her blood pressure in the normal range. Three hours after delivery of healthy male infant, the patient complained of nausea, increasing dyspnoea and palpitations. On physical examination tachycardia with ventricular extra systoles and pulmonary rales were detected. Her blood pressure was 80/40 mmHg and demanded the administration of inotropic agents (initially continuous infusion of norepinephrine 0.5 mg/h followed by dobutamine 7 μg/kg/min). Owing to worsening of oxygen saturation up to 70 % and gradual deterioration of consciousness, mechanical ventilation was applied and the patient was transferred to intensive care unit. Chest X ray indicated pulmonary congestion. Emergency computer tomography excluded pulmonary thromboembolism (PE) and confirmed severe pulmonary oedema (Fig. 1). The patient received loop diuretic, furosemide, at initial daily dose 80 mg, which was progressively reduced. The diuretic was discontinued after 12 days of treatment. The electrocardiogram disclosed sinus tachycardia with ST- segment elevation of 1,5 mm with negative T waves in aVL and ST- segment depression of 1 mm in II, III, aVF, V5-V6 (Fig. 2). Laboratory tests showed elevated troponin up to 908 pg/ml (normal value <14 pg/ml), NT- pro BNP 6236 pg/ml (normal value <125 pg/ml). The bedside transthoracic echocardiography (TTE) revealed severe left ventricular (LV) systolic dysfunction. Therefore the patient was transferred to Intensive Cardiac Therapy Clinic. Repeated TTE showed LV ejection fraction 30 % with hypokinesis of the mid and basal segments of posterior, anterior and lateral wall with preserved contractility of the apical segments. Urgent coronary angiography presented normal coronary arteries. The diagnosis of inverted stress- induced cardiomyopathy was set upon the overall clinical data. After 3 days the patient was weaned from respirator and extubated. Following hemodynamic improvement, inotropic agents were tapered gradually. Both TTE and magnetic resonance imaging (Figs. 3 and 4) performed on the fifth day showed complete recovery of myocardial function. The patient was discharged after 15 days in good overall condition. At 12- month follow- up she remained asymptomatic with no echocardiographic abnormalities.

## Discussion

It has been shown that SIC predominantly affects postmenopausal woman [1]. Although several cases of SIC in young woman have already been described, pregnancy associated SIC (P-SIC) appears to be rather unusual [3–7].

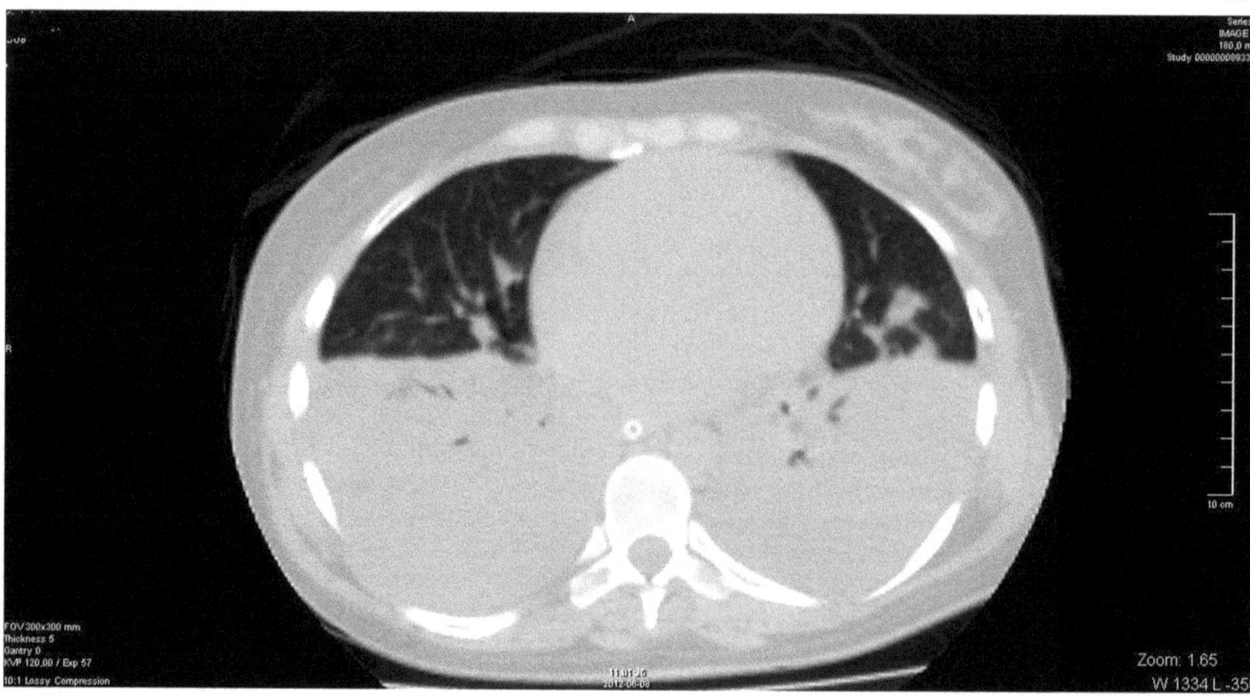


**Fig. 1** Chest computed tomography demonstrating severe pulmonary oedema

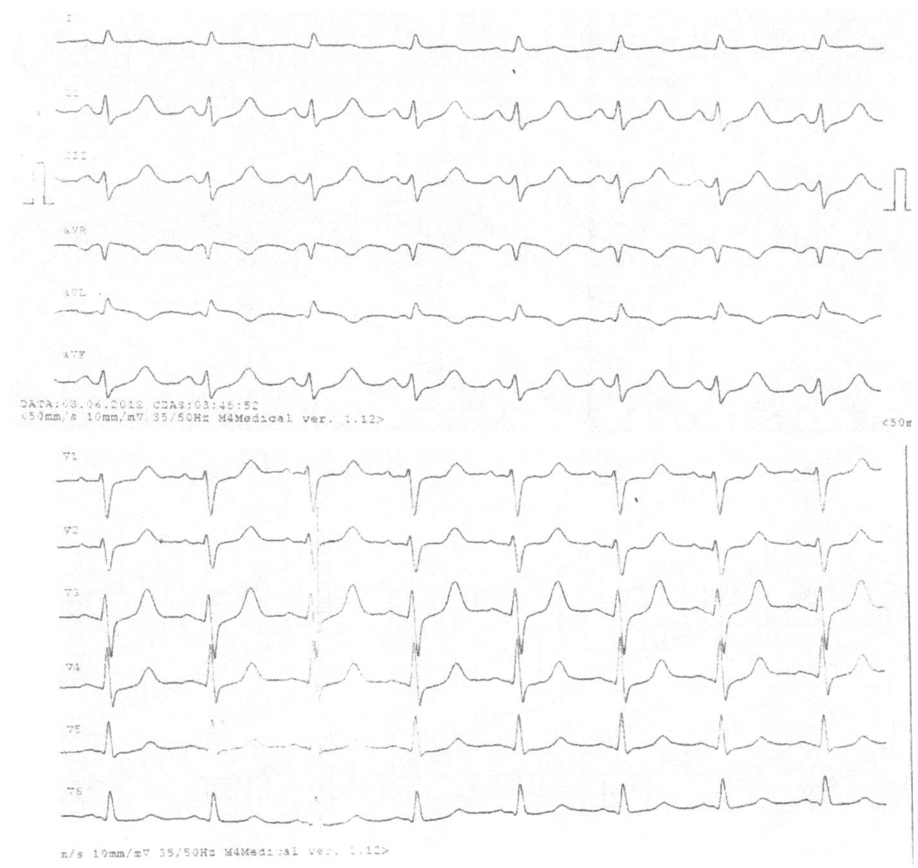

**Fig. 2** Electrocardiogram

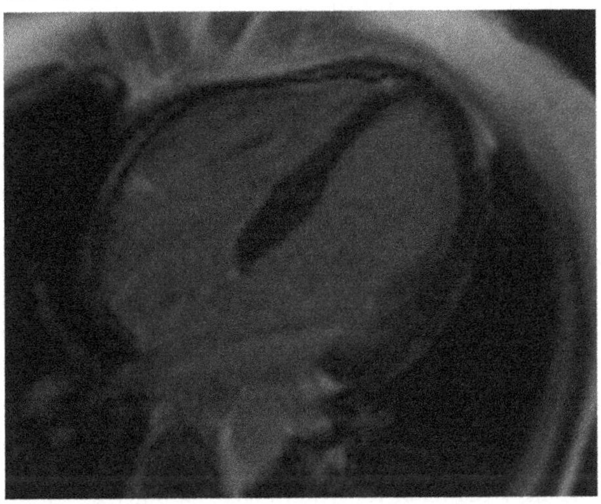

**Fig. 3** Cardiac magnetic resonance imaging with late gadolinium enhancement in four chamber view, without evidence of tissue abnormalities (scars, patchy fibrosis)

The pathophysiological mechanism of SIC is still not completely understood. Several possibilities have been discussed but increased levels of catecholamine and vasoconstrictive substances appear to play crucial role in triggering SIC [8]. It can be defined as a catecholamine- triggered myocyte injury caused by catecholamine- induced microvascular spasm or by direct catecholamine- associated myocardial toxicity. Cardiac troponins are elevated in almost all patients with SIC. However the elevation in serum troponin is disproportional in comparison to the extension of the akinetic myocardial regions. The pathophysiology of wall motion abnormalities in SIC is not well established. Reversible ventricular dysfunction may be also the result of epicardial coronary artery spasm and consequently regionally stunned myocardium [9]. This extended stunning is probably correlated with only slight elevation of cardiac necrosis markers. Moreover it has been reported that the risk of SIC can be reduced by blocking α- and β-adrenergic receptors [10, 11]. Furthermore, a difference in the distribution and density of adrenergic receptors in myocardium are responsible for the variance in SIC appearance in either the apical or mid- ventricular wall.

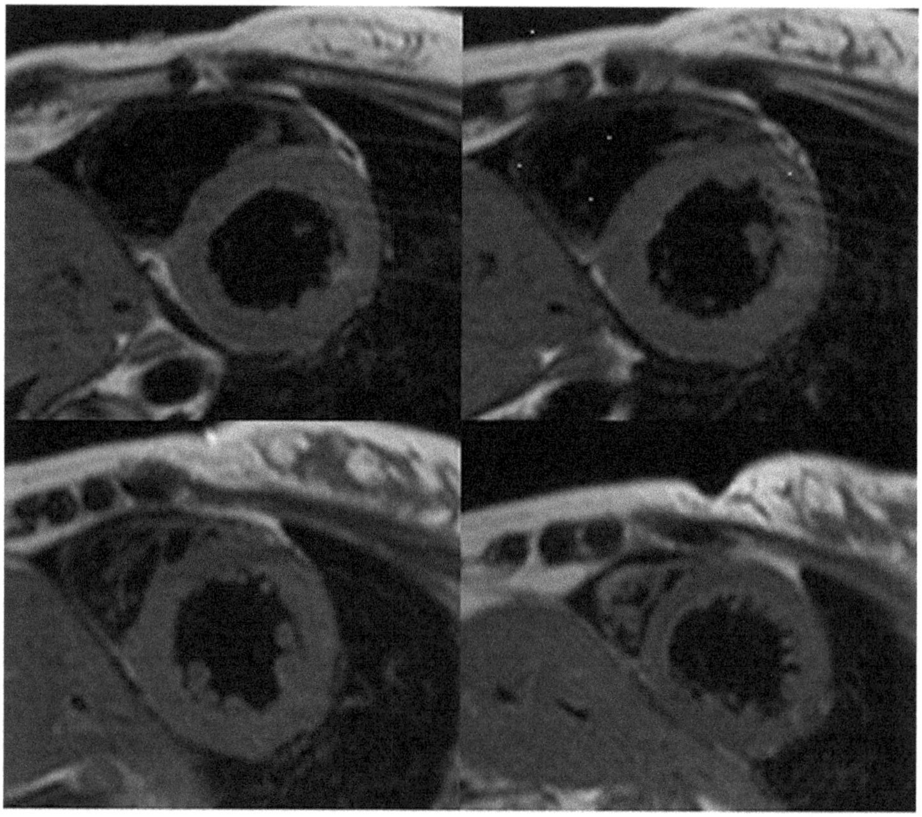

**Fig. 4** Short-axis, dark- blood T2- weighted cardiac magnetic resonance imaging demonstrating no signs of myocardial edema

Inverted SIC occurs mainly in younger females with higher prevalence of identifiable activating stress and possibly in relation to a larger distribution of adrenergic receptors in the basal segments of LV in this population [2, 12, 13]. The subjective experience of stress by woman in the course of delivery may be an additional factor contributing to occurrence of reverse SIC during caesarean section. SIC in the perioperative setting has been reported yet as well as vasoconstrictive substances such as ephedrine were suggested as triggering factors [14]. In our case, treatment of hypotension associated with spinal anaesthesia with ephedrine also appears to have precipitated SIC. Therefore adrenergic stimulants should be used with caution in treating maternal hypotension after spinal anaesthesia. However it is worth mentioning that hypotension is described as an undesirable result of central blockade and its prevalence is estimated as 30–90 % of all spinal anaesthesia. Standard methods of hypotension treatment in pregnancy are infusion of fluids and intravenous ephedrine administration, the use of corticosteroids is not recommended (their effect of action is too slow and weak). Ephedrine is easily adjustable and has a short duration of action so after all it appears to remain the first line option of treatment of hypotension associated with spinal anaesthesia. Moreover, taking into consideration that main aetiology of SIC appears to be the catecholamine- triggered myocyte injury, exogenous catecholamines in such patients with cardiogenic shock should be avoided. The use of inotropes and further activation of catecholamine receptors may worsen the clinical status and prognosis of these individuals. Unfortunately, due to persistent hypotension LV dysfunction, our patient received inotropic agents. This treatment could probably exacerbate or prolong the acute phase of the disease. According to current state of knowledge on Takotsubo syndrome of the Heart Failure Association of the European Society of Cardiology, in this case, treatment options should include mechanical support such as temporary LV assist devices, extracorporeal membrane oxygenation or if those option are not available low- dose of levosimendan infusion as a catecholamine sparing positive inotrope [15]. In the pathogenesis of SIC it is also suggested that lower estrogen levels may play a role [16]. In late pregnancy placenta produces high amounts of estradiol that decrease rapidly after placenta expulsion favouring a higher myocardium susceptibility to adrenergic stimuli. Consequently woman in the postpartum may represent another vulnerable group for SIC onset, especially inverted SIC.

Minatoguchi et al. identified a total of 18 (8 from Western countries) confirmed cases of symptomatic P-SIC [4]. Most women underwent caesarean delivery. Almost all electrocardiograms showed abnormalities and serum levels of cardiac enzymes were elevated. In 33 % cases, as well as in our, acute cardiopulmonary collapse occurred on the day of labour and symptoms were similar to those in ACS, PE or peripartum cardiomyopathy (PCM). In presented case computed tomography, as a diagnostic test of choice, excluded PE whereas coronary angiography has not confirmed ACS. PCM differs from typical SIC in terms of presentation and outcome and it does not present with a remarkable contraction pattern. Moreover recovery in PCM may be delayed of several months and is prevalent in less than 50 % of patients, whereas repeated TTE, among women with SIC, revealed normalized LV systolic function within 6 months in all reported cases [4, 17]. Furthermore in PCM myocardial late gadolinium enhancement can be present in cardiac magnetic resonance [18]. Therefore multimodality imaging may help to exclude or confirm the diagnosis of SIC. Echocardiography still remains preferred screening method to asses cardiac function. Bedside TTE seems to be a useful, non- invasive readily available diagnostic tool for the differential diagnosis of ACS, PE, PCM and SIC. Instantaneous recognition of SIC in the postpartum period has immediate therapeutic implications. Although SIC generally has a good prognosis, intensive heart failure therapy is required for successful convalescence.

## Conclusions

In conclusion, this case shows that inverted SIC may occur in young women, particularly in postpartum period, especially in combination with spinal anaesthesia and adrenergic stimulants administration.

On the basis of our experience we recommend the clinical awareness of possible diagnosis and further management of this unexpected variant of acute heart failure after caesarean delivery. Although initially the inverted stress- induced cardiomyopathy may seem dramatic, proper and accurate diagnosis usually leads to patients positive and successful outcome.

#### Abbreviations

ACS: acute coronary syndrome; LV: left ventricular; P-SIC: pregnancy associated stress- induced cardiomyopathy; PE: pulmonary thromboembolism; PMC: peripartum cardiomyopathy; SIC: stress- induced cardiomyopathy; TTE: transthoracic echocardiography.

#### Competing interests

The authors declare that they have no competing interests.

#### Authors' contributions

AL contributed in main conception and design of the current manuscript as well as in acquisition, analysis and interpretation of obtained data. AL have been also responsible for drafting the manuscript and revising it critically for important intellectual content. JB contributed in acquisition, analysis and interpretation of some essential data. AM contributed in acquisition, analysis and interpretation of some essential data. MZ contributed in conception and design of the current manuscript, interpretation of obtained data. MZ was also responsible for critical revision and final version acceptance for publication. All authors read and approved the final manuscript.

#### Author details

[1]Intensive Cardiac Therapy Clinic, Department of Cardiology and Cardiosurgery, Medical University, Pomorska 251, 92-213 Lodz, Poland. [2]Department of Anaesthesiology and Intensive Care, Jonscher Municipal Hospital, Lodz, Poland. [3]Department of Radiology, Medical University, Lodz, Poland.

#### References

1. Kawai S, Kitabatake A, Tomoike H, Takotsubo Cardiomyopathy Group. Guidelines for diagnosis of takotsubo (ampulla) cardiomyopathy. Circ J. 2007;71:990–2.
2. Ramaraj R, Movahed MR. Reverse or inverted takotsubo cardiomyopathy (reverse left ventricular apical ballooning syndrome) presents at a younger age compared with the mid or apical variant and is always associated with triggering stress. Congest Heart Fail. 2010;16:284–6.
3. Zdanowicz JA, Utz AC, Bernasconi I, Geier S, Corti R, Beinder E. "Broken heart" after cesarean delivery. Case report and review of literature. Arch Gynecol Obstet. 2011;283:687–94.
4. Minatoguchi M, Itakura A, Takagi E, Nishibayashi M, Kikuchi M, Ishihara O. Takotsubo cardiomyopathy after cesarean: a case report and published work review of pregnancy-related cases. J Obstet Gynaecol Res. 2014; 40:1534–9.
5. Crimi E, Baggish A, Leffert L, Pian-Smith MC, Januzzi JL, Jiang Y. Acute reversible stress-induced cardiomyopathy associated with cesarean delivery under spinal anesthesia. Circulation. 2008;117:3052–3.
6. Citro R, Pascotto M, Provenza G, Gregorio G, Bossone E. Transient left ventricular ballooning (tako-tsubo cardiomyopathy) soon after intravenous ergonovine injection following caesarean delivery. Int J Cardiol. 2010;138:e31–4.
7. Citro R, Giudice R, Mirra M, Bottiglieri G, Bossone E, Di Benedetto G, et al. Tako-tsubo syndrome soon after caesarean delivery: two case reports. Int J Cardiol. 2012;161:e48–9.
8. Ueyama T, Kasamatsu K, Hano T, Yamamoto K, Tsuruo Y, Nishio I. Emotional stress induces transient left ventricular hypocontraction in the rat via activation of cardiac adrenoceptors: a possible animal model of 'tako-tsubo' cardiomyopathy. Circ J. 2002;66:712–3.
9. Ono R, Falcao ML. Takotsubo cardiomyopathy systematic review: Pathophysiologic process, clinical presentation and diagnostic approach to takotsubo cardiomyopathy. Int J Cardiol. 2016;209:196–205.
10. Wittstein IS, Thiemann DR, Lima JA, Baughman KL, Schulman SP, Gerstenblith G, et al. Neurohumoral features of myocardial stunning due to sudden emotional stress. N Engl J Med. 2005;352:539–48.
11. Akashi YJ, Nakazawa K, Sakakibara M, Miyake F, Koike H, Sasaka K. The clinical features of takotsubo cardiomyopathy. QJM. 2003;96:563–73.
12. Hurst RT, Askew JW, Reuss CS, Lee RW, Sweeney JP, Fortuin FD, et al. Transient midventricular ballooning syndrome: a new variant. J Am Coll Cardiol. 2006;48:579–83.
13. Litvinov IV, Kotowycz MA, Wassmann S. Iatrogenic epinephrine-induced reverse Takotsubo cardiomyopathy: direct evidence supporting the role of catecholamines in the pathophysiology of the "broken heart syndrome". Clin Res Cardiol. 2009;98:457–62.
14. Bainbridge D, Cheng D. Stress-induced cardiomyopathy in the perioperative setting. Can J Anaesth. 2009;56:397–401.
15. Lyon AR, Bossone E, Schneider B, Sechtem U, Citro R, Underwood SR, et al. Current state of knowledge on Takotsubo syndrome: a position statement from task force on Takotsubo syndrome of the Heart Failure Association of the European Society of Cardiology. Eur J Heart Fail. 2016;18:8–27.

13

# Ischemic biomarker heart-type fatty acid binding protein (hFABP) in acute heart failure - diagnostic and prognostic insights compared to NT-proBNP and troponin I

Ursula Hoffmann[1], Florian Espeter[1], Christel Weiß[2], Parviz Ahmad-Nejad[3], Siegfried Lang[1], Martina Brueckmann[4,5], Ibrahim Akin[1], Michael Neumaier[6], Martin Borggrefe[1] and Michael Behnes[1*]

**Abstract**

**Background:** To evaluate diagnostic and long-term prognostic values of hFABP compared to NT-proBNP and troponin I (TnI) in patients presenting to the emergency department (ED) suspected of acute heart failure (AHF).

**Methods:** 401 patients with acute dyspnea or peripheral edema, 122 suffering from AHF, were prospectively enrolled and followed up to 5 years. hFABP combined with NT-proBNP versus NT-proBNP alone was tested for AHF diagnosis. Prognostic value of hFABP versus TnI was evaluated in models predicting all-cause mortality (ACM) and AHF related rehospitalization (AHF-RH) at 1 and 5 years, including 11 conventional risk factors plus NT-proBNP.

**Results:** Additional hFABP measurements improved diagnostic specificity and positive predictive value (PPV) of sole NT-proBNP testing at the cutoff <300 ng/l to "rule out" AHF. Highest hFABP levels (4th quartile) were associated with increased ACM (hazard ratios (HR): 2.1–2.5; $p = 0.04$) and AHF-RH risk at 5 years (HR 2.8–8.3, $p = 0.001$). ACM was better characterized in prognostic models including TnI, whereas AHF-RH was better characterized in prognostic models including hFABP. Cox analyses revealed a 2 % increase of ACM risk and 3–7 % increase of AHF-RH risk at 5 years by each unit increase of hFABP of 10 ng/ml.

**Conclusions:** Combining hFABP plus NT-proBNP (<300 ng/l) only improves diagnostic specificity and PPV to rule out AHF. hFABP may improve prognosis for long-term AHF-RH, whereas TnI may improve prognosis for ACM.

**Keywords:** Acute heart failure, hFABP, Mortality, NT-proBNP, Prognosis, Rehospitalisation, Troponin I

## Background

Human heart-type fatty acid binding protein (hFABP) is a 15 kDa small protein consisting of 132 amino acids [1]. It belongs to the FABP superfamily being characterized by relative tissue specificity [2]. hFABP is located primarily in the heart constituting 5–15 % of the cytosolic protein pool [3] and is assigned to transport fatty acids towards the mitochondria for ß-oxidation and energy expenditure [3–5]. Moreover it protects against free radical accumulation during myocardial ischemia [6–8] and influences signal transduction pathways for gene expression via peroxisome proliferator-activated receptors (PPAR) [9]. In healthy humans the normal range of hFABP in serum or plasma has been reported to vary between 0.0 and 5.5 ng/ml [10, 11]. Fatty acids represent the main source of energy in the heart accounting for 10 % of the total body turnover of fatty acids [4, 12–14].

The diagnostic value of hFABP has comprehensively been evaluated in patients suffering from acute myocardial infarction (AMI). Here, varying diagnostic area under the receiver-operating characteristic (ROC) curves and diagnostic goodness criteria (such as sensitives, specifities, positive and negative predictive values (NPV/PPV)) have

* Correspondence: michael.behnes@umm.de
[1]First Department of Medicine, University Medical Centre Mannheim (UMM), Faculty of Medicine Mannheim, University of Heidelberg, Theodor-Kutzer-Ufer 1-3, 68167 Mannheim, Germany
Full list of author information is available at the end of the article

been reported for hFABP measurements [15, 16]. Accordingly, combining hFABP with cardiac troponins revealed conflicting results [17–22]. In contrast, low specifities and PPVs have been reported for NT-proBNP to reliably diagnose acute heart failure (AHF). Therefore new biomarkers are increasingly focussed to improve both the diagnostic and prognostic assessement of AHF patients [23, 24]. hFABP was shown to be associated with chronic heart failure patients (CHF), whereas minor reports indicate a diagnostic role of hFABP in children developing concomitant acute heart failure (AHF) during pneumonia [25–28]. However, hFABP levels have never been primarily evaluated in patients suspected of AHF.

The present study evaluates the diagnostic and long term prognostic value of additional hFABP measurements compared to NT-proBNP and TnI in patients presenting with symptoms of acute dyspnea or peripheral edema to the emergency department.

## Methods

### Study patients, design and data collection

The present study represents a post hoc analysis of a specimen repository from patients enrolled in the Mannheim NT-proBNP Study (MANPRO, clinicaltrials.gov identifier: NCT00143793) [29], which was conducted as a single-centre prospective controlled study at the University Medical Centre Mannheim (UMM), Germany. The study was carried out according to the principles of the declaration of Helsinki and was approved by the medical ethics commission II of the Medical Faculty Mannheim, University of Heidelberg, Germany. Informed consent was obtained from all participating patients or their legal representatives.

Briefly, patients with symptoms of acute dyspnea and/or peripheral edema presenting to the emergency department were consecutively included from August 2005 until March 2006 and the underlying diseases such as AHF were diagnosed. Patients suffering from severe renal disease (defined as serum creatinine level greater than 2.8 mg/dl), anemia (hemoglobin concentrations below 8.0 g/dl), obvious traumatic causes of dyspnea, pregnancy, with a status after immediate cardiopulmonary resuscitation, participation in another clinical trial and patients with age under 18 years were excluded [29, 30].

### Diagnosis of acute heart failure

The investigators of the study were neither involved in therapeutic decisions nor in decisions regarding clinical examinations. To determine the main diagnosis of each patient, an independent study physician had unrestricted access to the records of the patients, but was blinded to the results of the biomarker measurements. Based on this approach all patients were classified into two categories: 1) Symptomatic patients because of AHF, 2) symptomatic patients due to any cause except for AHF.

Diagnosis of AHF was based on European Guidelines for the diagnosis of AHF [31, 32]. AHF diagnosis being a decompensated CHF or de-novo AHF, was based on the acute development of typical symptoms. Additionally, specific clinical signs made AHF diagnosis even more favourable, such as pulmonary rales, elevated jugular venous pressure or hepatojugular reflux. At least one of the following technical findings substantiated the diagnosis of AHF, such as radiographic evidence of pulmonary congestion and edema, abnormalities on the ECG (i.e. supraventricular tachycardia, ventricular arrhythmias, myocardial ischemia or infarction) or evidence of left ventricular (LV) systolic dysfunction (defined as LVEF <55 %) or diastolic dysfunction as assessed by echocardiography (see below). Patients not fulfilling AHF criteria were collected in the "no AHF" group. Diagnoses were not based on biomarker levels (such as hFABP or NT-proBNP) because patients and physicians were blinded to biomarker results.

Severity of symptoms were classified according to the functional New York Heart Association (NYHA) classification and structural ABCD classification of the American College of Cardiology/American Heart Association [31, 33]. Standard two-dimensional and colour Doppler imaging was performed by independent cardiologists during routine clinical care [30]. Parameters of LV systolic function comprised LV ejection fraction (Simpson's biplane) (LVEF) and fractional shortening by parasternal M-mode. A LVEF of <55 % was defined as LV systolic dysfunction. Diastolic function was routinely assessed by the E/A ratio during sinus rhythm (the ratio of the maximum velocities of early (E) to atrial (A) LV filling determined by pulsed-wave Doppler of the mitral valve), deceleration time, isovolumetric relaxation time and ratio of E/E' (which is used to estimate an increase in LV diastolic pressure, measured at the basal septum). Definitions of diastolic dysfunction corresponded to E/E' >15 or stages 1, 2 and 3 [34].

### Measurements of hFABP, NT-proBNP and troponin I

All samples were obtained by venipuncture into serum and ammonium heparin tubes for biomarker measurements, immediately at presentation to the emergency department. Within 30 min all blood samples were centrifuged at 2000 g for 10 min. Plasma was separated, aliquoted, frozen and stored at −80 °C.

hFABP was measured in serum, NT-proBNP and troponin I (TnI) were measured in ammonium heparin plasma in all 401 patients. hFABP measurement was performed with a commercially available immunoassay/ELISA (hFABP ELISA Catalog Number EA-0305, Signosis Inc., Sunnyvale, USA) [35]. hFABP was shown to be a stable protein even after repeated freezing and thawing [36]. NT-proBNP measurement was performed with a commercially available immunoassay on the Dimension® RxL clinical chemistry system (Flex reagent cartridge PBNP, Dimension System, Dade Behring Ltd., Atterbury Milton Keynes, United Kingdom) as previously described [29]. Contemporary sensitive TnI was measured with the SIEMENS Dimension® Vista intelligent lab system for contemporary sensitive cardiac troponin I testing. The lowest detection limit of the assay is 0.015 ng/ml. The 99th percentile measured at a healthy reference population is 0.045 ng/ml with a coefficient of variation (CV) of 10 % [37].

### Study endpoints

The first endpoint tested was whether the diagnostic value of combined hFABP plus NT-proBNP was comparable to NT-proBNP alone for diagnosis of AHF.

The second endpoint was to test the prognostic value of hFABP in patients admitted to the emergency department with symptoms of acute dyspnea and/or edema. Two prognostic outcomes were considered: all-cause mortality and AHF-related rehospitalization at 1 and 5 years.

Follow-up was performed in three successive steps: Firstly, our in-hospital electronic records were screened with regard to in-hospital all-cause mortality, AHF-related rehospitalization and last medical contact in our clinic over a follow-up period of at least 5 years. Secondly, family physicians of those patients with incomplete follow-up after step 1 (i.e. either patients without any re-admission or patients re-admitted for the last time before expiration of total 5 years follow-up) were contacted to complete survival status. Thirdly, survival status was completed by individual telephone visits with the remaining patients, who did not complete total 5 years follow-up after follow-up steps 1 and 2.

### Statistical methods

For normally distributed data, the Student $t$ test was applied. Otherwise, the Mann–Whitney $U$ test was used as nonparametric test. Deviations from a Gaussian distribution were tested by the Kolmogorov-Smirnov test. hFABP and NT-proBNP data were $\log_{10}$ transformed, thereby promoting normality, and the unpaired $t$-test was applied. Spearman's rank correlation for nonparametric data was used to test the association of hFABP blood levels with clinical parameters. Qualitative parameters were analyzed by use of a $2 \times 2$ contingency table and $Chi^2$ test or Fisher's exact test as appropriate. Quantitative data are presented as mean ± standard error of mean (SEM) or as median and interquartile range (IQR), depending on the distribution of the data. For qualitative parameters absolute and relative frequencies are presented. All analyses were exploratory and utilized a p value of 0.05 (2 tailed) for significance.

### Diagnostic value of combined hFABP plus NT-proBNP versus NT-proBNP alone

1) C-statistics: Receiver-operating characteristic curve (ROC) analyses with areas under the curves (AUC) were calculated for diagnosis of AHF. Two logistic regression models with AHF as dependent variable and the combined biomarkers hFABP plus NT-proBNP as well as NT-proBNP alone (reference biomarker) as independent variables were analyzed. The two areas under the ROC curves were compared using the method by Hanley [38]. The optimal cutoff for the combined biomarkers accorded to the probabilities being associated with hFABP and NT-proBNP to suffer from AHF as assessed by logistic regression models and was chosen where the Youden index (sensitivity + specificity − 1) yielded maximum values. Optimal cutoffs of single NT-proBNP measurements (i.e. reference) accorded to <300 pg/ml to "rule out AHF", as well as to "rule-in AHF" according to age-dependent cutoff levels of 450 ng/l (age <50 years), 900 ng/l (50–75 years), and 1800 ng/l (>75 years) [24]. Contingency tables were used to assess the individual diagnostic goodness criteria (i.e. accuracy, specificity, sensitivity, negative/positive predictive values (NPV/PPV)). Statistical accuracy was defined as the sum of true positives plus true negatives devided by the number of total measurements ($n = 401$). Accuracy, specificity, sensitivity were compared by McNemar tests.

### Prognostic value of hFABP versus troponin I

Kaplan Meyer curves according to hFABP quartiles were created and the corresponding hazard ratios (HRs) were calculated for each hFABP quartile in all patients for the two mentionend prognostic outcomes at 1 and 5 years (i.e. all cause mortality and AHF related rehospitalization).

Prognostic models were performed using Cox regression analyses including the following 12 variables to a reference model [39]: age, sex, left ventricular function, serum creatinine (mg/dl), NYHA functional class, presence of diabetes mellitus, the degree of coronary artery disease, haemoglobin (g/dl), serum sodium (mmol/l), beta-blocker treatment, angiotensin-converting enzyme inhibitor or angiotensin II receptor blocker treatment (ACEI/ARB) and logNT-proBNP levels. Variables of the reference model were chosen either because of univariate significant associations or because of commonly known prognostic effects [23, 39].

The biomarkers of interest, hFABP and troponin I, were subsequently added to this reference model as continuous variables.

To test whether the inclusion of hFABP and troponin I valuably improves prognosis of the reference model for all-cause mortality and AHF related rehospitalization, different established measurements of model performance were applied [23, 39–41].

Statistical measures of discrimination comprised C-statistics. C-statistics of models with additional hFABP or troponin I were compared using the Mann–Whitney *U* test. Statistical measures of model calibration comprise Hosmer-Lemeshow test, Bayesian information criterion (BIC), Akaike information criterion (AIK) and the Brier score. The global goodness of fit of the models was evaluated by likelihood ratio tests. Statistical measures of reclassification comprise integrated discrimination improvement (IDI) and net reclassification improvement (NRI) following Pencina [42].

In Cox regression models an increase of hazard ratio (HR) correspond to the logarithmic function of NT-proBNP (ng/l), hFABP per every 10 ng/ml and TnI per every µg/l change.

The calculations were performed with InStat and StatMate (GraphPad Software), SPSS software (SPSS Software GmbH), and SAS (SAS Institute Inc. Cary, NC, USA).

## Results

### Associations of hFABP levels with clinical parameters

Baseline characteristics of 401 study patients are summarized in Table 1. hFABP levels were able to differentiate patients with AHF (median = 28.8 ng/ml, IQR 20.3–48.1 ng/ml, $n = 122$) from those without (median = 16.9 ng/ml, IQR 7.2–24.4 ng/ml, $n = 279$) ($p = 0.0001$) (Fig. 1). hFABP levels were higher in NYHA class III/IV patients compared to NYHA class I/II patients (NYHA III/IV: median = 27.5 ng/ml, IQR 18.8–48.0 ng/ml, $n = 128$; NYHA I/II: median = 19.1 ng/ml, IQR 3.6–25.5 ng/ml, $n = 70$) ($p = 0.0001$) (Fig. 2, left) and higher in ACC/AHA class C/D patients compared to class A/B patients (class D/E: median = 22.6 ng/ml, IQR 13.8–39.2 ng/ml,

**Table 1** Baseline characteristics of 401 patients initially presenting with acute dyspnea or peripheral edema

| Variables | All patients ($n = 401$) | No AHF ($n = 279$) | AHF ($n = 122$) | *p* value* |
|---|---|---|---|---|
| Demographics | | | | |
| Age, mean (range) | 67 (18–96) | 65 (18–96) | 73 (36–96) | 0.0001 |
| Male, *n* (%) | 205 (51) | 131 (47) | 74 (61) | 0.7 |
| Cardiovascular risk factors, *n* (%) | | | | |
| Arterial hypertension | 268 (67) | 170 (61) | 98 (80) | 0.0001 |
| Hypercholesterinemia | 122 (30) | 207 (74) | 72 (59) | 0.003 |
| Cardiac family history | 132 (33) | 97 (35) | 35 (27) | 0.3 |
| Smoking | 206 (51) | 148 (53) | 58 (48) | 0.3 |
| Diabetes mellitus | 120 (30) | 67 (24) | 53 (43) | 0.0001 |
| Main diagnoses, *n* (%) | | | | |
| Chronic CHF | 143 (36) | 63 (23) | 80 (66) | 0.0001 |
| Atrial fibrillation | 90 (22) | 40 (14) | 50 (41) | 0.0001 |
| Coronary artery disease | 130 (32) | 73 (26) | 57 (47) | 0.0001 |
| Prior myocardial Infarction | 89 (22) | 47 (17) | 42 (34) | 0.0002 |
| Valvular heart disease | 118 (29) | 48 (17) | 70 (57) | 0.0001 |
| Acute exacerbated COPD | 31 (8) | 27 (10) | 4 (3) | 0.03 |
| Acute exacerbated asthma | 7 (2) | 7 (3) | 0 (0) | 0.1 |
| Pneumonia | 20 (5) | 19 (7) | 1 (1) | 0.01 |
| Pulmonary embolism | 12 (3) | 12 (4) | 0 (0) | 0.02 |
| Chronic kidney disease | 71 (17) | 30 (11) | 41 (34) | 0.0001 |
| Cancer | 19 (5) | 19 (7) | 0 (0) | 0.001 |
| Stroke | 10 (2) | 8 (3) | 2 (2) | 0.7 |
| LV EF (%), median (interquartile range) | 41 (30–52) | 50 (40–58) | 39 (27–50) | 0.04 |
| Symptoms and signs, *n* (%) | | | | |
| Peripheral edema | 46 (11) | 42 (15) | 4 (3) | 0.02 |
| Dyspnea | 235 (59) | 183 (66) | 52 (42) | 0.0001 |
| Both peripheral edema and dyspnea | 120 (30) | 54 (19) | 66 (54) | 0.0001 |

*p values for the comparison between AHF and no AHF group

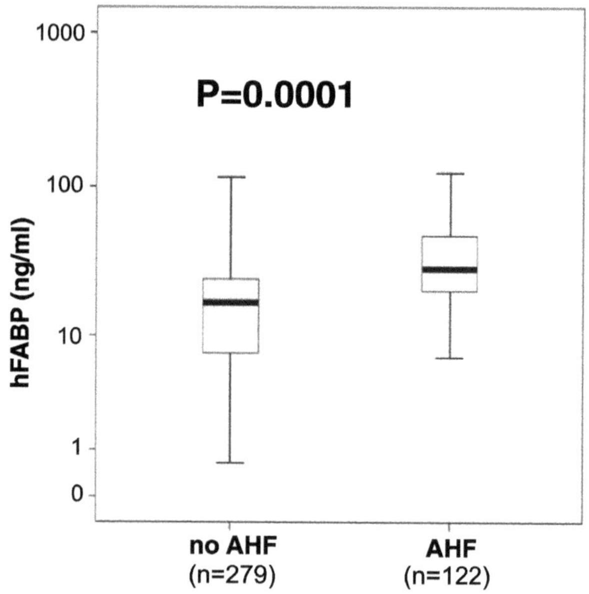


**Fig. 1** hFABP levels were significantly higher in patients suffering from acute heart failure (*AHF*) ($n = 122$) compared to those without ($n = 279$) ($p = 0.0001$). Data are presented as medians with 25th and 75th percentiles (boxes) and 5th and 95th percentiles (whiskers)

$n = 215$; class A/B: median = 18.1 ng/ml, IQ range 9.8–25.1 ng/ml, $n = 132$) ($p = 0.0001$) (Fig. 2, right). Patients with LV dysfunction being assessed by echocardiography (i.e. LVEF <55 %) had significantly higher levels of hFABP than patients with regular heart function (median = 27.0 ng/ml, IQR 17.3–50.9, $n = 91$ versus 19.2 ng/ml, 11.1–28.2, $n = 135$) ($p = 0.0001$). hFABP levels correlated significantly ($p < 0.05$) with several indices of cardiac function being assessed by echocardiography, such as fractional shortening ($r = -0.20$), E/A ($r = 0.23$), left atrial diameter ($r = 0.29$), LV enddiastolic diameter ($r = 0.34$) and LV endsystolic diameter ($r = 0.29$). hFABP

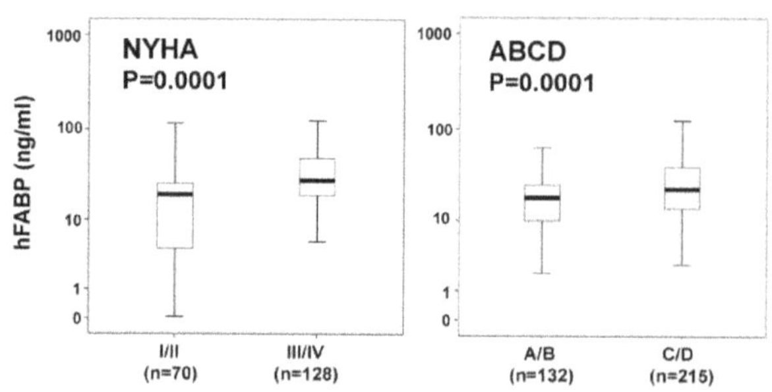


**Fig. 2** hFABP levels were significantly higher in patients of functional NYHA class III/IV ($n = 128$) compared to those of NYHA class I/II ($n = 70$) ($p = 0.01$) (*left*) and higher in patients of structural AHA/ACC stage C/D ($n = 215$) compared to those of stage A/B ($n = 132$) ($p = 0.0001$) (*right*). Data are presented as medians with 25th and 75th percentiles (boxes) and 5th and 95th percentiles (whiskers)

serum levels correlated significantly ($p < 0.05$) with creatinine ($r = 0.22$), hemoglobin ($r = -0.13$), NT-proBNP ($r = 0.32$) and TnI levels ($r = 0.23$).

### Diagnostic value of hFABP in combination with NT-proBNP

The AUC for the combined biomarkers hFABP plus NT-proBNP was equal to the AUC of NT-proBNP alone (hFABP plus NT-proBNP, AUC: 0.85; 95 % CI 0.79–0.87; NT-proBNP, AUC: 0.85; 95 % CI 0.81–0.89; AUC difference 0.0; $p > 0.05$), demonstrating that both AUCs valuable disriminate AHF patients from no AHF patients. The AUC of hFABP alone for diagnosis of AHF was 0.72 (95 % CI 0.67–0.78, $p = 0.0001$).

Combining hFABP plus NT-proBNP compared to single NT-proBNP at the "rule out AHF" cutoff of <300 ng/l revealed a significant increase in specificity, statistical accuracy and PPV ($p = 0.0001$): specificity (combined: 71 %, 95 % CI 66–77 %; NT-proBNP alone: 48 %, 95 % CI 42–54 %), PPV (combined: 58 %, 95 % CI 51–65 %; NT-proBNP alone: 45 %, 95 % CI 39–51 %), statistical accuracy (combined: 77 %, 95 % CI 73–81 %; NT-proBNP alone: 63 %, 95 % CI 58–68 %). Sensitivity (combined: 89 %, 95 % CI 84–95 %; NT-proBNP: 96 %, 95 % CI 92–99 %) and NPV (combined: 94 %, 95 % CI 91–97 %; NT-proBNP: 96 %, 95 % CI 93–99 %) were slightly decreased (at least 7 %).

Evaluation of hFABP plus NT-proBNP compared to NT-proBNP alone according to age-dependent cutoff levels to "rule-in AHF" (450 ng/l (age <50 years), 900 ng/l (50–75 years), and 1800 ng/l (>75 years)) did not reveal any improvements neither in AUC's, sensitivities, specificities, statistical accuracy nor predictive values (data not shown).

### Prognostic value of hFABP compared to troponin I

Non-survivors ($n = 57$) had a median hFABP value of 28.6 ng/ml (IQR 16.2–49.1 ng/ml) vs. 19.0 ng/ml (IQR 10.7–28.3 ng/ml) in survivors ($p = 0.0009$) at 1 year, and 26.2 pg/ml (IQR 16.2–44.9) in non-survivors ($n = 129$) vs. 17.8 ng/ml (IQR 10.3–24.9 ng/ml) in survivors at 5 years respectively ($p = 0.0001$). Patients being rehospitalized because of AHF had significantly higher hFABP levels than patients not being rehospitalized (1 year: AHF related rehospitalization, $n = 34$, median = 39.7 ng/ml (IQR 23.8–77.2 ng/ml), no AHF related rehospitalization, $n = 367$, median = 27.5 ng/ml (IQR 18.2–47.2 ng/ml), $p = 0.0001$; 5 years: AHF related rehospitalization, $n = 73$, median = 27.5 ng/ml (IQR 18.2–47.2 ng/ml), no AHF related rehospitalization, $n = 328$, median = 18.9 ng/ml (IQR 10.2–28.3 ng/ml), $p = 0.0001$).

### Kaplan Meier survival analyses

Kaplan Meier survival curves illustrate increasing risk of all-cause death at 1 and 5 years according to quartiles of hFABP. Patients with highest hFABP levels of the 4th quartile were up to 2.5 times more likely to die within follow-up periods (range of HRs: 2.1–2.5; $p = 0.04$) (Fig. 3, top). Additionally, patients with highest hFABP levels of the 4th quartile were up to 8.3 times more likely to be rehospitalized because of AHF within follow up periods (range of HRs 2.8–8.3, $p = 0.001$) (Fig. 3, bottom).

## Performance metrics of prognostic models

### *Discrimination*

Table 2 shows univariable associations of all variables with the prognostic outcomes. Either hFABP or TnI were adjusted in multivariable prognostic models relative to conventional assessment including 11 risk factors plus NT-proBNP. All-cause mortality and AHF related rehospitalization were significantly discriminated by including hFABP or TnI either in all ($n = 401$) or in AHF patients ($n = 122$), as indicated by individual significant AUCs above 0.7 ($p = 0.0001$, referring to each individual model) (Figs. 4 & 5).

When compared to the reference model, prognostic models including TnI revealed only numerically greatest, but not significantly different AUCs for all-cause mortality when applied in all ($n = 401$) as well as in AHF patients ($n = 122$) at 1 and 5 years (highlighted in blue, Figs. 4 & 5, top).

Accordingly, prognostic models including hFABP revealed only numerically greatest, but not significantly different AUCs for AHF-related rehospitalization when applied in all and AHF patients at 1 and 5 years (exception in all patients at 5 years) (highlighted in blue, Figs. 4 & 5, bottom).

### Calibration and reclassification

All-cause mortality was best calibrated in prognostic models including TnI (except all-cause mortality at 1 years in all patients). These models revealed favourable measures of calibration (such as Hosmer Lemshow, Brier Score, AIC, BIC and likelihood ratios) as well as beneficial NRIs (Figs. 4 & 5, top, highlighted in blue). AHF related rehospitalization was best calibrated in prognostic models including hFABP measurements. These models revealed favourable measures of calibration, such as Hosmer Lemshow, Brier Score, AIC, BIC and likelihood ratios as

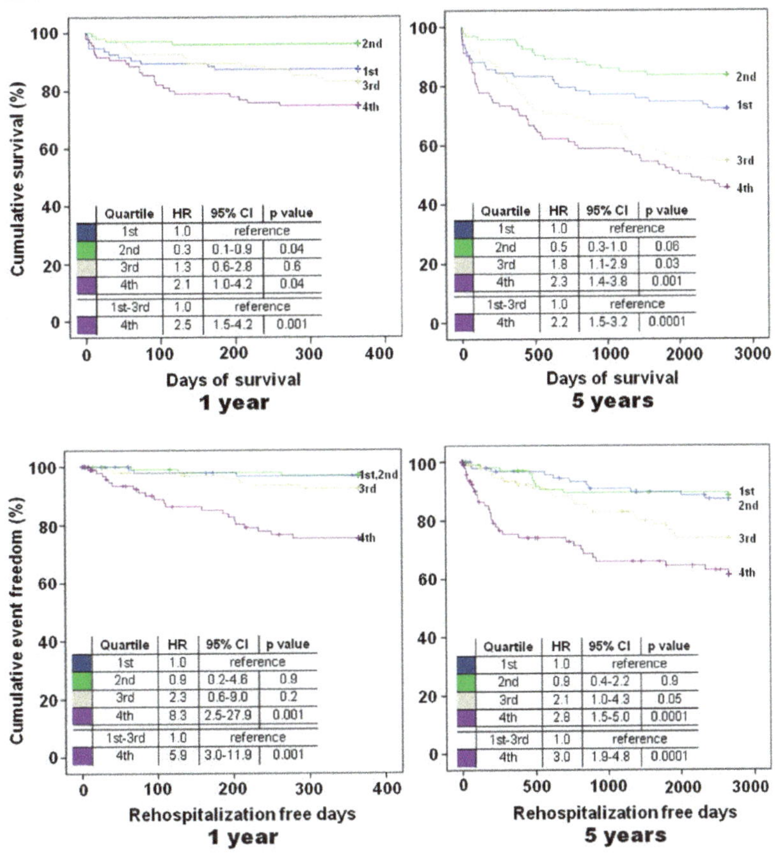


**Fig. 3** Kaplan-Meier curves evaluated by quartiles of hFABP after 1 (*left panel*) and 5 (*right panel*) years of follow-up in the total study cohort ($n = 401$). Increasing hFABP levels were significantly associated with long term all-cause mortality (**a**, *top*) and AHF related rehospitalization (**b**, *bottom*). Hazard Ratios (*HR*) were calculated for each risk group according to hFABP quartiles

**Table 2** Significance (*p* values) of univariate associations of prognostic variables for all-cause mortality and AHF related rehospitalization in all patients ($n = 401$)

| | All-cause mortality | | AHF related rehospitalization | |
|---|---|---|---|---|
| | 1 year | 5 years | 1 year | 5 years |
| Sex | 0.7174 | 0.9621 | 0.4660 | 0.9865 |
| Age | 0.0001* | 0.0001* | 0.0007* | 0.0001* |
| Diabetes | 0.9756 | 0.3776 | 0.0030* | 0.0001* |
| Left ventricular function | 0.0088* | 0.0002* | 0.0001* | 0.0001* |
| NYHA class | 0.2061 | 0.0029* | 0.0001* | 0.0001* |
| Coronary artery disease | 0.5443 | 0.4715 | 0.0203* | 0.0001* |
| Beta blocker | 0.9888 | 0.9876 | 0.0965 | 0.0008* |
| ACE inhibitor | 0.6988 | 0.2305 | 0.0002* | 0.0001* |
| Hemoglobin | 0.0001* | 0.0001* | 0.0182* | 0.1096 |
| Creatinine | 0.0554 | 0.0032* | 0.0001* | 0.0001* |
| Sodium | 0.0661* | 0.0099* | 0.3777 | 0.7839 |
| NTproBNP | 0.0001* | 0.0001* | 0.0001* | 0.0001* |
| hFABP | 0.0008* | 0.0001* | 0.0001* | 0.0001* |
| Troponin I | 0.0009* | 0.0001* | 0.0001* | 0.0002* |

*Level of significance, $p < 0.05$

well as beneficial NRIs (Figs. 4 and 5, bottom, highlighted in blue). In contrast, IDIs mostly revealed only low values and indicated none or insubstantial integrative improvements.

### Cox regression analyses

Multivariate prognostic Cox proportional hazard models, incorporating the same 12 risk factors as described above, revealed up to 2 % increase of all-cause mortality risk at 5 years alongside with increasing hFABP levels of 10 ng/ml being initially measured only once in the emergency department in all patients (HR 1.020; 95 % CI 1.020–0.998; statistical trend $p < 0.1$) (Table 3). In contrast, increasing TnI levels of 1 µg/l were not associated with an increased risk of all-cause mortality ($p > 0.1$) (Tables 3 and 4).

Accordingly, Cox models revealed up to 3–7 % increase of AHF related rehospitalization risk at 5 years alongside with increasing hFABP levels of 10 ng/ml (all patients: HR 1.034; 95 % CI 1.001–0.068; $p = 0.047$; AHF patients: HR 1.073; 95 % CI 1.018–0.132; $p = 0.008$). In contrast, increasing TnI levels of 1 µg/l were not associated with an increased risk of AHF related rehospitalization (Tables 3 and 4).

## Discussion

This post-hoc analysis of the MANPRO study evaluated the diagnostic and long-term prognostic values of hFABP levels in comparison to NT-proBNP and TnI in patients presenting to the emergency department with acute dyspnea and peripheral edema being suspected of acute heart failure (AHF). To the best of our knowledge, the present analysis is the first investigating the diagnostic and prognostic value of hFABP measurements in patients being suspected of AHF.

hFABP levels were able to differentiate AHF from other causes of dyspnea and/or edema, were associated with higher disease stages of CHF and correlated significantly with several indices of cardiac function being assessed by echocardiography. Combining hFABP with NT-proBNP increased specificity, statistical accuracy and PPV when compared to the age-independent cutoff of single NT-proBNP <300 pg/ml to "rule-out AHF". Secondly, highest hFABP levels measured initially in the emergency department were associated with all-cause mortality and AHF related rehospitalization at 1 and 5 years as assessed by Kaplan-Meyer analyses. Within multivariate adjustment in prognostic models containing 11 conventional prognostic risk factors plus NT-proBNP, all-cause mortality was better characterized in terms of statistical calibration and reclassification by additionally including TnI. In contrast, AHF-related rehospitalization was better characterized in multivariate models including hFABP.

In the context of heart failure syndromes, hFABP has mostly been evaluated in studies including adolescent patients suffering from CHF, thereby commonly focusing on the prognostic value of hFABP to predict both mortality and adverse cardiac events [43–45]. In contrast, increasing hFABP levels were shown to be associated with the severity of heart failure in children with chronic endocardial fibroelastosis or dilated cardiomyopathy [25]. Additionally it has been demonstrated that hFABP was even more sensitive than brain natriuretic peptide (BNP) to detect the development of secondary AHF in children primarily suffering from pneumonia [28].

The present study focused on the improvement of the weaknesses of the age-independent cutoff value of NT-proBNP <300 ng/l to "rule out AHF", such as the low specificity, accuracy and PPV [29]. As recently published for the presented study cohort [29], the NT-proBNP cutoff to "rule out AHF" was set at <300 ng/l with a corresponding sensitivity of 96 %, specificity of 48 %, PPV of 45 % and a NPV of 96 %.

As demonstrated in this study, increasing the specificity by additional hFABP measurements might detect even more patients as "no AHF", who truly do not suffer from AHF although presenting with dyspnea and/or peripheral in the emergency department. In contrast, additional hFABP measurements were not shown to reveal any improvements when applied for age-dependant NT-proBNP cutoffs to "rule in AHF" [24].

The usefulness of hFABP as a biomarker for the detection of AHF is mainly driven by the molecule's

**Performance of models for all-cause mortality (top) and AHF-related rehopitalization (bottom) at 1 and 5 yrs in all patients (n=401)**

| | all-cause mortality at 1 year | | | all-cause mortality at 5 years | | |
|---|---|---|---|---|---|---|
| | **reference model** | **with hFABP** | **with TnI** | **reference model** | **with hFABP** | **with TnI** |
| **Discrimination** | | | | | | |
| C-statistic | 0.8164<br>(0.7536 – 0.8792)<br>reference | 0.8182<br>(0.7558 – 0.8806)<br>p =0.7039<br>p=0.0001* | 0.8200<br>(0.7581 – 0.8819)<br>p = 0.1923<br>p=0.0001* | 0.8347<br>(0.7913 – 0.8781) | 0.8382<br>(0.7948 – 0.8816)<br>p =0.4345<br>p=0.0001* | 0.8427<br>(0.8004 – 0.8850)<br>p = 0.1411<br>p=0.0001* |
| **Calibration** | | | | | | |
| Hosmer | Chi² = 10.8299 | Chi² = 13.3290 | Chi² = 17.4374 | Chi² = 5.8820 | Chi² = 11.6683 | Chi² = 6.6280 |
| Lemeshow | p = 0.2115 | p = 0.1010 | p = 0.0259 | p = 0.6604 | p = 0.1666 | p = 0.5773 |
| Brier Score | 0.0973 | 0.0969 | 0.0967 | 0.1562 | 0.1532 | 0.1521 |
| AIC | 609.943 | 610.016 | 610.125 | 1335.556 | 1334.803 | 1329.800 |
| BIC | 638.298 | 640.396 | 640.505 | 1375.375 | 1377.466 | 1372.463 |
| Likelihood ratio | reference | p = 0.1651 | p = 0.1776 | reference | p = 0.0971 | p = 0.0054 |
| **Reclassification** | | | | | | |
| IDI – all | reference | +0.0052<br>(-0.0068 to +0.0171)<br>p = 0.3950 | +0.0046<br>(-0.0008 to +0.0100)<br>p = 0.0977 | reference | 0.0126<br>(-0.0005 to +0.0257)<br>p = 0.0592 | 0.0168<br>(0.0059 to 0.0277)<br>p = 0.0026 |
| NRI – all | reference | -0.1879<br>(-0.4715 to +0.0957)<br>p = 0.1940 | +0.4021<br>(0.1185 to 0.6857)<br>p = 0.0055 | reference | +0.1509<br>(-0.0668 to +0.3686)<br>p = 0.1744 | +0.6457<br>(0.4280 to +0.8635)<br>p = 0.0001 |
| NRI – death | reference | -0.3571<br>(-0.6191 to -0.0952)<br>p = 0.0075 | +0.3929<br>(0.1309 to 0.6548)<br>p = 0.0033 | reference | -0.2598<br>(-0.4338 to -0.0859)<br>p = 0.0034 | +0.5118<br>(0.3379 to 0.6857)<br>p = 0.0001 |
| NRI – survivor | reference | -0.1692<br>( -0.2780 to -0.0605)<br>p = 0.0023 | -0.0092<br>(-0.1180 to 0.0995)<br>p = 0.8678 | reference | -0.4107<br>(-0.5417 to -0.2798)<br>p < 0.0001 | -0.1339<br>(-0.2649 to -0.0030)<br>p = 0.0450 |

| | AHF-related rehospitalization at 1 year | | | AHF-related rehospitalization at 5 years | | |
|---|---|---|---|---|---|---|
| | **reference model** | **with hFABP** | **with TnI** | **reference model** | **with hFABP** | **with TnI** |
| **Discrimination** | | | | | | |
| C-statistic | 0.8869<br>(0.8404 – 0.9334)<br>reference | 0.8907<br>(0.8448 – 0.9366)<br>p = 0.5689<br>p=0.0001* | 0.8870<br>(0.8406 – 0.9334)<br>p = 0.9096<br>p=0.0001* | 0.8377<br>(0.7936 – 0.8819)<br>reference | 0.8381<br>(0.7936 – 0.8826)<br>p = 0.8935<br>p=0.0001* | 0.8393<br>(0.7955 – 0.8832)<br>p = 0.4680<br>p=0.0001* |
| **Calibration** | | | | | | |
| Hosmer | Chi² = 9.1593 | Chi² = 2.9295 | Chi² = 9.5700 | Chi² = 4.0088 | Chi² = 3.2968 | Chi² = 5.8918 |
| Lemeshow | p = 0.3290 | p = 0.9387 | p = 0.2965 | p = 0.8563 | p = 0.9144 | p = 0.6593 |
| Brier Score | 0.0612 | 0.0587 | 0.0612 | 0.1176 | 0.1165 | 0.1173 |
| AIC | 361.116 | 357.379 | 363.030 | 783.269 | 782.005 | 784.963 |
| BIC | 382.891 | 380.709 | 383.360 | 815.526 | 816.566 | 819.524 |
| Likelihood ratio | reference | p = 0.0166 | p = 0.7693 | reference | p = 0.0708 | p = 0.5802 |
| **Reclassification** | | | | | | |
| IDI | reference | 0.0262<br>(-0.0084 to +0.0608)<br>p= 0.1323 | 0.0005<br>(-0.0011 to +0.0012)<br>p = 0.9302 | reference | +0.0055<br>(-0.0042 to +0.0153)<br>p = 0.2683 | +0.0020<br>(-0.0026 to +0.0066)<br>p = 0.3888 |
| NRI – all | reference | +0.5615<br>(0.2145 to +0.9085)<br>p = 0.0015 | -0.0885<br>(-0.4355 to +0.2585)<br>p = 0.6172 | reference | +0.2328<br>(-0.0198 to +0.4885)<br>p = 0.0709 | +0.4036<br>(0.1509 to 0.6562)<br>p = 0.0017 |
| NRI – AHF-RH | reference | -0.0286<br>(-0.3599 to 0.3027)<br>p = 0.8658 | -0.0857<br>(-0.4170 to 0.2456)<br>p = 0.6121 | reference | -0.2703<br>(-0.4981 to -0.0424)<br>p = 0.0200 | +0.4595<br>(0.2316 to 0.6873)<br>p = 0.0001 |
| NRI – no AHF-RH | reference | -0.5900<br>(-0.6932 to -0.4869)<br>p = 0.0001 | +0.0028<br>(-0.1004 to 0.1059)<br>p = 0.9580 | reference | -0.5031<br>(-0.6123 to -0.3939)<br>p = 0.0001 | 0.0559<br>(-0.1651 to +0.0533)<br>p = 0.3158 |

Reference model includes age, sex, coronary artery disease, left ventricular function, NYHA functional class, diabetes mellitus, creatinine, ACEI or ARB treatment, beta blocker treatment, sodium, hemoglobin, NT-proBNP.
AIC = Akaike information criterion; BIC = Bayesian information criterion; IDI = integrated discrimation imrovement; NRI = net reclassification improvement. Definitions of statistical measures see methods section. Values in brackets are 95% confidence intervals (CI).
P values indicate differences versus the reference model (p<0.05 statistically significant, or p<0.01 statistical trend).
*P-values indicate level of significance of C-statistics referring to each individual model.
**Yellow boxes indicate improvements, blue boxes indicate best improvements compared to reference models.**

**Fig. 4** Performance of models for all-cause mortality (*top*) and AHF-related rehopitalization (*bottom*) at 1 and 5 years in all patients ($n = 401$)

biochemistry and pathophysiological behavior during myocardial injury. With a molecular size of 15 kDa hFABP is a small cytosolic protein, being highly present in the myocardium compared to skeletal muscle [4]. Besides this relative tissue specificity, hFABP is rapidly released into the serum within 2 h after myocardial injury, whereas it is usually not present in serum under healthy conditions. The development of acute heart failure is facilitated by myocardial ischemia and necrosis, cardiomyocyte damage from inflammatory cytokines, oxidative stress or apoptosis, thereby increasing the permeability of the cardiomyocyte membrane with consecutive release of cytosolic proteins [31, 46]. These conditions might also be the main stimulus for hFABP serum release in AHF [5, 10]. Therefore measurements of hFABP might be worth to be tested in a setting of patients being suspected of acute heart failure [31].

It is assumed that hospitalization because of recurrent AHF occurs in up to 30 % of heart failure patients within 90 % days post-discharge [47] and therefore has a major impact on the health care system. Conflicting data are available about the effectiveness of discharge planning, disease management programs and telemonitoring in heart failure patients, whereas it remains unclear, whether AHF readmissions are preventable and do necessarily indicate a suboptimal standard of care [47]. Yet the economic benefit implementing hFABP into clinical risk stratification has not been evaluated at

**Performance of models for all-cause mortality (top) and AHF-related rehopitalization (bottom) at 1 and 5 yrs in AHF patients (n=122)**

| | all-cause mortality at 1 year | | | all-cause mortality at 5 years | | |
|---|---|---|---|---|---|---|
| | reference model | with hFABP | with TnI | reference model | with hFABP | with TnI |
| **Discrimination** | | | | | | |
| C-statistic | 0.7961<br>(0.6898 – 0.9024)<br>reference | 0.8024<br>(0.6961 – 0.9087)<br>p = 0.3561<br>p = 0.0001* | 0.8123<br>(0.7061 – 0.9185)<br>p = 0.2007<br>p = 0.0001* | 0.8282<br>(0.7495 – 0.9070)<br>reference | 0.8292<br>(0.7503 – 0.9081)<br>p = 0.8483<br>p = 0.0001* | 0.8517<br>(0.7784 – 0.9240)<br>p = 0.1793<br>p = 0.0001* |
| **Calibration** | | | | | | |
| Hosmer Lemeshow | Chi$^2$ = 11.0225<br>p = 0.2004 | Chi$^2$ = 11.5415<br>p = 0.1729 | Chi$^2$ = 11.1609<br>p = 0.1927 | Chi$^2$ = 6.3283<br>p = 0.6105 | Chi$^2$ = 9.6666<br>p = 0.2892 | Chi$^2$ = 8.1612<br>p = 0.4179 |
| Brier Score | 0.1302 | 0.1295 | 0.1242 | 0.1683 | 0.1676 | 0.1521 |
| AIC | 228.390 | 229.659 | 226.879 | 487.349 | 489.324 | 479.840 |
| BIC | 244.883 | 247.330 | 244.549 | 515.952 | 519.969 | 510.486 |
| Likelihood ratio | reference | p = 0.3926 | p = 0.0610 | reference | p = 0.8744 | p = 0.0020 |
| **Reclassification** | | | | | | |
| IDI | reference | +0.0036<br>(-0.0143 to +0.0214)<br>p = 0.6966 | +0.0280<br>(0.0077 to 0.0483)<br>p = 0.0068 | reference | +0.0022<br>(-0.0059 to +0.0103)<br>p = 0.5883 | +0.0453<br>(0.0052 to 0.0854)<br>p = 0.0267 |
| NRI – all | reference | +0.5108<br>(0.0620 to +0.9595)<br>p = 0.0257 | +0.8522<br>(0.4034 to 1.3009)<br>p = 0.0002 | reference | -0.2794<br>(-0.6534 to +0.0946)<br>p = 0.1432 | +0.6005<br>(0.2265 to 0.9745)<br>p = 0.0017 |
| NRI - death | reference | +0.5000<br>(0.0999 to 0.9001)<br>p = 0.0143 | +0.5833<br>(0.1833 to 0.9834)<br>p = 0.0043 | reference | -0.2983<br>(-0.5579 to -0.0386)<br>p = 0.0243 | +0.5439<br>(0.2843 to 0.8035)<br>p = 0.0001 |
| NRI – survivor | reference | -0.0108<br>(-0.2140 to +0.1925)<br>p = 0.9174 | -0.2688<br>(-0.4721 to -0.0656)<br>p = 0.0095 | reference | -0.0189<br>(-0.2881 to +0.2504)<br>p = 0.8908 | -0.0566<br>(-0.3258 to +0.2126)<br>p = 0.6803 |

| | AHF-related rehospitalization at 1 year | | | AHF-related rehospitalization at 5 years | | |
|---|---|---|---|---|---|---|
| | reference model | with hFABP | With TnI | reference model | with hFABP | with TnI |
| **Discrimination** | | | | | | |
| C-statistic | 0.7436<br>(0.6378 – 0.8494)<br>reference | 0.7744<br>(0.6683 – 0.8804)<br>p = 0.2069<br>p = 0.0001* | 0.7447<br>(0.6392 – 0.8502)<br>p =0.7770<br>p = 0.0001* | 0.7616<br>(0.6742 – 0.8490)<br>reference | 0.7714<br>(0.6842 – 0.8587)<br>p = 0.4943<br>p = 0.0001* | 0.7619<br>(0.6746 – 0.8492)<br>p =0.9546<br>p = 0.0001* |
| **Calibration** | | | | | | |
| Hosmer Lemeshow | Chi$^2$ = 14.9047<br>p = 0.0610 | Chi$^2$ = 2.7392<br>p = 0.9496 | Chi$^2$ = 13.3978<br>p = 0.0989 | Chi$^2$ = 13.884<br>p = 0.0847 | Chi$^2$ = 10.8764<br>p = 0.2088 | Chi$^2$ = 12.4194<br>p = 0.1334 |
| Brier Score | 0.1560 | 0.1423 | 0.1559 | 0.1941 | 0.1875 | 0.1938 |
| AIC | 280.037 | 273.881 | 281.787 | 457.352 | 453.321 | 459.346 |
| BIC | 299.654 | 294.899 | 302.805 | 484.398 | 482.298 | 488.324 |
| Likelihood ratio | reference | p = 0.0043 | p = 0.6171 | reference | p = 0.0141 | p = 0.9383 |
| **Reclassification** | | | | | | |
| IDI | reference | +0.0703<br>(-0.0010 to 0.1417)<br>p = 0.0534 | +0.0004<br>(-0.0036 to +0.0044)<br>p = 0.8515 | reference | +0.0269<br>(-0.0054 to 0.0592)<br>p = 0.1028 | +0.0017<br>(-0.0051 to +0.0085)<br>p = 0.6228 |
| NRI – all | reference | +0.2740<br>(-0.1386 to 0.6866)<br>p = 0.1931 | +0.1854<br>(-0.2273 to +0.5980)<br>p = 0.3787 | reference | +0.0700<br>(-0.2908 to 0.4309)<br>p = 0.7037 | +0.0011<br>(-0.3597 to +0.3620)<br>p = 0.9951 |
| NRI - AHF-RH | reference | -0.0667<br>(-0.4245 to 0.2912)<br>p = 0.7150 | -0.1333<br>(-0.4912 to 0.2245)<br>p = 0.4652 | reference | -0.2157<br>(-0.4901 to 0.0588)<br>p = 0.1235 | +0.3726<br>(0.0981 to 0.6470)<br>p = 0.0078 |
| NRI -no AHF-RH | reference | -0.3407<br>(-0.5461 to -0.1352)<br>p = 0.0012 | -0.3187<br>(-0.5242 to -0.1132)<br>p = 0.0024 | reference | -0.2857<br>(-0.5200 to -0.0514)<br>p = 0.0168 | 0.3714<br>(0.1372 to 0.6057)<br>p = 0.0019 |

Reference model includes age, sex, coronary artery disease, left ventricular function, NYHA functional class, diabetes mellitus, creatinine, ACEI or ARB treatment, beta blocker treatment, sodium, hemoglobin, NT-proBNP.
AIC = Akaike information criterion; BIC = Bayesian information criterion; IDI = integrated discrimation imrovement; NRI = net reclassification improvement. Definitions of statistical measures see methods section. Values in brackets are 95% confidence intervals (CI).
P values indicate differences versus the reference model (p<0.05 statistically significant, or p<0.01 statistical trend).
*P-values indicate level of significance of C-statistics referring to each individual model.
Yellow boxes indicate improvements, blue boxes indicate best improvements compared to reference models.

**Fig. 5** Performance of models for all-cause mortality (*top*) and AHF-related rehopitalization (*bottom*) at 1 and 5 years in AHF patients ($n = 122$)

all. Additional costs due to the implementation of a new prognostic biomarkers can only be justified by an improvement of clinical outcomes themselves [23, 48, 49].

Based on our findings, the prognostic value of hFABP next to troponin I and NT-proBNP testing might identify those patients with an increased risk of upcoming AHF related rehospitalization or death. Within the present study, it was demonstrated that prognosis of all-cause mortality was better reclassified according to improved net reclassification improvements (NRI) due to additional measurements of TnI. Interestingly, patients without a future AHF related rehospitalization were more correctly reclassified due to additional measurements of hFABP. Each unit increase of hFABP by 10 ng/ml being measured only once in the emergency department was associated with a 2 % increase of all-cause mortality and 3–7 % increase of AHF related rehospitalization risk at 5 years. All prognostic models were calculated to current state-of-the-art statistics in order to receive valuable generalizing results [23, 39–41].

Therefore, our findings might help to further improve risk stratification of patients being suspected of AHF in order to reduce heart failure related mortality, readmissions and possibly health care costs after an initial emergency presentation and in-hospital treatment because of AHF [47, 48, 50, 51].

## Study limitations

The present study was conducted as a post-hoc non-randomized single-center study. The primary inclusion criteria have been patients presenting with acute dyspnea

**Table 3** Multivariable Cox Regression analyses for all-cause mortality and AHF related rehospitalization at 5 years in all patients ($n = 401$)

| | All-cause mortality | | | | | | AHF-related reospitalization | | | | | |
|---|---|---|---|---|---|---|---|---|---|---|---|---|
| | hFABP | | | Troponin I | | | hFABP | | | Troponin I | | |
| | HR | 95 % CI | *p* Value | HR | 95 % CI | *p* Value | HR | 95 % CI | *p* Value | HR | 95 % CI | *p* Value |
| Age | 1.033 | 1.016–1.050 | **0.001** | 1.036 | 1.019–1.054 | **0.001** | 1.012 | 0.989–1.034 | 0.301 | 1.012 | 0.989–1.034 | 0.296 |
| Sex | 1.261 | 0.844–1.884 | 0.259 | 1.193 | 0.788–1.804 | 0.405 | 1.012 | 0.593–1.726 | 0.966 | 0.989 | 0.574–1.705 | 0.968 |
| NYHA functional class | 1.107 | 0.826–1.485 | 0.496 | 1.091 | 0.816–1.458 | 0.556 | 1.799 | 1.257–2.576 | **0.001** | 1.765 | 1.236–2.519 | **0.002** |
| Left ventricular function | 1.227 | 0.964–1.562 | 0.096 | 1.267 | 0.993–1.616 | 0.057 | 1.013 | 0.756–1.359 | 0.930 | 0.995 | 0.745–1.329 | 0.973 |
| Coronary artery disease | 0.843 | 0.555–1.280 | 0.422 | 0.907 | 0.595–1.380 | 0.648 | 1.438 | 0.824–2.509 | 0.201 | 1.469 | 0.839–2.569 | 0.178 |
| Diabetes mellitus | 1.194 | 0.798–1.786 | 0.389 | 1.113 | 0.747–1.660 | 0.598 | 1.757 | 1.056–2.924 | **0.030** | 1.623 | 0.979–2.693 | 0.061 |
| Creatinine (mg/dl) | 0.783 | 0.470–1.305 | 0.348 | 0.849 | 0.515–1.398 | 0.519 | 0.797 | 0.414–1.533 | 0.496 | 0.859 | 0.451–1.636 | 0.643 |
| Sodium (mmol/l) | 0.974 | 0.939–1.011 | 0.160 | 0.976 | 0.941–1.012 | 0.183 | 1.039 | 0.978–1.104 | 0.212 | 1.039 | 0.978–1.103 | 0.218 |
| Hemoglobin (g/dl) | 0.860 | 0.776–0.954 | **0.005** | 0.868 | 0.782–0.962 | **0.007** | 1.000 | 0.874–1.145 | 0.997 | 0.996 | 0.870–1.141 | 0.957 |
| ACEI / ARB treatment | 0.707 | 0.478–1.045 | 0.082 | 0.714 | 0.484–1.052 | 0.089 | 1.647 | 0.969–2.799 | 0.066 | 1.651 | 0.967–2.820 | 0.066 |
| Beta-blocker treatment | 0.844 | 0.559–1.275 | 0.421 | 0.853 | 0.567–1.282 | 0.443 | 1.066 | 0.629–1.805 | 0.813 | 1.044 | 0.616–1.769 | 0.873 |
| LogNT-proBNP (ng/l) | 1.445 | 1.254–1.665 | **0.001** | 1.525 | 1.325–1.755 | **0.001** | 1.209 | 0.993–1.472 | 0.058 | 1.251 | 1.027–1.523 | **0.026** |
| hFABP (10 ng/ml) | 1.020 | 1.020–0.998 | 0.081 | - | - | - | 1.034 | 1.001–1.069 | **0.047** | - | - | - |
| Troponin I (µg/l) | - | - | - | 0.857 | 0.696–1.057 | 0.148 | - | - | - | 0.982 | 0.914–1.055 | 0.620 |

The logarithmic function of NT-proBNP and hFABP per every 10 ng/ml change were used in Cox Models. Significant p values (*p*<0.05) are written in bold type.
Dashes indicate non applicable
*HR* hazard ratio, *CI* confidence interval

**Table 4** Multivariable Cox Regression analyses for all-cause mortality and AHF related rehospitalization at 5 years in AHF patients ($n = 122$)

| | All-cause mortality | | | | | | AHF-related reospitalization | | | | | |
|---|---|---|---|---|---|---|---|---|---|---|---|---|
| | hFABP | | | Troponin I | | | hFABP | | | Troponin I | | |
| | HR | 95 % CI | *p* Value | HR | 95 % CI | *p* Value | HR | 95 % CI | *p* Value | HR | 95 % CI | *p* Value |
| Age | 1.056 | 1.025–1.088 | **0.001** | 1.060 | 1.029–1.092 | **0.001** | 1.027 | 0.997–1.058 | 0.079 | 1.032 | 1.002–1.062 | **0.039** |
| Sex | 1.096 | 0.573–2.098 | 0.783 | 0.657 | 0.317–1.362 | 0.259 | 1.354 | 0.651–2.815 | 0.418 | 1.548 | 0.742–3.230 | 0.244 |
| NYHA functional class | 0.942 | 0.619–1.433 | 0.780 | 0.501 | 0.075–3.333 | 0.475 | 1.610 | 1.001–2.592 | **0.049** | 0.798 | 0.059–10.61 | 0.864 |
| Left ventricular function | 1.263 | 0.926–1.724 | 0.141 | 1.450 | 1.040–2.021 | **0.028** | 1.227 | 0.875–1.720 | 0.236 | 1.167 | 0.836–1.628 | 0.364 |
| Coronary artery disease | 0.812 | 0.423–1.561 | 0.532 | 0.893 | 0.461–1.727 | 0.736 | 1.140 | 0.559–2.323 | 0.718 | 1.133 | 0.558–2.302 | 0.731 |
| Diabetes mellitus | 1.163 | 0.622–2.178 | 0.635 | 1.172 | 0.625–2.198 | 0.620 | 1.324 | 0.682–2.570 | 0.408 | 1.202 | 0.623–2.317 | 0.584 |
| Creatinine (mg/dl) | 0.952 | 0.463–1.954 | 0.892 | 1.234 | 0.597–2.547 | 0.571 | 0.400 | 0.159–1.003 | 0.051 | 0.448 | 0.187–1.073 | 0.072 |
| Sodium (mmol/l) | 0.978 | 0.920–1.039 | 0.463 | 0.967 | 0.910–1.026 | 0.264 | 1.113 | 1.023–1.211 | **0.013** | 1.123 | 1.030–1.225 | **0.008** |
| Hemoglobin (g/dl) | 0.836 | 0.701–0.998 | 0.047 | 0.827 | 0.694–0.986 | 0.034 | 0.949 | 0.792–1.139 | 0.576 | 0.934 | 0.780–1.117 | 0.453 |
| ACEI/ARB treatment | 0.919 | 0.498–1.701 | 0.790 | 1.005 | 0.544–1.859 | 0.987 | 1.425 | 0.722–2.812 | 0.307 | 1.501 | 0.758–2.974 | 0.244 |
| Beta-blocker treatment | 0.895 | 0.488–1.644 | 0.721 | 0.826 | 0.451–1.511 | 0.535 | 1.387 | 0.704–2.732 | 0.345 | 1.550 | 0.795–3.023 | 0.198 |
| LogNT-proBNP (ng/l) | 1.207 | 0.911–1.601 | 0.190 | 1.324 | 0.997–1.757 | 0.052 | 0.911 | 0.696–1.192 | 0.496 | 1.015 | 0.780–1.320 | 0.912 |
| hFABP (10 ng/ml) | 0.996 | 0.948–1.047 | 0.873 | - | - | - | 1.073 | 1.018–1.132 | **0.008** | - | - | - |
| Troponin I (µg/l) | - | - | - | 0.789 | 0.567–1.071 | 0.125 | - | - | - | 0.982 | 0.914–1.055 | 0.620 |

The logarithmic function of NT-proBNP and hFABP per every 10 ng/ml change were used in Cox Models. Significant p values (p<0.05) are written in bold type.
Dashes indicate non applicable
*HR* hazard ratio, *CI* confidence interval

and/or peripheral edema to the emergency department. AHF diagnosis was only made by one independent cardiologist as stated, while a triple panelist approach might have further increased the validity of AHF diagnosis [29]. Initial medical heart failure treatment (e.g. by nitrates and diuretics) might have influenced hemodynamic changes, the relief of clinical symptoms and heart function over time. Evaluable echocardiographic examinations were available in 210 of 401 patients with a median of 3 days after the inital emergency department presentation [30]. Assessment of hFABP performance in patients with HFpEF versus HFrEF has been beyond the scope of the present analysis. Patients with a history of cerebrovascular diseases (CVA or TIA) and atrial fibrillation were not excluded and might have influenced the range of hFABP levels. Cardiovascular mortality was not evaluated as a prognostic outcome in the present trial. Only index-hospital AHF-related rehospitalization was assessed. Competing AHF related rehospitalization at other hospitals was not evaluated. Prognostic event rates might have been under-estimated and might not reflect the complete clinical reality. Evaluating our results with ultra-sensitive troponin methods may allow better diagnostic and prognostic results compared to the contemporary TnI assay being used in this study. Notably, hFABP was measured by a manual, not standardized immunoassay, which might be time consuming and not cost effective in current clinical practice, as there is no automated bedside test currently available on the market. The diagnostic and prognostic values of hFABP, as well as its standardized and cost-effective measurement need to be confirmed by ongoing medical research within larger prospective clinical studies with AHF patients specifically taking into account the above mentioned limitations.

## Conclusions

Taken together, this post-hoc analysis demonstrates that (1) additional hFABP measurements improved diagnostic specificity of sole NT-proBNP testing at the cutoff <300 ng/l to "rule out" AHF. (2) In prognostic models containing 11 conventional risk factors plus NT-proBNP, hFABP mostly improved prognostic models for AHF-related rehospitalization at 1 and 5 years, whereas troponin I mostly improved prognostic models for all-cause mortality.

### Competing interests

The authors declare that they have no competing interests.

### Authors' contributions

UH conceived the study, participated in its design and coordination, participated in data analysis and interpretation and helped to draft and revise the manuscript for important intellectual content. All authors read and approved the final manuscript. FE carried out the immunoassays, performed statistical analysis, participated in data analysis and interpretation and helped to draft the manuscript. CW performed statistical analysis, participated in data analysis and interpretation and helped to draft and revise the manuscript for important intellectual content. PAN participated in the study design and coordination, data acquisition and analysis, carried out the immunoassays and helped to draft the manuscript. SL carried out the immunoassays, performed statistical analysis, participated in data analysis and interpretation, and helped to draft and revise the manuscript for important intellectual content. MBr conceived the study, participated in its design and coordination, participated in interpretation of data and critically revised the manuscript for important intellectual content. IA participated in the study design and coordination and helped to draft and revise the manuscript for important intellectual content. MN conceived the study, participated in its design and coordination, as well as data acquisition and revised the manuscript for important intelectual content. MBo participated in the study design and coordination, as well as data acquisition and revised the manuscript. MBe conceived the study, participated in its design and coordination, performed statistical analysis, participated in data analysis and interpretation and drafted the manuscript. All authors read and approved the final manuscript.

### Authors' information

Martina Brueckmann is an employee of Boehringer Ingelheim GmbH & Co. KG and a lecturer being associated to the Faculty of Medicine Mannheim, University of Heidelberg.

### Acknowledgements

Supported by the DZHK (Deutsches Zentrum für Herz-Kreislauf-Forschung–German Centre for Cardiovascular Research) and by the BMBF (German Ministry of Education and Research). None of the authors received any funding with respect to study design, collection, analysis, interpretation of data, writing of the manuscript or decision to submit the manuscript for publication.

### Author details

[1]First Department of Medicine, University Medical Centre Mannheim (UMM), Faculty of Medicine Mannheim, University of Heidelberg, Theodor-Kutzer-Ufer 1-3, 68167 Mannheim, Germany. [2]Department of Statistical Analysis, Faculty of Medicine Mannheim, University of Heidelberg, Mannheim, Germany. [3]Institute for Microbiology and Laboratory Medicine, HELIOS Klinikum Wuppertal, University of Witten/Herdecke, Wuppertal, Germany. [4]Boehringer Ingelheim GmbH & Co. KG, Ingelheim am Rhein, Germany. [5]Faculty of Medicine Mannheim, University of Heidelberg, Mannheim, Germany. [6]Institute for Clinical Chemistry, University Medical Centre Mannheim (UMM), Faculty of Medicine Mannheim, University of Heidelberg, Mannheim, Germany.

### References

1. Offner GD, Brecher P, Sawlivich WB, Costello CE, Troxler RF. Characterization and amino acid sequence of a fatty acid-binding protein from human heart. Biochem J. 1988;252(1):191–8.
2. Glatz JF, van der Vusse GJ. Nomenclature of fatty acid-binding proteins. Mol Cell Biochem. 1990;98(1–2):231–5.
3. Fournier NC, Richard MA. Role of fatty acid-binding protein in cardiac fatty acid oxidation. Mol Cell Biochem. 1990;98(1–2):149–59.
4. Alhadi HA, Fox KA. Do we need additional markers of myocyte necrosis: the potential value of heart fatty-acid-binding protein. QJM. 2004;97(4):187–98.
5. Smathers RL, Petersen DR. The human fatty acid-binding protein family: evolutionary divergences and functions. Hum Genomics. 2011;5(3):170–91.
6. Jones RM, Prasad MR, Das DK. Modulation of fatty acid-binding capacity of heart fatty acid-binding protein by oxygen-derived free radicals. Mol Cell Biochem. 1990;98(1–2):161–6.
7. Samanta A, Das DK, Jones R, George A, Prasad MR. Free radical scavenging by myocardial fatty acid binding protein. Free Radic Res Commun. 1989;7(2):73–82.
8. Otaki Y, Watanabe T, Takahashi H, Hirayama A, Narumi T, Kadowaki S, et al. Association of heart-type fatty acid-binding protein with cardiovascular risk factors and all-cause mortality in the general population: the Takahata study. PLoS One. 2014;9(5):e94834.
9. Wolfrum C, Borrmann CM, Borchers T, Spener F. Fatty acids and hypolipidemic drugs regulate peroxisome proliferator-activated receptors alpha-and gamma-mediated gene expression via liver fatty acid binding protein: a signaling path to the nucleus. Proc Natl Acad Sci U S A. 2001;98(5):2323–8.

10. Azzazy HM, Pelsers MM, Christenson RH. Unbound free fatty acids and heart-type fatty acid-binding protein: diagnostic assays and clinical applications. Clin Chem. 2006;52(1):19–29.
11. Colli A, Josa M, Pomar JL, Mestres CA, Gherli T. Heart fatty acid binding protein in the diagnosis of myocardial infarction: where do we stand today? Cardiology. 2007;108(1):4–10.
12. van der Vusse GJ, Glatz JF, Stam HC. Myocardial fatty acid homeostasis. Mol Cell Biochem. 1989;88(1–2):1–6.
13. Storch J, McDermott L. Structural and functional analysis of fatty acid-binding proteins. J Lipid Res. 2009;50(Suppl):S126–31.
14. Storch J, Thumser AE. Tissue-specific functions in the fatty acid-binding protein family. J Biol Chem. 2010;285(43):32679–83.
15. Dekker MS, Mosterd A, Van'tHof AW, Hoes AW. Novel biochemical markers in suspected acute coronary syndrome: systematic review and critical appraisal. Heart. 2010;96(13):1001–10.
16. Bruins Slot MH, Reitsma JB, Rutten FH, Hoes AW, van der Heijden GJ. Heart-type fatty acid-binding protein in the early diagnosis of acute myocardial infarction: a systematic review and meta-analysis. Heart. 2010;96(24):1957–63.
17. Kim KS, Lee HJ, Kim K, Jo YH, Kim TY, Lee JH, et al. Heart-type fatty acid binding protein as an adjunct to cardiac troponin-I for the diagnosis of myocardial infarction. J Korean Med Sci. 2011;26(1):47–52.
18. Lippi G, Mattiuzzi C, Cervellin G. Critical review and meta-analysis on the combination of heart-type fatty acid binding protein (H-FABP) and troponin for early diagnosis of acute myocardial infarction. Clin Biochem. 2013;46(1–2):26–30.
19. McMahon CG, Lamont JV, Curtin E, McConnell RI, Crockard M, Kurth MJ, et al. Diagnostic accuracy of heart-type fatty acid-binding protein for the early diagnosis of acute myocardial infarction. Am J Emerg Med. 2012;30(2):267–74.
20. Reiter M, Twerenbold R, Reichlin T, Mueller M, Hoeller R, Moehring B, et al. Heart-type fatty acid-binding protein in the early diagnosis of acute myocardial infarction. Heart. 2013;99(10):708–14.
21. Kilcullen N, Viswanathan K, Das R, Morrell C, Farrin A, Barth JH, et al. Heart-type fatty acid-binding protein predicts long-term mortality after acute coronary syndrome and identifies high-risk patients across the range of troponin values. J Am Coll Cardiol. 2007;50(21):2061–7.
22. Viswanathan K, Kilcullen N, Morrell C, Thistlethwaite SJ, Sivananthan MU, Hassan TB, et al. Heart-type fatty acid-binding protein predicts long-term mortality and re-infarction in consecutive patients with suspected acute coronary syndrome who are troponin-negative. J Am Coll Cardiol. 2010;55(23):2590–8.
23. Hlatky MA, Greenland P, Arnett DK, Ballantyne CM, Criqui MH, Elkind MS, et al. Criteria for evaluation of novel markers of cardiovascular risk: a scientific statement from the American Heart Association. Circulation. 2009;119(17):2408–16.
24. Thygesen K, Mair J, Mueller C, Huber K, Weber M, Plebani M, et al. Recommendations for the use of natriuretic peptides in acute cardiac care: a position statement from the Study Group on Biomarkers in Cardiology of the ESC Working Group on Acute Cardiac Care. Eur Heart J. 2012;33(16):2001–6.
25. Sun YP, Wang WD, Ma SC, Wang LY, Qiao LY, Zhang LP. [Changes of heart-type fatty acid-binding protein in children with chronic heart failure and its significance]. Zhongguo Dang Dai Er Ke Za Zhi. 2013;15(2):99–101.
26. Liu M, Zhou M, Bao Y, Xu Z, Li H, Zhang H, et al. Circulating adipocyte fatty acid-binding protein levels are independently associated with heart failure. Clin Sci (Lond). 2013;124(2):115–22.
27. Djousse L, Bartz TM, Ix JH, Kochar J, Kizer JR, Gottdiener JS, et al. Fatty acid-binding protein 4 and incident heart failure: the Cardiovascular Health Study. Eur J Heart Fail. 2013;15(4):394–9.
28. Wang WD, Sun YP, Cui XQ. [Serum levels of fatty acid-binding protein and brain natriuretic peptide in children with pneumonia complicated by acute congestive heart failure]. Zhongguo Dang Dai Er Ke Za Zhi. 2008;10(3):304–6.
29. Behnes M, Brueckmann M, Ahmad-Nejad P, Lang S, Wolpert C, Elmas E, et al. Diagnostic performance and cost effectiveness of measurements of plasma N-terminal pro brain natriuretic peptide in patients presenting with acute dyspnea or peripheral edema. Int J Cardiol. 2009;135(2):165–74.
30. Behnes M, Lang S, Breithardt OA, Kaden JJ, Haghi D, Ahmad-Nejad P, et al. Association of NT-proBNP with severity of heart valve disease in a medical patient population presenting with acute dyspnea or peripheral edema. J Heart Valve Dis. 2008;17(5):557–65.
31. McMurray JJ, Adamopoulos S, Anker SD, Auricchio A, Bohm M, Dickstein K, et al. ESC Guidelines for the diagnosis and treatment of acute and chronic heart failure 2012: The Task Force for the Diagnosis and Treatment of Acute and Chronic Heart Failure 2012 of the European Society of Cardiology. Developed in collaboration with the Heart Failure Association (HFA) of the ESC. Eur Heart J. 2012;33(14):1787–847.
32. Swedberg K, Cleland J, Dargie H, Drexler H, Follath F, Komajda M, et al. Guidelines for the diagnosis and treatment of chronic heart failure: executive summary (update 2005): The Task Force for the Diagnosis and Treatment of Chronic Heart Failure of the European Society of Cardiology. Eur Heart J. 2005;26(11):1115–40.
33. Hunt SA, Abraham WT, Chin MH, Feldman AM, Francis GS, Ganiats TG, et al. 2009 focused update incorporated into the ACC/AHA 2005 Guidelines for the Diagnosis and Management of Heart Failure in Adults: a report of the American College of Cardiology Foundation/American Heart Association Task Force on Practice Guidelines: developed in collaboration with the International Society for Heart and Lung Transplantation. Circulation. 2009;119(14):e391–479.
34. Nagueh SF, Appleton CP, Gillebert TC, Marino PN, Oh JK, Smiseth OA, et al. Recommendations for the evaluation of left ventricular diastolic function by echocardiography. Eur J Echocardiogr. 2009;10(2):165–93.
35. hFABP ELISA EA-0305; available online at: http://www.signosisinc.com/.
36. Pelsers MM, Hermens WT, Glatz JF. Fatty acid-binding proteins as plasma markers of tissue injury. Clin Chim Acta. 2005;352(1–2):15–35.
37. Apple FS, Collinson PO, Biomarkers ITFoCAoC. Analytical characteristics of high-sensitivity cardiac troponin assays. Clin Chem. 2012;58(1):54–61.
38. Hanley JA, McNeil BJ. A method of comparing the areas under receiver operating characteristic curves derived from the same cases. Radiology. 1983;148(3):839–43.
39. Bayes-Genis A, de Antonio M, Vila J, Penafiel J, Galan A, Barallat J, et al. Head-to-head comparison of 2 myocardial fibrosis biomarkers for long-term heart failure risk stratification: ST2 versus galectin-3. J Am Coll Cardiol. 2014;63(2):158–66.
40. Cook NR. Use and misuse of the receiver operating characteristic curve in risk prediction. Circulation. 2007;115(7):928–35.
41. Cook NR. Methods for evaluating novel biomarkers–a new paradigm. Int J Clin Pract. 2010;64(13):1723–7.
42. Pencina MJ, D'Agostino Sr RB, D'Agostino Jr RB, Vasan RS. Evaluating the added predictive ability of a new marker: from area under the ROC curve to reclassification and beyond. Stat Med. 2008;27(2):157–72. discussion 207-12.
43. Niizeki T, Takeishi Y, Arimoto T, Nozaki N, Hirono O, Watanabe T, et al. Persistently increased serum concentration of heart-type fatty acid-binding protein predicts adverse clinical outcomes in patients with chronic heart failure. Circ J. 2008;72(1):109–14.
44. Niizeki T, Takeishi Y, Arimoto T, Okuyama H, Takabatake N, Tachibana H, et al. Serum heart-type fatty acid binding protein predicts cardiac events in elderly patients with chronic heart failure. J Cardiol. 2005;46(1):9–15.
45. Niizeki T, Takeishi Y, Arimoto T, Takabatake N, Nozaki N, Hirono O, et al. Heart-type fatty acid-binding protein is more sensitive than troponin T to detect the ongoing myocardial damage in chronic heart failure patients. J Card Fail. 2007;13(2):120–7.
46. Kociol RD, Pang PS, Gheorghiade M, Fonarow GC, O'Connor CM, Felker GM. Troponin elevation in heart failure prevalence, mechanisms, and clinical implications. J Am Coll Cardiol. 2010;56(14):1071–8.
47. Butler J, Kalogeropoulos A. Hospital strategies to reduce heart failure readmissions: where is the evidence? J Am Coll Cardiol. 2012;60(7):615–7.
48. Kalogeropoulos AP, Georgiopoulou VV, Butler J. Clinical adoption of prognostic biomarkers: the case for heart failure. Prog Cardiovasc Dis. 2012;55(1):3–13.
49. Roger VL, Go AS, Lloyd-Jones DM, Benjamin EJ, Berry JD, Borden WB, et al. Heart disease and stroke statistics–2012 update: a report from the American Heart Association. Circulation. 2012;125(1):e2–220.
50. Behnes M, Brueckmann M, Lang S, Espeter F, Weiss C, Neumaier M, et al. Diagnostic and prognostic value of osteopontin in patients with acute congestive heart failure. Eur J Heart Fail. 2013;15(12):1390–400.
51. Behnes M, Brueckmann M, Lang S, Weiss C, Ahmad-Nejad P, Neumaier M, et al. Connective tissue growth factor (CTGF/CCN2): diagnostic and prognostic value in acute heart failure. Clin Res Cardiol. 2014;103(2):107–16.

# Solitary accessory and papillary muscle hypertrophy manifested as dynamic mid-wall obstruction and symptomatic heart failure: diagnostic feasibility by multi-modality imaging

Kuo-Tzu Sung[1], Chun-Ho Yun[2,3], Charles Jia-Yin Hou[1,3] and Chung-Lieh Hung[1,3,4*]

**Abstract**

**Background:** Solitary papillary muscle (PM) hypertrophy is an unique type of hypertrophic cardiomyopathy (HCM), which is characterized by predominant papillary muscle hypertrophy sparing the rest of other left ventricular segments. It has recently drawn our attention about the mechanism of left ventricular mid-cavity obstruction and the influence of pressure gradient in the left ventricular outflow tract (LVOT), thus carries clinical importance.

**Case presentation:** We reported a symptomatic, 83-year-old woman who presented with dynamic, high resting left ventricle (LV) mid-wall gradient without obvious septal hypertrophy or systolic anterior motion (SAM). Subsequent real-time (RT) three-dimensional echocardiography (3DE) and cardiac magnetic resonance imaging (MRI) demonstrated large, hypertrophic accessory papillary muscles squeezing mid-cavity of left ventricle producing dynamic pressure gradient during systole in the absence of left ventricular wall anomalies.

**Conclusion:** We proposed that combined use of echocardiography particularly RT-3DE and cardiac magnetic resonance imaging (MRI) can accurately identify this specific type of hypertrophic cardiomyopathy without remarkable traditional features.

**Keywords:** Solitary papillary muscle hypertrophy, LVOT obstruction, Hypertrophic cardiomyopathy

## Background

Hypertrophic obstructive cardiomyopathy (HOCM) refers to those subjects with significant dynamic left ventricular outflow tract (LVOT) obstruction due to mechanical causes, with most presents with asymmetrical septal hypertrophy resulting in dynamic systolic anterior motion (SAM) of mitral leaflets [1].

Solitary papillary muscle (PM) hypertrophy, a peculiar form of HCM manifested as predominant PM hypertrophy sparing the rest of other LV segments, has recently gained much attention owing to its mechanical consequences on left ventricular outflow tract (LVOT) pressure gradient formation [2,3].

## Case presentation

A 83-year-old woman with history of hypertension and hyperlipidemia. The blood pressure and hyperlipidemia were well-controlled with medication. She was admitted to our hospital with chest pain on effort and exertional shortness of breath. Her vital sign was stable with blood pressure 131/70 mmHg and heart rate 67 beats per minute at initial presentation. A mid-systolic ejection murmur was heard along the left sternal border with chest X-ray showed minor pulmonary congestion. Incidental high resting LV mid-wall pressure gradient (86 mmHg, Figure 1A) was shown by 2-dimensional echocardiography without LV septal wall thickness (8.5 mm). The LV end-diastolic volume was 90 ml, and LV end-systolic volume was 27 ml. Apparently hypertrophied anterolateral (A) and posteromedial (P) papillary muscles together with a large, third accessory PM were observed (Figure 1C). Neither aortic stenosis nor SAM was observed. Complete ECG disclosed obvious U wave

* Correspondence: jotaro3791@gmail.com
[1]Division of Cardiology, Department of Internal Medicine, Mackay Memorial Hospital, Taipei, Taiwan
[3]Department of Medicine, Mackay Medical College, and Mackay Medicine, Nursing and Management College, Taipei, Taiwan
Full list of author information is available at the end of the article

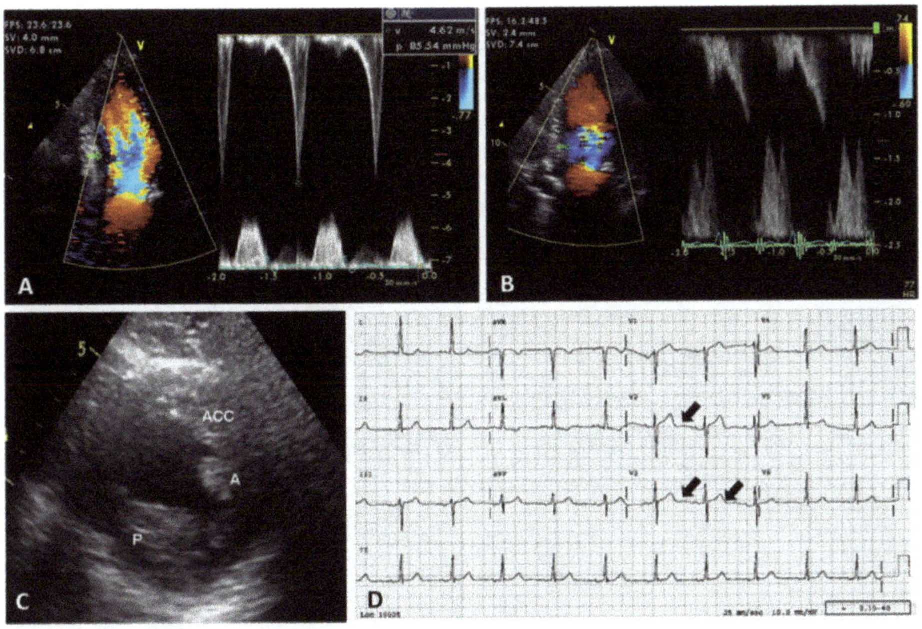


**Figure 1 2D Echocardiography and complete ECG. (A)** Continuous wave Doppler tracing of the LV mid-wall showed the peak pressure gradient was 85.5 mmHg at rest. **(B)** Subsequent continuous wave Doppler tracing eight hours later showed normal pressure gradient (estimated to be 5 mmHg). **(C)** In short axis view, apparently hypertrophied anterolateral and posteromedial papillary muscles together with a large, third accessory PM were observed (A: anterolateral papillary muscle, P: posteromedial papillary muscle, ACC: accessory papillary muscle). **(D)** Complete ECG showed prominent U wave in V1-V4.

(V1-V4) with normal QT interval (416ms, Figure 1D). Blood level of B-natriuretic peptide was obviously elevated (227 pg/ml).

Repeated 2D transthoracic echocardiogram during hospitalization revealed no more pressure gradient (plummeted to 5 mmHg) after holding diuretics (Figure 1B). Meanwhile, she was in euvolemic state with blood pressure 128/76 mmHg and heart rate 62 beats per minute. To further clarify the spatial relationships between these hypertrophied PMs and other LV wall segments, real-time 3D echocardiography (RT-3DE) was performed and showed nearly complete LV mid-wall cavity obliteration by the these morphological abnormal PMs during end-systolic phase (Figure 2A-B; Additional files 1, 2 and 3). Subsequent MRI study demonstrated normal LV volume (end-diastolic volume: 71.9 ml), unremarkable LV wall abnormalities, normal global LV mass index (79.9 gm/m$^2$) though significantly hypertrophied PMs (total PM mass: 20.2 gm; 13.4 gm/m$^2$ indexed to body surface area; Figure 2C-D) without visible perfusion defects or delayed hyperenhancement (DHE). High temporal resolution Tissue Doppler Imaging (>250 frames per second) further demonstrated markedly diminished diastolic mitral annulus relaxation velocities (1.8 cm/sec for basoseptal and 4.3 cm/sec for basolateral segments; Figure 2E-F). When PMs mass were taken into account (up to 16.8% LV mass; Figure 3A-B), the total LV mass may reach the echocardiographic criteria for LV hypertrophy [4] (defined as LV mass index >95 gm/m$^2$ in women and > 115 g/m$^2$ in men). Beta-blockade was then prescribed and the symptoms improved drastically during the subsequent follow up.

## Conclusions

So far, left ventricular hypertrophy remained the predominant and major phenotypic component of hypertrophied cardiomyopathy [1]. Few cases of dynamic LVOT or mid-cavity obstruction in relation to various morphological papillary muscle anomalies had been reported before, and these may include bifid [5] or octopus papillary muscle [6], accessory [7], single [2], or solitary papillary muscle hypertrophy [8]. Papillary muscle hypertrophy, when defined by at least one of the two papillary muscles is more than 1.1 cm in either vertical or horizontal diameter, had been recently shown to be a phenotypic variant of HCM [8,9]. Not until recently, morphological papillary muscle anomalies without features of phenotypic LV hypertrophy (isolated papillary muscle hypertrophy) had gradually been recognized to be an uncommon HCM variant [8,10]. The clinical features of LV mid-cavity obstruction caused by papillary muscle hypertrophy may vary greatly from asymptomatic to dyspnea, angina, syncope, and even sudden cardiac death [8-10], with prominent U wave and left ventricular hypertrophy by ECG [11,12], which is concordant with our current case findings.

While HCM subjects with concomitant morphological papillary muscle anomalies may present with

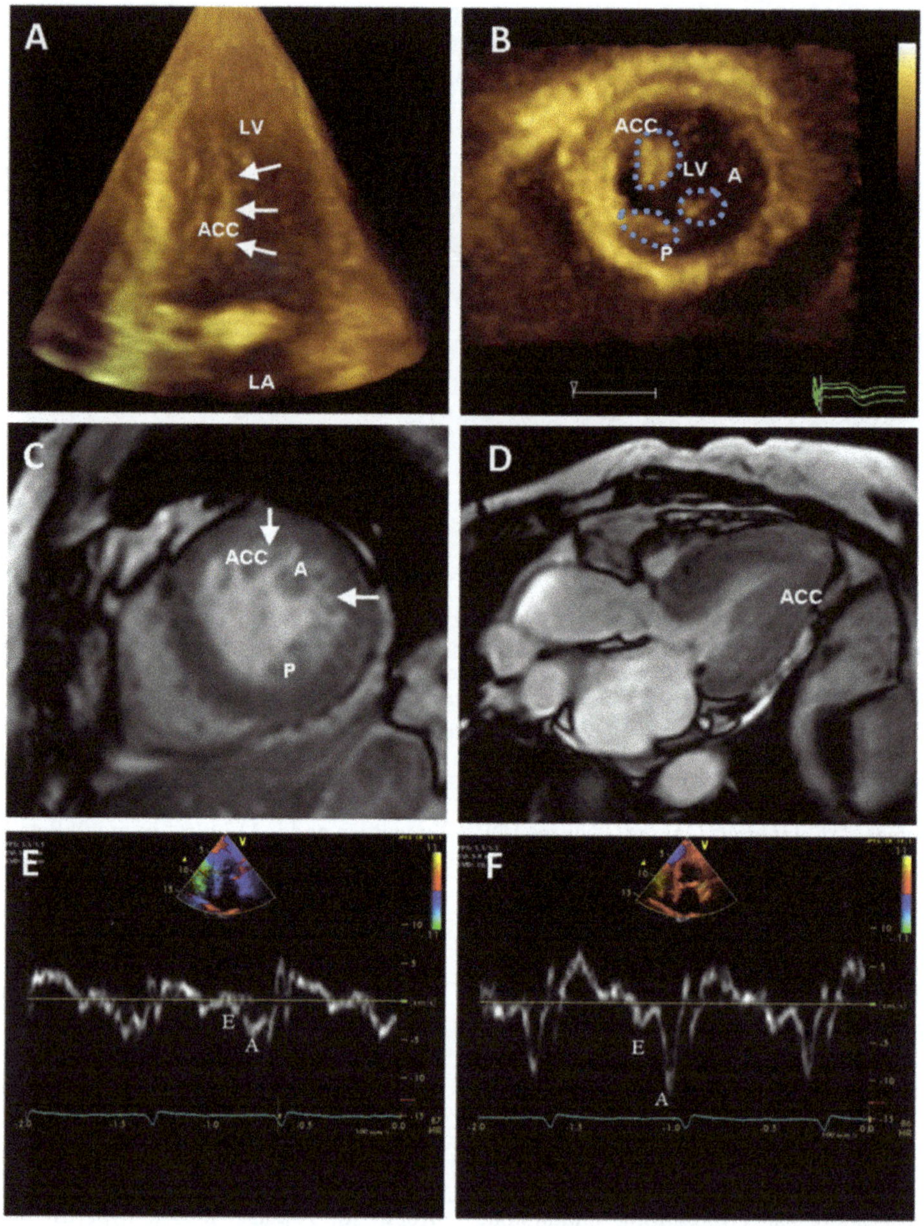


**Figure 2 Real 3D echocardiography, MRI, and tissue doppler imaging. (A)** 2D echocardiogram in the short-axis section of the left ventricle demonstrated uncommonly enlarged papillary muscles (A: anterolateral papillary muscle, P: posteromedial papillary muscle, ACC: accessory papillary muscle). **(B)** Real time 3D Echocardiography demonstrated that LV mid-cavity was almost obliterated during end-systolic phase from five chamber view (Additional file 1, movie 1). A: anterolateral papillary muscle, LA: left atrium, LV: left ventricle. **(C)** Contrast-enhanced MRI from LV short-axis showed two large papillary muscles as well as adjacent abundant muscular trabeculae producing mid-cavity obstruction during systolic phase. **(D)** MRI from long-views showed anterolateral papillary muscle squeezing left ventricular outflow tract against LV septum during systolic phase. High temporal resolution Tissue Doppler Imaging showed markedly diminished diastolic mitral annulus relaxation velocities, 1.8 cm/sec for basoseptal **(E)** and 4.3 cm/sec for basolateral segments **(F)**.

higher degree of resting LVOT gradient [13], it is not surprising that subjects with increasing number of hypertrophied papillary muscles with unchanged ventricular cavity size may have higher probability of causing LV chamber obliteration during systole. So far, there are reports presented with isolated papillary muscle hypertrophy and normal LV wall thickness. Herein, we report a case of morphological papillary muscle anomalies featured by dynamic LV mid-wall obstruction, with subjective exertional chest pain and dyspnea. We further observed in our case that severely impaired LV diastolic function and clinical

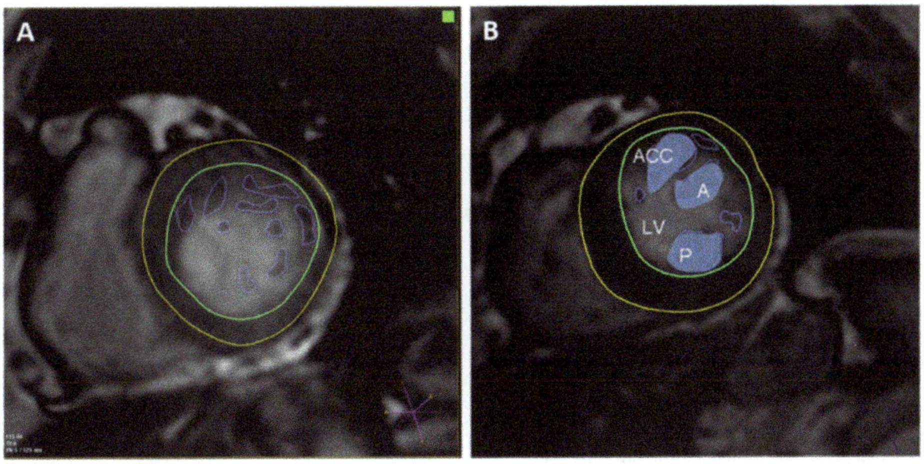


**Figure 3 Cardiac MRI, short axis view. (A)** Unremarkable LV wall abnormality with normal LV mass at end-diastolic phase by MRI; **(B)** Hypertrophy PMs as well as existence of accessory PM (ACC) shown.

heart failure [14] may occur as a consequence of excessive, redundant papillary muscle mass with normal LV mass [7].

Current guidelines for LV mass calculation do not take papillary muscle mass into account, while our relevant findings may suggest include papillary muscles in LV mass assessment, especially for these morphologically abnormal papillary muscle subjects.

Solitary papillary muscle hypertrophy as an uncommon variant form of HCM with coexisted additional, accessory papillary muscle may develop abnormally high resting LV mid-wall pressure gradient without SAM or significant regional LV wall hypertrophy. Cardiac MRI and RT-3DE may have their peculiar roles in uncovering these cardiac morphological/structural anomalies aiming for a more comprehensive analysis on their spatial relationships.

In conclusion, we recommended that for subjects with unusually high LV mid-wall or LVOT pressure gradient with unrevealing regional LV segment anomalies, RT-3DE and MRI should be considered as a screening tool to disclose these under-diagnosed, specific HCM subjects in daily routine.

## Consent

Written informed consent was obtained from the patient for publication of this Case report and any accompanying images. A copy of the written consent is available for review by the Editor-in-Chief of this journal.

### Abbreviations

LV: Left ventricle; RT: Real time; 3DE: three-dimensional echocardiography; MRI: magnetic resonance imaging; PM: Papillary muscle; HCM: Hypertrophic cardiomyopathy; HOCM: Hypertrophic obstructive cardiomyopathy; LVOT: Left ventricular outflow tract; SAM: Systolic anterior motion; DHE: Delayed hyperenhancement.

### Competing interests

The authors declare that they have no competing interests.

### Authors' contributions

KTS was the primary author of the text. CHY assisted in image acquisition and retouching. CLH conceived of the report, provided the images, and modified the manuscript. JYH provided additional supervision. All authors have read and approved the final manuscript.

### Author details

[1]Division of Cardiology, Department of Internal Medicine, Mackay Memorial Hospital, Taipei, Taiwan. [2]Department of Radiology, Mackay Memorial Hospital, Taipei, Taiwan. [3]Department of Medicine, Mackay Medical College, and Mackay Medicine, Nursing and Management College, Taipei, Taiwan. [4]Cardiovascular Medicine, Mackay Memorial Hospital, No. 92, Section 2, Chung Shan North Road, Taipei, Taiwan.

### References

1. Williams LK, Frenneaux MP, Steeds RP: **Echocardiography in hypertrophic cardiomyopathy diagnosis, prognosis, and role in management.** *Eur J Echocardiogr* 2009, **10**:iii9–iii14.
2. Austin BA, Kwon DH, Smedira NG, Thamilarasan M, Lever HM, Desai MY: **Abnormally thickened papillary muscle resulting in dynamic left ventricular outflow tract obstruction: an unusual presentation of hypertrophic cardiomyopathy.** *J Am Soc Echocardiogr* 2009, **22**(105):105–106.
3. Pacileo M, Cirillo P, Prastaro M, Chiariello M: **Latent left ventricular outflow tract obstruction induced by abnormal hypertrophic papillary muscle caused myocardial ischemia.** *Int J Cardiol* 2009, **132**:270–272.
4. Barbieri A, Bursi F, Mantovani F, Valenti C, Quaglia M, Berti E, Marino M, Modena MG: **Left ventricular hypertrophy reclassification and death: application of the Recommendation of the American Society of Echocardiography/European Association of Echocardiography.** *Eur Heart J Cardiovasc Imaging* 2012, **13**:109–117.
5. Ker J: **Bigeminy and the bifid papillary muscle.** *Cardiovasc Ultrasound* 2010, **8**:13.
6. Shah AS, Kukar A, Chaudhry FA, Sherrid MV: **Unusual anomalous single papillary muscle causing symptomatic mid left ventricular cavity obstruction: octopus papillary muscle.** *J Am Soc Echocardiogr* 2006, **19**:939.

7. Harrigan CJ, Appelbaum E, Maron BJ, Buros JL, Gibson CM, Lesser JR, Udelson JE, Manning WJ, Maron MS: **Significance of papillary muscle abnormalities identified by cardiovascular magnetic resonance in hypertrophic cardiomyopathy.** *Am J Cardiol* 2008, **101**:668–673.
8. Kobashi A, Suwa M, Ito T, Otake Y, Hirota Y, Kawamura K: **Solitary papillary muscle hypertrophy as a possible form of hypertrophic cardiomyopathy.** *Jpn Circ J* 1998, **62**:811–816.
9. Maron MS: **Clinical utility of cardiovascular magnetic resonance in hypertrophic cardiomyopathy.** *J Cardiovasc Magn Reson* 2012, **14**:13.
10. Correia AS, Pinho T, Madureira AJ, Araujo V, Maciel MJ: **Isolated papillary muscle hypertrophy: a variant of hypertrophic cardiomyopathy? Do not miss a hypertrophic cardiomyopathy.** *Eur Heart J Cardiovas Imaging* 2013, **14**:296.
11. Ker J: **Solitary papillary muscle hypertrophy: a new echo-electrocardiographic syndrome? A case report.** *Angiology* 2007, **58**:502–503.
12. Patil NP, Katti K: **Unusual papillary muscle hypertrophy in a septuagenarian.** *J Oscul Surg* 2011, **142**:704–705.
13. Kwon DH, Setser RM, Thamilarasan M, Popovic ZV, Smedira NG, Schoenhagen P, Garcia MJ, Lever HM, Desai MY: **Abnormal papillary muscle morphology is independently associated with increased left ventricular outflow tract obstruction in hypertrophic cardiomyopathy.** *Heart* 2008, **94**:1295–1301.
14. Kindermann M: **How to diagnose diastolic heart failure: a consensus statement on the diagnosis of heart failure with normal left ventricular ejection fraction by the Heart Failure and Echocardiography Associations of the European Society of Cardiology.** *Eur Heart J* 2007, **28**:2686. author reply 2686-2687.

# 15

# Efficacy and safety of mineralocorticoid receptor antagonists for patients with heart failure and diabetes mellitus

Meng-Die Chen[1], Si-Si Dong[1], Ning-Yu Cai[2], Meng-Di Fan[1], Su-Ping Gu[1], Jin-Jue Zheng[1], Hai-Min Yin[1], Xin-He Zhou[1], Liang-Xue Wang[1], Chun-Ying Li[1] and Chao Zheng[1*]

**Abstract**

**Background:** The aim of this study was to systematically assess the efficacy and safety of mineralocorticoid receptor antagonists (MRAs) for patients with heart failure (HF) and diabetes mellitus (DM).

**Methods:** We conducted a comprehensive search for controlled studies that evaluated the efficacy and safety of MRAs in patients with DM and HF. Medline, Embase and Cochrane databases were searched. Two reviewers independently identified citations, extracted data and evaluated quality. Risk estimations were abstracted and pooled where appropriate.

**Results:** Four observational studies were included. MRAs use was associated with reduced mortality compared with controls (RR = 0.78; 95 % CI: 0.69–0.88; $I^2 = 0$ %; $P < 0.001$). Increased risk of developing hyperkalaemia was observed in those patients taking MRAs (RR = 1.74; 95 % CI: 1.27–2.38; $I^2 = 0$ %; $P = 0.0005$).

**Conclusions:** The current cumulative evidence suggests that MRAs can improve clinical outcomes but increase the risk of hyperkalaemia in patients with DM and HF.

**Keywords:** Mineralocorticoid receptor antagonists, Heart failure, Diabetes mellitus

## Background

Diabetes mellitus (DM) and heart failure (HF) commonly coexist. About 40 % of hospitalized HF patients have DM, and these figures are expected to grow with the general aging of the population [1]. Results from more than 100,000 patients in the Acute Decompensated Heart Failure National Registry suggested that 44 % of HF patients had DM [2]. Results from a health maintenance organization show that about 12 of 10,000 patients with DM had HF at baseline, and 3.3 % of the rest developed HF during each year of follow-up [3]. There is now a large number of epidemiological and clinical data supporting the strong association between HF and DM [4]. Patients with HF can have insulin resistance, which increases their risk of developing type 2 DM [5]. It was shown in an Italian observational study that 28 % of elderly patients with HF developed new-onset type 2 DM in 3 years and HF is an independent risk factor for type 2 DM (OR 3.3; 95 % CI 2.6–4.0) [6]. Patients with HF are not only at increased risk of developing DM but patients with DM also have a greater probability of developing HF [7]. In patients with DM, every unit increase in glycosylated hemoglobin (HbA1c) is associated with a 10 % to 15 % increased risk of developing HF [8]. Recent literature suggested that co-existence of DM and HF can lead to increased morbidity and mortality [9]. Hospitalized HF patients with DM have an even worse prognosis with increased rates of cardiovascular (CV) mortality and post-discharge HF hospitalization [10]. Recently, a

* Correspondence: wallbb_1022@163.com
[1]Diabetes Center and Department of Endocrinology, The Second Affiliated Hospital of Wenzhou Medical University, No. 109 West Xueyuan Road, 325027, Wenzhou, Zhejiang, China
Full list of author information is available at the end of the article

subgroup analysis of the results indicated that during standard treatment, side effects were most likely to appear in hospitalized HF patients with DM compared to those without DM [11]. Thus, treating coincident HF and DM is still a challenge.

Mineralocorticoid receptor antagonists (MRAs) are powerful treatment agents for patients with cardiovascular disease [12]. Morbidity and mortality benefits from treatment with MRAs have been demonstrated in HF patient and MRAs have become part of standard medical therapy for HF [13, 14]. Similar to HF patients without DM, treatment with MRAs is associated with improved outcomes in patients with DM [15]. However, associated adverse events including hyperkalaemia, gynecomastia, menstrual irregularities, and acute kidney injury can not be ignored [16]. The effects of MRAs on glycaemic control are still uncertain. The results of some studies have demonstrated that spironolactone significantly elevated HbA1c levels or worsened glycaemic control [17, 18], while one study has shown that spironolactone may have a beneficial effect on serum insulin and HOMA-IR in patients with non-alcoholic fatty liver disease [19]. A few studies support the view that MRAs, whether spironolactone or eplerenone, did not have a significant effect on glucose levels [20–22]. Furthermore, results of a small direct comparative trial have shown that spironolactone increased HbA1c in patients with DM and HF, but eplerenone did not [23].

Aldosterone is a mineralocorticoid hormone that activates the apical epithelial sodium channel and the basolateral $Na^+$ /$K^+$ ATPase pump, and controls sodium excretion at the level of the distal tubules to exert an action on sodium homeostasis [24]. However aldosterone can have harmful effects on the cardiovascular system [25]. By blocking the mineralocorticoid receptor in the distal tubule of the kidney, MRAs prevent the activation of sodium channels and lead to diuresis with reduced excretion of potassium [26]. MRAs can prevent vascular inflammation, myocardial fibrosis and ventricular remodelling, and improve endothelial function [14]. HF and DM are characterized by a high level of oxidative stress and it has been reported that MRAs can reduce oxidative stress [18].

A better understanding of the efficacy and safety of MRAs in patients with HF and DM is needed. To date, no meta-analysis has been conducted concerning the relationship between treatment with MRAs and outcomes in those patients. Therefore, it is worth undertaking a systematic review to assess the efficacy and safety of treatment with MRAs in patients with concomitant HF and DM.

## Methods

This systematic review was conducted according to the Preferred Reporting Items for Systematic Reviews and Meta-Analyses (Additional file 1) guidelines [27].

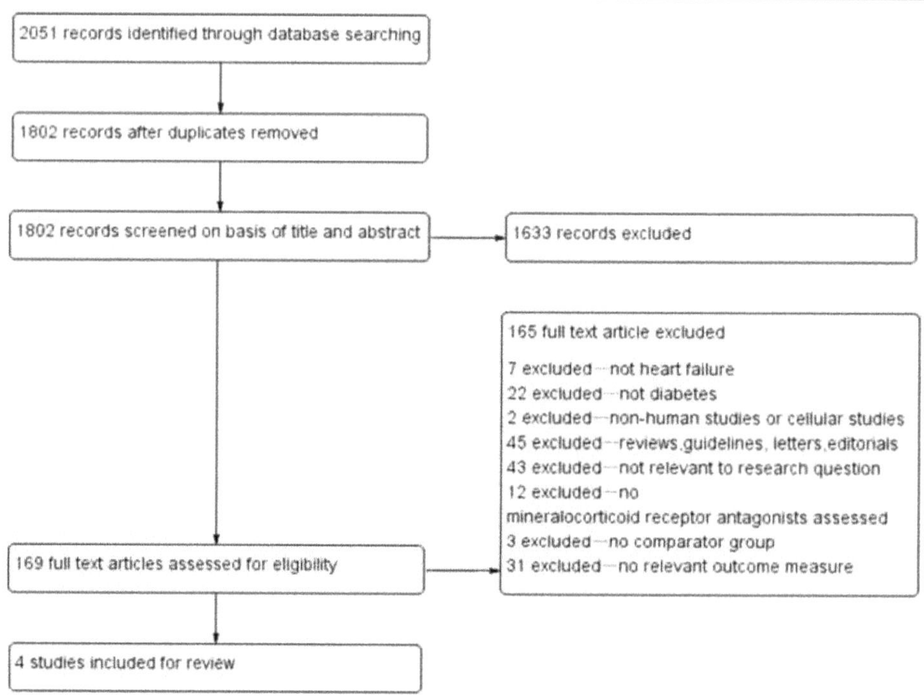


**Fig. 1** Flow diagram of study selection. Identified were 2051 potentially relevant articles; 1802 were excluded through screening of titles and abstracts, and 165 articles were excluded for not meeting our inclusion criteria. Finally, 4 studies were included

**Table 1** Characteristics of the included studies

| Study | Subjects (T/C) | Age (T/C) | Male (T/C) | Ejection fraction, (%) (T/ C) | Interventions (T/C) | Follow-up period | Outcomes | Crude events (T/C) |
|---|---|---|---|---|---|---|---|---|
| O'Keefe (2007) [29] | 749/734 | 66 ± 10/66 ± 10 | 63/64 | 32 ± 6 /32 ± 6 | Eplerenone/Placebo | Mean 16 months | ①all-cause mortality | ①153/175 |
| | | | | | | | ②Hyperkalaemia(>5.5 mmol/l) | ②42/22 |
| | | | | | | | ③Death from CV causes | ③131/152 |
| Eschalier (2013) [30] | 459/400 | 68.1 ± 7.4/N.r. | 356/N.r. | 26.44 ± 4.7/N.r. | Eplerenone/Placebo | N.r | ①Hyperkalaemia(>5.5 mmol/l) | ①63/33 |
| | | | | | | | ②CV mortality+HF hospitalization | ②99/141 |
| | | | | | | | ③Change in eGFR from baseline to final visit | ③- 4.94(17.4)/-2.93(18.9) |
| Vadugana than (2014) [31] | 444/306 | 65.1 ± 10.1/67.9 ± 10.7 | 320/242 | 26.7 ± 7.8/28.6 ± 8.8 | MRAs/no MRAs | Mean 9.9 months | ①all-cause mortality; | ①101/98 |
| | | | | | | | ②CV mortality+HF hospitalization | ②182/147 |
| | | | | | | | ③Death from CV causes | ③78/66 |
| Khosraviani (2014) [32] | 536/1114 | N.r. | N.r. | N.r. | Spironolactone/no spironolactone | 2 years | all-cause mortality | 79/223 |

Notes: *T* Trial Group, *C* Control Group, *N.r.* not report, *MRAs* mineralocorticoid receptor antagonists, *CV* cardiovascular, *HF* heart failure, *CI* confidence interval, *eGFR* estimated glomerular filtration rate

### Eligibility criteria

#### *Types of studies*

A study was included if it was either a randomised or non-randomised controlled trial, a prospective or retrospective cohort study, or a case–control study that evaluated the efficacy and safety of MRAs in patients with HF and DM.

#### *Types of participants*

Patients of any age, gender or race with HF and DM were included.

#### *Types of interventions*

Patients in the treatment groups were given MRAs while the control groups were given placebo or had no intervention. The studies were included regardless of the follow-up duration and dosage of treatment.

#### *Types of outcome measures*

The primary outcome measures were all-cause mortality and hyperkalaemia. The secondary outcome measures were CV mortality or HF hospitalization, death from CV causes and change in estimated glomerular filtration rate (eGFR).

### Literature search

A computerized literature search was conducted using Medline (1966–2015), Embase (1980–2015) and the Cochrane Central Register of Controlled Trials (1991–2015) from their inception to July 2015. The search strategy in Medline is shown in Additional file 2. In addition, we manually searched reference lists of all included studies and relevant review articles. Furthermore, we contacted experts and authors of included studies to retrieve potentially relevant published or unreported material. The retrieval was not restricted by language or quality of study.

### Study selection and data collection

Two reviewers (G.S.P. and Y.H.M.) independently screened the titles and abstracts to select potential references according to a data extraction form established above, including patients, methods, interventions and outcomes. For eligible studies, two reviewers (G.S.P. and Y.H.M.) extracted the data independently. Disagreements were settled through discussion or consultation with a third author (F.M.D.).

### Quality assessment

The quality of the included studies was evaluated using the nine-star Newcastle Ottawa scale (NOS) [28] by two investigators. Each study was evaluated based on eight items, and the scale ranged from zero to nine stars, the more stars the higher the methodological quality.

### Data synthesis and analysis

Data were analyzed using Review Manager (version 5.2). A fixed-effects model or random-effects model was used across the studies; relative risk (RR) and 95 % confidence intervals were calculated for dichotomous outcomes. A standard chi-square test and $I^2$ statistic were calculated to evaluate the heterogeneity between trial results. All P values were two sided and P values of less than 0.05 for any test were considered to be statistically significant.

## Results

### Study selection

There were 2051 potentially relevant articles retrieved of which 1802 were excluded because they were case reports, animal or basic research studies, or did not investigate any of outcomes of interest. After screening the titles and abstracts, we excluded 165 articles of the remaining 169 articles, for not meeting our inclusion criteria. No more eligible studies were found after manually searching reference lists. Ultimately a total of 4 studies that included 4742 participants were included in this systematic review. The screening process is summarized in a flow diagram (Fig. 1).

### Study characteristics

No randomized controlled trials were identified. Three [29–31] were post hoc subgroup analyses from randomized trials and one [32] was a prospective cohort study. A total of 4742 participants were included in the 4 studies, of whom 2188 were in treatment groups and 2554 were in control groups. In two studies [29, 30], the

**Table 2** Newcastle-Ottawa Scale (NOS) assessment of the quality of the studies

| | Selection | | | | Comparability | | | Outcome | | Score |
|---|---|---|---|---|---|---|---|---|---|---|
| Study | 1 | 2 | 3 | 4 | 5a | 5b | 6 | 7 | 8 | |
| O'Keefe, et al (2008) [29] | ★ | ★ | ★ | ★ | ★ | ★ | ★ | ☆ | ★ | 9 |
| Eschalier, et al (2013) [30] | ★ | ★ | ★ | ★ | ☆ | ☆ | ★ | ☆ | ★ | 6 |
| Vaduganathan, et al (2014) [31] | ★ | ★ | ★ | ★ | ★ | ★ | ★ | ☆ | ★ | 9 |
| Khosraviani, et al (2014) [32] | ★ | ★ | ★ | ★ | ☆ | ☆ | ★ | ☆ | ☆ | 5 |

Notes: *1* indicates exposed cohort truly representative, *2* the non exposed cohort drawn from the same community, *3* ascertainment of exposure by secure record or structured interview, *4* outcome of interest was not present at start of study, *5A* cohorts comparable on basis of sex and age, *5B* cohorts comparable on other factor(s), *6* quality of outcome assessment, *7* follow-up long enough for outcomes to occur, and *8* complete follow up, ★ yes, ☆ no

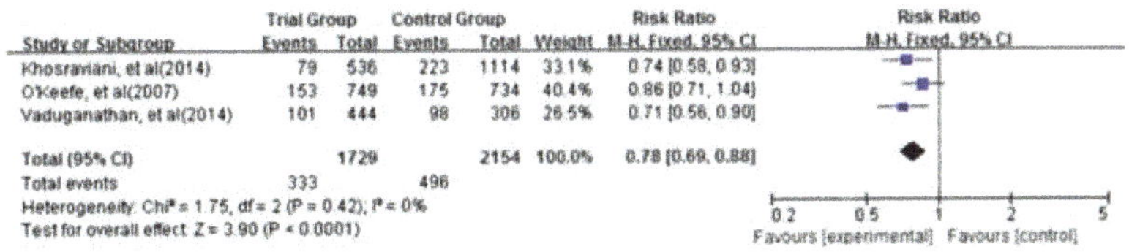


**Fig. 2** Forest plot of the comparison of treatment with MRAs versus without MRAs on all-cause mortality. Three of included studies evaluated the effect of MRAs on all-cause mortality. The mortality was 19 % in MRA groups compared with 23 % in control groups. The studies suggested that MRAs-based regimens reduced the risk of all-cause mortality in comparison to regimens without MRAs

control medicine was placebo ($n = 1134$); and the remaining two studies [31, 32] comparison groups without MRAs ($n = 1420$) were used.

Three studies [29–31] contained additional HF-specific information (e.g., New York Heart Association Functional Class or LVEF). These also included demographics, co-morbidities, other related drug therapies and additional laboratory determination data. One study [32] was an administrative analysis with no additional laboratory or clinical information. Detailed characteristics of included studies are listed in Table 1.

### Risk of bias in included studies

The methodological quality of the included studies is summarized in Table 2. The NOS results showed an average overall score of 7.25 (range 5–9).

### Effectiveness

#### *All-cause mortality*

Three of included studies [29, 31, 32] evaluated the effect of MRAs on all-cause mortality; 2-year, 16-month and 9.9-month mortality were evaluated respectively in these studies. Overall, the mortality was 19 % in the MRA treatment groups compared with 23 % in control groups (RR = 0.78, 95 % CI: 0.69–0.88, $I^2 = 0$ %, $P < 0.001$; Fig. 2). All studies suggested MRA-based regimens reduce the risk of all-cause mortality in comparison to regimens without MRAs.

In a study by O'Keefe et al. [29], which was a post hoc analysis from the EPHESUS trial, a reduction in all-cause mortality was observed in the eplerenone group that did not reach statistical significance. Khosraviani et al. [32] observed that spironolactone significantly reduced mortality compared to the control group without spironolactone (14.8 vs. 20.0 %, RR 0.74 [95 % CI 0.58–0.93]). Vaduganathan et al. [31] observed that MRA administration was associated with a 31 % reduction in all-cause mortality (RR 0.71 [95 % CI 0.56–0.90]) in unadjusted analyses, but the result turned to be negative after adjusting for baseline risk factors (adjusted HR 0.93; 95 % CI 0.75 to 1.15).

#### *CV mortality or HF hospitalization*

Two studies [30, 31] evaluated the effects of MRAs on CV mortality or HF hospitalization. Events occurred in 281 of the 903 participants treated with MRAs (31.1 %) compared with 288 of 706 (40.8 %) in the control group. Because significant heterogeneities were detected, we used a random-effect model to synthesize the data (RR = 0.73; 95 % CI: 0.52–1.01; $I^2 = 83$ %; $P < 0.06$; Fig. 3). However, these results did not reach statistical significance.

Eschalier et al. [30] observed that the HR as the primary outcome in the eplerenone group compared with the placebo group was 0.61 (95 % CI: 0.49 to 0.76). Vaduganathan et al. [31] observed that MRA treatment was associated with a 19 % reduction in the end point (RR 0.85; 95 % CI 0.73 to 1.00) in unadjusted analyses, but the results became negative after adjusting for baseline risk factors (adjusted HR 0.94; 95 % CI 0.80 to 1.10).

#### *Death from CV causes*

Two studies [29, 31] evaluated the effect of MRAs on death from cardiovascular causes. Treatment was

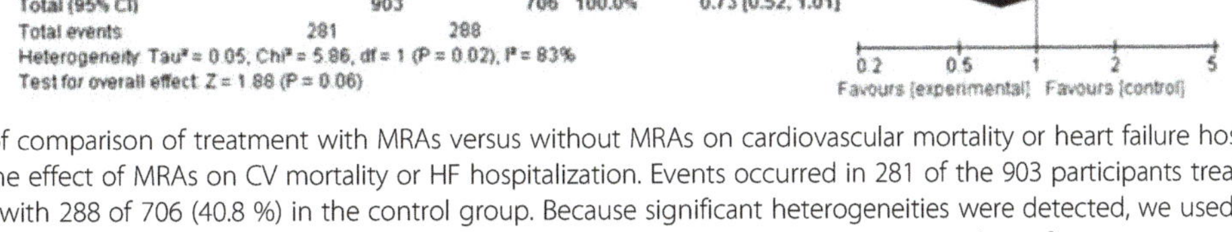


**Fig. 3** Forest plot of comparison of treatment with MRAs versus without MRAs on cardiovascular mortality or heart failure hospitalization. Two studies evaluated the effect of MRAs on CV mortality or HF hospitalization. Events occurred in 281 of the 903 participants treated with MRAs (31.1 %) compared with 288 of 706 (40.8 %) in the control group. Because significant heterogeneities were detected, we used a random-effect model to synthesize the data on the basis of the large population. These results did not reach statistical significance

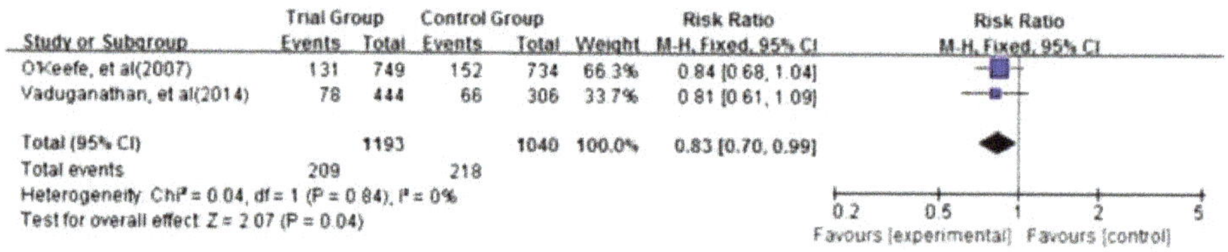


**Fig. 4** Forest plot of comparison of treatment with MRAs versus without MRAs on death from cardiovascular causes. Two studies evaluated the effect of MRAs on death from cardiovascular causes. Treatment with MRA-based regimens was associated with a statistically significant reduction in CV mortality compared with other treatments. Individually, in no study were observed statistically significant reductions in CV-cause mortality

associated with a statistically significant reduction in CV mortality compared with control group (17.5 % versus 20.9 %; RR = 0.83; 95 % CI: 0.70–0.99; $I^2 = 0$ %; $P = 0.04$; Fig. 4). Individually, no study observed statistically significant reductions in CV mortality.

## Safety

### *Hyperkalaemia*

Two studies [29, 30] evaluated the risk of developing hyperkalaemia caused by MRAs in patients with HF and DM. The occurrence of hyperkalaemia in the MRA group was higher than in the comparison group (8.7 % versus 4.9 %; RR = 1.74; 95 % CI: 1.27–2.38; $I^2 = 0$ %; $P = 0.0005$; Fig. 5).

Eschalier et al. [30] observed there was an increase in the incidence of potassium levels of >5.5 mmol/l with eplerenone (14.1 %) in patients with DM and HF compared with placebo (8.5 %), $P = 0.01$. O'Keefe et al. [29] also observed that hyperkalaemia occurred more frequently with eplerenone treatment than with placebo (5.6 vs. 3.0 %, $P = 0.015$).

### *Change in eGFR*

The change in eGFR from baseline to after the treatment period was reported in one study [30]. No significant difference was observed in the two groups ($P > 0.05$).

## Discussion

Four studies with 4742 individuals were identified. The main findings of the present study were that MRA treatment was associated with improved clinical outcomes compared with those regimens without MRAs in patients with DM and HF. From a safety perspective, the most serious adverse effect of MRAs (spironolactone and eplerenone) is the development of hyperkalaemia. However, as adverse effects were mentioned in only 50 % of the studies, there was not sufficient evidence to draw conclusions on the issue of safety.

There are a number of limitations in this study. First, only four studies were available; the included studies were all observational and none of them were randomized controlled trials. There were three post-hoc subanalyses of randomized controlled trials concerning MRAs in heart failure and just one prospective cohort study. Two students scored the quality of each of the articles, and quality scores for each study are shown in Table 2. However, the quality of individual research included in our analysis was not necessarily high. Eschalier et al. [30] did not provide the detailed information about characteristics of the subject investigated. Khosraviani et al. [32] failed to offer an elaborated description of the study design. Thus, the level of evidence for this meta-analysis does not seem to be high.

Secondly, any systematic review may suffer from publication or selection bias. Publication bias can be assessed graphically with a funnel plot, which could not be assessed owing to having just four available studies. Thirdly, methodology defects have been found in some of these studies, including failure to collect data prospectively and inadequate baseline comparisons. Some baseline characteristics were different among the studies. For example, studies used different MRAs (spironolactone, eplerenone), different controls (placebo control or blank control), different dosages of the active and control medicines, and different

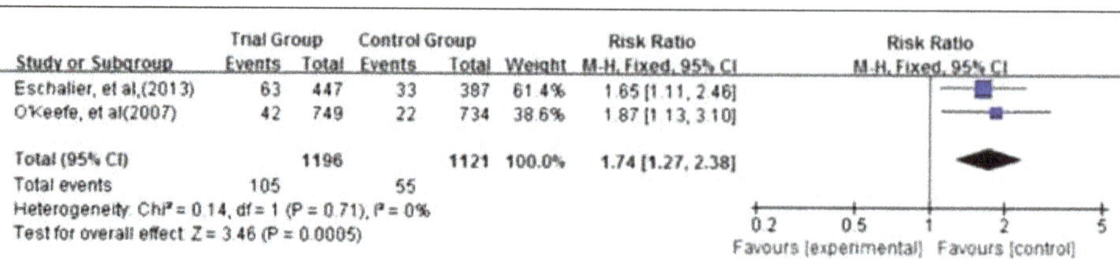


**Fig. 5** Forest plot of comparison of treatment with MRAs versus without MRAs on hyperkalaemia. Two studies evaluated the risk of developing hyperkalaemia caused by MRAs in patients with DM and HF. The occurrence of hyperkalaemia in the MRA group was higher than in the comparison group

follow-up times and background therapies. Lastly, significant heterogeneities were detected when the effects of MRAs on CV mortality or HF hospitalization were evaluated. The heterogeneity among the studies might be affected by various factors, such as study designs, study quality and patient characteristics. Therefore, a random-effect model was used to synthesize the data. But because only two studies reported these events, we could not perform meta-regression meta-analysis to examine the source of the heterogeneity.

Due to the limited quantity and quality of the included studies, it is premature to draw conclusion about the efficacy of MRAs in patients with HF and DM. However, it should be noted that the absence of sufficient scientific evidence does not mean that the treatment is ineffective. The safety of MRA therapy for those patients remains to be further determined. The possible electrolyte trouble could have a multifactorial origin. We observed that when using MRAs, many patients also used others drugs, including ACE inhibitors, angiotensin receptor blockers (ARBs), beta-blockers, and aspirin, but medical therapy was not different at baseline between the two groups. When the treatment with MRAs was undertaken, ACE inhibitors or ARBs were generally not discontinued, but patients underwent a modulation of their dosages or their dose was left unchanged. This suggests that ACE inhibitors or ARBs could be associated with the increased risk of hyperkalaemia; MRAs alone might not have caused this adverse effect. At the stage of the addition of MRA to therapy, a gradual uptitration of the MRA dose or a concomitant thoughtful reduction of the dose of ACE inhibitor or ARB could prevent the occurrence of hyperkalaemia, except in cases of severe impairment of kidney function. In addition, DM is an independent risk factor for the development of hyperkalaemia [33].

Several implications for research arise from this review. First, more randomized controlled trials of higher quality, with larger sample size and adequate follow up are needed to further evaluate the effect of MRAs. Second, the only extensively researched MRAs to date are spironolactone and eplerenone, further research on other MRAs such as canrenone is encouraged in these disease areas. Third, we should closely observe the incidence of adverse events, such as electrolyte abnormalities, gynecomastia, menstrual irregularities, acute kidney injury and the effects on serum glucose levels. Fourth, further study can focus on developing novel MRAs that have similar outcomes as spironolactone but lower rates of hyperkalaemia such as finerenone [34, 35]. Fifth, further study is needed with a focus on evaluating the outcomes of efficacy and safety in patients with heart failure associated with chronic renal failure, especially in patients with diabetic nephropathy, which are better represented in the literature regarding MRA efficacy and safety.

## Conclusions

The available evidence suggests that MRAs can reduce mortality risk in patients with HF and DM. However, the development of hyperkalaemia was reported in some of the reviewed studies. There is still a lack of convincing evidence for further evaluation of this treatment. More randomized controlled trials of higher quality, with a larger sample size, and long-term follow-up are needed in the future.

#### Abbreviations

MRAs: Mineralocorticoid receptor antagonists; DM: Diabetes mellitus; HF: Heart failure; EF: Ejection fraction; CV: Cardiovascular; HbA1c: Glycosylated hemoglobin; eGFR: Estimated glomerular filtration rate; RR: Relative risk.

#### Competing interests

The authors declare that they have no competing interests.

#### Authors' contributions

The following authors participated in various ways: in developing the idea into a concept (CMD, ZC), writing the initial protocol (DSS, CNY, ZJJ), developing the search strategy (GSP, FMD, YHM), identifying, selecting and appraising the included studies (ZXH, WLX, LCY), drafting the manuscript (CMD), reviewing and approving the final version of the manuscript (all authors).

#### Acknowledgments

This work is supported by the National Natural Science Foundation of China (NSFC)(No. 81200630), Natural Science Foundation of Zhejiang Province, China (No. LQ12H07001), Wenzhou City Science & Technology Bureau, China (No.Y20140033), Medical Technology Foundation of Zhejiang Province, China (No.2015KYA159), Opening Project of Zhejiang Provincial Top Key Discipline of Clinical Medicine.

#### Author details

[1]Diabetes Center and Department of Endocrinology, The Second Affiliated Hospital of Wenzhou Medical University, No. 109 West Xueyuan Road, 325027, Wenzhou, Zhejiang, China. [2]Department of Orthopedics, The Second Affiliated Hospital of Wenzhou Medical University, 325027, Wenzhou, Zhejiang, China.

#### References

1. Dei Cas A, Khan SS, Butler J, Mentz RJ, Bonow RO, Avogaro A, et al. Impact of diabetes on epidemiology, treatment, and outcomes of patients with heart failure. JACC Heart Fail. 2015;3(2):136–45.
2. Adams Jr KF, Fonarow GC, Emerman CL, LeJemtel TH, Costanzo MR, Abraham WT, et al. Characteristics and outcomes of patients hospitalized for heart failure in the United States: rationale, design, and preliminary observations from the first 100,000 cases in the Acute Decompensated Heart Failure National Registry (ADHERE). Am Heart J. 2005;149(2):209–16.
3. Nichols GA, Hillier TA, Erbey JR, Brown JB. Congestive heart failure in type 2 diabetes: prevalence, incidence, and risk factors. Diabetes Care. 2001;24(9):1614–9.

4. Khan MA, Deaton C, Rutter MK, Neyses L, Mamas MA. Incretins as a novel therapeutic strategy in patients with diabetes and heart failure. Heart Fail Rev. 2013;18(2):141–8.
5. Doehner W, Rauchhaus M, Ponikowski P, Godsland IF, von Haehling S, Okonko DO, et al. Impaired insulin sensitivity as an independent risk factor for mortality in patients with stable chronic heart failure. J Am Coll Cardiol. 2005;46(6):1019–26.
6. Amato L, Paolisso G, Cacciatore F, Ferrara N, Ferrara P, Canonico S, et al. Congestive heart failure predicts the development of non-insulin-dependent diabetes mellitus in the elderly. The Osservatorio Geriatrico Regione Campania Group. Diabetes Metab. 1997;23(3):213–8.
7. Dei Cas A, Spigoni V, Ridolfi V, Metra M. Diabetes and chronic heart failure: from diabetic cardiomyopathy to therapeutic approach. Endocr Metab Immune Disord Drug Targets. 2013;13(1):38–50.
8. Nichols GA, Gullion CM, Koro CE, Ephross SA, Brown JB. The incidence of congestive heart failure in type 2 diabetes: an update. Diabetes Care. 2004;27(8):1879–84.
9. Nasir S, Aguilar D. Congestive heart failure and diabetes mellitus: balancing glycemic control with heart failure improvement. Am J Cardiol. 2012;110(9 Suppl):50b–7b.
10. Sarma S, Mentz RJ, Kwasny MJ, Fought AJ, Huffman M, Subacius H, et al. Association between diabetes mellitus and post-discharge outcomes in patients hospitalized with heart failure: findings from the EVEREST trial. Eur J Heart Fail. 2013;15(2):194–202.
11. Dei Cas A, Fonarow GC, Gheorghiade M, Butler J. Concomitant diabetes mellitus and heart failure. Curr Probl Cardiol. 2015;40(1):7–43.
12. Parviz Y, Iqbal J, Pitt B, Adlam D, Al-Mohammad A, Zannad F. Emerging cardiovascular indications of mineralocorticoid receptor antagonists. Trends Endocrinol Metab. 2015;26(4):201–11.
13. Tirosh A, Garg R, Adler GK. Mineralocorticoid receptor antagonists and the metabolic syndrome. Curr Hypertens Rep. 2010;12(4):252–7.
14. Zannad F, Gattis Stough W, Rossignol P, Bauersachs J, McMurray JJ, Swedberg K, et al. Mineralocorticoid receptor antagonists for heart failure with reduced ejection fraction: integrating evidence into clinical practice. Eur Heart J. 2012;33(22):2782–95.
15. Gilbert RE, Krum H. Heart failure in diabetes: effects of anti-hyperglycaemic drug therapy. Lancet. 2015;385(9982):2107–17.
16. Danjuma MI, Mukherjee I, Makaronidis J, Osula S. Converging indications of aldosterone antagonists (spironolactone and eplerenone): a narrative review of safety profiles. Curr Hypertens Rep. 2014;16(2):414.
17. Matsumoto S, Takebayashi K, Aso Y. The effect of spironolactone on circulating adipocytokines in patients with type 2 diabetes mellitus complicated by diabetic nephropathy. Metabolism. 2006;55(12):1645–52.
18. Swaminathan K, Davies J, George J, Rajendra NS, Morris AD, Struthers AD. Spironolactone for poorly controlled hypertension in type 2 diabetes: conflicting effects on blood pressure, endothelial function, glycaemic control and hormonal profiles. Diabetologia. 2008;51(5):762–8.
19. Polyzos SA, Kountouras J, Zafeiriadou E, Patsiaoura K, Katsiki E, Deretzi G, et al. Effect of spironolactone and vitamin E on serum metabolic parameters and insulin resistance in patients with nonalcoholic fatty liver disease. J Renin Angiotensin Aldosterone Syst. 2011;12(4):498–503.
20. Krug AW, Stelzner L, Rao AD, Lichtman AH, Williams GH, Adler GK. Effect of low dose mineralocorticoid receptor antagonist eplerenone on glucose and lipid metabolism in healthy adult males. Metabolism. 2013;62(3):386–91.
21. Garg R, Rao AD, Adler G. Effect of spironolactone on glycemic control in patients with type 2 diabetes mellitus. Diabetes. 2015;64:A342–3.
22. McMurray EM, Wallace IR, Ennis C, Hunter SJ, Atkinson AB, Bell PM. Effect of eplerenone on insulin action in essential hypertension: a randomised, controlled, crossover study. J Hum Hypertens. 2014;28(10):575–8.
23. Yamaji M, Tsutamoto T, Kawahara C, Nishiyama K, Yamamoto T, Fujii M, et al. Effect of eplerenone versus spironolactone on cortisol and hemoglobin A(1)(c) levels in patients with chronic heart failure. Am Heart J. 2010;160(5):915–21.
24. Briet M, Schiffrin EL. Aldosterone: effects on the kidney and cardiovascular system. Nat Rev Nephrol. 2010;6(5):261–73.
25. Ferrario CM, Schiffrin EL. Role of mineralocorticoid receptor antagonists in cardiovascular disease. Circ Res. 2015;116(1):206–13.
26. Talatinian A, Chow SL, Heywood JT. Expanding role of mineralocorticoid receptor antagonists in the treatment of heart failure. Pharmacotherapy. 2012;32(9):827–37.
27. Moher D, Liberati A, Tetzlaff J, Altman DG, Group P. Preferred reporting items for systematic reviews and meta-analyses: the PRISMA statement. PLoS Med. 2009;6(7):e1000097.
28. Wells G, Shea B, O'connell D, Peterson J, Welch V, Losos M, et al. The Newcastle-Ottawa Scale (NOS) for assessing the quality of nonrandomised studies in meta-analyses. 2000.
29. O'Keefe JH, Abuissa H, Pitt B. Eplerenone improves prognosis in postmyocardial infarction diabetic patients with heart failure: results from EPHESUS. Diabetes Obes Metab. 2008;10(6):492–7.
30. Eschalier R, McMurray JJ, Swedberg K, van Veldhuisen DJ, Krum H, Pocock SJ, et al. Safety and efficacy of eplerenone in patients at high risk for hyperkalemia and/or worsening renal function: analyses of the EMPHASIS-HF study subgroups (Eplerenone in Mild Patients Hospitalization And Survival Study in Heart Failure). J Am Coll Cardiol. 2013;62(17):1585–93.
31. Vaduganathan M, Dei Cas A, Mentz RJ, Greene SJ, Khan S, Subacius HP, et al. Mineralocorticoid receptor antagonist use in hospitalized patients with heart failure, reduced ejection fraction, and diabetes mellitus (from the EVEREST trial). Am J Cardiol. 2014;114(5):743–50.
32. Khosraviani K, Eshtehardi P, Mojadidi MK, Zolty R. Mortality benefit of spironolactone in diabetic versus non-diabetic patients with congestive heart failure. J Am Coll Cardiol. 2014;63(12):A859.
33. Johnson ES, Weinstein JR, Thorp ML, Platt RW, Petrik AF, Yang X, et al. Predicting the risk of hyperkalemia in patients with chronic kidney disease starting lisinopril. Pharmacoepidemiol Drug Saf. 2010;19(3):266–72.
34. Pitt B, Kober L, Ponikowski P, Gheorghiade M, Filippatos G, Krum H, et al. Safety and tolerability of the novel non-steroidal mineralocorticoid receptor antagonist BAY 94–8862 in patients with chronic heart failure and mild or moderate chronic kidney disease: a randomized, double-blind trial. Eur Heart J. 2013;34(31):2453–63.
35. Kolkhof P, Flamme I, Perez SF, Baerfacker L, Hartmann E, Rinke M, et al. Cardiac and renal protection by a new mineralocorticoid receptor antagonist in salt-sensitive arterial hypertension. Eur Heart J. 2006;27:110–0.

# Prognostic significance of heart rate turbulence parameters in patients with chronic heart failure

De-Chun Yin[1], Zhao-Jun Wang[1], Shuai Guo[1], Hong-Yu Xie[1], Lin Sun[1], Wei Feng[1], Wei Qiu[1] and Xiu-Fen Qu[1,2*]

**Abstract**

**Background:** This study is aimed to evaluate the clinical significance of heart rate turbulence (HRT) parameters in predicting the prognosis in patients with chronic heart failure (CHF).

**Methods:** From June 2011 to December 2012, a total of 104 CHF patients and 30 healthy controls were enrolled in this study. We obtained a 24-hour Holter ECG recording to assess the HRT parameters, included turbulence onset (TO), turbulence slope (TS), standard deviation of N-N intervals (SDNN), and resting heart rate (RHR). The relationships between HRT parameters and the prognosis of CHF patients were determined.

**Results:** The assessment follow-up period lasted until January 31, 2013. The overall mortality of CHF patients was 9.6% (10/104). Our results revealed that CHF patients had higher levels of TO than those of healthy subjects, but the TS levels of CHF patients were lower than that of the control group. CHF patients with NYHA grade IV had higher $HRT_{1/2}$ rate than those with NYHA grade II/III. There were statistical differences in TS, LVEF, SDNN and RHR between the non-deteriorating group and the non-survivor group. Significant differences in TS among the three groups were also found. Furthermore, CHF patients in the non-survivor group had lower levels of TS than those in the deteriorating group. Correlation analyses indicated that TO negatively correlate with SDNN, while TS positively correlated with SDNN and left ventricular ejection fraction (LVEF). We also observed negative correlations between TS and left ventricular end-diastolic cavity dimension (LVEDD), RHR, homocysteine (Hcy) and C-reactive protein (CRP). Multivariate Cox regression analysis further confirmed that LVEF (≤30%), $HRT_2$, SDNN and RHR were independent risk factors which can indicate poor prognosis in CHF patients.

**Conclusions:** Our findings indicate that HRT may have good clinical predictive value in patients with CHF. Thus, quantifying HRT parameters could be a useful tool for predicting mortality in CHF patients.

**Keywords:** Heart rate turbulence, Chronic heart failure, Prognosis

## Background

Chronic heart failure (CHF), one of the most common forms of heart failure, is a pathophysiological state in which an abnormality of cardiac function is responsible for the failure of the heart to pump blood at a rate necessary to deliver nutrients to metabolizing tissues [1]. Despite advances in medical and surgical treatments, mortality in CHF patients remains high, and the five-year mortality rate in CHF patients averages 50%, whereas in the end-stage CHF, it may reach 75%; and the sudden death rate accounts for 30 ~ 50% of total mortality [2,3]. Recent studies have confirmed that the prognosis of CHF is uniformly poor, and the accuracy of diagnosis through clinical means alone is often inadequate, particularly in elderly obese people [4,5]. Currently, several studies have indicated that various indices or electrocardiographically derived parameters have been commonly used and tested as prognostic predictors for CHF [6,7].

Clinically, the currently accepted prognostic indicators for CHF mainly consist of heart rate variability (HRV) and LVEF, which may both have some limitations to their own extents [8]. HRV, as one of the oldest Holter-derived risk stratification parameters, is an established parameter for analyzing the performance of autonomic regulation in the sinus node [9]. Nevertheless, it is only mildly inclined to a series of physiological reflexes caused

* Correspondence: hbmu1h_qxf@163.com
[1]Department of Cardiology, The First Affiliated Hospital of Harbin Medical University, Harbin 150001, P.R. China
[2]Department of Cardiology, The First Affiliated Hospital of Harbin Medical University, Dazhi Street No.199, Nangang District, Harbin 150001, P.R. China

by the external environment and *in vitro* stimulation, and cannot reflect the instantaneous malignant arrhythmias. [10]. As for LVEF, it primarily reflects mechanical LV systolic function, however, in the clinical there were a large number of patients suffering from a high risk of sudden death who only detected a mild to moderate left ventricular function with CHF [11,12]. Therefore, it might be essential to actively explore other useful and valid predictors for CHF sufferers since the existing clinical techniques may be inappropriate to applied as a biomarker of high risk of sudden death in CHF.

Heart rate turbulence (HRT), modulated by the baroreceptor reflex, is a physiological biphasic response of the sinus node to premature ventricular contractions, which involves a short initial acceleration followed by a deceleration of the sinus rhythm due to the baroreflex. [13] There are two numeric descriptors that are usually employed to quantify HRT parameter: one is the turbulence onset (TO), which reflects the initial acceleration of heart rate after a ventricular premature beat (VPB); the other is the turbulence slope (TS), which is used to describe subsequent deceleration of heart rate following a ventricular premature beat [13,14]. Previous studies have shown that HRT assessment might be an important parameter in risk stratification after MI and has been suggested that it could be used as a measure of autonomic dysfunction [15,16]. Clinically, HRT can facilitate the predictive accuracy of nonsustained ventricular tachycardia (NSVT) in identifying patients at risk for serious arrhythmic events and in patients with left ventricular (LV) dysfunction [17]. Recent studies have proved more evidence that HRT parameters may be regarded as surrogate measures for baroreflex sensitivity in clinical and prognostic evaluation in patients with CHF [13,18]. In this study, we evaluated the clinical significance of HRT parameters in predicting prognosis in patients with CHF and determine whether HRT parameters could be considered as markers of the development and progression of CHF.

## Methods

### Ethics statement

The Ethics Committee of the First Affiliated Hospital of Harbin Medical University approved the study design. All patients gave informed consent in written to undergo diagnostic and therapeutic procedure at the time of hospitalization.

### Study design and subjects

The study was performed in patients diagnosed of CHF when admitted to the First Affiliated Hospital of Harbin Medical University from June 2011 to December 2012. Patients enrolled in this study must satisfy all of the following criteria: (1) all patients in the study had to meet the diagnostic criteria for CHF as specified by the 1995 World Health Organization/International Society and Federation Cardiology (WHO/ISFC); [19] (2) there must exist evidence for CHF, such as dyspnea, left/right heart failure, cardiac dilatation and left ventricular ejection fraction (LVEF) < 50%; (3) each patient presented with sinus rhythm also had > 5 ventricular premature beats (VPBs) measured; (4) patients diagnosed with CHF were graded II ~ IV according to the NYHA classification [20]. Patients were excluded based on the following criteria: (1) patients had chronic or persistent atrial fibrillation, an implanted permanent pacemaker or cardiac resynchronization therapy; (2) patients were in the acute phase of congestive heart failure or MI; (4) inability to perform a HRT determination or reliable data analysis; (5) patients had hypertrophic cardiomyopathy, myocarditis, diabetes, heart disease, pulmonary heart disease or history of myocardial infarction within 2 months; (6) patients had liver, kidney and other serious organs diseases; (7) patients took antiarrhythmia drugs other than β-blocker; (8) there existed too much interference in dynamic ECG.

In our present study, 104 CHF patients (72 males and 32 females) were enrolled with a mean age of 61.0 ± 10.0 years (range, 39 ~ 84 years). According to the NYHA classification, these patients were divided into grade II (16 males and 7 females), grade III (20 males and 27 females) and grade IV (27 males and 7 females) groups. There were 37 patients (28 males and 9 females) with ischemic heart disease and 67 patients (35 males and 32 females) with nonischemic heart disease. In addition, 30 healthy controls (21 males and 9 females) with a mean age of 58.0 ± 9.0 years (range, 40 ~ 83 years) were enrolled in the control group after detailed medical examination, which includes medical history taking, physical examination, chest X-ray, echocardiography, Holter monitoring and blood biochemical examination.

### Holter recording and evaluation of HRT parameters

All patients were managed under a uniform and standard assay method. HRT of CHF patients were quantified by TO and TS acquired through the 24-hour 3-lead Holter digital recordings (Syneflash recorder; ELA Medical, Le Plessis Robinson, France) according to a previously published method [13]. HRT was analyzed using the HRT Version 0.6 ~ 0.1 software program (Munich Germany). TO is the difference between the mean of the first two RR intervals after a VPB and the last two RR intervals before the VPB. Positive values for TO indicate deceleration, whereas negative values indicate acceleration of the sinus rhythm. TS, the maximum positive value of the slope of a regression line assessed over any sequence of five subsequent sinus-rhythm RR intervals within the first 20 sinus rhythm intervals after a VPB, are expressed in millisecond per interval RR (ms/RR). TO > or = 0%, TS < or = 2.5 ms/RR were considered abnormal

[18]. Based on the previous study, patients in our current study were stratified into three groups: $HRT_0$ group with TO < 0 and TS > 2.5 ms/normal-to-normal interval (both factors normal); $HRT_1$ group with either TO ≥ 0 or TS = 2.5 ms/RR (1 factor abnormal); $HRT_2$ group with TO ≥ 0 and TS ≤ 2.5 ms/RR (both factors abnormal) [18]. For the entire study population, time-domain measurements of heart rate variability (HRV), including mean N-N intervals, standard deviation of N-N intervals (SDNN), and resting heart rate (RHR), left ventricular end-diastolic dimension (LVEDD) were calculated from the 24-hour Holter ECG recording. The RHR was measured after 5 minutes rest while seated in a quiet room [21].

Two-dimensional and Doppler echocardiographic examinations were performed with a HP5500 ultrasound system (Hewlett Packard, Andover, Mass, USA). In the parasternal long-axis view, M-mode echocardiograms were made of left ventricle from the left hemithorax in short-axis.

### Follow-up

The median duration of the entire study follow-up was 10.5 ± 8.3 months (range, 6 ~ 18 months). All events recorded in the study were adjudicated blindly by an ad-hoc committee on the basis of pre-agreed definitions and procedures. Follow-up information was collected for all patients through outpatient service and phone calls. The end point was prospectively defined as the composite of heart failure and cardiac mortality.

The assessment follow-up period lasted until January 31, 2013. Finally, the overall mortality of CHF patients was 9.6% (10/104). There were 32 CHF patients (26 males and 6 females) exhibiting a deterioration of cardiac function and 62 patients showing no significant deterioration.

### Statistical analysis

Data were expressed as mean ± standard deviation (mean ± SD) unless otherwise specified and qualitative data are presented as percentages. Comparative analyses between the groups were performed with the Student's t-test for continuous variables and $\chi^2$ or Fisher's exact test for dichotomous parameters. Correlation between autonomic markers was assessed with Spearman correlation coefficient. Survival curves were estimated with the Kaplan-Meier method and compared by the log-rank test. Independent predictors of death were identified with multivariate Cox proportional hazards model and expressed as hazard ratio (HR) with 95% confidence interval (CI). A *P* value of less than 0.10 was considered statistically significant and all tests were two-sided. All analyses were performed using the SPSS 18.0 software (SPSS, Inc., Chicago, IL, USA).

## Results

### Comparison of heart rate turbulence

The differences in HRT between CHF patients and healthy subjects are summarized in Table 1. Our results revealed that CHF patients exhibited a significant reduction in HRT levels. CHF patients had higher levels of TO than those of healthy subjects (0.48 ± 1.58% vs. -1.73 ± 2.58%, $P < 0.001$), but the TS levels of CHF patients were lower than that of the control group (1.88 ± 1.99 vs. 4.41 ± 1.71 ms/RR, $P < 0.001$). There was a significant difference in the rate of $HRT_{1/2}$ between CHF patients and healthy controls (89/104 vs. 22/30, $P < 0.001$). Furthermore, CHF patients with NYHA grade IV had higher $HRT_{1/2}$ rate than those with NYHA grade II/III ($P = 0.013$, 0.051, respectively) (Figure 1).

### Relevance factors of HRT

Correlation analyses indicated that TO negatively correlated with SDNN ($r = -0.316$, $P < 0.001$), but no associations were found between TO and other factors (all $P > 0.05$). TS positively correlated with SDNN ($r = 0.270$, $P < 0.001$) and LVEF ($r = 0.365$, $P < 0.001$). However, there were negative associations between TS and LVEDD ($r = -0.313$, $P < 0.001$), RHR ($r = -0.299$, $P = 0.001$), Hcy ($r = -0.198$, $P < 0.001$) and CRP ($r = -0.278$, $P < 0.001$). We also observed no correlations with TS to age and TC levels (both $P > 0.05$). Correlations of TO and TS with relevance factors are shown in Table 2 and Figure 2.

### Comparison of CHF patients with different prognosis

Our results suggested that there were statistical differences in TS, LVEF, SDNN and RHR between the non-deteriorating group and the non-survivor group (all $P < 0.05$, as shown in Table 3). We observed a significant difference in TS among the three groups (all $P < 0.05$). Furthermore, CHF patients in the non-survivor group had lower levels of TS than those in the deteriorating group ($P < 0.001$).

### Survival analysis

Univariate survival analysis demonstrated that age (≥65), LVEF (≤30%), SDNN (≤100 ms), RHR (≥75 bpm), $HRT_1$

**Table 1 Difference in HRT Levels between CHF patients and healthy controls**

| Group | NYHA classification | $HRT_0$ | $HRT_{1/2}$ | |
|---|---|---|---|---|
| | | | $HRT_1$ | $HRT_2$ |
| CHF patients | Grade II (n = 23) | 6 | 13 | 5 |
| | Grade III (n = 47) | 8 | 23 | 16 |
| | Grade IV (n = 34) | 1 | 10 | 22 |
| Healthy controls | (n = 30) | 22 | 7 | 1 |

*HRT*, heart rate turbulence; *CHF*, chronic heart failure; *NYHA*, the New York Heart Association.

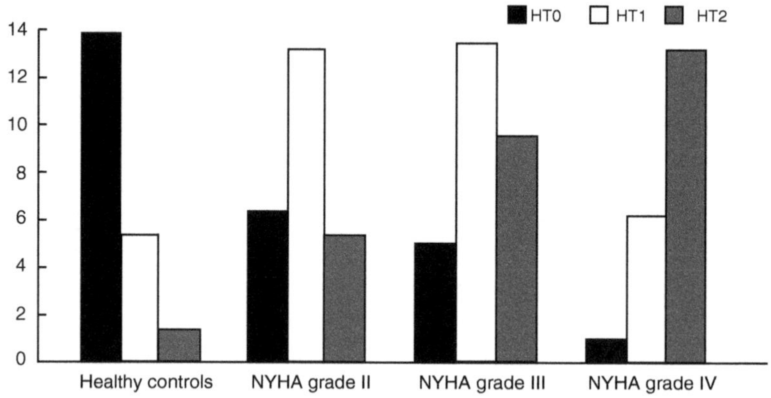


**Figure 1 Difference in HRT levels between CHF patients with different NYHA grade and healthy controls.**

and $HRT_2$ were associated with poor prognosis in CHF patients (all $P < 0.05$) (Table 4). Multivariate Cox regression analysis indicated that LVEF (≤30%), $HRT_2$, SDNN and RHR were independent risk factors for poor prognosis in CHF patients (all $P < 0.05$) (Table 5). Among these risk factors, $HRT_2$ was the strongest predictor of CHF with a high hazard risk of 5.12. The survival curve also showed that the survival rate of CHF patients with $HRT_0$ and $HRT_1$ were higher than those with $HRT_2$ (all $P < 0.05$) (Figure 3).

## Discussion

HRT is a baroreflex-mediated biphasic reaction of heart rate in response to premature ventricular beats [22]. Generally, abnormal HRT is widely accepted to be indicative of potential autonomic dysfunction or impaired baroreflex sensitivity in patients due to variety of disorders; it may also reflect changes in autonomic nervous system induced by different therapeutic modalities such as drugs, revascularization, or cardiac resynchronization therapy [15,23]. More importantly, impaired HRT has been demonstrated in identifying patients at high risk for all-cause mortality and sudden death, particularly in post-infarction and congestive heart failure patients [24]. Notably, HRT have a higher specificity and sensitivity as compared to some other detection methods since it is a bi-physiological response of the interaction between sinus and ventricular contraction that reflect the sensitive outcome of extremely weak endogenous stimuli triggering reflex regulation [25,26]. In recent decades, increasing number of clinical applications in HRT have gained global popularity as well as considerable successes, and it has been previously described as an independent predictor of mortality in patients with cardiovascular diseases [27,28].

Generally, HRT is described as the acceleration and subsequent deceleration of sinus rate [29]. Abnormal HRT has a well-established role in the stratification of post-infarction and heart failure in patients [30]. However, current emphasis on the medical application of HRT is far from perfect, and its function has not been fully assessed. In this study, we evaluated the relationships between HRT parameters and prognosis in CHF patients to explore the predictive values of HRT parameters in the development and progression of CHF. This study revealed that CHF patients exhibited a significant reduction in HRT levels with higher TO levels and lower TS levels than the healthy subjects, suggesting that the HRT levels may be closely related to the development and progression of CHF. Although the exact reasons for HRT reduction in patients with CHF are not fully understood, a potential explanation could be that CHF patients may suffer from myocardial deformation or damages in the terminal receptors, and abnormal sympathetic and vagal afferent stimulation, which may lead to dullness of baroreflex, cause decreased HRT or disappearance of HRT after VPBs in patients with organic heart disease [31]. Sredniawa et al. demonstrated that CHF patients were associated with more abnormal average values of HRT parameters, as a marker of the autonomic

**Table 2 Correlations of TO and TS with relevance factors**

| Factors | TO | | TS | |
|---|---|---|---|---|
| | *r* | *P* | *r* | *P* |
| Age | 0.760 | 0.401 | −0.600 | 0.505 |
| LVEDD | 0.152 | 0.090 | −0.313 | <0.001 |
| LVEF | −0.268 | 0.060 | 0.365 | 0.001 |
| SDNN | −0.316 | <0.001 | 0.270 | 0.020 |
| RHR | 0.211 | 0.180 | −0.299 | 0.010 |
| TC | 0.359 | 0.301 | −0.640 | 0.305 |
| Hcy | 0.314 | 0.062 | −0.198 | <0.001 |
| CRP | 0.218 | 0.052 | −0.278 | <0.001 |

*TO*, turbulence onset; *TS*, turbulence slope; *LVED*, left ventricular end-diastolic diameter; *LVEF*, left ventricular ejection fraction; *SDNN*, standard deviation of N-N intervals; *RHR*, resting heart rate; *TC*, total cholesterol; *Hcy*, homocysteine; *CRP*, C-reaction protein.

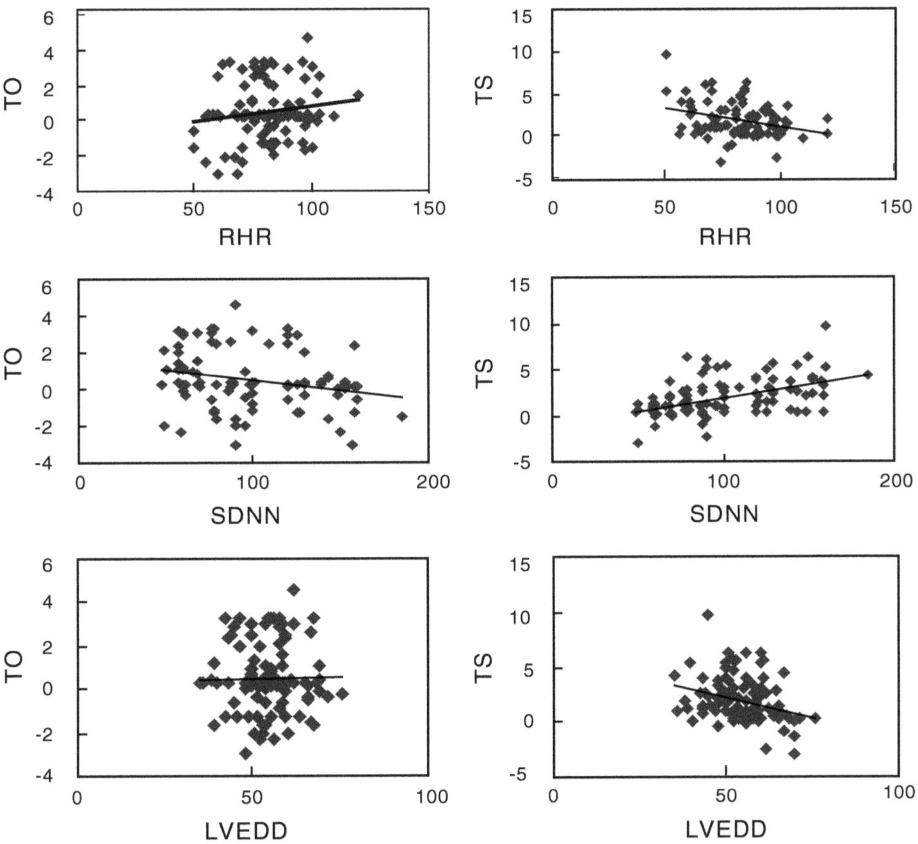


**Figure 2 Correlations of HRT parameters (TO and TS) with SDNN, RHR and LVEDD.**

**Table 3 Comparison of CHF patients with different prognosis**

| Factors | Non-deteriorating group (n = 62) | Deteriorating group (n = 32) | Non-survivor group (n = 10) |
|---|---|---|---|
| Age | 64.78 ± 11.92 | 60.63 ± 10.25 | 60.12 ± 10.34 |
| TO | 0.33 ± 1.64 | 0.23 ± 1.53 | 0.95 ± 1.63 |
| TS | 2.50 ± 2.61 | 2.15 ± 1.82※ | 0.87 ± 1.33※# |
| LVEDD | 44.58 ± 10.12 | 41.24 ± 7.24 | 26.82 ± 8.86※ |
| LVEF | 56.15 ± 7.17 | 53.31 ± 9.01 | 61.01 ± 9.40 |
| SDNN | 102.88 ± 36.98 | 97.28 ± 34.88 | 95.57 ± 31.66※ |
| RHR | 76.65 ± 15.23 | 83.48 ± 12.76 | 89.58 ± 14.07※ |
| TC | 4.56 ± 4.36 | 4.16 ± 0.16 | 3.16 ± 0.62 |
| Hcy | 8.59 ± 2.06 | 14.55 ± 4.11 | 16.95 ± 6.30 |
| CRP | 7.71 ± 1.22 | 11.84 ± 2.96 | 12.67 ± 5.67 |

*CHF*, chronic heart failure; *TO*, turbulence onset; *TS*, turbulence onset; *LVEDD*, left ventricular end-diastolic diameter; *LVEF*, left ventricular ejection fraction; *SDNN*, standard deviation of N-N intervals; *RHR*, resting heart rate; *TC*, total cholesterol; *Hcy*, homocysteine; *CRP*, C-reaction protein; ※$P < 0.05$ compared with the non-deteriorating group; #$P < 0.05$ compared with the non-deteriorating group.

regulation in the heart, might play important roles in the progression toward end-stage heart failure or all-cause mortality of CHF patients [18]. Analysis of HRT is an easy and innocuous way to assess the parasympathetic nervous system, and it can be used as a prognostic marker both in ischemic heart disease and heart failure; in some cases, it even has a better correlation than LVEF [32]. We also found a significant difference in $HRT_{1/2}$ rate between CHF

**Table 4 Univariate survival analysis of HRT parameters with prognosis of CHF patients**

| | HR (95% CI) | *P* value |
|---|---|---|
| Age | 3.91 (1.03, 19.56) | 0.048 |
| $HRT_0$ | 1.34 (0.50, 3.38) | 0.648 |
| $HRT_1$ | 3.78 (1.86, 7.01) | 0.010 |
| $HRT_2$ | 5.40 (2.65, 25.48) | 0.015 |
| LVEF | 4.96 (1.83, 17.20) | 0.020 |
| LVEDD | 2.70 (1.08, 7.36) | 0.038 |
| SDNN | 3.95 (1.11, 14.02) | 0.034 |
| RHR | 4.04 (1.39, 20.95) | 0.015 |

*HRT*, heart rate turbulence; *CHF*, chronic heart failure; *HR*, hazard risk; *LVEF*, left ventricular ejection fraction; *LVEDD*, left ventricular end-diastolic diameter; *SDNN*, standard deviation of N-N intervals; *RHR*, resting heart rate.

**Table 5 Multivariate cox regression analysis of HRT parameters with prognosis of CHF patients**

| | HR (95% CI) | *P* value |
|---|---|---|
| $HRT_1$ | 5.12 (1.53, 16.37) | 0.022 |
| $HRT_2$ | 4.68 (1.54, 16.78) | 0.030 |
| LVEF | 1.37 (0.84, 2.13) | 0.123 |
| LVEDD | 3.69 (1.32, 11.46) | 0.046 |
| SDNN | 3.18 (1.69, 17.43) | 0.034 |
| RHR | 1.84 (0.77, 2.46) | 0.152 |

*HRT*, heart rate turbulence; *CHF*, chronic heart failure; *HR*, hazard risk; *LVEF*, left ventricular ejection fraction; *LVEDD*, left ventricular end-diastolic diameter; *SDNN*, standard deviation of N-N intervals; *RHR*, resting heart rate.

patients and healthy controls. Furthermore, CHF patients with NYHA grade IV had a higher positive rate of $HRT_{1/2}$ than those with NYHA grade II/III, revealing that HRT was correlated with the severity of CHF. The observation of more depressed HRT in patients with advanced NYHA functional class is also consistent with previous reports and studies [33]. In addition, our study also found statistical differences in TS, LVEF, SDNN and RHR between the non-deteriorating group and the non-survivor group; significant differences in TS among the three groups were also observed. Moreover, correlation analyses indicated that both the TS and TO were significantly correlated with SDNN and that only TS was significantly correlated with LVEF. These findings revealed that TS could be considered as a stronger predictor of hospitalization for worsening heart failure and death in CHF patients than LVEF, SDNN and RHR. The mechanisms of the decreased TS in CHF patients are not clear; it is likely that the TS is more susceptible to CHF events because it correlates with both the left ventricular function and the cardiac autonomic status [34]. Consistent with our results, a previous study suggested that the TS appears to be a more suitable prognostic marker for CHF death and hospitalization than LVEF and SDNN, which further confirmed that HRT serves great predictive value in the prognosis of CHF [35]. Univariate survival analysis demonstrated that age (≥65), LVEF (≤30%), SDNN (≤100 ms), RHR (≥75 bpm), $HRT_1$ and $HRT_2$ were associated with poor prognosis of CHF patients. Multivariate Cox regression analysis indicated that LVEF (≤30%), $HRT_2$, SDNN and RHR were independent risk factors for poor prognosis of CHF patients. Among these risk factors, $HRT_2$ (the combination of abnormal TO and TS) was the strongest predictor of CHF with a high hazard risk of 5.12 after CHF and remained highly significant after adjustment for LVEF and other clinical risk factors. The combination of abnormal TO and TS may result in tachycardia which would cause decreased heart efficiency in increased myocardial oxygen consumption, decreased myocardial perfusion during myocardial relaxation and diastolic, thereby leading to myocardial injury and aggravating or worsening heart failure [36]. Nevertheless, some limitations of this study should be acknowledged. Firstly, a lack of image analysis software to automatically identify and analyze the matched VPBs, as well as HRT, limited the accuracy in the prognostic significance of HRT in CHF patients. Secondly, HRT level is easily affected by various factors, therefore certain limitations still remain in the sensitivity, specificity and positive predictive value of HRT in CHF patients.

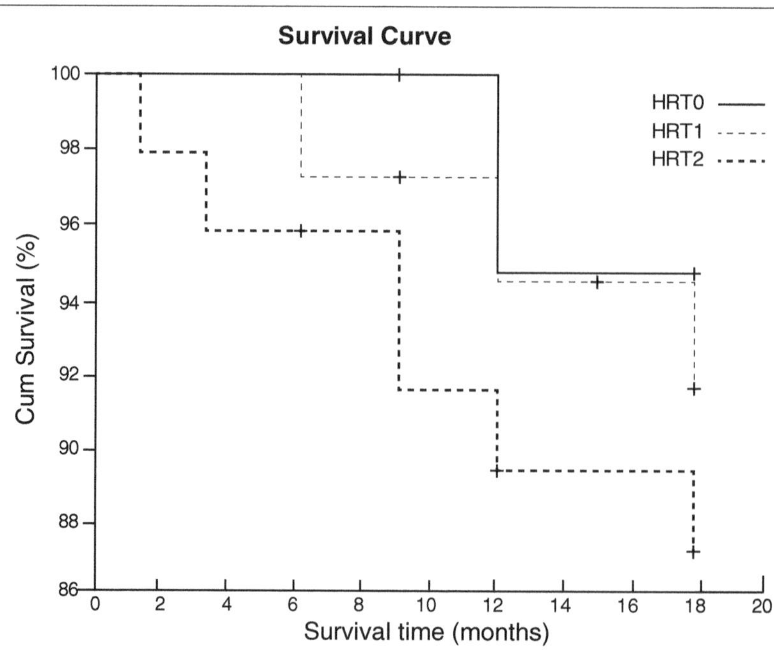


**Figure 3** Survival curve for the survival rate of CHF patients with $HRT_0$, $HRT_1$ and $HRT_2$.

Thirdly, due to the short follow-up time and the relatively small sample size, the correlation between HRT and CHF requires further verification.

## Conclusions

Our findings indicated that HRT may have good clinical predictive values in patients with CHF. Thus, quantifying HRT parameters could be useful tool in predicting mortality in CHF patients. However, due to the limitations mentioned above, further detailed studies with larger sample size and longer follow-up periods are still required to confirm our results.

### Competing interests

The authors have declared no competing interests among themselves.

### Authors' contribution

YDC carried out the experiments and drafted the manuscript. WSJ, GS and FW analyzed the data. XHY, SL and QW contributed the material and the analysis tools. YDC and QXF participated in the design of the study and performed the statistical analysis. QXF conceived the study, and participated in its design and coordination and helped draft the manuscript. All authors read and approved the final manuscript.

### Acknowledgments

This work was supported by the Department of Health Project of Heilongjiang Province (2013025). We would also like to thank our colleagues at the Department of Cardiology, the First Affiliated Hospital of Harbin Medical University.

### References

1. Melillo P, Fusco R, Sansone M, Bracale M, Pecchia L: **Discrimination power of long-term heart rate variability measures for chronic heart failure detection.** *Med Biol Eng Comput* 2011, **49**:67–74.
2. Bui AL, Horwich TB, Fonarow GC: **Epidemiology and risk profile of heart failure.** *Nat Rev Cardiol* 2011, **8**:30–41.
3. Ramani GV, Uber PA, Mehra MR: **Chronic heart failure: contemporary diagnosis and management.** *Mayo Clin Proc* 2010, **85**:180–195.
4. Barrios V, Escobar C, De La Sierra A, Llisterri JL, Gonzalez-Segura D: **Detection of unrecognized clinical heart failure in elderly hypertensive women attended in primary care setting.** *Blood Press* 2010, **19**(5):301–307.
5. Bozkurt B, Mann DL, Deswal A: **Biomarkers of inflammation in heart failure.** *Heart Fail Rev* 2010, **15**:331–341.
6. Parissis JT, Ikonomidis I, Rafouli-Stergiou P, Mebazaa A, Delgado J, Farmakis D, Vilas-Boas F, Paraskevaidis I, Anastasiou-Nana M, Follath F: **Clinical characteristics and predictors of in-hospital mortality in acute heart failure with preserved left ventricular ejection fraction.** *Am J Cardiol* 2011, **107**:79–84.
7. Routledge FS, Campbell TS, McFetridge-Durdle JA, Bacon SL: **Improvements in heart rate variability with exercise therapy.** *Can J Cardiol* 2010, **26**:303–312.
8. Smilde TD, van Veldhuisen DJ, van den Berg MP: **Prognostic value of heart rate variability and ventricular arrhythmias during 13-year follow-up in patients with mild to moderate heart failure.** *Clin Res Cardiol* 2009, **98**:233–239.
9. Thayer JF, Yamamoto SS, Brosschot JF: **The relationship of autonomic imbalance, heart rate variability and cardiovascular disease risk factors.** *Int J Cardiol* 2010, **141**:122–131.
10. Xhyheri B, Manfrini O, Mazzolini M, Pizzi C, Bugiardini R: **Heart rate variability today.** *Prog Cardiovasc Dis* 2012, **55**(3):321–331.
11. Clavel MA, Dumesnil JG, Capoulade R, Mathieu P, Senechal M, Pibarot P: **Outcome of patients with aortic stenosis, small valve area, and low-flow, low-gradient despite preserved left ventricular ejection fraction.** *J Am Coll Cardiol* 2012, **60**(14):1259–1267.
12. Pellicori P, Kallvikbacka-Bennett A, Khaleva O, Carubelli V, Costanzo P, Castiello T, Wong K, Zhang J, Cleland JG, Clark AL: **Global longitudinal strain in patients with suspected heart failure and a normal ejection fraction: does it improve diagnosis and risk stratification?** *Int J Cardiovasc Imaging* 2014, **30**(1):69–79.
13. La Rovere MT, Maestri R, Pinna GD, Sleight P, Febo O: **Clinical and haemodynamic correlates of heart rate turbulence as a non-invasive index of baroreflex sensitivity in chronic heart failure.** *Clin Sci (Lond)* 2011, **121**(6):279–284.
14. D'Addio G, Cesarelli M, Corbi G, Romano M, Furgi G, Ferrara N, Rengo F: **Reproducibility of heart rate turbulence indexes in heart failure patients.** *Conf Proc IEEE Eng Med Biol Soc* 2010, **2010**:2573–2576.
15. Bienias P, Ciurzynski M, Glinska-Wielochowska M, Szewczyk A, Korczak D, Kalinska-Bienias A, Gliński W, Pruszczyk P: **Heart rate turbulence assessment in systemic sclerosis: the role for the detection of cardiac autonomic nervous system dysfunction.** *Rheumatology (Oxford)* 2010, **49**(2):355–360.
16. Szymanowska K, Piatkowska A, Nowicka A, Michalski M, Dankowski R, Kandziora M, Biegalski W, Wierzchowiecki M, Poprawski K: **Clinical significance of heart rate turbulence assessment in patients with chronic heart failure.** *Kardiol Pol* 2008, **66**(12):1289–1295.
17. Miwa Y, Yoshino H, Hoshida K, Miyakoshi M, Tsukada T, Yusu S, Ikeda T: **Risk stratification for serious arrhythmic events using nonsustained ventricular tachycardia and heart rate turbulence detected by 24-hour holter electrocardiograms in patients with left ventricular dysfunction.** *Ann Noninvasive Electrocardiol* 2012, **17**(3):260–267.
18. Sredniawa B, Cebula S, Kowalczyk J, Batchvarov VN, Musialik-Lydka A, Sliwinska A, Wozniak A, Zakliczynski M, Zembala M, Kalarus Z: **Heart rate turbulence for prediction of heart transplantation and mortality in chronic heart failure.** *Ann Noninvasive Electrocardiol* 2010, **15**(3):230–237.
19. Pankuweit S, Hufnagel G, Eckhardt H, Herrmann H, Uttecht S, Maisch B: **Cardiotropic DNA viruses and bacteria in the pathogenesis of dilated cardiomyopathy with or without inflammation.** *Med Klin (Munich)* 1998, **93**(4):223–228.
20. Shi ZH, Gao CY, Liu LG, Zhang RR, Xu RH: **The effect of ventricular fibrillation time and NYHA classification on defibrillation in intensive care unit patients.** *Chin Crit Care Med* 2013, **25**(2):99–101.
21. Fox K, Borer JS, Camm AJ, Danchin N, Ferrari R, Lopez Sendon JL, Steg PG, Tardif JC, Tavazzi L, Tendera M: **Resting heart rate in cardiovascular disease.** *J Am Coll Cardiol* 2007, **50**(9):823–830.
22. Lenis G, Dossel O: **T Wave Morphology during Heart Rate Turbulence in Patients with Chronic Heart Failure.** *Biomed Tech (Berl)* 2013, **58**(Suppl. 1):1.
23. Stein PK, Barzilay JI: **Relationship of abnormal heart rate turbulence and elevated CRP to cardiac mortality in low, intermediate, and high-risk older adults.** *J Cardiovasc Electrophysiol* 2011, **22**(2):122–127.
24. Lorvidhaya P, Addo K, Chodosh A, Iyer V, Lum J, Buxton AE: **Sudden cardiac death risk stratification in patients with heart failure.** *Heart Fail Clin* 2011, **7**(2):157–174. vii.
25. Bauer A, Barthel P, Muller A, Ulm K, Huikuri H, Malik M, Schmidt G: **Risk prediction by heart rate turbulence and deceleration capacity in postinfarction patients with preserved left ventricular function retrospective analysis of 4 independent trials.** *J Electrocardiol* 2009, **42**(6):597–601.
26. Cozzolino D, Furlan R, Gruosso D, Maggio CD, Giudice EM, Torella R, Giugliano D: **Effects of a mixed meal on hemodynamics and autonomic control of the heart in patients with type 1 diabetes.** *J Clin Endocrinol Metabol* 2010, **95**(1):194–200.
27. Francis J, Watanabe MA, Schmidt G: **Heart rate turbulence: a new predictor for risk of sudden cardiac death.** *Annals Noninvasive Electrocardiology* 2005, **10**(1):102–109.
28. Manzano-Fernandez S, Pastor-Perez FJ, Barquero-Perez O, Pascual-Figal DA, Goya-Esteban R, Rojo-Alvarez JL, Caamaño-Fernández A, Martínez Martínez-Espejo MD, Januzzi JL, Valdés M, García-Alberola A: **Short-term variability of heart rate turbulence in chronic heart failure.** *J Card Fail* 2011, **17**(9):735–741.
29. Lewis MJ, Annandale J, D'Silva LA, Davies RE, Reed Z, Lewis KE: **Influence of long-term oxygen therapy on cardiac acceleration and deceleration capacity in hypoxic patients with chronic obstructive pulmonary disease.** *Clin Physiol Funct Imaging* 2011, **31**(4):258–265.
30. Stein PK, Deedwania P: **Usefulness of abnormal heart rate turbulence to predict cardiovascular mortality in high-risk patients with acute myocardial infarction and left ventricular dysfunction (from the EPHESUS study).** *Am J Cardiol* 2009, **103**(11):1495–1499.
31. Trzos E, Krzeminska-Pakula M, Rechcinski T, Drozdz J, Kurpesa M: **Heart rate turbulence in patients with chronic heart failure.** *Kardiol Pol* 2008, **66**(11):1183–1190. discussion 1191–1183.

32. Piotrowicz E, Baranowski R, Piotrowska M, Zielinski T, Piotrowicz R: **Variable effects of physical training of heart rate variability, heart rate recovery, and heart rate turbulence in chronic heart failure.** *Pacing Clin Electrophysiol* 2009, **32**(Suppl 1):S113–115.
33. Hadase M, Azuma A, Zen K, Asada S, Kawasaki T, Kamitani T, Kawasaki S, Sugihara H, Matsubara H: **Very low frequency power of heart rate variability is a powerful predictor of clinical prognosis in patients with congestive heart failure.** *Circ J* 2004, **68**(4):343–347.
34. Kindermann M: **How to diagnose diastolic heart failure: a consensus statement on the diagnosis of heart failure with normal left ventricular ejection fraction by the Heart Failure and Echocardiography Associations of the European Society of Cardiology.** *Eur Heart J* 2007, **28**(21):2686. author reply 2686–2687.
35. Fox K, Ferrari R, Tendera M, Steg PG, Ford I: **Rationale and design of a randomized, double-blind, placebo-controlled trial of ivabradine in patients with stable coronary artery disease and left ventricular systolic dysfunction: the morBidity-mortality EvAlUaTion of the I(f) inhibitor ivabradine in patients with coronary disease and left ventricULar dysfunction (BEAUTIFUL) study.** *Am Heart J* 2006, **152**(5):860–866.
36. Nul DR, Doval HC, Grancelli HO, Varini SD, Soifer S, Perrone SV, Prieto N, Scapin O: **Heart rate is a marker of amiodarone mortality reduction in severe heart failure. The GESICA-GEMA Investigators. Grupo de Estudio de la Sobrevida en la Insuficiencia Cardiaca en Argentina-Grupo de Estudios Multicentricos en Argentina.** *J Am Coll Cardiol* 1997, **29**(6):1199–1205.

# 17

# Galectin-3 and fibulin-1 in systolic heart failure - relation to glucose metabolism and left ventricular contractile reserve

Pernille Holmager[1,2,11*], Michael Egstrup[3], Ida Gustafsson[4], Morten Schou[2,5], Jordi S. Dahl[6], Lars Melholt Rasmussen[7,8], Jacob E. Møller[9], Christian Tuxen[10], Jens Faber[1,2] and Caroline Kistorp[1,2]

## Abstract

**Background:** Heart failure (HF) patients with diabetes (DM) have an adverse prognosis and reduced functional capacity, which could be associated with cardiac fibrosis, increased chamber stiffness and reduced left ventricular (LV) contractile reserve. Galectin-3 (Gal-3) and fibulin-1 are circulating biomarkers potentially reflecting cardiac fibrosis. We hypothesize that plasma levels of Gal-3 and fibulin-1 are elevated in HF patients with DM and are associated with reduced LV contractile reserve in these patients.

**Methods:** A total of 155 patients with HF with reduced ejection fraction underwent a low-dose dobutamine echocardiography and blood sampling for biomarker measurements. Patients were classified according to history of DM and an oral glucose tolerance test (OGTT) as: normal glucose tolerance (NGT) ($n = 70$), impaired glucose tolerance (IGT) ($n = 25$) and DM ($n = 60$).

**Results:** Galectin-3 levels were elevated in DM patients as compared to non-diabetic patients ($P = 0.02$), while higher fibulin-1 levels were observed in HF patients with IGF and DM ($P = 0.07$). Reduced LV contractile reserve was associated with increasing Gal-3 levels ($\beta = -0.19$, $P = 0.03$) although, this association was attenuated after adjustment for estimated glomerular filtration rate ($P = 0.66$). Fibulin-1 was not associated with LV contractile reserve ($P = 0.71$).

**Conclusions:** Galectin-3 and fibulin-1 levels were elevated in HF patients with impaired glucose metabolism. However, reduced LV contractile reserve among HF patients with DM does not to have an independent impact on plasma Gal-3 and fibulin-1 levels.

**Keywords:** Diabetes, Myocardial fibrosis, Galectin-3, Fibulin-1, Left ventricular contractile reserve

## Background

Patients with heart failure with reduced ejection fraction (HFrEF) and concomitant diabetes (DM) have a considerably increased mortality rate and reduced exercise capacity compared to non-diabetic HFrEF patients [1]. It is well-established that in HFrEF DM is frequent, and screening with an oral glucose tolerance test (OGTT) reveals a prevalence of more than 30% [2]. We have previously reported that the co-existence of DM, whether it is by history or newly diagnosed is associated with a reduced left ventricular (LV) contractile reserve assessed by low-dose dobutamine echocardiography (LDDE) among HFrEF patients [3]. Further, reduced LV contractile reserve is predictive of prognosis and thus could contribute to the unfavorable outcome of diabetic HFrEF patients [4]. The pathophysiological processes leading to reduced LV contractile reserve remain to be fully elucidated but have been associated with myocardial fibrosis in patients with cardiomyopathy [5].

Galectin-3 (Gal-3) is a galactoside-binding protein which is released to the circulation by activated macrophages and is considered a biomarker of cardiac fibrosis and remodeling [6]. In the myocardium, Gal-3 is primarily expressed in the fibroblasts and in macrophages and plays an important role in the formation of myocardial fibrosis

* Correspondence: holmager@dadlnet.dk
[1]Department of Medicine, Endocrine Unit, Herlev University Hospital, Herlev, Denmark
[2]Faculty of Health and Medical Sciences, Copenhagen University, Copenhagen, Denmark
Full list of author information is available at the end of the article

through activation of fibroblasts [6]. In DM increased plasma Gal-3 levels have been associated with both macro- and microvascular complications [7]. Moreover, high levels of Gal-3 are reported in patients with chronic HFrEF and renal dysfunction [8]. Hence, we hypothesize that elevated Gal-3 is associated with reduced LV contractile reserve found among HFrEF patients with DM.

The novel promising biomarker fibulin-1 is emerging as a potential biomarker of cardiomyopathy [9]. Fibulin-1 is an extracellular matrix glycoprotein and is considered to reflect pathological accumulation of extracellular matrix components surrounding vascular smooth muscle cells [10]. To our knowledge no previous studies of fibulin-1 in HFrEF patients have been performed. In patients with chronic renal dysfunction high levels of fibulin-1 are associated with increasing age, HbA1c and creatinine [11]. Plasma fibulin-1 levels have been investigated in patients with aortic stenosis, where an association with decreased longitudinal systolic LV function has been observed [12]. The effects of HFrEF and abnormal glucose metabolism on circulating fibulin-1 levels have, to our knowledge, not been examined previously.

Therefore, the aims of this study were to evaluate the impact of DM and abnormal glucose metabolism on plasma Gal-3 and fibulin-1 concentrations, and further to investigate whether Gal-3 and fibulin-1 levels were associated with LV contractile reserve in HFrEF patients according to presence of DM.

## Methods

### Study population

Between May 2008 and June 2010 155 patients were recruited from the HF clinic at Frederiksberg University Hospital, Copenhagen, Denmark. The cohort has previously been described in detail [3]. Patients were enrolled in the present study if LV ejection fraction (LVEF) was ≤ 45% by echocardiography and baseline measurements of Gal-3 and fibulin-1 were available.

Patients were classified as having DM either by history or DM newly diagnosed by an oral glucose tolerance test (OGTT). The OGTT was performed in patients without known DM within 2 weeks after the baseline visit by ingestion of 75 g glucose dissolved in 250 mL water. Plasma glucose was measured in the fasting state (fasting plasma glucose, FPG) and after 2 h (2hPG). Glycemic status was defined according to WHO diagnostic criteria: Normal glucose tolerance (NGT): FPG <6.1 mmol/L and 2hPG <7.8 mmol/L. Impaired glucose tolerance (IGT): FPG <7.0 mmol/L and 2hPG between 7.8 and 11.1 mmol/L. DM: FPG >7.0 mmol/L and/or 2hPG >11.1 mmol/L.

### Echocardiography

Resting echocardiography and LDDE (as described in detail previously [3]) was performed within 2 weeks after referral to the outpatient clinic on a standard ultrasound machine (IE-33, Philips Inc.) and stored for later analysis [3]. The Doppler analyses were based on an average of five beats for patients with sinus rhythm and 10 beats for patients with atrial fibrillation (AF). LVEF was calculated by the biplane method from apical four- and two-chamber views [13].

### Laboratory analysis

After a minimum 8-h overnight fast and 20 min of supine rest, venous blood was obtained for measurement. Blood was drawn into EDTA tubes, promptly centrifuged at 4 °C, and plasma was frozen at −80 °C in aliquots until laboratory analyses were performed. Insulin resistance was estimated using the Homeostasis Model of Assessment-Insulin Resistance (HOMA-IR): Fasting Glucose (mmol/L) x Insulin (mU/L)/22.5. Galectin-3 was determined using an ELISA kit (BG Medicine, Waltham, USA) [14]. The lower detection limit was 1.32 ng/mL, intra- and interassay coefficient of variation (CV) <6% and <10%, respectively [14]. The fibulin-1 double-antibody sandwich ELISA has previously been described extensively [15]. Antibodies are a mouse anti-fibulin monoclonal 5D12/H7 IgG and goat anti-rabbit IgG alkaline phosphatase [16]. The assay has a lower detection limit of 1.56 μg/mL, an intra- and interassay CV <8% and ~10%, respectively [15].

### Statistical analysis

Distribution of the biomarkers Gal-3 and fibulin-1 in the total study population is depicted in histograms. Continuous variables are presented as mean (SD) or as median (interquartile range), as appropriate. The groups were compared using independent sample *T*-test or Kruskall-Wallis' test if the assumption of Gaussian distribution was not met. Fibulin-1 levels were normally distributed, while GAL-3 levels were not. The IGT group was small, and we previously demonstrated that LV contractile reserve is reduced in patients with known or new DM but not affected by IGT. Hence, we divided the population in two groups: DM (new or known), and non-DM (NGT or IGT) in the multivariable linear regression analysis. The associations between Gal-3, fibulin-1 and HbA1c were depicted in scatter plots. Multivariable linear regression analyses examining the association between Gal-3 and fibulin-1 levels with LV function were performed. The multivariable regression analyses included co-variables considered of having potential impact of LV contractile reserve in univariable analysis: Age, sex, presence of ischemic heart disease (IHD), estimated glomerular filtration rate (eGFR), atrial fibrillation (AF) and DM status [3]. Further, the relationship between Gal-3, fibulin-1 and parameters of glucose metabolism as HbA1c and DM were examined in multivariable models including confounders associated with Gal-3 and fibulin-1 at the $P$ <0.1 level in univariable analysis. Multivariable linear regression analysis was performed as stepwise analyses with backward elimination. Logarithmic transformation of Gal-3 and fibulin-1 were used in the linear regression analyses to meet the assumptions of linearity. Statistical analyses were performed using the SPSS 22 package.

## Results

According to the OGTT and history of DM, 70 (45%) of the HF patients had NGT, 25 (16%) had IGT, and 60 (39%) DM, of these 28 (18%) were newly diagnosed. Baseline characteristics according to DM status are presented in Table 1. There were no significant differences with regard to age, gender distribution, eGFR, and IHD between HF patients with and without DM. LVEF at rest ($P = 0.003$), LV contractile reserve ($P = 0.01$), and systolic longitudinal tissue velocity (S') during LDDE ($P = 0.03$) were reduced among patients with DM compared to the non-diabetic patients. Distributions of Gal-3 and of fibulin-1 are displayed in Fig. 1. Median (IQR) Gal-3 was 16.0 (12.8–21.0) ng/mL, and mean fibulin-1 was 57 ± 16 μg/mL. The univariable associations between the biomarkers and clinical parameters are shown in Table 2. Galectin-3 levels were strongly associated with impaired renal function (eGFR) ($\beta = -0.49$, $P < 0.001$) and ($\beta = -0.46$, $P < 0.001$) after full adjustment. Fibulin-1 levels were correlated to eGFR, NT-proBNP, presence of AF, and age (Table 2) and remained correlated to eGFR ($\beta = -0.26$, $P < 0.001$) after full adjustment.

### Galectin-3, fibulin-1 and relationship with glucose metabolism

Plasma Gal-3 levels were elevated among HF patients with DM (17.9 (12.9 26.1) ng/mL) and IGT (16.8 (14.1–22.1) ng/mL) as compared with NGT patients 15.2 (11.6–18.3) ng/mL ($P = 0.02$) (Table 1). No difference was found in patients classified as IGT compared to NGT ($P = 0.38$). The relationship between the presence of DM and Gal-3 levels was further investigated in a multivariable model adjusting for age, eGFR, AF, and NYHA functional class, being confounders associated with Gal-3 at the $P < 0.1$ level. In this model DM was independently associated with elevated Gal-3 ($\beta = 0.17$, $P = 0.02$). An impact of glucose metabolism on Gal-3 levels was further observed by a positive association with HbA1c ($\beta = 0.25$, $P = 0.02$) (Fig. 2), and FPG ($P = 0.02$), but only borderline significantly associated with 2hPG and HOMA (Table 2). HbA1c was entered in a multivariable model, and demonstrated to have an independent relation with increasing Gal-3 levels ($\beta = 0.16$, $P = 0.02$). After full adjustment, no association between Gal-3 and FPG ($P = 0.56$, data not shown) was observed.

**Table 1** Baseline characteristics according to diabetes status

| Demographics | DM ($n = 60$) | Non-DM ($n = 95$) | $P$ value |
|---|---|---|---|
| Age, years | 70.8 (9.6) | 69.7 (10.8) | 0.54 |
| Sex (female/male), % | 32/68 | 33/67 | 0.90 |
| IHD, n (%) | 40 (67) | 52 (55) | 0.20 |
| NYHA I + II vs. III + IV, % | 77/23 | 85/15 | 0.21 |
| AF, n (%) | 18 (30) | 21 (22) | 0.30 |
| Systolic BP, mmHg | 134 (110–151) | 135 (120–146) | 0.58 |
| Heart rate, beats/min | 73 (66–81) | 69 (60–81) | 0.03 |
| *Metabolism* | | | |
| BMI, kg/m$^2$ | 28.1 (5.4) | 26.3 (5.0) | 0.05 |
| FPG, mmol/L | 6.9 (1.4) | 5.7 (0.5) | <0.001 |
| 2hPG (mmol/l) | 11.7 (2.9) | 6.6 (1.9) | <0.001 |
| HbA1C, mmol/mol | 49 (12) | 40 (4) | <0.001 |
| HOMA-IR | 2.8 (1.5–5.8) | 1.7 (1.0–2,8) | <0.001 |
| Total cholesterol, mmol/L | 4.0 (1.0) | 4.4 (1.1) | 0.02 |
| Estimated GFR, ml/min/1.73 m$^2$ | 68 (26) | 74 (19) | 0.10 |
| *Biomarkers* | | | |
| NT-proBNP, pg/mL | 1111 (418–2227) | 771 (310–1854) | 0.08 |
| Gal-3, ng/ml | 17.9 (12.9–26.1) | 15.6 (12.6–19.3) | 0.02 |
| Fibulin-1, μg/ml | 60 (19) | 55 (13) | 0.07 |
| *Echocardiographic variables* | | | |
| LVEF rest, % | 34 (29–41) | 39 (33–45) | 0.003 |
| S' (rest), cm/s | 5.2 (4.5–6.5) | 5.7 (4.8–6.4) | 0.10 |
| E, cm/s | 81.6 (62.2–99.7) | 72.9 (60.0–92.4) | 0.31 |
| e', cm/s | 5.9 (4.6–7.5) | 6.6 (5.5–8.7) | 0.03 |
| E/e' (rest) per unit | 12.2 (9.6–16.5) | 10.2 (8.1–15.4) | 0.007 |
| LVEF stress, % | 40 (34–47) | 49 (40–57) | <0.001 |
| LV contractile reserve, % | 7 (2–10) | 10 (4–15) | 0.01 |
| S' (stress), cm/s | 8.3 (6.3–9.6) | 7.3 (5.7–8.5) | 0.03 |
| *Medical treatment* | | | |
| ACE/AngII-inhibitors, n, (%) | 85 (89) | 48 (80) | 0.10 |
| β-blocker, n (%) | 53 (88) | 72 (76) | 0.05 |
| Loop diuretic dose, mg/24 h | 60 (0–80) | 0 (0–60) | 0.001 |

Oral glucose tolerance test was only performed in the non-diabetic HF patient. 2hPG: 2 h plasma glucose. *AF* Atrial fibrillation; *BMI* Body mass index; *BSA* Body surface area *E* Peak early diastolic transmitral flow velocity; *e'*; early diastolic longitudinal tissue velocities; *FPG* Fasting plasma glucose; *Gal-3* Galectin-3; *GFR* Glomerular filtration rate; *HOMA-IR* Homeostatic model assessment of Insulin Resistance. *IHD* Ischemic heart disease; *LV* left ventricular; *LVEF* Left ventricular ejection fraction; *NT-proBNP* N-terminal pro B-natriuretic peptide; *NYHA* NYHA functional class; *S'* Systolic longitudinal tissue velocity

There was only a trend towards increased plasma fibulin-1 levels when comparing in HF patients with DM vs non DM ($P = 0.07$), although impaired glucose metabolism assessed by presence of IGT and DM were associated with equivalent elevated mean fibulin-1 levels 61 ± 16 μg/mL vs. 60 ± 19 μg/mL, respectively compared to HF patients with NGT 52 ± 13 μg/mL ($P = 0.01$). Further, HbA1c was associated with increasing fibulin-1

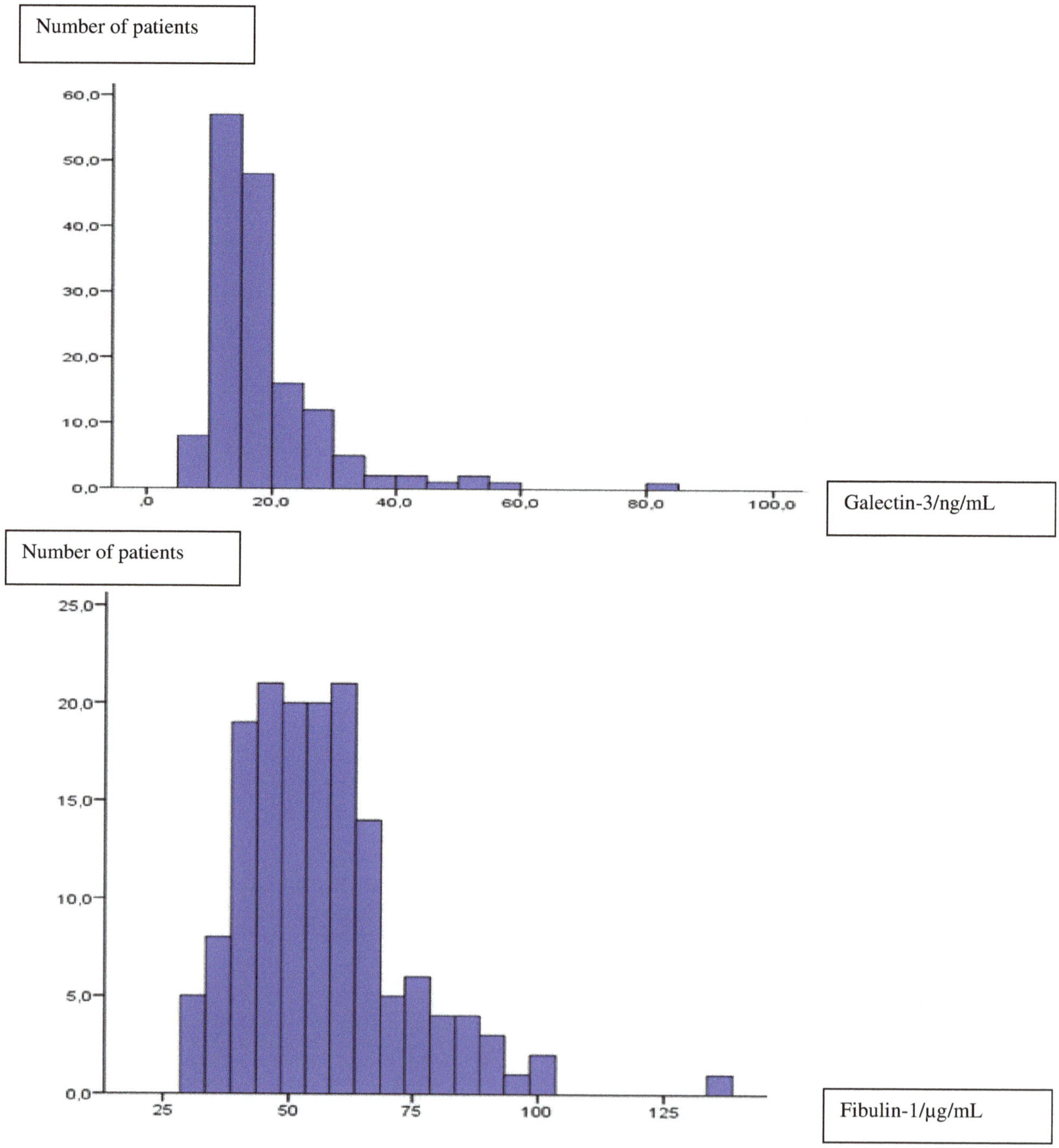


**Fig. 1** Histograms of Galectin-3 and Fibulin-1

concentrations (β = 0.21, $P = 0.009$) (Fig. 2), and this relation was not markedly attenuated after adjustment for the confounders age, AF, and eGFR (β = 0.15, $P = 0.05$). Fibulin-1 levels which were more than 2SD from mean Finulin-1 levels were considered outliers. Hence, we excluded 3 measurements of Fibulin-1 levels which were considered outliers. The exclusion of the outliers did not change the results (data not shown).

#### Galectin-3, fibulin-1 and relationship with LV function

The univariable associations between plasma Gal-3 and fibulin-1 levels with echocardiographic parameters

**Table 2** Associations of galectin-3 and fibulin-1 levels with clinical and glucometabolic parameters

| | Galectin-3 | | Fibulin-1 | |
|---|---|---|---|---|
| Parameter | β (SE) | *P*-Value | β (SE) | *P*-Value |
| Age, per year | 0.16 (0.23) | 0.05 | 0.36 (0.12) | <0.001 |
| Sex | 0.04 (0.07) | 0.59 | −0.09 (2.75) | 0.29 |
| Ischemic heart disease | −0.01 (0.07) | 0.90 | −0.009 (2.71) | 0.92 |
| NYHA I + II vs. III + IV | 0.16 (0.09) | 0.06 | 0.08 (3.37) | 0.34 |
| Atrial fibrillation | 0.17 (0.07) | 0.03 | 0.17 (2.83) | 0.03 |
| Diabetes mellitus | 0.27 (0.07) | 0.001 | 0.16 (2.62) | 0.05 |
| eGFR, per ml/min/1.73 $m^2$ | −0.49 (0.10) | <0.001 | −0.33 (0.06) | <0.001 |
| *Metabolism* | | | | |
| BMI, per kg/$m^2$ | −0.04 (0.006) | 0.63 | −0.12 (0.25) | 0.14 |
| FPG, per mmol/L | 0.19 (0.02) | 0.02 | −0.07 (1.37) | 0.44 |
| 2hPG, per mmol/L | 0.15 (0.01) | 0.09 | 0.26 (0.42) | 0.004 |
| HbA1C, per mmol/mol | 0.25 (0.16) | 0.02 | 0.21 (0.14) | 0.009 |
| HOMA-IR, per unit | 0.17 (0.01) | 0.06 | −0.08 (0.52) | 0.36 |
| *Biomarkers* | | | | |
| NT-proBNP per pg/mL | 0.30 (0.12) | <0.001 | 0.38 (2.24) | <0.001 |

Univariable regression models

*2hPG* 2 h plasma glucose, *BMI* Body mass index, *FPG* Fasting plasma glucose, *GFR* Glomerular filtration rate, *HOMA-IR* Homeostatic model assessment of insulin resistance, *NT-proBNP* N-terminal pro B-natriuretic peptide, *NYHA* NYHA functional class

obtained at rest and during LDDE are displayed in Table 3. There was an association between Gal-3 and LV contractile reserve (β = −0.19, $P = 0.03$) and Gal-3 and LVEF during stress (β = −0.25, $P = 0.003$). In a multivariable regression model the association with LV contractile reserve was no longer significant ($P = 0.66$), as only DM (β = −0.20, $P = 0.03$) and eGFR (β = −0.18, $P = 0.04$) remained predictive of LV contractile reserve after complete adjustment (data not shown).

Finally, the patients were divided into two groups; normal and low eGFR (<60 mL/min/1.73 $m^2$). In both groups, no association between Gal-3 and LV contractile reserve (β = −0.06, $P = 0.57$ in patients with normal eGFR vs. β = −0.02, $P = 0.95$ in patients with low eGFR) was demonstrated. With regard to fibulin-1, resting LVEF, LVEF and S' during stress were all associated with increasing levels of this biomarker in a univariable analysis, as presented in Table 3. Yet, after adjustment for relevant co-variables including eGFR no independent associations between fibulin-1 and these LV systolic measures were found. An independent relation of fibulin-1 with decreasing eGFR (β = −0.24, $P = 0.004$) and with age (β = 0.22, $P = 0.008$) was observed. Again, the patients were divided into two groups; normal and low eGFR (<60 mL/min/1.73 $m^2$). In both groups, no association between fibulin-1 and LV contractile reserve (β = 0.06, $P = 0.55$ in patients with normal eGFR vs. β = 0.02, $P = 0.89$ in patients with low eGFR) was presented. We have performed analyses where the patients with known diabetes were separated from the patients with newly diagnosed diabetes. This, however, did not influence the results.

## Discussion

The primary findings of the present study were that plasma Gal-3 and fibulin-1 levels were elevated in HFrEF patients with abnormal glucose metabolism compared to HFrEF patients with NGT. The impact of impaired glucose metabolism on both Gal-3 and fibulin-1 levels was underlined by an independent association with increasing HbA1c. However, increased Gal-3 and fibulin-1 levels were not associated with the reduced contractile reserve observed among diabetic HFrEF patients.

Median Gal-3 level was 16.0 ng/mL, which is similar to findings in comparable HFrEF populations and clearly increased compared to healthy subjects [17, 18]. The mean fibulin-1 level in our HF population was 57 ± 16 μg/mL, which is slightly higher than the mean level observed in a DM population (46 ± 1.3 μg/mL [19]). Fibulin-1 is a novel biomarker and high concentrations have primarily been reported in patients with aortic stenosis and DM compared to a level of 5.6 (4.1–8.4) μg/mL reported in healthy men [11, 20, 21].

The current results suggest that glucose metabolism is associated with circulating Gal-3 concentrations in HF, as elevated levels were found in patients with DM and an association with increasing HbA1c was demonstrated. The observations were supported by two previous

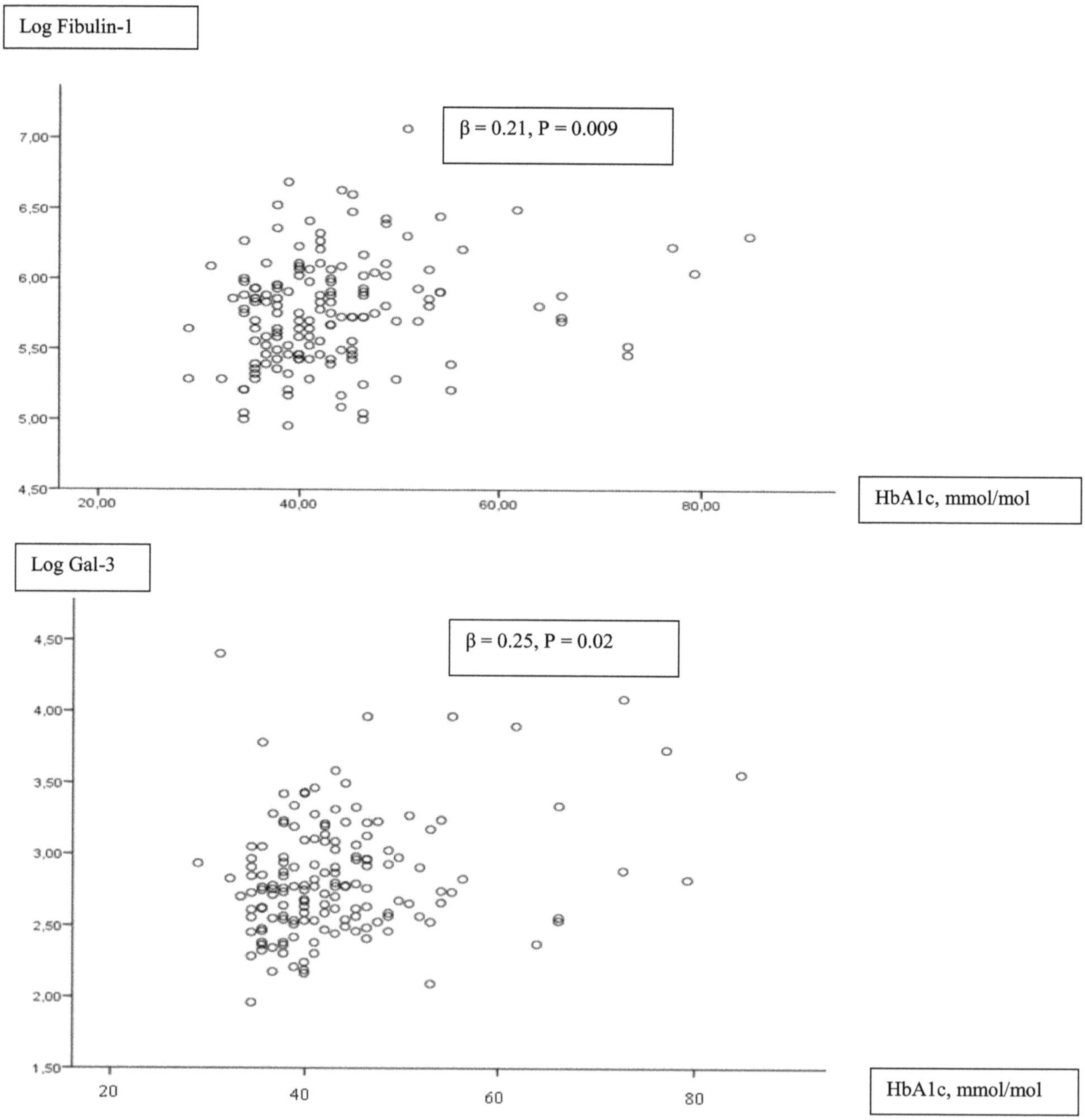


**Fig. 2** Scatter plot of HbA1c, Galectin-3 and fibulin-1 levels

studies reporting increased concentrations in patients with type 2 DM [18, 21]. However, we found a significant impact of renal function on plasma Gal-3 levels suggesting that other parameters, such as DM complications like diabetic nephropathy were more predictive of Gal-3 levels in HFrEF patients.

With regard to fibulin-1 we found elevated concentrations among patients with IGT and DM compared to NGT and a positive association with HbA1c, which corresponds with previous findings among type 2 DM reporting elevated circulating levels and of an upregulation of fibulin-1 in the arterial walls [19, 22].

To our knowledge, the present study is the first to evaluate the relation between circulating Gal-3 and fibulin-1 levels and cardiac function evaluated by LDDE. Galectin-3 was not associated with LV contractile reserve and LVEF during low dose dobutamine infusion after adjusting for relevant confounders, especially eGFR. The present study demonstrated that impaired renal function was a strong and independent predictor of

**Table 3** Associations of galectin-3 and fibulin-1 levels with echocardiographic parameters

| | Galectin-3 | | Fibulin-1 | |
|---|---|---|---|---|
| | β (SE) | *P*-Value | β (SE) | *P*-Value |
| *Resting echocardiography* | | | | |
| LVEF, per % | −0.15 (0.14) | 0.08 | −0.24 (0.14) | 0.004 |
| S', per cm/s | −0.15 (0.14) | 0.07 | −0.25 (0.02) | 0.002 |
| *Stress echocardiography* | | | | |
| LVEF stress, per % | −0.25 (0.14) | 0.003 | −0.20 (0.003) | 0.02 |
| LV contractile reserve, per % | −0.19 (0.06) | 0.03 | −0.03 (0.005) | 0.71 |
| S' (stress), per cm/s | −0.15 (0.14) | 0.07 | −0.24 (0.01) | 0.004 |

Univariable regression analyses
*LV* left ventricular/left ventricle, *LVEF* Left ventricular ejection fraction, *S'* Systolic longitudinal tissue velocity

elevated Gal-3 levels, which is in line with previous studies in patients with DM and in a community cohort [8, 23]. The elimination of Gal-3 has to our best knowledge not been described, but the present findings indicate a renal component. The gold standard for evaluation of myocardial fibrosis requires an endomyocardial biopsy, which is a high-risk procedure. Cardiac magnetic resonance imaging (CMR) is another method that seems to provide a good estimate of myocardial fibrosis [24, 25]. However, it is technically difficult to perform CMR in patients with AF and devices; which are highly prevalent in HFrEF patients. Furthermore, the association between cardiac fibrosis estimated by CMR and Gal-3 levels is not well described. In patients with previous myocardial infarction Gal-3 was moderately associated with LVEF and infarct size [26]. We report no association of the biomarkers Gal-3 with IHD. A proposed mechanism could be that former MI in our HFrEF patients are not associated with persisting increased activity of the fibrotic tissue and thereby secretion to the circulation of these biomarkers.

Myocardial fibrosis evaluated by histomorphometry and LV contractile reserve seems associated in patients with dilated cardiomyopathy [5]. In patients with acute decompensated HF, the PRIDE study reported a relationship between Gal-3 and resting echocardiographic parameters related to diastolic function [27]. In the current cohort of patients with chronic HFrEF we found no independent association with parameters related to diastolic function (data not shown).

We found no association between fibulin-1 levels and LV contractile reserve, while univariable associations were demonstrated between fibulin-1 and resting parameters LVEF and S'. However, no association was shown in the multivariable analyses. This is partly in accordance with data from patients with aorta stenosis, where fibulin-1 levels were related with S', but not with LVEF [10]. Furthermore, we demonstrated a moderate, inverse association with eGFR which could blunt a potential weaker association with LV contractile reserve.

### Limitations

This is a cross-sectional study. Hence, conclusion regarding causality is not possible. A larger sample size would have allowed us to investigate the IGT group in more detail.

## Conclusion

Galectin-3, but not fibulin-1 levels are elevated in diabetic compared to non-diabetic HFrEF patients. Both Gal-3 and fibulin-1 levels are independently and positively associated with HbA1c, but not with LV contractile reserve in HF patients.

#### Abbreviations

2hPG: 2 h plasma glucose; AF: Atrial fibrillation; BMI: Body mass index; BSA: Body surface area; CMR: Cardiac magnetic resonance imaging; DM: Diabetes mellitus; E: Peak early diastolic transmitral flow velocity; e': Early diastolic longitudinal tissue velocities; eGFR: Estimated glomerular filtration rate; FPG: Fasting plasma glucose; Gal-3: Galectin 3; GFR: Glomerular filtration rate; HF: Heart failure; HFrEF: Heart failure with reduced ejection fraction; HOMA-IR: Homeostasis Model of Assessment-Insulin Resistance; IGT: Impaired glucose tolerance; IHD: Ischemic heart disease; LDDE: Low dose dobutamine echocardiography; LV: Left ventricular; LVEF: Left ventricular ejection fraction; MI: Myocardial infarction; NGT: Normal Glucose tolerance; NT-proBNP: N-terminal pro B-natriuretic peptide; NYHA: NYHA functional class; OGTT: Oral Glucose Tolerance Test; S': Systolic longitudinal tissue velocity; SD: Standard deviation

#### Acknowledgements

Ulla Kjaerulff-Hansen, Hanne Dorthe Mogensen, Susanne Månsson, Marianne Sørensen and Anne-Marie Jakobsen are thanked for assistance with biomarker analyses. Department of Clinical Biochemistry at Frederiksberg Hospital is thanked for conducting the OGTTs.

#### Funding

The study was financed from a research grant from Herlev University Hospital.

#### Authors' contributions

PH: Acquisition of data, interpretation of data, drafting the manuscript, final approval of the version. ME: acquisition of data, analysis of data, final approval of the version. IG: hypothesis generating, revising manuscript critically for important intellectual content, final approval of the version. MS: Interpretation of data, final approval of the version. JD and LMR: interpretation of data (especially regarding fibulin-1), final approval of the version. JME and CDT: interpretation of data, revising manuscript critically, final approval of the version. JF and CK: Hypothesis generating, revising manuscript critically for important intellectual content, final approval of the version. All authors read and approved the final manuscript.

**Competing interests**

None of the authors have reported any conflicts of interest with regard to the present study.

**Author details**

[1]Department of Medicine, Endocrine Unit, Herlev University Hospital, Herlev, Denmark. [2]Faculty of Health and Medical Sciences, Copenhagen University, Copenhagen, Denmark. [3]Department of Cardiology, Rigshospitalet, Copenhagen, Denmark. [4]Department of Cardiology, Hvidovre University Hospital, Hvidovre, Denmark. [5]Department of Cardiology, Herlev University Hospital, Herlev, Denmark. [6]Department of Cardiology and Cardiothoracic Surgery, Odense University Hospital, Odense, Denmark. [7]Department of Clinical Biochemistry and Pharmacology, Odense University Hospital, Odense, Denmark. [8]Centre of Individualized Medicine in Arterial Diseases, Odense University Hospital, Odense, Denmark. [9]Department of Cardiology, Odense University Hospital, Odense, Denmark. [10]Department of Cardiology, Bispebjerg University Hospital, Copenhagen, Denmark. [11]Department of Endocrinology, Herlev Hospital, Herlev, Denmark.

**References**

1. Gustafsson I, Brendorp B, Seibaek M, et al. Influence of diabetes and diabetes-gender interaction on the risk of death in patients hospitalized with congestive heart failure. J Am Coll Cardiol. 2004;43:771–7.
2. Egstrup M, Schou M, Gustafsson I, et al. Oral glucose tolerance testing in an outpatient heart failure clinic reveals a high proportion of undiagnosed diabetic patients with an adverse prognosis. Eur J Heart Fail. 2011;13(3):319–26.
3. Egstrup M, Kistorp CN, Schou M, et al. Abnormal glucose metabolism is associated with reduced left ventricular contractile reserve and exercise intolerance in patients with chronic heart failure. Eur Heart J Cardiovasc Imaging. 2013;14(4):349–57.
4. Williams MJ, Odabashian J, Lauer MS, et al. Prognostic value of dobutamine echocardiography in patients with left ventricular dysfunction. J Am Coll Cardiol. 1996;27(1):132–9.
5. Otasevic P, Popovic ZB, Vasiljevic JD, et al. Relation of myocardial histomorphometric features and left ventricular contractile reserve assessed by high-dose dobutamine stress echocardiography in patients with idiopathic dilated cardiomyopathy. Eur J Heart Fail. 2005;7(1):49–56.
6. Sharma UC, Pokharel S, van Brakel TJ, et al. Galectin-3 marks activated macrophages in failure-prone hypertrophied hearts and contributes to cardiac dysfunction. Circulation. 2004;110(19):3121–8.
7. Jin QH, Lou YF, Li TL, et al. Serum galectin-3: a risk factor for vascular complications in type 2 diabetes mellitus. Chin Med J (Engl). 2013;126(11):2109–15.
8. Gopal DM, Kommineni M, Ayalon N et al. Relationship of plasma galectin-3 to renal fuinction in patients with heart failure: effects of clinical status, pathophysiology of heart failure, and presence or abscence of heart failure. J Am Heart Assoc. 2012;1(5):e000760. doi: 10.1161/JAHA.112.000760. Epub 2012 Oct 25.
9. Beisvag V, Lehre PK, Midelfart H, et al. Aetiology-sepcific patterns in end-stage heart failure patients identified by functional annotation and classification of microarray data. Eur J Heart Fail. 2006;8:381–9.
10. Hansen ML, Dahl JS, Argraves WS, et al. Aortic valve stenosis and atrial fibrillation influence plasma fibulin-1 levels in patients treated with coronary bypass surgery. Cardiology. 2013;126(3):202–6.
11. Schoze A, Bladbjerg EM, Sidelmann Jj et al. Plasma concentrations of extracellular matrix protein fibulin-1 are related to cardiovascular risk markers in chronic kidney disease and diabetes. Cardiovascl. Diabetol 2013 Jan 7;12:6. Doi: 10.1186/1475-2840-12-6
12. Dahl JS, Moller JE, Videbaek L, et al. Plasma fibulin-1 is linked to restrictive filling of the left ventricle and to mortality in patients with aortic valve stenosis. J Am Heart Assoc. 2012;1(6):e003889.
13. Lang RM, Bierig M, Devereux RB, et al. Recommendations for chamber quantification. Eur J Echocardiogr. 2006;7(2):79–108.
14. Christenson RH, Duh SH, Wu AH, et al. Multi-center determination of galectin-3 assay performance characteristics: Anatomy of a novel assay for use in heart failure. Clin Biochem. 2010;43(7–8):683–90.
15. Cangemi C, Skov V, Poulsen MK, et al. Fibulin-1 is a marker for arterial extracellular matrix alterations in type 2 diabetes. Clin Chem. 2011;57(11):1556–65.
16. Argraves WS, Tran H, Burgess WH, et al. Fibulin is an extracellular matrix and plasma glycoprotein with repeated domain structure. J Cell Biol. 1990;111(6 Pt 2):3155–64.
17. Tang WH, Shrestha K, Shao Z, et al. Usefulness of plasma galectin-3 levels in systolic heart failure to predict renal insufficiency and survival. Am J Cardiol. 2011;108(3):385–90.
18. Weigert J, Neumeier M, Wanninger J, et al. Serum galectin-3 is elevated in obesity and negatively correlates with glycosylated hemoglobin in type 2 diabetes. J Clin Endocrinol Metab. 2010;95(3):1404–11.
19. Skov V, Cangemi C, Gram J, et al. Metformin, but not rosiglitazone, attenuates the increasing plasma levels of a new cardiovascular marker, fibulin-1, in patients with type 2 diabetes. Diabetes Care. 2014;37(3):760–6.
20. Hansen ML, Rasmussen LM. Associations between plasma fibulin-1, pulse wave velocity and diabetes in patients with coronary heart disease. J Diabetes Complications. 2015;29(3):362–6. doi:10.1016/j.jdiacomp.2015.01.003. Epub 2015 Jan 13.
21. Paapstel K, Zilmer M, Eha J, et al. Association between fibulin-1 and aortic augmentation index in male patients with peripheral arterial disease. Eur J Vasc Endovasc Surg. 2016;51(1):76–82. doi:10.1016/j.ejvs.2015.09.004. Epub 2015 Oct 21.
22. Skov V, Knudsen S, Olesen M, et al. Global gene expression profiling displays a network of dysregulated genes in non-atherosclerotic arterial tissue from patients with type 2 diabetes. Cardiovasc Diabetol. 2012;11:15.
23. Ho JE, Liu C, Lyass A, et al. Galectin-3, a marker of cardiac fibrosis, predicts incident heart failure in the community. J Am Coll Cardiol. 2012;60(14):1249–56.
24. Mewton N, Liu CY, Croisille P, et al. Assessment of myocardial fibrosis with cardiovascular magnetic resonance. J Am Coll Cardiol. 2011;57(8):891–903.
25. Karamitsos TD, Francis JM, Myerson S, et al. The role of cardiovascular magnetic resonance imaging in heart failure. J Am Coll Cardiol. 2009;54(15):1407–24.
26. Singsaas EG, Manhenke CA, Dickstein K, et al. Circulation Galectin-3 levels are increased in patients with ischemic heart disease, but are not influenced by acute myocardial infarction. Cardiology. 2016;134:398–405. doi:10.1159/000445103.
27. Shah RV, Chen-Tournoux AA, Picard MH, et al. Galectin-3, cardiac structure and function, and long-term mortality in patients with acutely decompensated heart failure. Eur J Heart Fail. 2010;12(8):826–32.

# Is there a C-reactive protein value beyond which one should consider infection as the cause of acute heart failure?

Joana Pereira[1,6*], Ana Ribeiro[1], João Ferreira-Coimbra[1], Isaac Barroso[2], João-Tiago Guimarães[3,4], Paulo Bettencourt[4,5] and Patrícia Lourenço[1,4]

**Abstract**

**Background:** Heart Failure (HF) is a low grade inflammatory condition. High sensitivity C-reactive protein (hsCRP) is an established marker of inflammation. A cut-off value of hsCRP beyond which an infection should be sought has never been studied in HF. We aimed to determine the best hsCRP cut-off for infection prediction in acute HF.

**Methods:** We analyzed patients included in an acute HF registry – EDIFICA (Estratificação de Doentes com InsuFIciência Cardíaca Aguda). Admission hsCRP measurement was available as part of the registry's protocol. Patients with acute coronary syndrome as the cause of acute HF were excluded from the registry. Infection was considered according to the diagnosis registered in the discharge record. A receiver-operating characteristic (ROC) curve was used to determine the best hsCRP cut-off for infection prediction.

**Results:** We studied 615 patients. Mean age was 76 years, 45.2% were male, 60.3% had systolic dysfunction. Median admission hsCRP was 20.3 (9.5–55.5)mg/L; in 41.6% the cause of decompensation was an infection. The area under the ROC curve for admission hsCRP in the prediction of infection was 0.79 (0.76–0.83); the best hsCRP cut-off was 25 mg/L with a sensitivity of 72.7%, specificity 77.2%, positive predictive value 69.4% and negative predictive value 79.9%. Age and elevated hsCRP independently associated with an infection as the precipitant of acute HF.

**Conclusions:** We suggest 25 mg/L as a cut-off beyond which an infection should be sought underlying acute HF. Almost 80% of the patients with hsCRP< 25 mg/L are not infected and 69.4% of those with higher hsCRP have a concomitant infection.

**Keywords:** Acute heart failure, C-reactive protein, Infection, Cut-off

## Background

Inflammation appears to play a central role in the pathophysiology of heart failure (HF) [1, 2]. Several studies have corroborated this inflammatory hypothesis, which stands that endogenous cytokine cascades are implicated in the development and progression of HF [1, 3–8]. Inflammatory biomarkers are elevated in the blood of patients with HF [9, 10]. C-reactive protein is an acute-phase protein mainly synthesized in the liver; it is the most widely used and accepted marker to assess inflammation in everyday clinical practice [9].

HF can be considered a low-grade inflammatory condition. Chronic HF patients have increased levels of high-sensitivity C-reactive protein (hsCRP), regardless of the HF aetiology, and its levels increase with the severity of the disease [4, 9, 11–14].There is also clear evidence that a systemic inflammatory response is activated in acute HF [10, 15, 16]. Most studies demonstrating this inflammatory response in acute HF excluded patients with infection or other inflammatory conditions in order to prove the independent role of inflammation in HF [10, 17]. Notwithstanding, infection is well known to frequently underlie HF decompensation [18–20].

* Correspondence: joanaalmeidapereira@gmail.com
[1]Department of Internal Medicine, São João Hospital, Porto, Portugal
[6]Serviço de Medicina Interna, Hospital S. João, Alameda Professor Hernâni Monteiro, 4202-451 Porto, Portugal
Full list of author information is available at the end of the article

For the general population and patients with stable coronary artery disease, an also well established low-grade inflammatory condition [8], the hsCRP cut-offs proposed for future risk of cardiovascular events are < 1 mg/L (low risk), 1-3 mg/L (intermediate risk) and > 3 mg/L (high risk). Levels > 10 mg/l should be disregarded and repeated after 2 weeks to allow any inflammation to resolve and if repeated levels persist > 10 mg/L, a non cardiovascular aetiology for such hsCRP elevation should be considered [21, 22]. No hsCRP value beyond which an inflammatory or infectious condition has to be excluded as ever been proposed for HF, neither acute, nor chronic. The knowledge of such a cut-off would be particularly useful in the acute setting in which an infection is often the precipitant of HF decompensation.

The aim of our work was to determine the best cut-off value of hsCRP to predict infection in patients presenting with acute HF.

## Methods

We conducted a retrospective cohort study in a group of patients that had been included in an acute HF registry - EDIFICA (Estratificação de Doentes com InsuFIciência Cardíaca Aguda) - that took place in the Internal Medicine department of São João Hospital Center between January 2009 and December 2010. Patients eligible for inclusion were all patients admitted to our department with the primary diagnosis of acute HF during such period; both de novo and worsening chronic HF were eligible. The 2008 European Society of Cardiology guidelines were used for the diagnosis of HF [20] and both patients with reduced and preserved ejection fraction were included; patients with ejection fraction≥50% were considered to have HF with preserved ejection fraction (HFpEF). Patients with acute coronary syndrome as the cause of acute HF were excluded from the registry. A complete physical examination at admission and in the discharge day was performed to all patients. A 12-lead electrocardiogram was also performed at admission. As part of the registry's protocol, patients were drawn a venous blood sample within the first 48 h of hospital admission. An echocardiogram was performed to all patients during hospitalization, images were obtained with a standard ultrasound equipment (System 6, GE Vingmed, Horten, Norway) with a 2.5-MHz probe. The patient's treatment strategy, timing of discharge and discharge medication were at the discretion of the attending physician. The attending physicians were aware of the ongoing registry.

B-type natriuretic peptide (BNP) determination is a routine laboratory procedure in our hospital; an Abbott chemiluminescentmicroparticle immunoassay (2-step immunoassay) is used. Serum creatinine was measured using conventional methods with an Olympus AU5400® automated clinical chemistry analyzer Beckman-Coulter®. Haemoglobin was obtained using an automated blood counter Sysmex® XE-5000 (Hyogo, Japan), differential blood counts were also performed in accordance with routine clinical practice.

Serum hsCRP was assayed using particle-enhanced immunonephelometric assays on a BN™II laser nephelometer (Siemens, Erlangen, Germany). The manufacturer claims, for three different hs-CRP concentrations, 2.39 mg/L, 6.50 mg/L, 7.72 mg/L, intra-assay coefficients of variation (CV) of 5.2%, 5.0% and 4.6%, respectively, and inter-assay CV of 5.2%, 5.7% and 5.4%. The normal range of hsCRP is < 3.00 mg/L.

The glomerular filtration rate was estimated using the Modification of Diet in Renal Disease (MDRD) Study Equation.

All patients provided written informed consent to participate in the study. The registry's protocol conformed to the ethical guidelines of the declaration of Helsinki and it was approved by the local ethics committee.

A retrospective analysis was conducted in this patient cohort to determine the admission hsCRP beyond which an infectious condition should be sought. Patients with missing data regarding admission hsCRP (26 patients) were excluded from the analysis. The study flow chart is depicted in Fig. 1.

An infectious condition at admission and underlying acute HF was considered according to the discharge diagnosis list as judge by the attending physician and also according to the information in the discharge record.

### Statistical analysis

We used a receiver-operating characteristic (ROC) curve to define the best hsCRP cut-off for association with an infectious condition. The area under the ROC curve (AUC) was determined.

Patients with an infectious condition underlying acute HF and those without concomitant infection were compared; and patients with hsCRP< 25 mg/L and those with ≥25 mg/L were also compared: Chi square test for categorical variables, Student's t test to compare continuous variables and a Mann-Whitney U test when continuous variables had a highly skewed distribution. Variables independently associated with infection upon admission and underlying HF decompensation and variables independently associated with elevated hsCRP were assessed using multivariate logistic regression analysis. Models were built taking into consideration variables with a differential distribution between the groups compared.

The $p$ value considered for statistical significance was 0.05. Data was stored and analyzed using SPSS® software (IBM corp, Armonk, NY, version 20.0).

## Results

We studied 615 acute HF patients (Fig. 1). Mean patient's age was 76 (±12) years, 278 (45.2%) patients were male,

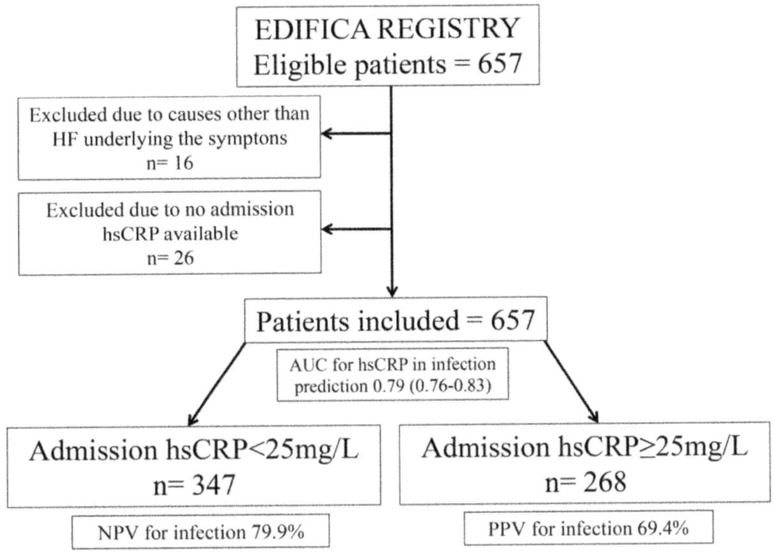


**Fig. 1** Study flow chart and main results

60.3% had left ventricular systolic dysfunction and 42.4% (261 patients) had ejection fraction< 35%. The percentage of patients with devices was modest, 7.3% of the patients with severe dysfunction; however we were dealing with an acute HF cohort of old and very old fragile patients. Median (interquartile range) admission hsCRP was 20.3 (9.5–55.5) mg/L. In 256 (41.6%) patients, an infection was considered as the factor precipitating or decompensating HF [68.0% had a respiratory infection, 15.2% a urinary infection, 7.8% a cutaneous infection, in 2.0% of the patients there were other, rarer, foci of infection (abdominal, cardiovascular, bones/joints), and in 7.0% the infectious focus remained unknown]. Table 1 compares patients according to infection status upon admission.

**Table 1** Comparison between acute HF patients with and without an infectious condition underlying cardiac decompensation

| Characteristics | Non-infected patients ($n = 359$) | Infected patients ($n = 256$) | *p*-value |
|---|---|---|---|
| Male sex, n (%) | 175 (48.7) | 103 (40.2) | 0.04 |
| Age, mean (SD) | 75 (12) | 79 (11) | < 0.001 |
| Atrial fibrillation, n (%) | 173 (48.2) | 107 (41.8) | 0.12 |
| Diabetes *mellitus*, n (%) | 159 (44.3) | 94 (36.7) | 0.06 |
| Coronary heart disease, n (%) | 159 (44.4) | 92 (36.0) | 0.04 |
| Admission NYHA IV (vs II/III) | 209 (58.2) | 162 (63.3) | 0.29 |
| Admission heart rate (bpm), mean (SD) | 90 (25) | 88 (21) | 0.34 |
| Admission systolic blood pressure (mmHg), mean (SD) | 136 (31) | 130 (28) | 0.01 |
| Left ventricular systolic dysfunction, n (%) | 234 (65.1) | 137 (53.5) | 0.003 |
| Haemoglobin (mmol/L), mean (SD) | 7.4 (1.4) | 7.1 (1.3) | 0.001 |
| Leukocytes (cells/μL) | 7934 (3056) | 9704 (4122) | < 0.001 |
| Neutrophils (cells/μL) | 5774 (2511) | 7733 (3815) | < 0.001 |
| Monocyte-to-Lymphocyte Ratio, mean (SD) | 0.54 (0.37) | 0.65 (0.40) | 0.001 |
| Glomerular filtration rate (mL/min/1.73m$^2$) | 48.3 (20.9) | 44.9 (20.7) | 0.05 |
| C-reactive protein (mg/L), median (IQR) | 12.8 (7.1–24.2) | 53.1 (22.8–116.0) | < 0.001 |
| C-reactive protein ≥25 mg/L | 82 (22.8) | 186 (72.7) | < 0.001 |
| BNP (pmol/L), median (IQR) | 458.8 (257.2–783.5) | 547.4 (293.7–858.1) | 0.08 |
| Acetylsalicylic acid, n (%) | 174 (48.5) | 119 (46.5) | 0.65 |
| Statin, n (%) | 188 (52.4) | 120 (46.9) | 0.19 |
| 1-year death | 130 (36.2) | 102 (39.8) | 0.36 |

*BNP* B-type natriuretic peptide, *hsCRP* high sensitivity C-reactive protein, *IQR* interquartile range, *NYHA* New York Heart Association, *SD* standard deviation

Apart an expected higher admission hsCRP (median value 53.1 mg/L in infected patients against 12.8 mg/L median value in non-infected) and neutrophil count, patients with a concomitant infection at admission were more often older women, with higher proportion of patients with HF with preserved ejection fraction and were more often admitted with lower systolic blood pressure, lower haemoglobin and worse renal function. Acute HF patients with a concomitant infection less frequently had coronary artery disease and there was also a non-significant trend for them to have higher BNP levels and less often to have diabetes.

The AUC for hsCRP in the prediction of infection as the cause underlying cardiac decompensation was of 0.79 (0.76–0.83), $p < 0.001$. Figure 2 depicts the ROC curve of the association of hsCRP with an infectious condition. The hsCRP value of 25 mg/L corresponded to the best cut-off for associated infection prediction. Using the cut-off of 25 mg/L, infection would be detected with a sensitivity of 72.7% and a specificity of 77.2%. The positive predictive value for infection when hsCRP ≥25 mg/L was 69.4% and the negative predictive value for infection when hsCRP< 25 mg/L was 79.9% (Fig. 1). If the classically accepted cut-off of 10 mg/L used in the general population and stable coronary heart disease was to be applied in this study sample of acute HF patients, the sensitivity would be of 91.4% and the specificity of 38.7%; this 10 mg/L cut-off would show a higher negative predictive value of 86.3%, however the positive predicted value would result unacceptably low – 51.5%.

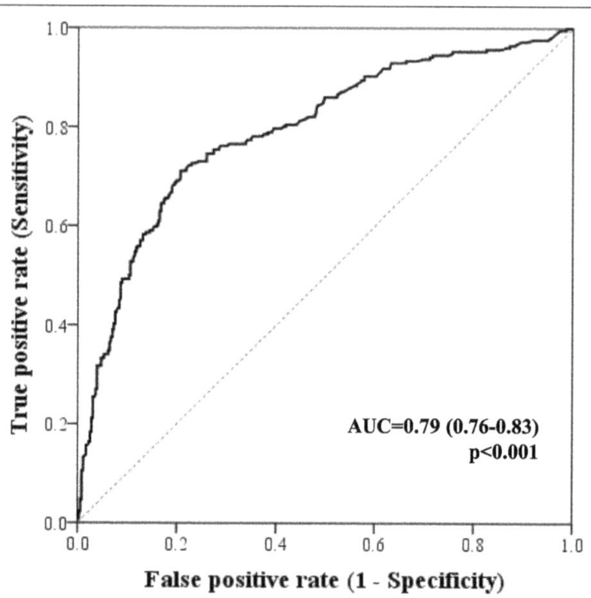


**Fig. 2** Receiver-operating characteristic (ROC) curve of the ability of admission hsCRP for infection prediction in patients hospitalized with acute HF. The AUC is of 0.79 (0.76–0.83), $p < 0.001$

Table 2 shows the comparison between patients admitted with hsCRP< 25 mg/L and those with hsCRP≥25 mg/L. Patients with higher admission hsCRP more often had an infectious condition underlying acute HF, were more often male, with lower admission systolic blood pressure, lower admission haemoglobin, higher BNP, and expectedly higher neutrophil count.

Despite the different distribution of variables according to the coexistence of infection upon admission, the only variables independently associated with an infectious condition complicating acute HF were age, neutrophil count and hsCRP, both analysed as a continuous and as a categorical variable (cut-off 25 mg/L). Table 3 shows the multivariate regression models for infection prediction in acute HF, with hsCRP analysed as a continuous and as a categorical variable. Increasing age, neutrophil count and admission hsCRP were independently associated with the coexistence of an infection upon admission with acute HF. Patients admitted with acute HF who presented with a hsCRP≥25 mg/L had an approximately 8-fold higher risk of having an infection as the cause of cardiac decompensation than when admission hsCRP was lower.

Independent predictors of elevated hsCRP at admission (≥25 mg/L) were male gender (OR = 1.87, 95% CI: 1.20–2.91) and haemoglobin (OR = 0.76, 95% CI: 0.64–0.90 per each mmol/L increase). An infectious condition was also an independent predictor of elevated hsCRP with a 8-fold higher risk. Adjustments were made accounting for age, diabetes, coronary artery disease, admission systolic blood pressure, admission glomerular filtration rate, BNP, leukocyte and neutrophil counts, monocyte to linfocyte ratio and left ventricular systolic dysfunction (data not shown).

## Discussion

Our results add some important findings to the current knowledge on the role of hsCRP and inflammation in acute HF. In our 615 patients' cohort, 25 mg/L value appears to be the best hsCRP cut-off for prediction of concomitant infection in the acute HF setting. In 72.7% of the patients presenting with acute HF, in whom an underlying infection decompensates HF, the hsCRP value was ≥25 mg/L. On the other hand, if a patient presented with acute HF and had an admission hsCRP ≥25 mg/L he had an almost 70% probability of having an infectious condition causing the cardiac decompensation. Our results also suggest that patients hospital-admitted with acute HF that have a hsCRP< 25 mg/L we are almost 80% certain that no infection complicates the clinical scenario.

In accordance with previous publications [18, 19, 23], we report a high prevalence of concomitant infection in patients presenting with acute HF and reinforce

**Table 2** Comparison between acute HF patients admitted with hsCRP below and above 25 mg/L

| Characteristics | hsCRP< 25 mg/L (*n* = 347) | hsCRP≥25 mg/L (*n* = 268) | p-value |
|---|---|---|---|
| Male sex, n (%) | 144 (41.5) | 134 (50.0) | 0.04 |
| Age, mean (SD) | 76 (12) | 77 (12) | 0.53 |
| Atrial fibrillation, n (%) | 159 (45.8) | 121 (45.1) | 0.88 |
| Diabetes *mellitus*, n (%) | 149 (42.9) | 104 (38.8) | 0.30 |
| Coronary heart disease, n (%) | 143 (41.2) | 108 (40.3) | 0.83 |
| Admission NYHA IV (vs II/III) | 207 (59.6) | 164 (61.2) | 0.87 |
| Admission heart rate (bpm), mean (SD) | 88 (24) | 89 (23) | 0.58 |
| Admission systolic blood pressure (mmHg), mean (SD) | 137 (29) | 130 (29) | 0.01 |
| Left ventricular systolic dysfunction, n (%) | 215 (62.0) | 156 (58.2) | 0.22 |
| Haemoglobin (mmol/L), mean (SD) | 7.4 (1.3) | 7.1 (1.3) | < 0.001 |
| Leukocytes (cells/μL) | 7918 (3172) | 9645 (3972) | < 0.001 |
| Neutrophils (cells/μL) | 5861 (2830) | 7534 (3543) | < 0.001 |
| Monocyte-to-Lymphocyte Ratio, mean (SD) | 0.53 (0.36) | 0.67 (0.40) | < 0.001 |
| Glomerular filtration rate (mL/min/1.73m$^2$) | 48.0 (20.7) | 45.4 (21.0) | 0.13 |
| Infectious condition at admission, n (%) | 70 (20.2) | 186 (69.4) | < 0.001 |
| BNP (pmol/L), median (IQR) | 446.8 (252.2–797.0) | 549.0 (304.4–848.8) | 0.05 |
| Acetylsalicylic acid, n (%) | 167 (48.1) | 126 (47.0) | 0.69 |
| Statin, n (%) | 165 (47.6) | 143 (53.4) | 0.19 |
| 1-year death | 130 (37.5) | 102 (38.1) | 0.88 |

*BNP* B-type natriuretic peptide, *hsCRP* high sensitivity C-reactive protein, *IQR* interquartile range, *NYHA* New York Heart Association, *SD* standard deviation

infection as an important precipitant of acute HF. Procalcitonin, another inflammatory biomarker, was found to be higher in patients with HF in comparison with control subjects and patients in whom acute HF and infection coexisted presented even higher levels of procalcitonin [24]. The recognition that an often life threatening infection precipitates acute HF and that the diagnosis of superimposed infections is sometimes difficult in this context has led to the development of strategies to more accurately identify coexistent infection. Procalcitonin has emerged as a promising tool for the early and accurate diagnosis of pneumonia and for guiding antibiotic therapy in acute HF patients [25, 26]. However, hsCRP is an inflammatory marker more widely available, more extensively studied, and much more familiar to physicians treating HF patients. Moreover, the AUC reported for procalcitonin in the diagnosis of pneumonia was of 0.72, which is lower than the one we report for the association of hsCRP with an infection underlying HF decompensation – AUC = 0.79 [27]. HsCRP has additional recognized prognostic information in the HF context rendering it a perhaps more useful biomarker in acute HF [17, 28–30].

Despite the differences between groups of patients with hsCRP below and above the 25 mg/L cut-off, the only variables independently associated with higher hsCRP were male gender, lower hemoglobin and concomitant infection. The relationship between gender and hsCRP is still controversial; however, inflammatory activation and the role of inflammation are clearly gender influenced. Depending on the population studied higher hsCRP values either in male or in female have been reported [31, 32]. Anemia is a common comorbidity in inflammatory conditions – anemia of chronic diseases [33]. Despite differences between groups of acute HF patients with and without a concomitant infection upon admission, the only independent predictors of infection were older age, higher neutrophil count and higher hsCRP. Older patients become progressively immune incompetent in one hand and have higher comorbidity burden in the other hand and, therefore, are more prone to infectious complications of their chronic diseases [34]. HsCRP is a well studied and accepted non-specific biomarker of inflammatory and infectious conditions [35]. Of note that the monocyte-to-lymphocyte ratio was not independently associated with the coexistence of an infectious condition; this eventually reflects the fact that the monocyte-to-lymphocyte ratio is probably more associated with chronic inflammatory burden and cardiovascular risk [36, 37] and less a mirror of acute changes in response to infection.

As a low-grade inflammatory disorder we would expect patients with HF, and particularly those with acute HF, to present with elevated hsCRP. In fact, in our patient population, those with acute HF and no infectious condition had a median hsCRP value at admission

**Table 3** Predictors of an infectious condition underlying decompensated HF: multivariate models

| | OR (95% CI) | *P*-value | Wald |
|---|---|---|---|
| Age, per year | 1.03 (1.01–1.05) | 0.01 | 6.60 |
| hsCRP≥25 mg/L | 8.05 (5.24–12.36) | < 0.001 | 90.82 |
| Male sex | 0.68 (0.43–1.08) | 0.10 | 2.72 |
| Diabetes *mellitus* | 0.89 (0.72–1.10) | 0.27 | 1.22 |
| Coronary heart disease | 0.73 (0.47–1.12) | 0.15 | 2.05 |
| Admission systolic blood pressure, per mmHg | 1.00 (0.99–1.00) | 0.18 | 1.77 |
| Haemoglobin, per mmol/L | 0.87 (0.74–1.03) | 0.11 | 2.53 |
| BNP per 100 pmol/L | 1.02 (0.98–1.06) | 0.30 | 1.09 |
| Leukocytes per 1000 cells/μL | 0.90 (0.76–1.06) | 0.21 | 1.58 |
| Neutrophils per 1000 cells/μL | 1.32 (1.09–1.60) | 0.005 | 7.88 |
| Monocyte-to-Lymphocyte Ratio | 0.96 (0.53–1.74) | 0.88 | 0.02 |
| Glomerular filtration rate per 10 mL/min/1.73 m2 | 1.08 (0.96–1.21) | 0.22 | 1.48 |
| Left ventricular systolic dysfunction | 0.76 (0.48–1.22) | 0.26 | 1.28 |
| | OR (95% CI) | *P*-value | |
| Age, per year | 1.02 (1.00–1.04) | 0.02 | 5.51 |
| hsCRP per 1 mg/L | 1.02 (1.01–1.02) | < 0.001 | 44.85 |
| Male sex | 0.84 (0.54–1.30) | 0.44 | 0.60 |
| Diabetes *mellitus* | 0.90 (0.73–1.10) | 0.31 | 1.02 |
| Coronary heart disease | 0.77 (0.51–1.17) | 0.23 | 1.46 |
| Admission systolic blood pressure, per mmHg | 0.99 (0.99–1.00) | 0.11 | 2.51 |
| Haemoglobin, per mmol/L | 0.86 (0.73–1.02) | 0.08 | 3.17 |
| BNP per 100 pmol/L | 1.01 (0.98–1.05) | 0.48 | 0.50 |
| Leuckoytes per 1000 cells/μL | 0.88 (0.72–1.08) | 0.22 | 1.51 |
| Neutrophils per 1000 cells/μL | 1.33 (1.06–1.66) | 0.01 | 6.31 |
| Monocyte-to-Lymphocyte Ratio | 0.84 (0.45–1.55) | 0.57 | 0.32 |
| Glomerular filtration rate per 10 mL/min/1.73m$^2$ | 1.05 (0.94–1.17) | 0.41 | 0.67 |
| Left ventricular systolic dysfunction | 0.77 (0.49–1.20) | 0.25 | 1.34 |

*BNP* B-type natriuretic peptide, *CI* Confidence Interval, *hsCRP* high sensitivity C-reactive protein, *OR* Odds Ratio

of 12.8 mg/L. It is important to remember that inflammatory and oxidative acute and chronic conditions may affect the electrophysiological functions, and the electrical/anatomical properties of cardiac function [38]. This could have been addressed by device interrogation; however, the number of patients with devices was low. This issue is even more pertinent if we consider this is a cohort of old HF patients and that 41.1% of them were diabetic, factors known to affect patients' response to device implantation and HF prognosis [39, 40].

The prognostic significance of hsCRP is documented in HF, mainly in the chronic context [9, 13, 41]; but also in the acute setting [29]. The interpretation of hsCRP in acute HF patients may be more intricate precisely because infectious intercurrences frequently underlie the HF worsening and hsCRP in a non-specific marker of inflammation. Part of the acute HF treatment implies addressing the decompensating factor and a clear recognition of an infection and its treatment may be crucial [42]. This is even more important if we consider that clinical manifestations of infection can be very mild and atypical in this group of classically old and very old patients.

Previous studies have shown that hsCRP has a prognostic role in acute HF patients and that higher levels of this acute-phase protein are associated with higher mortality [29]. Most studies that demonstrated an inflammatory response in acute HF excluded patients with concurrent infection or other inflammatory conditions in order to prove the independent role of inflammation in HF [10, 17]. The exact value that could help distinguishing patients with elevated hsCRP in relation with the inflammatory process underlying HF and those with elevated hsCRP due to a concomitant infectious process was never studied in HF. This is important, particularly in acute HF, not only to help defining the treatment strategy but also for clinicians to be able to interpret the prognostic value of hsCRP.

To the best of our knowledge this is the first study proposing a cut-off value beyond which an infection is highly prevalent in acute HF patients and therefore needs to be sought. The existence of such a cut-off can eventually help clinicians treating acute HF patients in their everyday clinical practice, representing a major advantage in the management of these patients with unquestionable clinical implications.

We propose the cut-off of 25 mg/L as the one beyond which hsCRP elevation should be considered as not totally attributable to low grade inflammation in acute HF. This value is higher than the arbitrary value of 10 mg/L accepted for the general population and patients with stable coronary artery disease.

This 25 mg/L cut-off value for hsCRP that we propose is grown out of a relatively large population of "real world" acute HF patients. The fact that it is significantly higher than the one for the general population is not totally unexpected since acute HF patients are experiencing a decompensation/exacerbation of an inflammatory condition. The use of the classical cut-off of 10 mg/L would have an elevated sensitivity (over 90%), but an also extremely elevated false positive rate of 61.3% and a low positive predictive value with only approximately half of the patients having an infectious condition when hsCRP value at acute HF presentation was ≥10 mg/L.

Our study has some limitations that need to be noted. The single center nature of the study implies generalisability concerns. The retrospective nature of the study has known inherent problems, namely concerning the availability and quality of the data collected. A treatment and general approach bias related to the fact that physicians treating HF patients were aware of the ongoing registry should also be kept in mind. It would have also been interesting to have included in the multivariate models other inflammatory markers, such as cytokines or TNF-α, however, no such data were available. Perhaps the most important setback comes from the definition of infection. We relied on the clinical evaluation of the attending physician and its registry in the discharge diagnosis list or in the discharge record. Criteria could be different between the physicians but, consulting the discharge notes, there were clinical and laboratory or radiologic criteria to support the diagnosis of infection.

Apart these limitations we were able to show that in the setting of acute HF, clinicians can rely on hsCRP values to adequately diagnose infection as the trigger of the decompensation and to treat it in accordance. Acute HF patients represent a group with a low grade inflammatory condition experiencing an episode of decompensation and an elevation of hsCRP is already expected. We have documented such hsCRP elevation in non-infected patients as well as an even higher elevation in infected ones. We have as well documented the ability of hsCRP to predict a concurrent infectious condition in acute HF decompensations.

## Conclusions

In patients with acute HF presenting with a hsCRP≥25 mg/L, an infectious condition complicating or underlying cardiac decompensation should be sought. Almost 80% of the patients with hsCRP< 25 mg/L are not infected and 69.4% of those with higher hsCRP have a concomitant infection.

### Abbreviations

AUC: Area under the curve; BNP: B-type natriuretic peptide; BPM: Beats per minute; CI: Confidence Interval; HF: Heart Failure; HFpEF: Heart Failure with preserved ejection fraction; hsCRP: High sensitivity C-reactive protein; IQR: Interquartile range; NYHA: New York Heart Association; OR: Odds Ratio; ROC: Receiver-operating characteristic; SD: Standard deviation

### Acknowledgements

This article is a result of the project DOCnet (NORTE-01-0145-FEDER-000003), supported by Norte Portugal Regional Operational Programme (NORTE 2020), under the PORTUGAL 2020 Partnership Agreement, through the European Regional Development Fund (ERDF).

### Funding

This article is a result of the project DOCnet (NORTE-01-0145-FEDER-000003), supported by Norte Portugal Regional Operational Programme (NORTE 2020), under the PORTUGAL 2020 Partnership Agreement, through the European Regional Development Fund (ERDF).

### Authors' contributions

JP: conception and design of the research, analysis and interpretation of the data, and drafting the manuscript. AR; JFC; IB; JTG: data interpretation and critical revision of the manuscript for important intellectual content. PB: obtained funding for the study, data acquisition and interpretation, and critical revision of the manuscript for important intellectual content. PL: conception and design of the research; acquisition, analysis and interpretation of the data; statistical analysis; supervised the work; and critical revision of the manuscript for important intellectual content. All authors read and approved the final manuscript.

### Competing interests

The authors declare that they have no competing interests.

**Author details**
[1]Department of Internal Medicine, São João Hospital, Porto, Portugal. [2]Department of Biochemistry, São João Hospital, Porto, Portugal. [3]Department of Clinical Pathology, São João Hospital, Porto, Portugal. [4]Unidade de Investigação e Desenvolvimento Cardiovascular do Porto, Faculty of Medicine of University of Porto, Porto, Portugal. [5]Hospital da CUF, Porto, Portugal. [6]Serviço de Medicina Interna, Hospital S. João, Alameda Professor Hernâni Monteiro, 4202-451 Porto, Portugal.

**References**

1. Seta Y, Shan K, Bozkurt B, et al. Basic mechanisms in heart failure: the cytokine hypothesis. J Card Fail. 1996;2(3):243–9.
2. Sharma R, Coats AJ, Anker SD. The role of inflammatory mediators in chronic heart failure: cytokines, nitric oxide, and endothelin-1. Int J Cardiol. 2000;72(2):175–86.
3. Mann DL. Mechanisms and models in heart failure: a combinatorial approach. Circulation. 1999;100(9):999–1008.
4. Chirinos JA, Zambrano JP, Chakko S, et al. Usefulness of C-reactive protein as an independent predictor of death in patients with ischemic cardiomyopathy. Am J Cardiol. 2005;95(1):88–90.
5. Lagrand WK, Visser CA, Hermens WT, et al. C-reactive protein as a cardiovascular risk factor: more than an epiphenomenon? Circulation. 1999; 100(1):96–102.
6. Testa M, Yeh M, Lee P, et al. Circulating levels of cytokines and their endogenous modulators in patients with mild to severe congestive heart failure due to coronary artery disease or hypertension. J Am Coll Cardiol. 1996;28(4):964–71.
7. Rauchhaus M, Doehner W, Francis DP, et al. Plasma cytokine parameters and mortality in patients with chronic heart failure. Circulation. 2000;102(25):3060–7.
8. Barbero U, D'Ascenzo F, Nijhoff F, et al. Assessing risk in patients with stable coronary disease: when should we intensify care and follow-up? Results from a meta-analysis of observational studies of the COURAGE and FAME era. Scientifica. 2016;2016:3769152.
9. Yin WH, Chen JW, Jen HL, et al. Independent prognostic value of elevated high-sensitivity C-reactive protein in chronic heart failure. Am Heart J. 2004; 147(5):931–8.
10. Boulogne M, Sadoune M, Launay JM, et al. Inflammation versus mechanical stretch biomarkers over time in acutely decompensated heart failure with reduced ejection fraction. Int J Cardiol. 2016;226:53–9.
11. Ronnow BS, Reyna SP, Muhlestein JB, et al. C-reactive protein predicts death in patients with non-ischemic cardiomyopathy. Cardiology. 2005;104(4):196–201.
12. Steele IC, Nugent AM, Maguire S, et al. Cytokine profile in chronic cardiac failure. Eur J Clin Investig. 1996;26(11):1018–22.
13. Tanner H, Mohacsi P, Fuller-Bicer GA, et al. Cytokine activation and disease progression in patients with stable moderate chronic heart failure. J Heart Lung Transplant. 2007;26(6):622–9.
14. Kaneko K, Kanda T, Yamauchi Y, et al. C-reactive protein in dilated cardiomyopathy. Cardiology. 1999;91(4):215–9.
15. Sato Y, Takatsu Y, Kataoka K, et al. Serial circulating concentrations of C-reactive protein, interleukin (IL)-4, and IL-6 in patients with acute left heart decompensation. Clin Cardiol. 1999;22(12):811–3.
16. Peschel T, Schonauer M, Thiele H, et al. Invasive assessment of bacterial endotoxin and inflammatory cytokines in patients with acute heart failure. Eur J Heart Fail. 2003;5(5):609–14.
17. Villacorta H, Masetto AC, Mesquita ET. C-reactive protein: an inflammatory marker with prognostic value in patients with decompensated heart failure. Arq Bras Cardiol. 2007;88(5):585–9.
18. Ghali JK, Kadakia S, Cooper R, et al. Precipitating factors leading to decompensation of heart failure. Traits among urban blacks. Arch Intern Med. 1988;148(9):2013–6.
19. Opasich C, Febo O, Riccardi PG, et al. Concomitant factors of decompensation in chronic heart failure. Am J Cardiol. 1996;78(3):354–7.
20. Dickstein K, Cohen-Solal A, Filippatos G, et al. ESC guidelines for the diagnosis and treatment of acute and chronic heart failure 2008: the task force for the diagnosis and treatment of acute and chronic heart failure 2008 of the European Society of Cardiology. Developed in collaboration with the heart failure association of the ESC (HFA) and endorsed by the European Society of Intensive Care Medicine (ESICM). Eur Heart J. 2008; 29(19):2388–442.
21. Pearson TA, Mensah GA, Alexander RW, et al. Markers of inflammation and cardiovascular disease: application to clinical and public health practice: a statement for healthcare professionals from the Centers for Disease Control and Prevention and the American Heart Association. Circulation. 2003; 107(3):499–511.
22. Sabatine MS, Morrow DA, Jablonski KA, et al. Prognostic significance of the centers for disease control/American Heart Association high-sensitivity C-reactive protein cut points for cardiovascular and other outcomes in patients with stable coronary artery disease. Circulation. 2007;115(12):1528–36.
23. Wang CC, Chang HY, Yin WH, et al. TSOC-HFrEF registry: a registry of hospitalized patients with decompensated systolic heart failure: description of population and management. Acta Cardiologica Sinica. 2016;32(4):400–11.
24. Wang W, Zhang X, Ge N, et al. Procalcitonin testing for diagnosis and short-term prognosis in bacterial infection complicated by congestive heart failure: a multicenter analysis of 4,698 cases. Crit Care. 2014;18(1):R4.
25. Mollar A, Minana G, Villanueva MP, et al. Utility of Procalcitonin for diagnosis of superimposed infections in patients with acute heart failure. Rev Cardiovasc Med. 2016;17(3–4):144–8.
26. Sager R, Kutz A, Mueller B, et al. Procalcitonin-guided diagnosis and antibiotic stewardship revisited. BMC Med. 2017;15(1):15.
27. Maisel A, Neath SX, Landsberg J, et al. Use of procalcitonin for the diagnosis of pneumonia in patients presenting with a chief complaint of dyspnoea: results from the BACH (biomarkers in acute heart failure) trial. Eur J Heart Fail. 2012;14(3):278–86.
28. Siirila-Waris K, Lassus J, Melin J, et al. Characteristics, outcomes, and predictors of 1-year mortality in patients hospitalized for acute heart failure. Eur Heart J. 2006;27(24):3011–7.
29. Mueller C, Laule-Kilian K, Christ A, et al. Inflammation and long-term mortality in acute congestive heart failure. Am Heart J. 2006;151(4):845–50.
30. Kalogeropoulos AP, Tang WH, Hsu A, et al. High-sensitivity C-reactive protein in acute heart failure: insights from the ASCEND-HF trial. J Card Fail. 2014;20(5):319–26.
31. Lee YJ, Lee JH, Shin YH, et al. Gender difference and determinants of C-reactive protein level in Korean adults. Clin Chem Lab Med. 2009;47(7):863–9.
32. Ishii S, Karlamangla AS, Bote M, et al. Gender, obesity and repeated elevation of C-reactive protein: data from the CARDIA cohort. PLoS One. 2012;7(4):e36062.
33. Weiss G, Goodnough LT. Anemia of chronic disease. N Engl J Med. 2005; 352(10):1011–23.
34. Yoshikawa TT. Epidemiology and unique aspects of aging and infectious diseases. Clin Infect Dis. 2000;30(6):931–3.
35. Clyne B, Olshaker JS. The C-reactive protein. J Emerg Med. 1999;17(6):1019–25.
36. Gijsberts CM, Ellenbroek G, Ten Berg MJ, et al. Effect of monocyte-to-lymphocyte ratio on heart failure characteristics and hospitalizations in a coronary angiography cohort. Am J Cardiol. 2017;120(6):911–6.
37. o Hartaigh B, Bosch JA, Thomas GN, et al. Which leukocyte subsets predict cardiovascular mortality? From the LUdwigshafen RIsk and cardiovascular health (LURIC) study. Atherosclerosis. 2012;224(1):161–9.
38. Sardu C, Santamaria M, Funaro S, et al. Cardiac electrophysiological alterations and clinical response in cardiac resynchronization therapy with a defibrillator treated patients affected by metabolic syndrome. Medicine. 2017;96(14):e6558.
39. Sardu C, Barbieri M, Santamaria M, et al. Multipolar pacing by cardiac resynchronization therapy with a defibrillators treatment in type 2 diabetes mellitus failing heart patients: impact on responders rate, and clinical outcomes. Cardiovasc Diabetol. 2017;16(1):75.
40. Sardu C, Marfella R, Santulli G. Impact of diabetes mellitus on the clinical response to cardiac resynchronization therapy in elderly people. J Cardiovasc Transl Res. 2014;7(3):362–8.
41. Ishikawa C, Tsutamoto T, Fujii M, et al. Prediction of mortality by high-sensitivity C-reactive protein and brain natriuretic peptide in patients with dilated cardiomyopathy. Circ J. 2006;70(7):857–63.
42. Ponikowski P, Voors AA, Anker SD, et al. ESC guidelines for the diagnosis and treatment of acute and chronic heart failure. Rev Esp Cardiol. 2016; 69(12):1167.

# 19

# Cardiorenal Anemia Syndrome and Survival among Heart Failure Patients in Tanzania

Pedro Pallangyo[1*], Francis Fredrick[2], Smita Bhalia[1], Paulina Nicholaus[1], Peter Kisenge[1], Benjamin Mtinangi[2], Mohamed Janabi[1] and Stephen Humphrey[2]

**Abstract**

**Background:** Cardiorenal anemia syndrome (CRAS) is an evolving global epidemic associated with increased morbimortality and cost of care. The management of patients with CRAS remains a challenging undertaking worldwide and the lack of evidence-based clinical guidelines adds to the challenge. We aimed to explore the prevalence and survival rates of heart failure patients with CRAS in Tanzania.

**Methods:** We screened 789 patients and consecutively recruited 463 who met the inclusion criteria. Each participant underwent an interview, physical examination, anthropometric measurements, anemia, renal functions and echocardiographic assessment. All participants were followed until death or for up-to 180 days, whichever came first. Bivariate comparison and subsequent Cox proportional-hazards regression model were used to compare the CRAS and non-CRAS groups with respect to the primary end point.

**Results:** The mean age of participants was 46.4 ± 18.9 years, and 56.5% were women. Overall, 51.9% of participants had renal insufficiency, 72.8% were anemic and 44.4% had CRAS. During a mean follow-up of 103 ± 75 days, 57.8% of participants died. Patients with CRAS displayed a higher mortality rate (73.5%) compared to those free of CRAS (45.8%), ($p < 0.001$). During multivariate analysis in a cox regression model of 21 potential predictors of mortality; renal dysfunction (HR 1.9; 95% CI 1.0–3.5; $p = 0.03$), severe anemia (HR 1.8; 95% CI 1.0–3.1; $p = 0.04$), hyponatremia (HR 2.2; 95% CI 1.3–3.7; $p = 0.004$) and rehospitalization (HR 4.3; 95% CI 2.2–8.4; $p < 0.001$) proved to be the strongest factors.

**Conclusion:** Cardiorenal anemia syndrome is considerably prevalent and is associated with an increase in mortality amongst patients with heart failure. In view of this, timely, aggressive and collaborative measures to improve renal functions and/or correct anemia are crucial in the management of CRAS patients. Furthermore, these findings call for guideline committees to revise and/or develop evidence-based recommendations for management of patients with CRAS.

**Keywords:** CRAS, Heart failure, Renal insufficiency, Anemia, Mortality

## Background

Comorbid heart failure, renal failure and anemia commonly referred to as cardiorenal anemia syndrome (CRAS) is an evolving epidemic encountered by health-care professionals worldwide. The interactive links between the CRAS triad are complex and multi-factorial with high potential for increased morbidity, mortality, complexity and cost of care. Studies have reported CRAS prevalence ranging from 19 to 62% and mortality rates of up-to 51% amongst heart failure patients [1–8].

The management of patients with CRAS remains a challenging undertaking largely due to the complexity and heterogeneity of this syndrome. Furthermore, the present clinical guidelines lack evidence-based recommendations for managing patients with CRAS. Despite the evidence of increasing hospitalizations due to heart failure and renal dysfunction, CRAS has not been thoroughly explored in Tanzania. To investigate on this subject, we performed a prospective cohort study to determine the prevalence and survival rates of heart failure patients with CRAS.

* Correspondence: pedro.pallangyo@gmail.com
[1]Department of Cardiovascular Medicine, Jakaya Kikwete Cardiac Institute, P.O Box 65141, Dar es Salaam, Tanzania
Full list of author information is available at the end of the article

## Methods

### Recruitment process and definition of terms

From March through October 2014, we screened for and consecutively enrolled patients with clinical diagnosis of heart failure who were admitted to Muhimbili National Hospital and the Jakaya Kikwete Cardiac Institute in Dar es Salaam, Tanzania. Demographic, clinical, laboratory, and echocardiographic data were gathered during the hospital admission of enrollment. We employed the following prospective selection criteria. Patients were included if they had symptoms of heart failure as per the Framingham criteria and later patients underwent a 2-dimensional echocardiography for diagnosis confirmation. We used an ejection fraction (EF) of below 45% to denote a systolic dysfunction. Renal dysfunction and anemia were diagnosed using the serum creatinine (sCr) and hemoglobin (Hb) measurements respectively. We estimated the renal functions with the Modification of Diet in Renal Disease (MDRD) equation, where estimated glomerular filtration rate (eGFR) (mL/min/1.73 $m^2$) = 186.3 × sCr - 1.154 × age - 0.203 × 0.742 (if female). No correction for race was necessary as all participants were of African descent. Renal dysfunction was defined by an eGFR value of <60 mL/min/1.73 $m^2$. WHO criteria for anemia i.e. Hb concentration of <13.0 g/dL for males and <12.0 g/dL for females was used to diagnose anemia. Participants were categorized as having CRAS if they had both renal dysfunction and anemia.

### Follow-up and study outcomes

Follow-up continued through April 2015, data was censored at the time of death or after the completion of the 180-day follow-up period, whichever occurred first. Follow-up was conducted through weekly phone calls and a participant was deemed lost to follow-up when all of the 3 phone numbers given during enrollment were not reachable in 3 different occasion 7-days apart, with at least 3 attempts on each occasion. The primary outcome measure was the all-cause mortality within 180 days after enrollment.

### Statistical analysis

STATA v11.0 software was utilized in all statistical analyses. We compared categorical variables using the Pearson Chi square tests or Fisher's exact tests; Student's T-test was used in comparison of continuous variables. Bivariate comparison and subsequent Cox proportional-hazards regression model were used to compare the CRAS and non-CRAS groups with respect to the primary end point. Statistically significant variables maintained in the regression final model underwent stepwise and backward selection procedures. The multivariate models were fitted with baseline covariates associated with mortality by bivariate analysis at the <0.05 significance level. Wald Chi-Square tests was used to assess for the interaction terms, with $p < 0.1$ considered significant. We did not include patients with missing data or those lost to follow-up in the regression analyses. Differences in survival between the two groups were compared using the log-rank test. Hazard ratios with 95% confidence intervals and $p$-values are reported. All tests were 2-sided, and statistical significance was defined by $p < 0.05$.

## Results

### Study population

Figure 1 shows the study profile (enrollment, follow-up and survival). During the study period, 463 of the 789 screened patients met the inclusion criteria and were recruited into this study. The baseline demographic characteristics were similar amongst study participants regardless of their CRAS status; however, their baseline clinical and laboratory characteristics displayed a different pattern, Table 1. The mean age of participants was

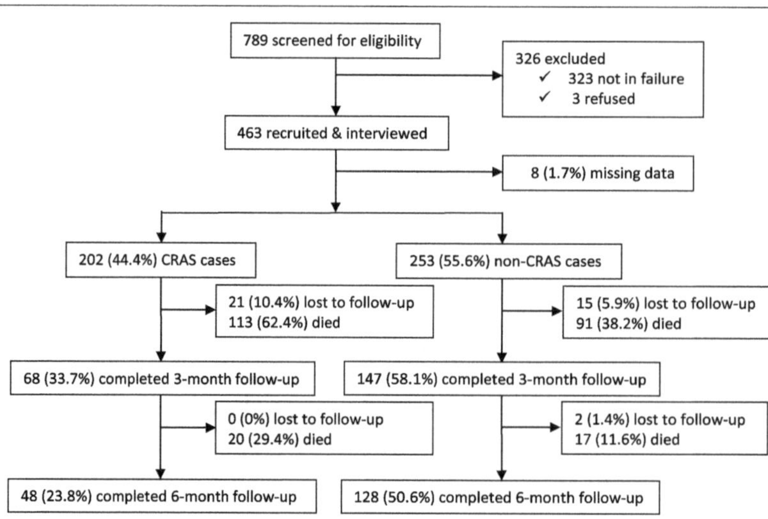


**Fig. 1** Study Profile

**Table 1** Baseline Demographic & Clinical Characteristics of the Study Population

| Characteristic | All Patients ($n = 455$) | CRAS ($n = 202$) | Non-CRAS ($n = 253$) | *p*-Value |
|---|---|---|---|---|
| **Demographics** | | | | |
| - Age, mean (SD), years | 46.4 (18.9) | 48.1 (17.8) | 45.0 (19.7) | |
| - Age groups | | | | 0.09 |
| < 30 | 112 (24.6) | 42 (20.8) | 70 (27.7) | 0.09 |
| 30–50 | 140 (30.8) | 65 (32.2) | 75 (29.6) | 0.56 |
| > 50 | 203 (44.6) | 95 (47.0) | 108 (42.7) | 0.35 |
| - Female sex, no (%) | 257 (56.5) | 124 (61.4) | 133 (52.6) | 0.06 |
| - Primary education (%) | 319 (70.1) | 136 (67.3) | 183 (72.3) | 0.25 |
| - Self-employment (%) | 226 (49.7) | 99 (49.0) | 127 (50.2) | 0.80 |
| - Urban residence (%) | 303 (66.6) | 132 (65.4) | 171 (67.6) | 0.61 |
| - Ever smoker (%) | 49 (10.8) | 22 (10.9) | 27 (10.7) | 0.95 |
| - Health insurance (%) | 97 (21.3) | 41 (20.3) | 56 (22.1) | 0.64 |
| **Vital sign,** mean (SD) | | | | |
| - Respiratory Rate, breaths/min | 24.1 (6.5) | 23.9 (6.5) | 24.3 (6.5) | 0.48 |
| - Heart rate, beats/min | 98.5 (22.2) | 94.5 (21.0) | 101.7 (22.7) | **<0.001** |
| - Systolic BP, mmHg | 132.4 (35.9) | 144.7 (40.2) | 122.5 (28.5) | **<0.001** |
| - Diastolic BP, mmHg | 82.3 (24.7) | 87.2 (26.6) | 78.4 (22.3) | **<0.001** |
| - Oxygen saturation, % | 96.3 (7.6) | 96.5 (7.6) | 96.2 (7.6) | 0.64 |
| - NYHA III&IV (%) | 420 (92.3) | 188 (93.1) | 232 (91.7) | 0.58 |
| - BMI, kg/m$^2$ | 25.1 (5.2) | 25.6 (4.7) | 24.8 (5.6) | 0.13 |
| **Serum concentration**, mean (SD) | | | | |
| - Hemoglobin, g/dL | 10.3 (3.1) | 8.3 (2.3) | 9.9 (2.1)[a] | **<0.001** |
| - Mean Cell Volume, fL | 82.9 (9.0) | 81.5 (8.4) | 84.0 (9.4) | **<0.01** |
| - Mean Cell Hemoglobin, pg/cell | 26.6 (3.6) | 25.9 (3.1) | 27.1 (4.0) | **<0.001** |
| - Creatinine, µmol/L | 446.3 (679.1) | 870.1 (838.2) | 278.2 (224.0)[b] | **<0.001** |
| - Total cholesterol, mg/dl | 4.2 (2.2) | 5.0 (2.4) | 3.6 (1.8) | **<0.001** |
| - LDL cholesterol, mg/dl | 3.2 (2.0) | 3.9 (2.1) | 2.5 (1.7) | **<0.001** |
| - HDL cholesterol, mg/dl | 1.0 (0.4) | 0.9 (0.5) | 1.0 (0.4) | 0.25 |
| - Sodium, mmol/L | 132.0 (8.3) | 131.3 (8.8) | 132.6 (7.9) | 0.9 |
| Hyponatremia (%) | 232 (54.7) | 112 (59.3) | 120 (51.1) | 0.09 |
| - Potassium, mmol/L | 4.4 (1.3) | 4.9 (1.5) | 4.1 (1.0) | 0.9 |
| Hypokalemia (%) | 80 (18.4) | 28 (14.5) | 52 (21.6) | 0.06 |
| Hyperkalemia (%) | 130 (30.0) | 87 (45.1) | 43 (17.8) | **<0.001** |
| - Calcium, mmol/L | 2.1 (0.3) | 2.1 (0.3) | 2.1 (0.2) | 1 |
| Hypocalcemia (%) | 169 (48.8) | 94 (54.3) | 75 (43.4) | **0.04** |
| - Magnesium, mmol/L | 0.9 (0.2) | 0.9 (0.2) | 0.8 (0.1) | 1 |
| Hypomagnesemia (%) | 41 (16.1) | 14 (11.0) | 27 (21.1) | **0.03** |
| **Comorbid conditions** | | | | |
| - Hypertension (%) | 246 (54.1) | 143 (70.8) | 103 (40.7) | **<0.001** |
| - Diabetes (%) | 67 (14.7) | 42 (20.8) | 25 (9.9) | **<0.01** |
| - HIV (%) | 31 (6.8) | 18 (8.9) | 13 (5.1) | 0.11 |
| **Admission Duration**, mean, days (SD) | 13.9 (13.0) | 14.4 (11.0) | 13.5 (14.5) | 0.42 |

[a] and [b] represents anemic ($n = 129$) and renal insufficiency ($n = 34$) subgroups amongst non-CRAS participants respectively

46.4 ± 18.9 years, and 257 (56.5%) were women. Ninety two point three percent (92.3%) of patients were in New York Heart Association (NYHA) functional class III/IV on admission. A total of 246 (54.1%) participants had a history of hypertension, 67 (14.7%) had diabetes and 31 (6.8%) were HIV infected (Additional file 1).

### Prevalence and associated factors for CRAS

Of the 455 participants with complete data, 236 (51.9%) had renal insufficiency and 331 (72.8%) had anemia. We found that 202 (44.4%) of our heart failure cohort had the CRAS. Participants with CRAS displayed a higher likelihood for both end-stage renal disease (ESRD) (eGFR < 15) and the severe form of anemia (Hb < 8 g/dL) compared to their non-CRAS counterparts with renal dysfunction or anemia, (both $p < 0.001$). Comorbid diabetes or hypertension was associated with higher rates of CRAS compared to those free from either condition, ($p < 0.01$ & $p < 0.001$ respectively).

Overall, hypertensive heart diseases (40.9%) was the leading cause of heart failure, followed by cardiomyopathies (26%) and valvular heart diseases (23%). Of the valvular etiology, 82.6% were attributable to rheumatic heart disease. We observed that 114/236 (48.3%) of participants with renal insufficiency were in ESRD and 14 (12.3%) of these were on dialysis. Normocytic normochromic anemias constituted 180/331 (54.4%) of anemias, while the microcytic hypochromic form was found in 107/331 (32.3%) of anemic subjects.

### Primary outcome

During a mean follow-up of 103 ± 75 days, 241/417 (57.8%) participants died, with 21.6% of these fatalities occurring either at home or on the way to a health facility. Patients with CRAS had a significantly higher mortality rate 133/181 (73.5%) compared to those free of CRAS 108/236 (45.8%), ($p < 0.001$), Fig. 2. Mortality rate was observed to increase with worsening of heart failure i.e. 33.3%, 54.2%, and 63.2% in NYHA class II, III, and IV respectively. Presence of anemia and/or renal insufficiency was observed to independently and synergistically increase the mortality rate, Table 2. During multivariate analysis in a cox regression model of 21 potential associated factors for mortality; renal dysfunction (HR 1.9; 95% CI 1.0–3.5; $p = 0.03$), severe anemia (HR 1.8; 95% CI 1.0–3.1; $p = 0.04$), hyponatremia (HR 2.2; 95% CI 1.3–3.7; $p = 0.004$) and rehospitalization (HR 4.3; 95% CI 2.2–8.4; $p < 0.001$) proved to be the strongest factors.

### Subgroup analysis

The superior rate of death observed in participants with CRAS was consistent across all major subgroup analyses we conducted, (Fig. 3). Overall, patients with CRAS displayed a two times mortality rate compared to non-CRAS participants, (HR 2.1, 95% CI 1.6–2.6, $p < 0.001$).

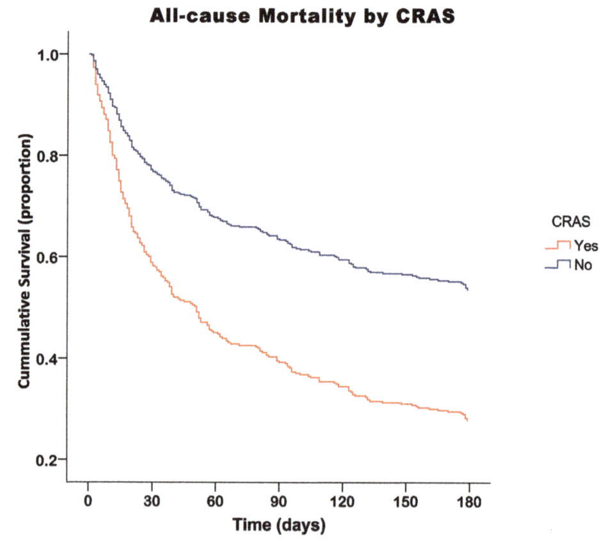


**Fig. 2** Cox Proportional Hazard Model Survival Curve by CRAS

## Discussion

The present study shows that CRAS is considerably prevalent and is associated with increased mortality among hospitalized patients with heart failure. These observations are in unison with the previously published data [1–8]. Compared to participants without comorbid renal dysfunction and anemia, patients with CRAS had a 2-fold mortality hazard. Contrary to previous studies, we observed very high mortality rates within a short period of follow-up. These findings were independent of demographic confounders and established risk factors. Over one fifth of the deceased participants died before reaching a health facility. The authors believe this is so because of the weak emergency systems, poor infrastructure and extreme poverty which hinder a timely access to healthcare services in low and medium countries like Tanzania.

The mean age of our heart failure cohort was 46 years. This is a relatively young age compared to the mean of >70 years reported in the western world [9–11]. Such

**Table 2** Mortality Rates (%) by CRAS Triad Components at 30, 90 & 180 Days

| | 30-day | 90-day | 180-day |
|---|---|---|---|
| HF | 22.7 | 31.3 | 39.0 |
| HF + Anemia | 24.6 | 39.7 | 47.5 |
| HF + CKI | 33.3 | 50.0 | 55.9 |
| HF + CKI + Anemia | 41.4 | 62.4 | 73.5 |

Key: *HF* Heart Failure, *CKI* Chronic Kidney Insufficiency

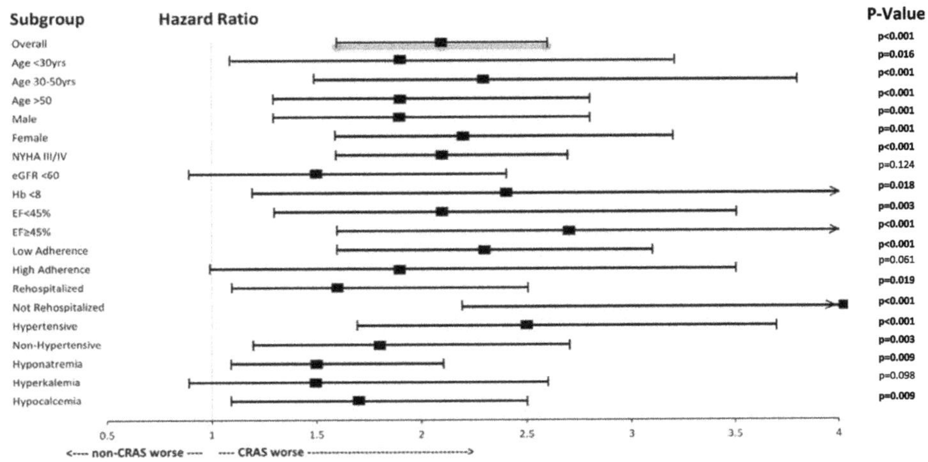


**Fig. 3** Hazard Ratios for All-cause Mortality by CRAS. This forest plot shows the hazard ratios (*black squares*), 95% CIs (*horizontal lines*), and *p*-values for the interaction between the all-cause mortality and any subgroup variable by CRAS-status

young onset of heart failure has been reported in a number of developing nations and remain a major concern. Hypertension continues to be the leading cause of heart failure in resource limited settings. We observed that hypertensive patients had a doubled risk of having CRAS compared to their hypertension-free counterparts, (RR = 2.1, 95% CI 1.6–2.6, $p < 0.001$).

Renal insufficiency was present in over a half of the study participants. These findings are in consonance with a number of previous studies [12, 13]. Anemia prevalence and severity was found to increase with worsening of renal functions. These findings are in keeping with our current understanding of anemia's potential in causing renal insufficiency as well as worsening it. Only 12% of patients in ESRD were on dialysis, this is probably due to the remaining high cost of dialysis despite an increasing number of service providers in this setting.

Almost three-quarters of patients in this present study were anemic. The reported anemia rates among heart failure patients have a wide range among studies and our rate falls within [1]. This variability is partly attributable to the use of inconsistent definitions of anemia (i.e. Hb cut-off points) and/or different inclusion criteria for age among studies. In this set-up however the anemia prevalence is reportedly high even in the general population almost certainly due to a significant burden of malnutrition and infectious diseases. We therefore hypothesize that a good number of heart failure patients were primarily anemic even before the onset of heart failure.

Our study has several strengths. First, our diagnosis of heart failure though initially utilized a screening tool (Framingham criteria), the diagnostic confirmation relied on a 2-dimensional echocardiography. Enrolled patients were admitted in a tertiary hospital with a national status receiving cases from the whole country and thus our findings are perhaps generalizable to Tanzania and similar resource limited settings. We reported the all-cause mortality which is a relatively unbiased and the most valid endpoint.

This study was observational with obvious limitations. The absence of serial measurements of hemoglobin and creatinine in this study implies that we missed new cases and trends of progression of anemia and renal insufficiency that occurred during the follow-up period. Moreover, with a single creatinine measurement taken, we were not in a position to qualify whether the renal insufficient participants were in acute or chronic phase.

## Conclusion

The CRAS is considerably prevalent and is associated with an increase of mortality amongst patients with heart failure. Our results suggest that in patients with heart failure; timely, aggressive and collaborative measures to improve renal functions and/or correct anemia might improve survival of heart failure patients. Furthermore, these findings call for guideline committees to revise and/or develop evidence-based recommendations for management of patients with CRAS.

### Abbreviations

CRAS: Cardiorenal anemia syndrome; EF: Ejection fraction; eGFR: Estimated glomerular filtration rate; ESRD: End stage renal disease; Hb: Hemoglobin; HIV: Human immunodeficiency virus; HR: Hazard ratio; MDRD: Modification of diet in renal disease; NYHA: New York Heart Association; RR: Relative risk; sCr: serum creatinine

### Acknowledgement

We thank the nursing and medical staffs of the Muhimbili National Hospital medical wards and the Jakaya Kikwete Cardiac Institute for their cooperation in this study. We extend our gratitude to all the study participants and their relatives for their willingness, tolerance and cooperation offered during the study duration.

**Funding**

This study was possible through a research grant from the Commission for Science and Technology (COSTECH) of Tanzania. The investigators and the study sponsor never had confidentiality agreement.

**Authors' contributions**

PP, FF, BM, and SH conceived the study. PP, SB and PN conducted all the patient recruitment, interviews, and physical examinations. PK and MJ assisted with performing and interpreting echocardiography. PP performed all data entry and analysis. The corresponding author wrote the first draft of the manuscript, and other authors contributed to and approved it. All the authors made the decision to submit the manuscript for publication. All the authors assume responsibility for the accuracy and integrity of the analysis.

**Competing interests**

The authors declare that they have no competing interests.

**Author details**

[1]Department of Cardiovascular Medicine, Jakaya Kikwete Cardiac Institute, P.O Box 65141, Dar es Salaam, Tanzania. [2]Muhimbili University of Health and Allied Sciences, P.O Box 65001, Dar es Salaam, Tanzania.

**References**

1. Scrutinio D, Passantino A, Santoro D, Catanzaro R. The cardio-renal anemia syndrome in systolic heart failure: prevalence, clinical correlates, and long-term survival. Eur J Heart Fail. 2011;13:61–7.
2. Efstratiadis G, Konstantinou D, Chytas I, Vergoulas G. Cardio-renal anemia syndrome. Hippokratia. 2008;12(1):11–6.
3. Schrier R, et al. Cardiorenal syndrome in acute decompensated heart failure. Clin J Am Soc Nephrol. 2009;4:2013–26.
4. Lu KJ, Kearney LG, Hare DL, et al. Cardiorenal Anemia Syndrome as a Prognosticator for Death in Heart Failure. Am J Cardiol. 2013;111(8):1187–91.
5. NP Singh, Kumar A, Sarkar T. cardiorenal syndrome: an overview. Chapter 132. http://www.apiindia.org/medicine_update_2013/chap132.pdf.
6. Geisberg C, Butler J. Addressing the challenges of cardiorenal syndrome. Cleve Clin J Med. 2006;73(5):485–91.
7. Liu PP. Cardiorenal syndrome in heart failure: a cardiologist's perspective. Can J Cardiol. 2008;24:25B–9B.
8. Anand IS. Cardiorenal syndrome: a cardiologist's perspective of pathophysiology. Clin J Am Soc Nephrol. 2013;8(10):1800–7.
9. Gustafsson F, Torp-Pedersen C, Brendorp B, et al. Long-term survival in patients hospitalized with congestive heart failure: relation to preserved and reduced left ventricular systolic function. Eur Heart J. 2003;24:863–70.
10. Cowie MR, Fox KF, Wood DA, et al. Hospitalization of Patients with Heart Failure: A Population Based Study. Eur Heart J. 2002;23:877–85.
11. Lee DS, Austin PC, Rouleau JL, Liu PP, Naimark D, Tu JV. Predicting Mortality Among Patients Hospitalized for Heart Failure: Derivation and Validation of a Clinical Model. JAMA. 2003;290:2581–7.
12. McAlister FA, Ezekowitz J, Tonelli M, Armstrong PW. Renal Insufficiency and Heart Failure – Prognostic and Therapeutic Implications from a Prospective Cohort Study. Circulation. 2004;109:1004–9.
13. Silva R, Nikitin NP, Witte KK, et al. Incidence of Renal Dysfunction over 6 months in Patients with Chronic Heart Failure due to left ventricular systolic dysfunction; contributing factors and relationship to prognosis. Eur Heart J. 2006;27:569–81.

# 20

# The clinical epidemiology of fatigue in newly diagnosed heart failure

Brent A. Williams

**Abstract**

**Background:** Fatigue is a common and distressing but poorly understood symptom among patients with heart failure (HF). This study sought to evaluate the prevalence, predictors, and prognostic value of clinically documented fatigue in newly diagnosed HF patients from the community.

**Methods:** This retrospective cohort study consisted of 12,285 newly diagnosed HF patients receiving health care services through the Geisinger Health System, with passive data collection through electronic medical records (EMR). Incident HF, fatigue, and other study variables were derived from coded data within EMRs. A collection of 87 candidate predictors were evaluated to ascertain the strongest independent predictors of fatigue using logistic regression. Patients were followed for all-cause mortality for an average of 4.8 years. The associations between fatigue and 6-month, 12-month, and overall mortality were evaluated via Cox proportional hazards regression models.

**Results:** Clinically documented fatigue was found in 4827 (39%) newly diagnosed HF patients. Depression demonstrated the strongest association with fatigue. Fatigue was often part of a symptom cluster, as other HF symptoms including dyspnea, chest pain, edema, syncope, and palpitations were significant predictors of fatigue. Volume depletion, lower body mass index, and abnormal weight loss were also strong predictors of fatigue. Fatigue was not significantly associated with either 6-month (HR = 1.12, $p = 0.16$) or overall mortality (HR = 1.00, $p = 0.89$) in adjusted models.

**Conclusions:** Fatigue is a commonly documented symptom among newly diagnosed HF patients, and its origins may lie in both psychologic and physiologic factors. Though fatigue did provide a prognostic signal in the short-term, this was largely explained by physiologic confounders. Proper therapeutic remediation of fatigue in HF relies on identifying underlying factors.

**Keywords:** Heart failure, Symptoms, Fatigue, Prognosis, Quality of life

## Background

Heart failure (HF) is often a highly symptomatic condition, with shortness of breath, fatigue, chest pain, edema, and syncope being the most commonly reported symptoms [1–7]. These symptoms impair quality of life, drive the need for HF-related hospitalizations, inhibit individuals' ability to function physically and perform activities of daily living, and in many cases signal a poor prognosis in the HF condition [1, 8]. Fatigue in particular has often been cited as the most common and distressing symptom associated with HF [3, 5–7, 9]. However, as instruments for measuring the quantitative and qualitative aspects of fatigue have not been studied extensively in HF nor reached widespread incorporation in clinical practice, the true burden imposed by fatigue in HF has been challenging to assess [5]. Furthermore, the origins of fatigue in HF are not well understood and several contributing etiologies are possible which confounds proper application of therapy [3–7, 9–12]. Previous studies have had limited ability to evaluate these several potential etiologic factors collectively. Lastly, whether fatigue signals a hastened mortality independent of other clinical factors remains unresolved.

Accordingly, the current study sought to expand knowledge on the clinical epidemiology of fatigue in a community-based cohort of newly diagnosed HF patients receiving primary care and other health care services through a single health care system. In particular,

Correspondence: bawilliams2@geisinger.edu
Geisinger Health System, 100 N. Academy Avenue, Danville, PA 17822, USA

this study employed the extensive electronic medical record (EMR) data repository of the study institution to (1) estimate the prevalence of clinically documented fatigue in a large cohort of patients with newly diagnosed HF; (2) identify independent predictors of fatigue with a goal of better understanding possible etiologies; and (3) determine whether fatigue is independently associated with post-diagnosis mortality and whether the prognostic effect varies by time since diagnosis.

## Methods

### Geisinger Health System

This study consists of 12,285 individuals with newly diagnosed HF receiving primary care and other health care services through the Geisinger Health System (Geisinger) between January 1, 2001, and December 31, 2013. The parent study was approved by the Geisinger Institutional Review Board who allowed a waiver of patient consent due to the retrospective nature of the study. Geisinger consists of numerous ambulatory clinics providing both primary and specialty care, several community hospitals, and a full-service insurance company. Since 2001, Geisinger has provided health care services to over three million people throughout central and northeast Pennsylvania. In recent years, Geisinger physicians and advanced practitioners have served approximately 500,000 patients annually through its network of clinics and hospitals. All outpatient and inpatient facilities are linked through the EMR system, EpicCare. The Geisinger EMR data repository contains information on all 3+ million patients including detailed demographics, vital signs, social history (e.g. smoking, alcohol), diagnoses, procedures, problem lists, medical history, medications, laboratory results, and billing information from nearly all outpatient and inpatient encounters at Geisinger since 2001. Importantly, the aforementioned data elements are contained within fixed fields with a standardized structure and content across all Geisinger facilities, facilitating data extraction and organization for large research data sets as described here.

### Heart failure patient population

All patients meeting the following criteria were included in this study: (1) receiving health care services through Geisinger for at least a 2-year period between January 2001 and December 2013; (2) being free of HF for at least 2 years following the first Geisinger encounter as judged by the absence of HF diagnosis codes at all encounters during this interval; (3) having at least one primary care encounter at Geisinger during the HF-free period; and (4) developing incident HF as defined by the presence of HF diagnosis codes at either one inpatient or two outpatient encounters after the HF-free period. These inclusion criteria are designed to capture a representative, community-based sample of HF patients receiving all or most of their health care through Geisinger. For this study, *primary care* encounters are defined as clinical visits to a department of family medicine or general internal medicine within Geisinger. The 2-year HF-free period is considered an optimum blanking period for valid exclusion of pre-existing HF among individuals entering the Geisinger EMR system. HF diagnoses are based on the following International Classification of Diseases – Ninth Revision (ICD-9) codes: 398.91, 402.X, 404.X, or 428.X. ICD-9 codes can be found within multiple EMR domains, including encounter diagnoses (primary or secondary), problems lists, and billing. The date of HF diagnosis was defined as the first day an HF diagnosis code was found.

### Other study variables

Fatigue status (yes/no) as of the date of diagnosis was determined by the presence of any of the following ICD-9 codes at any encounter either prior to, or up to 90 days following the diagnosis date: 780.7; 780.71; 780.79. Fatigue was documented in the EMR as a discrete diagnosis either by clinical staff directly interacting with the patient, or by billing coding specialists during post-encounter review of clinical notes. Other medical history variables were defined in an analogous manner according to appropriate ICD-9 codes. Age and smoking status were determined as of the diagnosis date. Vital signs and laboratory results included were those measured closest, but prior to, the diagnosis date. Medications include those with an active prescription on the diagnosis date or within 90 days following. All-cause mortality was derived by cross-referencing the master list of Geisinger patients with files from the Social Security Administration. Deceased patients are flagged and date of death recorded.

### Data analysis strategy

Baseline characteristics at the diagnosis date, including demographics, physical examination findings, medical history, laboratory results, and medications are reported across fatigue status as percentages for categorical variables and medians with interquartile ranges for continuous variables. Differences in categorical variables were tested for statistical significance by chi-square tests, and differences in continuous variables by Wilcoxon rank sum tests as many of the continuous variables were not normally distributed.

Independent predictors of fatigue were determined by multivariable logistic regression with fatigue status as the binary dependent variable. A forward stepwise variable selection algorithm was employed to identify those variables with the strongest independent associations with fatigue. The 87 candidate variables considered for inclusion in the final model are those listed in Tables 1, 2 and 3. The collection of candidate variables was

**Table 1** Baseline characteristics of newly diagnosed heart failure patients stratified by fatigue status at baseline

| | All patients ($n$ = 12,285) | No Fatigue ($n$ = 7458) | Fatigue ($n$ = 4827) | $p$-value |
|---|---|---|---|---|
| Demographics | | | | |
| Age, years | 76 (66, 83) | 75 (65, 82) | 77 (67, 84) | <0.001 |
| Female, % | 51 | 47 | 57 | <0.001 |
| Smoking history, % | 56 | 56 | 54 | 0.030 |
| Physical examination | | | | |
| Body mass index, kg/m$^2$ | 30 (26, 35) | 30 (26, 36) | 29 (25, 35) | <0.001 |
| Systolic BP, mm Hg | 128 (117, 142) | 130 (118, 144) | 128 (116, 142) | 0.005 |
| Diastolic BP, mm Hg | 70 (62, 80) | 70 (62, 80) | 70 (60, 78) | <0.001 |
| Heart rate, bpm | 75 (66, 84) | 74 (64, 84) | 76 (66, 84) | 0.042 |
| Medical history | | | | |
| Abnormal weight loss, % | 11 | 8 | 15 | <0.001 |
| Anemia, % | 48 | 41 | 59 | <0.001 |
| Anxiety disorder, % | 11 | 9 | 15 | <0.001 |
| Aortic aneurysm, % | 7 | 6 | 8 | <0.001 |
| Atrial fibrillation, % | 37 | 35 | 40 | <0.001 |
| Cancer, % | 30 | 27 | 33 | <0.001 |
| Cardiomyopathy, % | 14 | 14 | 14 | 0.272 |
| Cerebrovascular disease, % | 34 | 29 | 42 | <0.001 |
| Chest pain, % | 53 | 47 | 63 | <0.001 |
| Chronic lung disease, % | 39 | 36 | 43 | <0.001 |
| Conduction disorder, % | 16 | 14 | 19 | <0.001 |
| Coronary atherosclerosis, % | 60 | 59 | 61 | 0.012 |
| Dementia, % | 6 | 5 | 8 | <0.001 |
| Depression, % | 26 | 19 | 36 | <0.001 |
| Diabetes, % | 44 | 44 | 44 | 0.616 |
| Dyspnea, % | 62 | 55 | 71 | <0.001 |
| Edema, % | 43 | 39 | 50 | <0.001 |
| Gastroesophageal reflux, % | 43 | 37 | 53 | <0.001 |
| Gout, % | 12 | 12 | 13 | 0.006 |
| Hypercholesterolemia, % | 76 | 74 | 80 | <0.001 |
| Hyperpotassemia, % | 8 | 7 | 11 | <0.001 |
| Hypertension, % | 88 | 86 | 90 | <0.001 |
| Hyperthyroidism, % | 3 | 2 | 3 | 0.003 |
| Hypopotassemia, % | 17 | 13 | 22 | <0.001 |
| Hypothyroidism, % | 26 | 22 | 31 | <0.001 |
| Kidney disease, % | 31 | 28 | 36 | <0.001 |
| Liver disease, % | 4 | 3 | 5 | <0.001 |
| Myocardial infarction, % | 25 | 24 | 26 | <0.001 |
| Palpitations, % | 11 | 9 | 15 | <0.001 |
| Peripheral vascular disease, % | 27 | 23 | 33 | <0.001 |
| Pulmonary embolism, % | 5 | 5 | 7 | <0.001 |
| Pulmonary hypertension, % | 14 | 13 | 16 | <0.001 |

**Table 1** Baseline characteristics of newly diagnosed heart failure patients stratified by fatigue status at baseline *(Continued)*

| | | | | |
|---|---|---|---|---|
| Sleep apnea, % | 15 | 13 | 17 | <0.001 |
| Syncope, % | 31 | 23 | 43 | <0.001 |
| Tachycardia, % | 9 | 8 | 12 | <0.001 |
| Valve disease, % | 39 | 36 | 43 | <0.001 |
| Venous thromboembolism, % | 7 | 6 | 9 | <0.001 |
| Vitamin D deficiency, % | 12 | 8 | 18 | <0.001 |
| Volume depletion, % | 11 | 7 | 17 | <0.001 |

*BP* Blood pressure

**Table 2** Laboratory values of newly diagnosed heart failure patients stratified by fatigue status at baseline

| | All patients ($n$ = 12,285) | No Fatigue ($n$ = 7458) | Fatigue ($n$ = 4827) | $p$-value |
|---|---|---|---|---|
| Alanine aminotransferase, IU/L | 20 (15, 30) | 21 (15, 30) | 20 (14, 29) | <0.001 |
| Albumin, g/dl | 4.0 (3.6, 4.2) | 4.0 (3.7, 4.2) | 3.9 (3.6, 4.2) | <0.001 |
| Alkaline phosphatase, U/L | 78 (63, 99) | 78 (64, 98) | 77 (63, 99) | 0.43 |
| Aspartate aminotransferase, U/L | 25 (20, 32) | 25 (20, 32) | 25 (20, 32) | 0.51 |
| Bicarbonate, mEq/l | 27 (25, 30) | 27 (25, 30) | 27 (25, 30) | <0.01 |
| Bilirubin, mg/dl | 0.5 (0.3, 0.7) | 0.5 (0.4, 0.7) | 0.5 (0.3, 0.7) | <0.001 |
| Blood urea nitrogen, mg/dl | 21 (16, 28) | 21 (16, 28) | 21 (16, 28) | 0.32 |
| Calcium, mg/dl | 9.2 (8.9, 9.6) | 9.2 (8.9, 9.6) | 9.2 (8.8, 9.5) | <0.001 |
| Chloride, mmol/l | 102 (99, 105) | 102 (99, 105) | 102 (99, 105) | 0.04 |
| Creatinine, mg/dl | 1.0 (0.8, 1.3) | 1.0 (0.8, 1.3) | 1.0 (0.8, 1.3) | 0.64 |
| Glucose, mg/dl | 110 (95, 141) | 111 (95, 142) | 110 (95, 139) | 0.23 |
| HDL cholesterol, mg/dl | 47 (38, 57) | 46 (38, 56) | 47 (38, 58) | <0.001 |
| Hematocrit, % | 38.2 (34.3, 41.8) | 38.8 (34.8, 42.3) | 37.5 (33.6, 41.1) | <0.001 |
| Hemoglobin, g/dl | 12.8 (11.4, 14.1) | 13.0 (11.6, 14.3) | 12.6 (11.2, 13.8) | <0.001 |
| LDL cholesterol, mg/dl | 87 (66, 111) | 87 (67, 110) | 86 (66, 111) | 0.17 |
| MCH, pg | 30.5 (29.2, 31.8) | 30.5 (29.2, 31.8) | 30.5 (29.1, 31.8) | 0.63 |
| MCHC, g/dl | 33.7 (32.9, 34.3) | 33.7 (32.9, 34.3) | 33.6 (32.8, 34.3) | <0.001 |
| Mean corpuscular volume, $mcm^3$ | 90.7 (87.3, 94.2) | 90.6 (87.2, 94.0) | 90.7 (87.3, 94.4) | 0.07 |
| Mean platelet volume, fl | 9.4 (8.2, 10.6) | 9.4 (8.3, 10.6) | 9.4 (8.1, 10.5) | <0.01 |
| Neutrophil:lymphocyte | 3.6 (2.3, 6.2) | 3.6 (2.3, 6.0) | 3.6 (2.4, 6.3) | 0.19 |
| Platelet count, $\times 10^3$/mcl | 223 (178, 279) | 224 (179, 278) | 222 (178, 280) | 0.18 |
| Potassium, mEq/l | 4.2 (3.9, 4.6) | 4.3 (3.9, 4.6) | 4.2 (3.9, 4.6) | <0.001 |
| Protein, g/dl | 6.9 (6.4, 7.2) | 6.9 (6.5, 7.3) | 6.8 (6.4, 7.2) | <0.001 |
| RDW, % | 14.2 (13.4, 15.3) | 14.1 (13.4, 15.2) | 14.3 (13.5, 15.5) | <0.001 |
| Red blood cell count, $\times 10^6$/mcl | 4.24 (3.77, 4.65) | 4.30 (3.85, 4.70) | 4.15 (3.68, 4.56) | <0.001 |
| Sodium, mmol/l | 139 (137, 141) | 139 (137, 141) | 139 (137, 141) | <0.001 |
| Total cholesterol, mg/dl | 165 (139, 194) | 165 (139, 194) | 165 (138, 195) | 0.34 |
| Triglycerides, mg/dl | 125 (89, 178) | 125 (89, 180) | 123 (89, 175) | 0.04 |
| White blood cell, $\times 10^3$/mcl | 7.82 (6.36, 9.87) | 7.85 (6.40, 9.84) | 7.79 (6.27, 9.94) | 0.43 |

*HDL* High density lipoprotein, *LDL* Low density lipoprotein, *MCH* Mean corpuscular hemoglobin, *MCHC* Mean corpuscular hemoglobin concentration, *RDW* Red cell distribution width

**Table 3** Medications of newly diagnosed heart failure patients stratified by fatigue status at baseline

| | All patients ($n$ = 12,285) | No Fatigue ($n$ = 7458) | Fatigue ($n$ = 4827) | $p$-value |
|---|---|---|---|---|
| ACE inhibitor, % | 68 | 67 | 68 | 0.34 |
| Angiotensin receptor blocker, % | 21 | 19 | 24 | <0.001 |
| Antiarrhythmic type III, % | 19 | 18 | 21 | <0.001 |
| Anticoagulants, % | 38 | 36 | 40 | <0.001 |
| Antiplatelet, % | 27 | 25 | 29 | <0.001 |
| Aspirin, % | 76 | 74 | 79 | <0.001 |
| Beta blocker, % | 80 | 78 | 82 | <0.001 |
| Calcium channel blocker, % | 45 | 43 | 49 | <0.001 |
| Digoxin, % | 19 | 19 | 19 | 0.61 |
| Diuretic, % | 88 | 86 | 90 | <0.001 |
| Nitrates, % | 47 | 45 | 50 | <0.001 |
| Statin, % | 66 | 65 | 68 | <0.001 |
| Antidepressant, % | 41 | 34 | 54 | <0.001 |

*ACE* Angiotensin Converting Enzyme

chosen based on a combination of potential relevance in explaining fatigue, typical comorbid conditions which accompany HF, and data availability. For this analysis, laboratory values were divided into multi-level nominal categories to ease interpretation while accounting for possible non-linear associations with fatigue status. Separate categories were created for missing lab values. Multivariable models developed from a large data set such as considered here tend to find an abundance of predictors statistically significant at typical $p$-value thresholds despite having relatively small effect sizes and thus questionable clinical relevance. To circumvent this potential difficulty, a more stringent $p$-value threshold of 0.001 for model inclusion was employed. Furthermore, a model term for the number of days between the first EMR-documented Geisinger encounter and the HF diagnosis date (encounter time) was forced into the final model as a control term. Encounter time introduces a potential information bias into the study design as a positive correlation exists between encounter time and many diagnoses. This information bias is partly controlled by including encounter time in the final model. Upon achieving a final model, significant predictors are reported according to the rank order of their associated Wald chi-square test statistic (from highest to lowest) which is qualitatively equivalent but more quantitatively informative than ranking according to $p$-value magnitude (from lowest to highest). The discriminatory ability of the final model was evaluated by the c-statistic.

For evaluating the prognostic impact of fatigue, a time-to-event variable was created as the number of days from the HF diagnosis date until death or December 31, 2013, the last date survival status was known with confidence. Patients not known to have died were censored on this date. Kaplan-Meier survival estimates were calculated at various time points following diagnosis both overall and stratified by fatigue status. Differences in survival by fatigue status were evaluated for statistical significance by the log rank test. Visual inspection of crude survival curves suggested an early divergence within the first six to 12 months following diagnosis which did not appreciably worsen beyond 12 months, suggesting fatigue may portend a poor short-term prognosis but lose its predictive ability long-term. Accordingly, two additional survival endpoints were considered: death within 6 months of diagnosis and death within 12 months of diagnosis. Cox proportional hazards models were developed to evaluate the association between fatigue and mortality endpoints. Hazard ratios and 95% confidence intervals are reported for all models. An adjusted Cox model included all independent predictors of fatigue as identified by the aforementioned logistic regression model. In survival models, interactions between fatigue-gender and fatigue-depression were evaluated given the strong associations between these variables.

## Results

### Characteristics of incident HF at diagnosis

Among 12,285 newly diagnosed HF cases, 4195 (34%) were inpatient diagnoses and 8090 (66%) were outpatient diagnoses. The average (SD) number of years between the first Geisinger encounter and diagnosis date was 6.6 (3.1) years. The median age of new HF cases was 76 years and 51% were female. HF cases had large amounts of cardiovascular comorbidity with 60% having coronary atherosclerosis, 25% prior myocardial infarction, 34% cerebrovascular disease, and 37% atrial fibrillation. Clinically documented symptoms near, or prior to, the HF diagnosis date were highly prevalent with 62% having documented dyspnea, 53% chest pain, 43% edema, and 31% syncope.

Fatigue was clinically documented in 4827 (39%) of the incident HF cases. Patients with fatigue were on average older, more likely to be female, had more cardiovascular and non-cardiovascular comorbidity, and more additional symptoms including dyspnea, chest pain, edema, syncope, and palpitations (Table 1). Though absolute differences were small, patients with fatigue had several worse laboratory parameters, including markers of nutrition (albumin, protein) and multiple red blood cell indices (hemoglobin, hematocrit, red blood cell count) (Table 2). Patients with fatigue were also more likely to be prescribed several medications, though absolute differences across fatigue status groups were small (Table 3).

### Predictors of fatigue

Out of 87 candidate predictors, 18 were independently associated with fatigue at a multivariable *p*-value threshold of 0.001 (Table 4). Significant predictors of fatigue are listed in Table 4 from strongest to weakest according to the Wald chi-square statistic from the final multivariable model. Depression had the strongest association with fatigue, being associated with an 80% increased likelihood of fatigue. Other symptoms were also strongly associated with fatigue including syncope (61% increased likelihood of fatigue), dyspnea (33%), chest pain (31%), palpitations (32%), and edema (19%). Several possible indicators of volume regulation, cachexia, and/or frailty were also strongly associated with fatigue including volume depletion (56%), abnormal weight loss (39%), and body mass index (7% higher likelihood of fatigue per 5 kg/m$^2$ lower BMI). Female gender (37%) and anemia (32%) were also among the strongest predictors of fatigue. The c-statistic for the full model was 0.734 (95% CI: 0.725, 0.743).

**Table 4** Multivariable predictors of fatigue among newly diagnosed heart failure patients

| | Odds ratio[a] (95% CI) | Wald chi-square |
|---|---|---|
| 1) Depression | 1.80 (1.64, 1.97) | 152.9 |
| 2) Syncope | 1.61 (1.47, 1.76) | 110.4 |
| 3) Female | 1.37 (1.26, 1.50) | 50.6 |
| 4) Volume depletion | 1.56 (1.37, 1.78) | 44.3 |
| 5) Dyspnea | 1.33 (1.22, 1.46) | 39.8 |
| 6) Gastroesophageal reflux | 1.30 (1.20, 1.42) | 38.7 |
| 7) Chest pain | 1.31 (1.20, 1.43) | 37.6 |
| 8) Anemia | 1.32 (1.21, 1.45) | 37.2 |
| 9) BMI (per 5 kg/m$^2$ increase) | 0.93 (0.90, 0.96) | 25.0 |
| 10) Abnormal weight loss | 1.39 (1.21, 1.59) | 23.0 |
| 11) Sleep apnea | 1.35 (1.19, 1.53) | 23.0 |
| 12) Palpitations | 1.32 (1.16, 1.49) | 18.2 |
| 13) Cerebrovascular disease | 1.20 (1.10, 1.31) | 17.0 |
| 14) Vitamin D deficiency | 1.30 (1.15, 1.48) | 16.8 |
| 15) Edema | 1.19 (1.09, 1.30) | 16.2 |
| 16) Hematocrit (H-NL v. NL) | 1.34 (1.06, 1.70) | 15.6 |
| 17) Hypopotassemia | 1.21 (1.09, 1.35) | 11.9 |
| 18) Age (per 5 year increase) | 1.03 (1.02, 1.05) | 11.1 |

*H-NL* High-Normal, *NL* Normal, *BMI* Body Mass Index
[a]Adjusted for number of days from first encounter to diagnosis date

### Prognostic value of fatigue

Among the 12,285 incident HF cases, 5679 (46%) were known to have died by December 31, 2013. Average follow-up time among known survivors was 4.8 (±3.1) years. Kaplan-Meier survival estimates at 6 months, 1 year, 5 years, and 10 years following diagnosis were 93%, 88, 57 and 31%, respectively. Survival curves stratified by fatigue status at time of diagnosis showed early divergence within the first year following diagnosis with little additional divergence over subsequent follow-up (Fig. 1). Unadjusted hazard ratios for fatigue at diagnosis were 1.49 (1.31, 1.70; $p < 0.001$), 1.39 (1.26, 1.54; $p < 0.001$), and 1.20 (1.14, 1.27; $p < 0.001$) for 6-month, 12-month, and overall mortality, respectively. After adjustment for the predictors of fatigue identified earlier, hazard ratios were greatly attenuated: 1.12 (0.96, 1.30; $p = 0.16$) for 6-month mortality; 1.07 (0.95, 1.21; $p = 0.26$) for 12-month mortality; and 1.00 (0.94, 1.06; $p = 0.89$) for overall mortality (Table 5). Much of the attenuation in adjusted models could be attributed to anemia, dyspnea, lower body mass index, volume depletion, and abnormal weight loss, as these variables were strongly associated with both fatigue and short-term mortality (Tables 4 & 5). No significant interactions were observed between fatigue-gender and fatigue-depression on any survival endpoints (all $p > 0.4$).

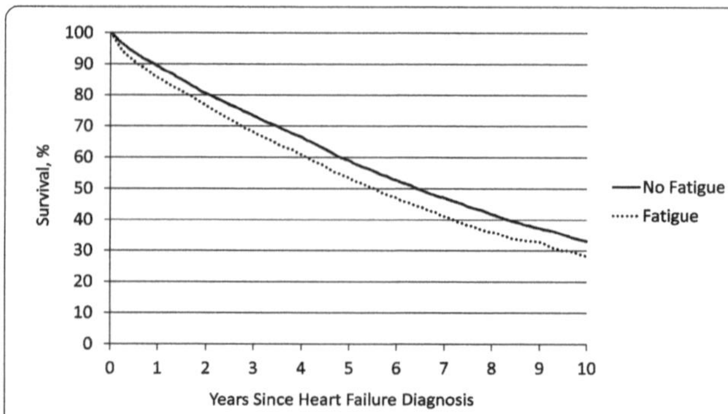


**Fig. 1** Post-diagnosis survival by fatigue status among newly diagnosed heart failure patients

**Table 5** Multivariable Cox proportional hazards models for 6-month, 12-month, and overall mortality

| | 6-Month HR (95% CI) | 12-Month HR (95% CI) | Overall HR (95% CI) |
|---|---|---|---|
| Fatigue | | | |
| Unadjusted | 1.49 (1.31, 1.70) | 1.39 (1.26, 1.54) | 1.20 (1.14, 1.27) |
| Adjusted | 1.12 (0.96, 1.30) | 1.07 (0.95, 1.21 | 1.00 (0.94, 1.06) |
| 1) Age (per 5 year increase) | 1.19 (1.15, 1.25) | 1.19 (1.15, 1.23) | 1.25 (1.23, 1.26) |
| 2) Anemia | 1.60 (1.35, 1.90) | 1.46 (1.28, 1.67) | 1.18 (1.11, 1.26) |
| 3) Dyspnea | 1.62 (1.37, 1.92) | 1.48 (1.30, 1.69) | 1.18 (1.12, 1.26) |
| 4) BMI (per 5 kg/m$^2$ increase) | 0.84 (0.79, 0.90) | 0.82 (0.77, 0.86) | 0.92 (0.89, 0.94) |
| 5) Hypopotassemia | 1.41 (1.20, 1.67) | 1.32 (1.15, 1.50) | 1.17 (1.08, 1.26) |
| 6) Volume depletion | 1.43 (1.19, 1.72) | 1.35 (1.16, 1.56) | 1.28 (1.18, 1.39) |
| 7) Abnormal weight loss | 1.40 (1.16, 1.68) | 1.41 (1.22, 1.63) | 1.34 (1.23, 1.46) |
| 8) Cerebrovascular disease | 1.24 (1.07, 1.43) | 1.28 (1.14, 1.44) | 1.25 (1.18, 1.32) |
| 9) Palpitations | 0.73 (0.58, 0.94) | 0.71 (0.59, 0.86) | 0.72 (0.65, 0.80) |
| 10) Female | 0.84 (0.72, 0.98) | 0.84 (0.75, 0.95) | 0.81 (0.77, 0.86) |
| 11) Syncope | 0.86 (0.73, 1.00) | 0.87 (0.77, 0.99) | 0.93 (0.87, 0.99) |
| 12) Sleep apnea | 0.77 (0.59, 1.00) | 0.89 (0.73, 1.08) | 0.96 (0.87, 1.06) |
| 13) Depression | 1.14 (0.97, 1.34) | 1.20 (1.05, 1.36) | 1.18 (1.10, 1.26) |
| 14) Edema | 1.12 (0.97, 1.30) | 1.24 (1.10, 1.38) | 1.21 (1.14, 1.28) |
| 15) Chest pain | 0.92 (0.79, 1.07) | 0.97 (0.86, 1.09) | 0.88 (0.83, 0.93) |
| 16) Vitamin D deficiency | 0.90 (0.74, 1.10) | 0.94 (0.81, 1.11) | 1.12 (1.01, 1.23) |
| 17) Hematocrit (H-NL vs. NL) | 0.79 (0.45, 1.40) | 0.93 (0.62, 1.39) | 1.04 (0.87, 1.25) |
| 18) Gastroesophageal reflux | 0.98 (0.85, 1.14) | 0.92 (0.82, 1.04) | 0.94 (0.89, 1.00) |

*H-NL* High-Normal, *NL* Normal, *BMI* Body Mass Index

## Discussion

This study sought to evaluate the clinical epidemiology of fatigue in a large cohort of newly diagnosed HF patients from a non-clinical trial, community-based setting. The extensive EMR data repository of the Geisinger Health System was utilized to provide a detailed perspective on the prevalence, predictors, and prognostic value of clinically documented fatigue in a large HF population receiving primary care and other health care services through a single health care system. We found that 39% of incident HF patients had clinically documented fatigue at the time of diagnosis. Fatigue was often part of a symptom cluster, as individuals with fatigue were also significantly more likely to have documented dyspnea, chest pain, edema, syncope, and palpitations. The variable showing the strongest association with fatigue was depression, suggesting a strong psychological component to fatigue in HF. Fatigue was also strongly associated with other factors possibly indicative of fluid homeostasis, cachexia, and/or frailty, such as volume depletion, lower body mass index, and abnormal weight loss. Fatigue was not independently associated with either short- or long-term mortality after considering the strongest correlates of fatigue.

Heart failure is often a very symptomatic condition, and the presence and severity of symptoms often contribute to its diagnosis [4]. Fatigue in particular has been noted as a very common symptom in HF, but estimating its true prevalence is challenging as the fatigue construct is intrinsically difficult to define in an objective manner and no fatigue measurement tool exists that has gained widespread popularity in either the clinical or research settings [2, 5–7]. Prior studies have reported that the prevalence of fatigue in HF ranges from 28 to 59% with variation likely attributable to the method of measurement, specific characteristics of the HF population studied, timing of the measurement with respect to disease exacerbations, and other factors [10, 13–17]. Our estimate of fatigue prevalence in a newly diagnosed HF population (39%) falls within the range observed in previous studies. The definition of fatigue employed in the current study involved observing any one of three fatigue-related ICD-9 codes either near, or prior to, the HF diagnosis date. Of note, fatigue had to be either directly coded into the EMR by clinical staff or abstracted from a clinical note reviewed by a billing coding specialist. Given the ubiquity of fatigue, it seems likely that fatigue documented in the clinical environment resulted from the fatigue being *greater than what is typical or expected* with respect to frequency, severity, duration, and/or ease of provocation, but we are unable to validate this supposition. Evaluating prevalence estimates from prior studies in concert with the employed fatigue definition may help clarify the meaning of clinically documented fatigue in our study population. For instance, Ingle et al. reported that 27% of HF patients had some, a lot, or very much fatigue at rest, while 38% reported fatigue limited their daily activity some, a lot, or very much [15]. Perez-Moreno et al. noted that 43% of HF patients reported fatigue at rest or with slight exertion [10]. Ekman et al. found that 50% of HF patients reported fatigue either walking at normal pace on a flat surface, walking slowly on a flat surface or during washing or dressing, or at rest [17]. Finally, Barnes et al. found that 59% of chronic HF patients were moderately to extremely troubled by fatigue [16].

Identifying the origin(s) of fatigue in HF can also be challenging as fatigue may be a consequence of one or more underlying etiologies. In the context of HF, fatigue may be attributable to peripheral sequelae of the cardiac dysfunction itself, psychological morbidity which often accompanies HF, any of several additional comorbidities often coexisting with HF, or aging [2, 4]. Our analysis of a large number of candidate predictors of fatigue serves not only to identify potential etiologic origins of fatigue but also suggests possible therapeutic opportunities for its alleviation. The variable with the strongest association with fatigue in our analysis was depression, suggesting a strong psychological component to fatigue in HF. Depression is common in HF (26% in our study), and depressive symptoms have significant overlap with several HF-related symptoms, including fatigue [3, 5, 18]. Several previous studies have noted an association between depression and fatigue in HF, but the nature of the causal relationship is not clear and may be bidirectional [6, 18, 19]. In the current study, depression was documented prior to fatigue in 59% of patients with both conditions documented, while fatigue was documented first in 36% (5% on same day). Our results also revealed that fatigue was often part of a symptom cluster, as dyspnea, chest pain, edema, syncope, and palpitations were all independently associated with fatigue. Recognition of symptom clusters in HF is increasing, along with their potential to impact adversely both life quality and expectancy [20–23]. Symptom clusters may reflect a common underlying etiology (e.g. volume overload) causing multiple somatic manifestations and/or an increased awareness of additional symptoms by patient or provider once an initial problematic symptom has been identified [20–24].

We also found volume depletion, lower body mass index, and abnormal weight loss to be among the strongest predictors of fatigue. These factors may reflect some combination of volume dysregulation, cachexia, and/or frailty, all of which are not infrequent in the HF population and signal an advanced stage of disease and an adverse prognosis [4]. These traits may be a direct result of catabolic processes in the skeletal musculature believed to be activated in HF, leading to structural and functional alterations which impede oxygen delivery and utilization in the working muscle, causing muscle weakness, atrophy, and wasting [7, 9, 25, 26]. These aberrations have been hypothesized as a direct cause of fatigue and other symptoms in HF, and importantly, both the muscle abnormalities and fatigue have been shown to improve with exercise training [4, 9, 25–27]. Beyond depression and markers of volume regulation and frailty, other notable independent predictors of fatigue were female gender, anemia, sleep apnea, vitamin D deficiency, and higher age – female gender and anemia in particular have shown to be predictors of fatigue in prior studies [4, 6, 17, 28, 29].

The logic behind evaluating the independent prognostic effect of fatigue (or any symptom) lies in its potential as a signal of some prognostically relevant pathophysiologic process not captured by usual clinical measures. In this regard, our results are largely consistent with prior studies showing that fatigue has at most a small, but perhaps no, independent association with all-cause mortality after adjusting for the strongest correlates of fatigue [10, 11, 15, 17, 29, 30]. Though our results showed fatigue was associated with a 49% increased risk of short-term death within 6 months following HF diagnosis, the effect diminished greatly (HR = 1.12, $p$ = 0.16) after controlling for the strongest correlates of fatigue. Notably, this small effect diminished further when evaluating 12-month (HR = 1.07, $p$ = 0.26) and overall (HR = 1.00, $p$ = 0.97) mortality, suggesting that any prognostic signal provided by fatigue wanes over time. Importantly, our results suggest that the presence of dyspnea (often a marker of congestion), anemia, volume depletion, and a lower body mass index explain much of the increased risk associated with fatigue in unadjusted models. Multiple prior studies have observed no to modest increased mortality risk with various measures of fatigue. In a recent secondary analysis of the CORONA trial (Controlled Rosuvastatin Multinational Trial in Heart Failure), Perez-Moreno et al. showed that the highest level of fatigue was associated with a non-significant 17% increased risk of all-cause mortality ($p$ = 0.26) in patients with systolic HF of ischemic origin, while Ekman et al. reported no independent prognostic effect of fatigue among systolic HF patients enrolled in COMET (Carvedilol or Metoprolol European Trial) [10, 17]. Notably, these two studies did show that fatigue was associated with an increased risk of HF hospitalization and worsening HF, respectively [10, 17]. Our work confirms and extends the mortality findings to a community-based cohort with HF of various origins and ejection fractions.

Study limitations derive largely from the retrospective nature of this study originating from EMRs. Study data is derived from usual clinical practice, thus there was no standardized assessment of fatigue or other study variables and variability in inter-coder practices is inevitable. The patient had to either spontaneously report fatigue as a concern during a clinical encounter or clinical staff had to specifically query about fatigue in the absence of any stimulus. Furthermore, clinical staff had to either explicitly document fatigue with an appropriate ICD-9 code or within a clinical note with subsequent abstraction by a coding specialist. These factors may have led to an underestimation of fatigue prevalence. We also had no information on fatigue severity, frequency, duration, or ease of provocation, and thus were unable to evaluate whether predictors or the prognostic relevance of these fatigue attributes differ from what was observed for our binary definition of fatigue. Furthermore, data elements necessarily were restricted to diagnostic codes and other fixed-field elements which restricted data availability. For instance, New York Heart Association class is a popular metric for assessing the symptomatic impact of HF and likely overlaps with fatigue, but was not available in the current study. Nonetheless, this study was able to include a large, real-world community-based cohort with newly diagnosed HF and evaluate a large number of potential correlates of fatigue well in excess of prior studies.

## Conclusion

Fatigue was a commonly documented symptom among individuals with newly diagnosed HF, but less so than other HF symptoms such as dyspnea, chest pain, and edema. Though fatigue does not appear to signal an adverse prognosis independent of other clinically documented attributes in HF, the symptom is common and capable of imposing a significant adverse impact on life enjoyment. Thus, fatigue may be a meritorious therapeutic target in itself. Indeed, HF guidelines and performance measures note regular symptom assessment and management as important components of HF care, but to our knowledge the efficacy of established HF therapies has not been evaluated with respect to fatigue in particular, perhaps related in part to the difficulty in its measurement [4, 31]. Therapeutic remediation of fatigue requires correctly identifying its etiologic origins, and our results suggest depression, volume regulation, cachexia/frailty, and anemia are the strongest potentially modifiable contributors to fatigue in HF. A standardized, extensively validated instrument for measuring the qualitative and quantitative aspects of fatigue may be valuable in both clinical and research settings, especially in the evaluation of new HF therapies.

### Abbreviations

EMR: Electronic medical record; HF: Heart failure; HR: Hazard ratio; ICD-9: International classification of diseases – 9th revision

### Acknowledgements

Not applicable.

### Funding

Not applicable.

### Author's contributions

BW was the sole data analyst and author of this manuscript.

### Competing interests

The author declares that he has no competing interests.

### References

1. Allen LA, Spertus JA. End points for comparative effectiveness research in heart failure. Heart Fail Clin. 2013;9:15–28.
2. Lam C, Smeltzer SC. Patterns of symptom recognition, interpretation, and response in heart failure patients: an integrative review. J Cardiovasc Nurs. 2013;28:348–59.
3. Sears SF, Woodrow L, Cutitta K, et al. A Patient's guide to living confidently with chronic heart failure. Circulation. 2013;127:e525–8.
4. Yancy CW, Jessup M, Bozkurt B, et al. 2013 ACCF/AHA guideline for the Management of Heart Failure. J Am Coll Cardiol. 2013;62:e147–239.
5. Jones J, McDermott CM, Nowels CT, et al. The experience of fatigue as a distressing symptom of heart failure. Heart Lung. 2012;41:484–91.
6. Fink AM, Sullivan SL, Zerwic JJ, Piano MR. Fatigue with systolic heart failure. J Cardiovasc Nurs. 2009;24:410–7.
7. Witte KK, Clark AL. Why does chronic heart failure cause breathlessness and fatigue? Prog Cardiovasc Dis. 2007;49:366–84.
8. Lainscak M, Keber I. Patient's view of heart failure: from the understanding to the quality of life. Eur J Cardiovasc Nurs. 2003;2:275–81.
9. Drexler J, Coats A. Explaining fatigue in congestive heart failure. Annu Rev Med. 1996;47:241–56.
10. Perez-Moreno AC, Jhund PS, Macdonald MR, et al. Fatigue as a predictor of outcome in patients with heart failure: analysis of CORONA (controlled Rosuvastatin multinational trial in heart failure). J Am Coll Cardiol HF. 2014;2:187–97.
11. Song EK, Moser DK, Rayens MK, Lennie TA. Symptom clusters predict event-free survival in patients with heart failure. J Cardiovasc Nurs. 2010;25:284–91.
12. Falk K, Swedberg K, Gaston-Johansson F, Ekman I. Fatigue is a prevalent and severe symptom associated with uncertainty and sense of coherence in patients with chronic heart failure. Eur J Cardiovasc Nurs. 2007;6:99–104.
13. Alehagen U, Dahlstrom U, Rehfeld JF, Goetze JP. Pro-A-type Natriuretic peptide, Proadrenomedullin, and N-terminal pro-B-type Natriuretic peptide used in a Multimarker strategy in primary health Care in Risk Assessment of patients with symptoms of heart failure. J Card Fail. 2013;19:31–9.
14. Edelmann F, Wachter R, Schmidt AG, et al. Effect of Spironolactone on diastolic function and exercise capacity in patients with heart failure with preserved ejection fraction: the Aldo-DHF randomized controlled trial. JAMA. 2013;309:781–91.
15. Ingle L, Rigby AS, Carroll S, et al. Prognostic value of the 6 min walk test and self-perceived symptom severity in older patients with chronic heart failure. Eur Heart J. 2007;28:560–8.
16. Barnes S, Gott M, Payne S, et al. Prevalence of symptoms in a community-based sample of heart failure patients. J Pain Symptom Manag. 2006;32: 208–16.
17. Ekman I, Cleland J, Swedberg K, et al. Symptoms in patients with heart failure are prognostic predictors: insights from COMET. J Card Fail. 2005;11:288–92.
18. Moudgil R, Haddad H. Depression in heart failure. Curr Opin Cardiol. 2013; 28:249–58.

19. Smith O, Michielsen HJ, Pelle AJ, et al. Symptoms of fatigue in chronic heart failure patients: clinical and psychological predictors. Eur J Heart Fail. 2007;9:922–7.
20. Yu DS, Chan HY, Leung DY, et al. Symptom clusters and quality of life among patients with advanced heart failure. J Geriatr Cardiol. 2016;13:408–14.
21. Park J, Johantgen ME. A cross-cultural comparison of symptom reporting and symptom clusters in heart failure. J Transcult Nurs. 2016; (in press)
22. Herr JK, Salyer J, Flattery M, et al. Heart failure symptom clusters and functional status – a cross-sectional study. J Adv Nurs. 2015;71:1274–87.
23. Hwang SY, Kim J. Cluster dyads of risk factors and symptoms are associated with major adverse cardiac events in patients with acute myocardial infarction. Int J Nurs Pract. 2015;21:166–74.
24. Jurgens CY, Lee CS, Reitano JM, Riegel B. Heart failure symptom monitoring and response training. Heart Lung. 2013;42:273–80.
25. Middlekauff HR. Making the case for skeletal Myopathy as the major limitation of exercise capacity in heart failure. Circ Heart Fail. 2010;3:537–46.
26. Clark AL. Origin of symptoms of chronic heart failure. Heart. 2006;92:12–6.
27. Pozehl B, Duncan K, Hertzog M. The effects of exercise training on fatigue and dyspnea in heart failure. Eur J Cardiovasc Nurs. 2008;7:127–32.
28. Doehner W, Von Haehling S, Anker SD. Anemia predicts health related quality of life in heart failure patients. Int J Cardiol. 2013;162:67–8.
29. Ngo K, Kotecha D, Walters JA, et al. Erythropoiesis-stimulating agents for anemia in chronic heart failure patients. Cochrane Database Syst Rev. 2010; 1:CD007613.
30. Hobbs F, Roalfe AK, Davis RC, et al. Prognosis of all-cause heart failure and borderline left ventricular systolic dysfunction: 5 year mortality follow-up of the Echocardiographic heart of England screening study (ECHOES). Eur Heart J. 2007;28:1128–34.
31. Bonow RO, Ganiats TG, Beam CT, et al. ACCF/AHA/AMA-PCPI 2011 performance measures for adults with heart failure. Circulation. 2012;125: 2382–401.

# Blood lactate is a predictor of short-term mortality in patients with myocardial infarction complicated by heart failure but without cardiogenic shock

Grunde Gjesdal, Oscar Ö. Braun*, J. Gustav Smith, Fredrik Scherstén and Patrik Tydén

## Abstract

**Background:** Mortality in patients with acute myocardial infarction (AMI) has improved substantially with modern therapy including percutaneous coronary interventions (PCI) but remains high in certain subgroups such as patients presenting with overt cardiogenic shock. However, the risk for AMI in patients presenting acutely with signs of heart failure but without cardiogenic shock is less well described. We aimed to identify risk factors for mortality in AMI patients with heart failure without overt cardiogenic shock.

**Methods:** Using data from the Swedish Coronary Angiography and Angioplasty Registry (SCAAR), we identified patients with operator-registered heart failure (Killip class II-IV), and evaluated predictors of mortality based on clinical factors from review of patient records.

**Results:** A total of 1260 unique patients with acute myocardial infarction underwent PCI in 2014, of which 77 patients (7%) showed signs of heart failure (Killip II-IV) Overall 30-day mortality in patients with Killip class II-IV was 20% ($N = 15$). In patients classified Killip IV (1%), 30-day mortality was 50% ($N = 6$). In patients presenting with mild to moderate heart failure (Killlip class II-III), 30-day mortality was 14% ($N = 9$). In patients with Killip class II-III, lactate ≥2.5 mmol/L was associated with 30-day mortality, whereas systolic blood pressure < 90 mmHg, age, sex and BMI were not. In patients with lactate < 2.5 mmol/L 30-day mortality was 5% ($N = 2$) whereas mortality was 28% ($N = 7$) with lactate ≥2.5 mmol/L. This cut-off provided discriminative information on 30-day mortality (area under ROC curve 0.74).

**Conclusions:** In patients with AMI and signs of mild to moderate heart failure, lactate ≥2.5 mmol/L provides additional prognostic information. Interventions to reduce risk may be targeted to these patients.

**Keywords:** Lactate, Acute coronary syndrome, Myocardial infarction, Killip class, Cardiogenic shock

## Background

Since Thomas Killip and John T Kimball proposed a classification for heart failure in patients with acute myocardial infarction (AMI) [1] (Table 1), mortality in AMI has improved significantly [1, 2]. Although prognosis for stable patients has improved, mortality remains high in patients with impaired hemodynamics and especially in those with cardiogenic shock [3–5]. For these patients, the only treatment proven to improve mortality is early revascularization [6, 7] while use of mechanical support devices such as intra-aortic balloon pump counterpulsation and left ventricular assist devices such as the Impella pump™ has not been proven to reduce mortality [8, 9].

While patients presenting with cardiogenic shock in the context of AMI have been thoroughly investigated [4, 5, 10], less attention has been paid to prognostic markers of short term mortality in patients with AMI and signs of heart failure but without overt cardiogenic shock. Factors such as age, previous myocardial infarction, cardiothoracic ratio on chest X-ray, blood urea and

* Correspondence: Oscar.Braun@med.lu.se
Department of Cardiology, Clinical Sciences, Lund University and Skåne University Hospital, SE-221 81 Lund, Sweden

**Table 1** Killip classification

| | |
|---|---|
| Killip class I: | Individuals with no clinical signs of heart failure. |
| Killip class II: | Individuals with rales or crackles in the lungs, an S3, and elevated jugular venous pressure. |
| Killip class III: | Individuals with frank acute pulmonary edema. |
| Killip class IV: | Individuals in cardiogenic shock or hypotension (measured as systolic blood pressure lower than 90 mmHg) and evidence of peripheral vasoconstriction (oliguria, cyanosis or sweating). |

lactate concentrations have all been shown to influence mortality in patients with AMI [11], but there may still be subgroups within these apparently stable patients with mortality rates worthy of extra attention.

Blood lactate is an established prognostic marker in septic shock [12, 13] and in intensive care unit patients in general [14, 15]. In septic patients with stable hemodynamics, elevated lactate concentrations have been associated with future need for vasopressor support [16]. In patients presenting with AMI and cardiogenic shock, several studies have shown the usefulness of lactate as a prognostic marker [17, 18]. Furthermore, elevated blood lactate at presentation has even been associated with increased mortality in patients with acute decompensated heart failure in general [19]. In 1991 Mavric et al [11] showed a relationship between elevated blood lactate and later development of shock even in patients with Killip classes I and II, but such a relationship has not yet been proven after the introduction of percutaneous coronary intervention (PCI).

In this study, our aim was to identify whether blood lactate concentration could be used as a prognostic marker in patients presenting with AMI with signs of heart failure but without pronounced hemodynamic impact and absence of hypotension.

## Methods

### Study design

Using data from the Swedish Coronary Angiography and Angioplasty Registry (SCAAR), we identified patients treated for primary AMI at Skåne University Hospital in Lund during the period of January 1st to December 31st 2014. For patients who underwent more than one angiography during the time-period, the analysis was restricted to the first occasion. Prior to data extraction, the institutional review board exempted the study from formal review.

### Inclusion criteria and data collection

On admission to the catheter lab, patients had blood drawn for various analyses including lactate, according to clinical routine, and were assigned to Killip classes I-IV according to absence or grade of heart failure. Patients presenting with some degree of operator-classified heart failure (Killip class II-IV) were selected. Patients classified in Killip class I, i.e. no signs of no heart failure, were excluded from the analysis,.

In all patients in Killip class II and above, data on age, sex, BMI and mortality at 30 and 365 days were collected from the SCAAR registry. Systolic blood pressure and blood lactate on arrival was collected from the electronic medical records.

### Statistical analysis

Normal distribution was confirmed by visual inspection of histograms. Results are presented as numbers (N) and percentages (%). Difference in mortality was assessed by Kaplan-Meier survival curves and the log rank test. Cox regression analyses were performed to assess statistical significance of lactate and known variables affecting survival (hypotension, age, sex, BMI), and clinical significance was demonstrated by ROC-analysis. A threshold value for elevated blood lactate was set at $> 2.5$ mmol/L for the statistical analysis. All statistical analyses were performed in SPSS version 24 (IBM Corporation, Armonk, NY, USA).

## Results

A total of 1260 patients with acute primary MI underwent PCI in Lund 2014. Patients with ST-segment elevation complicated by out of hospital cardiac arrest ($N =$ 27), and patients with AMI seeking care more than 24 h after symptom debut ($N = 28$) and rescue PCI ($N = 1$) were excluded from the analysis on the basis of well-established high baseline mortality. For 46 patients, Killip classification was not available and these patients were excluded from further analysis (Fig. 1). Baseline characteristics are presented in Table 2. Angiographic findings for patients with Killip II-III are presented in Table 3.

We identified 1081 (93%) patients classified in the catheterization laboratory as being free from signs of heart failure (Killip class I). 30-day mortality in this group was 3% ($N = 32$) and 1-year mortality was 8% ($N = 85$).

Seventy-seven patients (7%) showed signs of heart failure (Killip II-IV), and had an overall mortality at 30 days and 1 year of 20% ($N = 15$) and 25% ($N = 19$) respectively (Fig. 2).

Patients who had signs of heart failure, but were not in shock and did not have symptomatic hypotension (Killip class II-III) had an overall 30-day mortality of 14% ($N = 9$). 1-year mortality in this group was 20% ($N = 13$) (Fig. 2). Two patients registered as Killip class II or III presented with systolic blood pressure below 90 mmHg. Both were alive after 1 year.

In patients with cardiogenic chock at presentation, defined as Killip class IV (1%), mortality was 50% ($N = 6$) both after 30 days and 1 year.

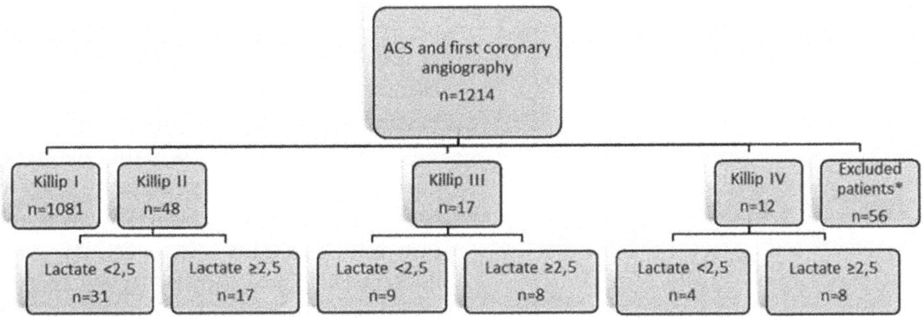


**Fig. 1** Patient flow-chart showing patient population and selection. ACS = acute coronary syndrome

In patients with Killip class II-IV, but blood lactate < 2.5 mmol/L, 30-day mortality was 7% ($N = 3$) compared to 36% ($N = 12$) in patients presenting with blood lactate ≥2.5 mmol/L. Mortality in the same groups at 1 year were 9% ($N = 4$) and 46% ($N = 15$) respectively (Fig. 3).

In these groups, blood lactate at arrival was associated with both 30-day and 1-year mortality ($p = 0.021$ and $p = 0.029$ respectively) when analysed as a continuous variable. As a dichotomous variable with cut-of ≥2.5 mmol/L, blood lactate was associated with both 30-day ($p = 0.006$) and 1-year ($p = 0.002$) mortality. This association was significant even when excluding patients presenting in Killip class IV (Table 4, Fig. 4).

In patients with Killip class II-III but lactate < 2.5 mmol/L, 30-day mortality was 5% ($N = 2$) and 1-year mortality was 8% ($N = 3$) (Fig. 3). In the comparable group with elevated lactate, mortality was 28% ($N = 7$) at 30 days and 40% ($N = 10$) after 1 year (Fig. 3). This cut-off provided discriminative information on both 30-day ($p = 0.026$ and area under ROC curve 0.73) and 1-year mortality ($p = 0.002$ and area under the ROC curve 0.74).

Systolic blood pressure at presentation was associated with mortality when including all patients with signs of heart failure ($p = 0.013$ and 0.025 at 30-days and 1-year respectively). This relationship was not seen in patients with Killip class II and III.

Regarding hypotension analysed as a dichotomous parameter of systolic blood pressure below, as compared to higher than or equal to 90 mmHg, no association to mortality was found. Neither age, sex nor BMI showed a positive correlation to mortality ($p > 0.05$).

## Discussion

Evaluation of heart failure by Killip classification has been an important adjunct in prognostic evaluation since first described by Killip and Kimball in the early 1960's [1]. It's clinical usefulness has been demonstrated several times, most recently by DeGeare et al., in a modern post-revascularization setting in 2001 [3]. The present study extends these observations, and demonstrates that even in patients with AMI presenting with

**Table 2** Baseline patient characteristics

| | Killip I ($n = 1081$) | Killip II ($N = 48$) | Killip III ($N = 17$) | Killip IV ($N = 12$) | Total ($N = 1158$) |
|---|---|---|---|---|---|
| BMI (mean/range) $p = 0.29$ | 27 (12–51) | 27 (15–37) | 25 (20–36) | 27 (22–31) | 27 (12–51) |
| Age (mean/range) $p = 0.49$ | 67 (28–95) | 72 (47–93) | 73 (45–86) | 67 (45–82) | 67 (28–95) |
| Male sex $p = 0.15$ | 698 (65%) | 32 (67%) | 11 (65%) | 9 (75%) | 750 (65%) |
| Smoker $p = 0.79$ | 314 (29%) | 7 (15%) | 3 (18%) | 4 (33%) | 328 (28%) |
| Former smoker $p = 0.66$ | 412 (38%) | 15 (31%) | 6 (35%) | 4 (33%) | 437 (38%) |
| Diabetes Mellitus $p = 0.74$ | 207 (19%) | 16 (33%) | 8 (47%) | 3 (25%) | 234 (20%) |
| Hypertension $p = 0.31$ | 565 (52%) | 27 (56%) | 12 (71%) | 8 (67%) | 612 (53%) |
| Hyperlipidaemia $p = 0.37$ | 352 (33%) | 14 (29%) | 7 (41%) | 3 (25%) | 376 (33%) |
| Prior ACS $p = 0.10$ | 209 (19%) | 11 (23%) | 3 (18%) | 2 (17%) | 225 (19%) |
| Prior PCI $p = 0.33$ | 168 (16%) | 7 (15%) | 1 (6%) | 0 | 176 (15%) |
| Prior CABG $p = 0.25$ | 62 (6%) | 5 (10%) | 2 (12%) | 0 | 69 (6%) |
| Creatinine clearance $p = 0.66$ | 87 | 72 | 78 | 62 | 86 |

For BMI and age data are presented as mean and range within brackets
For Creatinine clearance data are presented as mean
*P*-value from Cox regression analysis regarding the parameters relation to 30-day mortality stratified by Killip group
*ACS* acute coronary syndrome, *BMI* body mass index, *CABG* coronary artery bypass graft, *PCI* percutaneous coronary intervention

**Table 3** Angiographic finds in patients Killip class II-III

| | Frequency | Percentage |
|---|---|---|
| 1-VD without mainstem | 11 | 17 |
| 2-VD without mainstem | 13 | 20 |
| 3-VD without mainstem | 15 | 23 |
| Main stem stenosis | 21 | 32 |
| Normal/atheromatosis | 5 | 8 |
| Total | 65 | 100 |

*VD* vessel disease

Killip class II and III, lactate levels ≥ 2.5 mmol/L confers a worse prognosis.

In our material, lactate analysed as a continuous variable was significantly related both to short- and long term mortality in patients with acute coronary syndrome and signs of heart failure.

Further, in patients presenting with clinical light to moderate heart failure, defined as Killip class II and III, we found that an increased blood lactate level analysed as a dichotomous parameter with threshold ≥2.5 mmol/L, was associated with increased mortality at both 30 and 365 days even when excluding patients with known negative prognostic factors such as overt cardiogenic shock, hypotension, and out of hospital cardiac arrest, patients seeking care more than 24 h after symptom debut and undergoing rescue PCI.

A control sample of 20 patients classified as Killip class I was analysed, from which 4 patients presented with blood lactate > 2.5 mmol/L. Three of these patient had MI, while one healthy individual underwent a coronary angiography on behalf of suspected unstable angina pectoris with normal result. All where alive after 365 days. Even though several patients classified as Killip I had lactate levels above normal, the mortality of the group as a whole remained as low as 3% after 30 days. This could suggest that an elevated lactate level can be used a predictor of mortality, only when clinical signs of heart failure is present, a question that lies beyond the scope of this study.

It is established that patients presenting with acute coronary syndrome but without overt signs of congestive heart failure (Killip class I) have a relatively favourable outcome (mortality 3% at 30-days in our material, and 2.4% in De Geare and colleagues' material from 2001) [3]. On the other hand, mortality in cardiogenic shock remains high in spite of historical efforts to improve outcome with means such as inotrope agents, [20] intra-aortic balloon pumps [8], ventricular assist devices [9] and extra corporeal membrane oxygenation (ECMO) [21]. Our data showed a 30-day mortality of 50% in patients with ACS and cardiogenic shock. This level is consistent with comparable international data [5].

Earlier studies on blood lactate have proved its role in risk stratification regarding patients in need of intensive care in general [14, 15] and specifically in patients suffering of sepsis [12, 13, 16]. In patients suffering of acute coronary disease, data have been more inconsistent. Lazzeri and colleagues [18] showed in 2010 that an increased lactate was associated with early mortality in patients presenting with STEMI and advanced Killip class, but could not identify a relationship in patients in Killip class I and II. To the best of our knowledge, though, this study did not separate patients with no signs of heart failure from those with low-grade heart failure, and lactate level was tested as a continuous variable, and not as a dichotomous parameter with a low cut-of point. The same year, Vermeulen et al [22] demonstrated a relationship between blood lactate and

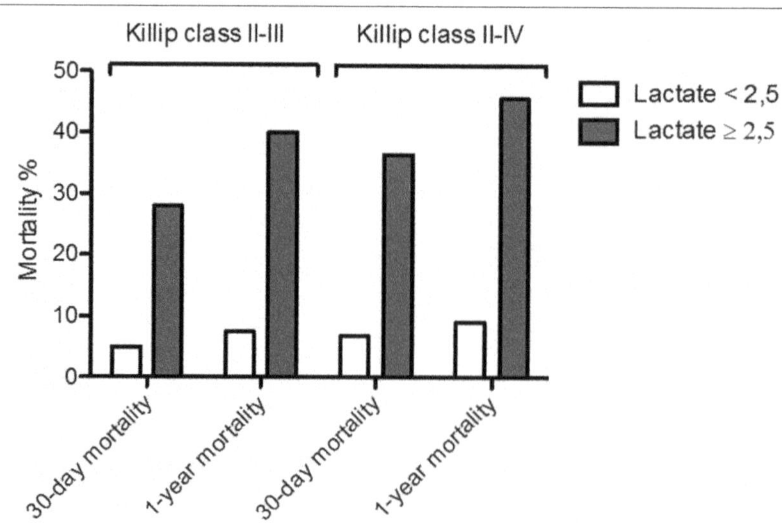


**Fig. 2** 30-day and 1-year mortality in patients with AMI and Killip class II-III presenting with normal (< 2.5 mmol/L) compared to elevated (≥2.5 mmol/L) blood lactate

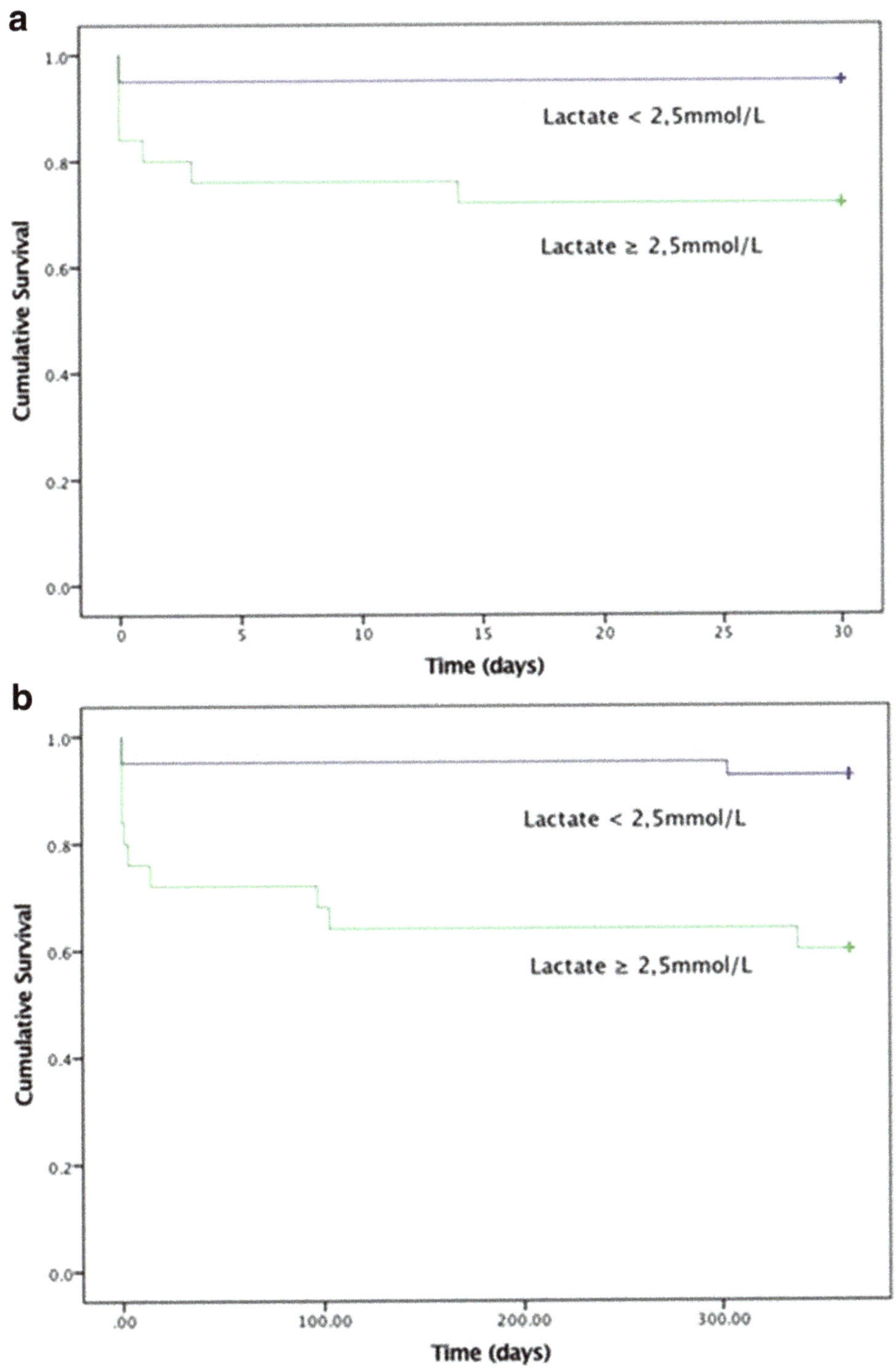


**Fig. 3** **a** Kaplan-Meier curve showing 30-day mortality in patients presenting in Killip class II-III with and without elevated lactate defined as blood lactate ≥2.5 mmol/L. **b** Kaplan-Meier curve: 1-year mortality in patients presenting in Killip class II-III with and without elevated lactate defined as blood lactate ≥2.5 mmol/L

short-term mortality in STEMI, but did not exclude patients with advanced Killip class (however, intubated patients were excluded).

Blood pressure analysed as a semi-continuous variable (by steps of 10mHg), was statistically associated with mortality only when including patients classified as Killip class IV. When excluding patients with overt shock or hypotension with signs of peripheral vasoconstriction (Killip class IV), this association was no longer seen. The same result was seen when analysing systolic

**Table 4** Cox Regression Analysis, Killip class II-III

| | 30-day mortality | 1-year mortality |
|---|---|---|
| Lactate (per 1 mmol/L) | HR = 1.14<br>CI = 0.93–1.4 | HR = 1.12<br>CI = 0.94–1.33 |
| Lactate ≥2.5 mmol/L | HR = 5.94<br>CI = 1.23–28.64* | HR = 6.20<br>CI = 1.70–22.61* |
| SBP (per 10 mmHg) | HR = 0.86<br>CI = 0.67–1.09 | HR = 0.89<br>CI = 0.73–1.08 |
| SBP ≤ 90 mmHg | N.A | N.A |
| Male sex | HR = 0.61<br>CI = 0.16–2.28 | HR = 0.77<br>CI = 0.25–2.35 |
| Age (per 5 years) | HR = 1.16<br>CI = 0.83–1.62 | HR = 1.20<br>CI = 0.91–1.59 |
| BMI (per 5 units) | HR = 0.98<br>CI = 0.52–1.83 | HR = 0.90<br>CI = 0.52–1.55 |

*$P < 0,05$
*HR* hazard ratio, *CI* 95% confidence interval, *BMI* body mass index, *SBP* systolic blood pressure

blood pressure as a dichotomous parameter with threshold 90 mmHg.

The relationship between systolic blood pressure and mortality in the case of acute heart failure has been established previously [5], and lack of significance in this study may have several explanations. Mainly, one could suspect it to be type I error due to few hypotensive patients. Among 77 patients in Killip class II and higher only 6 (8%) were hypotensive at arrival. This number is lower than expected from previous studies, but might be attributed to relatively short transport times and well-developed infrastructure in southern Sweden, and hence relatively short time from symptom debut to arrival at the hospital. Secondly, when analysing blood pressure as a dichotomous parameter, we disregard any differences between moderate and more severe hypotension.

The main limitation of this study is the relatively small number of available subjects from a single centre. The SCAAR registry consists of data manually recorded by the responsible angiography operator, and for a total of 46 (4%) patients were excluded from the study on ground of missing Killip classification. All data were reviewed retrospectively. Data on blood pressure and blood lactate were derived from first recorded values in the patient journal on arrival, but the exact time of measurement or sampling relating to the angiographic procedure cannot accurately be decided retrospectively. In addition, time from symptom debut could possibly affect lactate levels, but is not available in our data. Collecting peak lactate and lactate development could have given additional information. Furthermore, lactate levels are possibly affected by presence of diabetes. Analysing this relationship would have been interesting to analyse further, if not limited by our data number.

Compared with equivalent data from earlier studies [3, 23], the data in our material included relatively

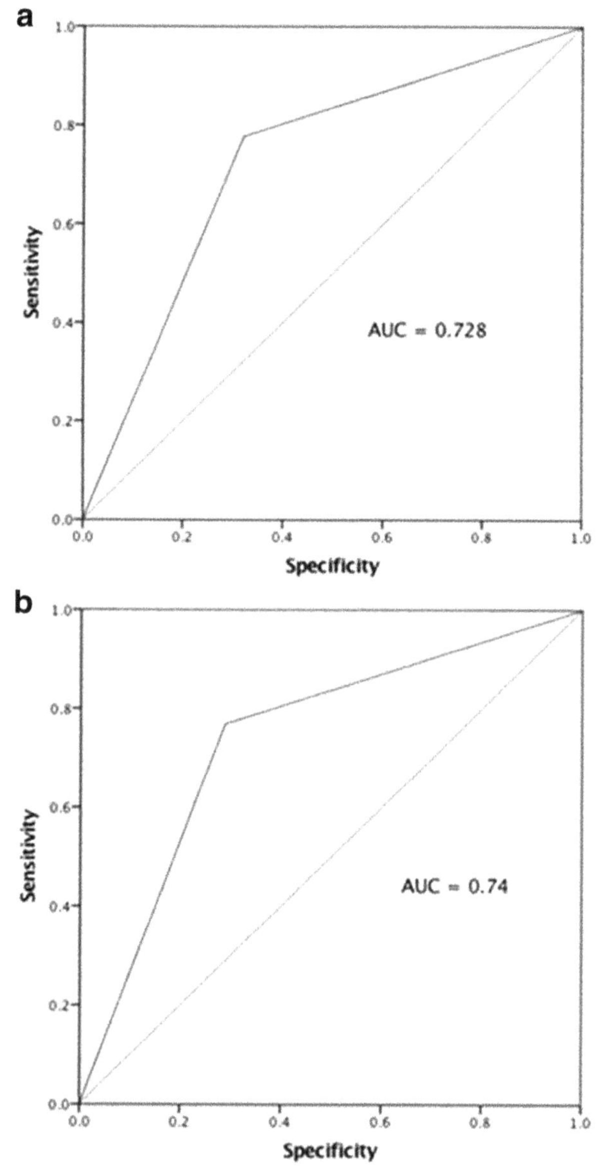


**Fig. 4** **a** ROC-curve showing relationship between elevated blood lactate (≥ 2.5 mmol/L) and 30-day mortality in patients presenting with heart failure Killip class II-III. **b** ROC-curve showing relationship between elevated blood lactate (≥ 2.5 mmol/L) and 1-year mortality in patients presenting with heart failure Killip class II-III. AUC = area under the curve

few patients presenting with signs of heart failure as a whole, as well as far developed heart failure. Notably, the mortality in patients in Killip class II was higher than those in Killip class III. This difference is probably due to few available data, but could also be a result of imprecise classification. Despite this, the mortality rates in both Killip class IV and Killip classes II/II when assessed together, are in parity or even lower than similar data from previous studies [3, 23].

Patients with acute coronary syndrome and evaluated heart failure in Killip class IV or hypotension have a high mortality rate. In this material, we have identified patients with clinical heart failure without affected hemodynamics, which despite adequate blood pressure have high mortality rates. Rising lactate in these patients could be a marker of tissue hypoxia as a result of peripheral vasoconstriction, as adrenergic compensation still maintains the blood pressure despite an increase in preload and falling cardiac output (CO). Could lactate in these cases in fact be a marker of insipient but still compensated cardiogenic shock? Mortality in established cardiogenic shock is still severe. If lactate indeed is an early marker, it might be a useful adjunct in early detection and initiation of treatment to prevent escalation into overt cardiogenic shock.

## Conclusion

Our study suggests that in patients suffering from acute myocardial infarction, a blood lactate level of over or equal to 2.5 mmol/l obtained in the angiographic catheter lab may be used as an adjunct in identifying patients with higher risk of short term death, even in the absence of apparent signs of cardiogenic shock and hypotension. The study was, however, small, and should be regarded as a hypothesis-generating pilot study.

#### Abbreviations

AMI: Acute myocardial infarction; BMI: Body mass index; CO: Cardiac output; MI: Myocardial infarction; PCI: Percutaneous coronary interventions; SCAAR: Swedish Coronary Angiography and Angioplasty Registry

#### Acknowledgements

Not applicable.

#### Funding

This research received no specific grant from any funding agency in the public, commercial, or for non-profit sectors.

#### Authors' contributions

GG analysed and interpreted the patient data from the SCAAR registry and electronic medical records. OÖB, JGS, FS and PT contributed in analysing the data and writing the manuscript. All authors read and approved the final manuscript.

#### Competing interests

The authors declare that they have no competing interests.

#### References

1. Killip T, Kimball JT. Treatment of myocardial infarction in a coronary care unit. A two year experience with 250 patients. Am J Cardiol. 1967;20(4):457–64.
2. McManus DD, Gore J, Yarzebski J, Spencer F, Lessard D, Goldberg RJ. Recent trends in the incidence, treatment, and outcomes of patients with STEMI and NSTEMI. Am J Med. 2011;124(1):40–7. doi: 10.1016/j.amjmed.2010.07.023.
3. DeGeare VS, Boura JA, Grines LL, O'Neill WW, Grines CL. Predictive value of the Killip classification in patients undergoing primary percutaneous coronary intervention for acute myocardial infarction. Am J Cardiol. 2001; 87(9):1035–8.
4. Harjola V-P, Lassus J, Sionis A, Køber L, Tarvasmäki T, Spinar J, et al. Clinical picture and risk prediction of short-term mortality in cardiogenic shock. Eur J Heart Fail. 2015;17(5):501–9. doi: 10.1002/ejhf.260.
5. Jeger RV, Radovanovic D, Hunziker PR, Pfisterer ME, Stauffer J-C, Erne P, et al. Ten-year trends in the incidence and treatment of cardiogenic shock. Ann Intern Med. 2008;149(9):618–26.
6. Lee KL, Woodlief LH, Topol EJ, Weaver WD, Betriu A, Col J, et al. Predictors of 30-day mortality in the era of reperfusion for acute myocardial infarction. Results from an international trial of 41,021 patients. GUSTO-I Investigators. Circ. 1995;91(6):1659–68.
7. Hochman JS, Sleeper LA, Webb JG, Sanborn TA, White HD, Talley JD, et al. Early revascularization in acute myocardial infarction complicated by cardiogenic shock. SHOCK Investigators. Should We Emergently Revascularize Occluded Coronaries for Cardiogenic Shock. N Engl J Med. 1999;341(9):625–34. doi: 10.1056/NEJM199908263410901.
8. Thiele H, Zeymer U, Neumann F-J, Ferenc M, Olbrich H-G, Hausleiter J, et al. Intra-aortic balloon counterpulsation in acute myocardial infarction complicated by cardiogenic shock (IABP-SHOCK II): final 12 month results of a randomised, open-label trial. Lancet (London, England). 2013;382(9905): 1638–45. doi: 10.1016/S0140-6736(13)61783-3.
9. Lauten A, Engström AE, Jung C, Empen K, Erne P, Cook S, et al. Percutaneous left-ventricular support with the Impella-2.5-assist device in acute cardiogenic shock: results of the Impella-EUROSHOCK-registry. Circulation Heart Fail. 2013;6(1):23–30. doi: 10.1161/CIRCHEARTFAILURE.112. 967224.
10. Goldberg RJ, Samad NA, Yarzebski J, Gurwitz J, Bigelow C, Gore JM. Temporal trends in cardiogenic shock complicating acute myocardial infarction. N Engl J Med. 1999;340(15):1162–8. doi: 10.1056/ NEJM199904153401504.
11. Mavrić Z, Zaputović L, Zagar D, Matana A, Smokvina D. Usefulness of blood lactate as a predictor of shock development in acute myocardial infarction. Am J Cardiol. 1991;67(7):565–8.
12. Shapiro NI, Howell MD, Talmor D, Nathanson LA, Lisbon A, Wolfe RE, Weiss JW. Serum lactate as a predictor of mortality in emergency department patients with infection. Ann Emerg Med. 2005;45(5):524–8. doi: 10.1016/j. annemergmed.2004.12.006.
13. Rimachi R, Bruzzi de Carvahlo F, Orellano-Jimenez C, Cotton F, Vincent JL, De Backer D. Lactate/pyruvate ratio as a marker of tissue hypoxia in circulatory and septic shock. Anaesth Intensive Care. 2012;40(3):427–32.
14. Jansen TC, van Bommel J, Bakker J. Blood lactate monitoring in critically ill patients: a systematic health technology assessment. Crit Care Med. 2009; 37(10):2827–39. doi: 10.1097/CCM.0b013e3181a98899.
15. Khosravani H, Shahpori R, Stelfox HT, Kirkpatrick AW, Laupland KB. Occurrence and adverse effect on outcome of hyperlactatemia in the critically ill. Critical Care (London, England). 2009;13(3):R90. doi: 10.1186/cc7918.
16. Musikatavorn K, Thepnimitra S, Komindr A, Puttaphaisan P, Rojanasarntikul D. Venous lactate in predicting the need for intensive care unit and mortality among nonelderly sepsis patients with stable hemodynamic. Am J Emerg Med. 2015;33(7):925–30. doi: 10.1016/j.ajem.2015.04.010.
17. Attaná P, Lazzeri C, Chiostri M, Picariello C, Gensini GF, Valente S. Lactate clearance in cardiogenic shock following ST elevation myocardial infarction: A pilot study. Acute Card Care. 2012;14(1):20–6. doi: 10.3109/17482941.2011. 655293.
18. Lazzeri C, Valente S, Chiostri M, Picariello C, Gensini GF. Lactate in the acute phase of ST-elevation myocardial infarction treated with mechanical revascularization: a single-center experience. Am J Emerg Med. 2012;30(1): 92–6. doi: 10.1016/j.ajem.2010.10.008.
19. Kawase T, Toyofuku M, Higashihara T, Okubo Y, Takahashi L, Kagawa Y, et al. Validation of lactate level as a predictor of early mortality in acute decompensated heart failure patients who entered intensive care unit. J Cardiol. 2015;65(2):164–70. doi: 10.1016/j.jjcc.2014.05.006.
20. Belletti A, Castro ML, Silvetti S, Greco T, Biondi-Zoccai G, Pasin L, et al. The Effect of inotropes and vasopressors on mortality: a meta-analysis of randomized clinical trials. Br J Anaesth. 2015;115(5):656–75.
21. Rihal CS, Naidu SS, Givertz MM, Szeto WY, Burke JA, Kapur NK, et al. 2015 SCAI/ACC/HFSA/STS Clinical Expert Consensus Statement on the Use of Percutaneous Mechanical Circulatory Support Devices in Cardiovascular Care: Endorsed by the American Heart Assocation, the Cardiological Society of India, and Sociedad Latino Americana de Cardiologia Intervencion; Affirmation of Value by the Canadian Association of Interventional Cardiology-Association Canadienne de Cardiologie d'intervention. J Am Coll Cardiol. 2015;65(19):e7–e26.

# Aortic stiffening precedes onset of heart failure with preserved ejection fraction in patients with asymptomatic diastolic dysfunction

Ilya Karagodin[1*], Omer Aba-Omer[1], Rodney Sparapani[2] and Jennifer L. Strande[1,3]

**Abstract**

**Background:** Identifying which patients with diastolic dysfunction will progress to heart failure with preserved ejection fraction (HFpEF) remains challenging. The goal of this study is to determine whether increased vascular stiffness as identified on 2D transthoracic echocardiography (TTE) serves as a biomarker for the development of HFpEF in patients with diastolic dysfunction.

**Methods:** The study design is a matched retrospective case–control study. Subjects with diastolic dysfunction were divided into two groups based on whether they had a clinical diagnosis of HFpEF. The two groups were matched based on age, gender, race and body surface area, resulting in 77 matched pairs ($n = 154$). Data from the first TTE that documented diastolic dysfunction prior to the development of HFpEF was extracted along with baseline demographic and clinical data. Indices of vascular stiffness were measured and compared. A sub-group analysis was performed to compare diabetic subjects in Group 1 ($n = 43$) to those in Group 2 ($n = 21$).

**Results:** Group 1 had significantly decreased aortic distensibility as measured on the initial TTE when compared to Group 2 ($1.9 \pm 1.0$ vs. $2.8 \pm 1.8$ $cm^2 dyne^{-1} 10^{-3}$, $p = 0.01$). In the diabetic subset, Group 1 had significantly less aortic strain ($6.9 \pm 3.3$ vs. $9.7 \pm 5.6\%$, $p = 0.02$) and aortic distensibility ($1.8 \pm 1.0$ vs. $3.5 \pm 2.6$ $cm^2 dyne^{-1} 10^{-3}$, $p = 0.02$) compared to Group 2. Other indices of vascular stiffness did not differ significantly between groups.

**Conclusions:** This study demonstrates that increased proximal aortic stiffness is associated with the development of HFpEF in patients with asymptomatic diastolic dysfunction. Larger prospective studies are needed to further investigate this relationship.

**Keywords:** Heart Failure, Heart Failure with Preserved Ejection Fraction (HFpEF), Diabetes, Echocardiography, Cardiomyopathy, Biomarker

## Background

Diastolic dysfunction is known to be an important contributor to the development of heart failure with preserved ejection fraction (HFpEF) [1]. The pathophysiologic mechanisms that contribute to the continuum between diastolic dysfunction and HFpEF have yet to be fully elucidated. Patients with HFpEF have been shown to have arterial stiffening beyond that associated with normal aging and hypertension [2]. The recoil of the ascending aorta during each cardiac cycle may facilitate early diastolic left ventricular filling [3]. Aortic stiffening, as indicated by decreased aortic distensibility, has been associated with more severe symptoms of heart failure in patients with HFpEF [4]. We therefore hypothesize that increased vascular stiffness in the setting of diastolic dysfunction is associated with the development of HFpEF.

Hypertension, coronary artery disease (CAD), obesity, atrial fibrillation (AF), chronic kidney disease (CKD) and diabetes mellitus (DM) have all been shown to be

* Correspondence: ikaragodin@mcw.edu
[1]Department of Medicine, Medical College of Wisconsin, 9200 Wisconsin Ave, Milwaukee, WI 53226, USA
Full list of author information is available at the end of the article

associated with HFpEF [5–8]. A recent systematic meta-analysis of 27 studies found a significant correlation between arterial stiffness and diastolic dysfunction. Even though it has been speculated that diastolic dysfunction and arterial stiffness may be an important mechanism in the development of HFpEF in these patient populations [9], there has been no study to date that has correlated arterial or aortic stiffness and diastolic dysfunction with the development of HFpEF. DM in particular has been shown to be an independent predictor of morbidity and mortality in patients with heart failure, with the relative risk of cardiovascular death or heart failure hospitalization conferred by DM greater in patients with HFpEF compared to heart failure with reduced ejection fraction [10]. One hypothesis is that increased advanced glycation end product deposition and collagen cross-linking in the diabetic myocardium leads to endothelial dysfunction and increased vascular stiffness, thereby increasing cardiac afterload and myocardial oxygen requirements, ultimately leading to diastolic dysfunction and the subsequent development of HFpEF [11].

Pulse-wave velocity, as measured by applanation tonometry, remains the gold-standard non-invasive method for measuring vascular stiffness. Velocity-encoded magnetic resonance imaging (MRI) has also been shown to have excellent correlation with invasive hemodynamic measurements of aortic stiffness [12]. In addition, non-invasive measurement of aortic distensibility using TTE has been shown to have a high degree of accuracy when compared with invasive measurements in different populations [12, 13]. TTE is widely available at most medical centers and measurements of vascular stiffness can be performed from a routine comprehensive TTE without the need to follow special protocols or obtain additional images, making it an attractive alternative approach to evaluating aortic stiffness in subjects at risk for developing HFpEF.

The goal of this study is to determine whether increased vascular stiffness serves as a biomarker for the subsequent development of HFpEF in patients with diastolic dysfunction and whether this can be identified on TTE. We hypothesize that those patients who progress from asymptomatic diastolic dysfunction to HFpEF, both diabetic and non-diabetic, have a greater degree of vascular stiffness at baseline compared to those that remain asymptomatic.

## Methods

### Study design and patient selection

The study design is a matched case–control study in which data was retrospectively reviewed and collected. The study protocol was approved by the Medical College of Wisconsin Institutional Review Board. Human subject research data was de-identified and stored electronically on a secure, password-protected computer server (REDCap). REDCap servers are securely housed in an on-site limited access data center managed by the Medical College of Wisconsin. All web-based information transmission is encrypted. The data is stored on a private, firewall-protected network. All users are given individual user IDs and passwords and their access is restricted on a role-specific basis. REDCap was developed specifically around HIPAA-security guidelines and is implemented and maintained per Medical College of Wisconsin guidelines.

The echocardiogram database at Froedtert Memorial Lutheran Hospital (FMLH) was used to screen TTEs between 7/1/2003 and 7/1/2013. The search terms included (1) diastolic dysfunction and (2) preserved ejection fraction ($EF > 50\%$) and excluded (1) systolic dysfunction, (2) normal diastolic function, (3) E/A fusion, (4) mitral valve abnormalities, (5) severe aortic stenosis, (6) severe mitral regurgitation, (7) annuloplasty and/or (8) bioprosthetic valves. After accounting for serial studies, 561 subjects qualified for the study. Subjects were further excluded if they had missing clinical data ($n = 63$) in the EHR, any serial TTE report that included an EF of <50% ($n = 40$), non-diagnostic echocardiograms ($n = 10$), or if they had previously undergone heart transplantation ($n = 1$).

Among the remaining subjects ($n = 447$), the electronic health record (EHR) was reviewed to identify those subjects who had heart failure with preserved ejection fraction. Subjects were assigned to Group 1 ($n = 107$) if their EHR contained an ICD-9 diagnosis of congestive heart failure and clinical documentation of at least one of the following signs or symptoms of heart failure by the end of the study period: shortness of breath, weight gain, orthopnea, paroxysmal nocturnal dyspnea or increased leg swelling. Subjects were placed into Group 2 ($n = 340$) if they remained free of heart failure throughout the study period. After information on gender, race, age and body surface area (BSA) was collected, the subjects were optimally matched for these variables to yield 77 matched pairs ($n = 154$) of subjects which were ultimately included in our study (Fig. 1).

For each subject, TTE reports were screened in a retrospective fashion until the earliest study that documented diastolic dysfunction was identified, from which echocardiographic data was extracted. Echocardiographic data was initially extracted from the clinical report which was generated by a board-certified cardiologist. This data included: blood pressure (BP), left ventricular posterior wall thickness at end-diastole (LVPWd) and end-systole (LVPWs), left ventricular (LV) mass, LV mass index, LV ejection fraction (LVEF) as measured by Simpson's equation, fractional shortening (FS), LV internal diameter at end-diastole (LVIDd) and

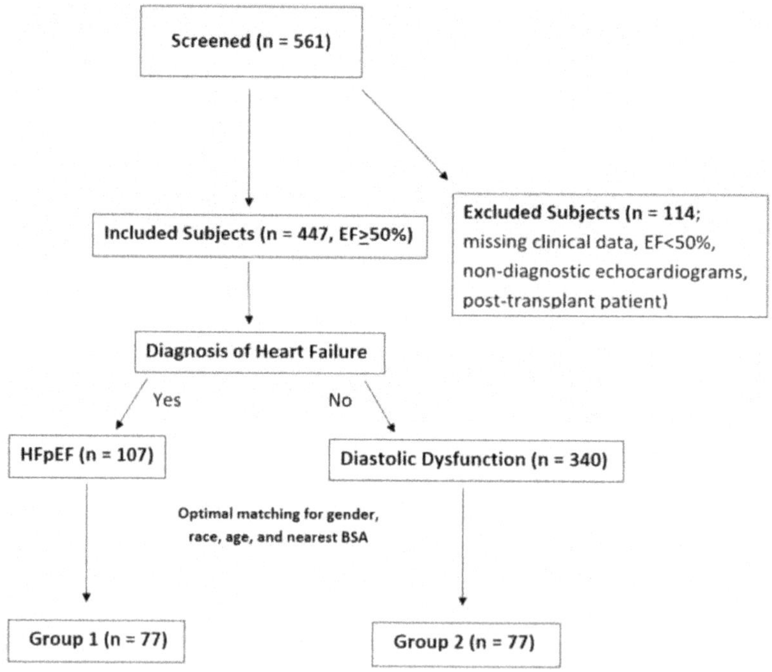


**Fig. 1** Flow diagram of study. Flow diagram illustrating method of subject selection, including exclusion and matching criteria

end-systole (LVIDs), LV end-diastolic volume (LVEDV) and index, LV end-systolic volume (LVESV) and index, relative wall thickness (RWT), left atrial linear dimension, left atrial volume index, mitral peak E velocity, mitral peak A velocity, E/A ratio, stroke volume (SV) and stroke volume index (SVI). Left ventricular volumes (EDV and ESV) were calculated using the biplane method of disks (modified Simpson's rule). SV, LVEF and FS were determined based on the American Society of Echocardiography/European Association of Cardiovascular Imaging (ASE/EACVI) guidelines [14] and reported in Table 1. Diastolic function was determined and graded by the interpreting cardiologist according to the recommendation of the American Society of Echocardiography 2002 and 2009 guidelines. The 2002 guidelines identified diastolic dysfunction as having a lower E than A-wave velocity with a prolonged isovolumic relaxation time and shortened deceleration time [15]. Mitral annular tissue e' and a' velocities were not routinely measured or reported until 2009 when diastolic function grading was further defined as: normal diastolic function: E/A ≥1, average e' >9 cm/s; mild diastolic dysfunction: E/A < 1, average e' ≤ 9 cm/s, moderate diastolic dysfunction: E/A ≥ 1, average e' ≤ 9 cm/s, severe diastolic dysfunction: E/A ≥ 2, average e' ≤ 9 [16]. Because mitral annular tissue velocities were not included on the reports until 2009, we did not report this data in the study.

**Table 1** Study calculations [12, 34–37]

| Variable | Formula |
|---|---|
| Pulse Pressure (PP; mmHg) | systolic blood pressure (SBP) – diastolic blood pressure (DBP) |
| Diastolic Wall Strain (%) | (LVPWs-LVPWd)*100/LVPWs |
| End Systolic Pressure (mmHg) | 0.9*SBP |
| Arterial Stiffness (mmHg/mL/$m^2$) | PP/SVI |
| Arterial Elastance (mmHg/mL) | ESP/SV |
| Aortic Strain (%) | (AoS-AoD)*100/AoD |
| Aortic Distensibility ($cm^2$ $dyne^{-1}10^{-3}$) | 2* [(AoS-AoD)/(AoD*PP)] * 1000 |
| Relative Wall Thickness (cm) | 2*(LVPWd)/LVIDd |
| LV Mass (g) | 0.8* [1.04 * (IVSd + LVIDd + LVPWd) $^3$ - $LVIDd^3$] + 0.6 g |
| Fractional Shortening (%) | (LVIDd-LVIDs)/LVIDd*100 |
| Stroke Volume (mL) | EDV - ESV |
| Ejection Fraction (%) | (SV/EDV) * 100 |

Additional clinical data including hypertension, CAD, DM, AF, CKD (estimated GFR <60 mL/min/1.73 $m^2$ for 3 months or more), alcohol and tobacco use, N-terminal pro-hormone brain natriuretic peptide (NT-proBNP) level, glomerular filtration rate (GFR, estimated by the CKD-EPI equation [17]), and data on medication use (beta blockers, calcium channel blockers, ACE inhibitors and angiotensin receptor blockers) was extracted from the EHR at FMLH.

### Assessment of arterial and aortic stiffness

From the earliest TTE documenting diastolic dysfunction in study subjects and prior to Group 1 subjects developing heart failure, the dimensions of the ascending aorta were measured. Ascending aortic diameters were measured three centimeters above the aortic valve at end-diastole (AoD) and end-systole (AoS) in the 2D parasternal view (Fig. 2). These measurements were used to calculate aortic distensibility and aortic strain using formulas reported in Table 1. Arterial stiffness and arterial elastance were calculated as reported in Table 1 and included the SV as determined from the same TTE that was used to measure aortic dimensions.

### Additional calculations

The following calculations that were not included in the clinical report were performed, as outlined in Table 1: pulse pressure (PP), diastolic wall strain (DWS), end systolic pressure (ESP), arterial stiffness, arterial elastance, aortic strain, aortic distensibility and relative wall thickness (RWT). Missing blood pressure recordings at the time of the earliest echocardiogram documenting diastolic dysfunction prevented the calculation of some indices of vascular stiffness in 48/77 subjects in Group 1 and 28/77 subjects in Group 2.

For reference, we used previous literature that published mean adult values for aortic distensibility (in $cm^2 dyne^{-1} 10^{-3}$) and aortic strain (%) in control subjects (10 ± 5.1 and 18 ± 8.0, respectively), hypertensive subjects (3.1 ± 1.5 and 11 ± 7.0, respectively), diabetic subjects (5.1 ± 2.8 and 9 ± 3.0, respectively) and subjects with both hypertension and diabetes (2.0 ± 0.9 and 8 ± 3.0, respectively) [18].

### Statistical analysis

The data analysis was performed using Statistical Analysis System (SAS) software, version 9.3. Continuous variables are expressed in the Tables as mean ± standard deviation and categorical variables as a percentage. For the matched pairs in our study (Group 1 vs. Group 2), McNemar's statistic was used to compare qualitative variables and a one-sample t-test was used to compare quantitative variables. A $p$-value of $<0.0125$ was considered statistically significant, based on the Bonferroni correction for multiple comparisons.

We performed a multiple logistic regression analysis to determine whether aortic distensibility is associated with higher predictive risk when adjusting for age, gender, race, BSA, hypertension, DM and CKD. To calculate the optimal cut-off value for aortic distensibility, we fit a simple logistic regression and generated a receiver operating characteristic (ROC) curve to achieve the highest possible level of sensitivity and specificity, and to maximize the area under the curve (AUC).

We also performed simple linear regressions, eliminating outliers more than two standard deviations outside of the mean, to evaluate whether aortic distensibility is correlated to other clinical or echocardiographic parameters, specifically age, gender, race, body surface area, hypertension, DM, CKD, LV mass, LV mass index, LV internal diameter end-diastole, LV-end diastolic volume and index, relative wall thickness and E/A velocity.

An unmatched sub-group analysis was also performed to compare the diabetic patients in each group (Group 1 vs. Group 2). A one-way analysis of variance (ANOVA) was used to compare the differences between groups. A $p$-value of $<0.05$ was considered statistically significant for the sub-group analysis.

## Results

### Baseline characteristics

The baseline characteristics of the two groups are shown in Table 2. Subjects in Group 1 had significantly more hypertension ($p = 0.02$), DM ($p = 0.0002$), CAD ($p = 0.01$), and AF ($p = 0.003$), and subjects in Group 1 had significantly lower GFRs ($p = 0.002$) and significantly

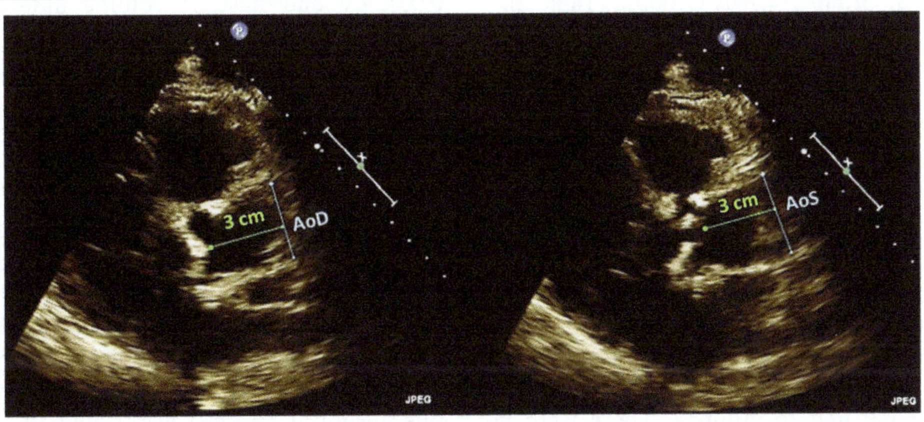


**Fig. 2** Ascending aortic diameter measurements. Ascending aortic diameters were measured three centimeters above the aortic valve at end-diastole (AoD) and end-systole (AoS) in the 2D parasternal view

**Table 2** Baseline characteristics

| Variable | Group 1: HFpEF ($n = 77$) | Group 2: Diastolic Dysfunction ($n = 77$) | *P*-value |
|---|---|---|---|
| Age (years) | 68.6 ± 9.9 | 68.5 ± 9.9 | 0.96 |
| Gender (% Female) | 67.5 | 67.5 | 1.0 |
| Race (% African American) | 30.5 | 30.5 | 1.0 |
| Body Surface Area ($m^2$) | 1.97 ± 0.31 | 1.93 ± 0.24 | 0.31 |
| Tobacco Use (%) | 56.2 | 60.3 | 0.61 |
| Alcohol Use (%) | 49.3 | 58.0 | 0.27 |
| Hypertension (%) | 88.3 | 72.7 | 0.02 |
| Diabetes (%) | 55.8 | 27.3 | 0.0002 |
| Coronary Artery Disease (%) | 61.0 | 39.0 | 0.01 |
| Atrial Fibrillation (%) | 40.3 | 16.9 | 0.003 |
| Chronic Kidney Disease (%) | 63.6 | 24.7 | <0.0001 |
| NT-proBNP (pg/mL) | 9810 ± 14308 | 2148 ± 3026 | 0.07 |
| GFR (mL/min/1.73 $m^2$) | 44.8 ± 20.0 | 57.9 ± 23.6 | 0.002 |
| Systolic BP (mmHg) | 145.9 ± 29.7 | 140.9 ± 21.0 | 0.73 |
| Diastolic BP (mmHg) | 70.7 ± 15.7 | 74.6 ± 10.9 | 0.37 |
| Pulse Pressure (mmHg) | 75.6 ± 21.5 | 66.3 ± 16.7 | 0.17 |
| Beta Blockers (%) | 62.3 | 72.7 | 0.21 |
| Calcium Channel Blockers (%) | 28.6 | 28.6 | 1.0 |
| ACE Inhibitors (%) | 16.9 | 26.0 | 0.13 |
| Angiotensin Receptor Blockers (%) | 18.2 | 23.4 | 0.45 |

*Note*: Continuous data expressed as mean ± standard deviation. Categorical variables expressed as percentage

more clinical diagnoses of CKD ($p < 0.0001$) compared to those in Group 2.

In the overall cohort, there were no significant differences between the number of patients on beta blockers, calcium channel blockers, ACE inhibitors or angiotensin receptor blockers in Group 1 versus Group 2 (Table 2).

### Echocardiographic measurements

The echocardiographic measurements of the two groups are shown in Table 3. Group 1 had significantly increased left ventricular posterior wall thickness at end-diastole ($p = 0.03$) and end-systole ($p = 0.0001$), as well as increased left ventricular mass ($p = 0.0004$), left ventricular mass index ($p = 0.001$), left ventricular internal diameter at end-diastole ($p = 0.006$), and left ventricular internal diameter at end-systole ($p = 0.02$) compared to Group 2. Group 1 also had significantly increased left atrial linear dimension ($p = 0.028$) and mitral peak A velocity ($p = 0.048$) compared to group 2. There were no significant differences in diastolic wall strain ($p = 0.23$). No significant differences were observed with respect to other TTE measurements including severity of diastolic dysfunction (Table 3).

### Assessment of arterial and aortic stiffness

Group 1 ($n = 29$) had a significant decrease in aortic distensibility compared to Group 2 ($n = 48$; $p = 0.01$). No significant differences were observed with respect to arterial stiffness, arterial elastance and aortic strain (Table 4).

To further explore the predictive value of decreased aortic distensibility as an independent risk factor for the development of HFpEF, we performed a multiple logistic regression analysis corrected for age, BSA, gender, race, HTN, DM and CKD. The measure of aortic distensibility was a significant predictor of the development of HFpEF [odds ratio = 0.61 and 95% confidence interval (0.39–0.96)].

ROC curves were generated for aortic distensibility as an indicator of future HFpEF development. If aortic distensibilty was not included in the model but all other independent variables (age, BSA, gender, race, HTN, DM and CKD) remained the same, the area under the ROC curve was 0.796. Adding aortic distensibility to the predictive model boosted the area under the curve to 0.815. Therefore, at the time diastolic dysfunction is first detected by echocardiogram, the addition of aortic distensibilty increases the predictive value of the underlying co-morbidities for HFpEF development. To determine an optimal cutoff for aortic distensibility, we fit a simple logistic regression to arrive at a cutoff of 1.84 $cm^2 dyne^{-1} 10^{-3}$ with 62.1% sensitivity and 68.8% specificity (Fig. 3).

Furthermore, using simple linear regressions that eliminated outliers more than two standard deviations outside of the mean, aortic distensibility was poorly correlated to age ($r^2 = 0.007$), gender ($r^2 = 0.003$), race ($r^2 = 0.004$), BSA ($r^2 = 0.00002$), hypertension ($r^2 = 0.11$), DM ($r^2 = 0.02$), CKD ($r^2 = 0.08$), LV mass ($r^2 = 0.04$), LV mass index ($r^2 = 0.05$), LV internal diameter end-diastole ($r^2 = 0.03$), LV end-diastolic volume ($r^2 = 0.03$), LV end-diastolic volume index ($r^2 = 0.04$), relative wall thickness ($r^2 = 0.03$), and E/A velocity ($r^2 = 0.07$).

### Diabetic sub-group analysis

A sub-group analysis was performed to compare diabetic subjects in Group 1 ($n = 43$) to diabetic subjects in Group 2 ($n = 21$). There were no significant differences observed between groups in terms of age, gender, race, BSA, tobacco use, alcohol use, CAD, hypertension, AF or cardiac medication usage (Table 5). The vascular stiffness measurements, as in the main cohort, were limited by missing blood pressure recordings. Despite this, Group 1 ($n = 43$) was noted to have significantly decreased aortic strain compared to Group 2 ($n = 9$; $p = 0.02$). Aortic distensibility was also significantly

**Table 3** Transthoracic echocardiogram measurements

| Measurement | Group 1: HFpEF ($n = 77$) | Group 2: Diastolic Dysfunction ($n = 77$) | *P*-value (matched pairs only) |
|---|---|---|---|
| LV posterior wall thickness end-diastole (cm) | 1.20 ± 0.25 - (77) | 1.11 ± 0.22 - (77) | 0.03 |
| LV posterior wall thickness end-systole (cm) | 1.85 ± 0.38 - (75) | 1.64 ± 0.26 - (72) | 0.0001 |
| LV mass (g) | 217.9 ± 72.7 - (72) | 177.9 ± 58.5 - (74) | 0.0004 |
| LV mass index (g/m$^2$) | 110.9 ± 34.5 - (44) | 91.3 ± 26.8 - (71) | 0.001 |
| LVEF – Simpson's (%) | 61.8 ± 6.37 - (59) | 60.3 ± 5.52 - (66) | 0.25 |
| Fractional shortening index (%) | 33.5 ± 9.36 - (76) | 34.5 ± 10.3 - (74) | 0.48 |
| LV internal diameter end-diastole (cm) | 4.67 ± 0.70 - (77) | 4.40 ± 0.57 - (76) | 0.006 |
| LV internal diameter end-systole (cm) | 3.09 ± 0.60 - (77) | 2.88 ± 0.61 - (76) | 0.02 |
| LV end-diastolic volume (mL) | 87.8 ± 34.5 - (63) | 84.9 ± 30.4 - (67) | 0.99 |
| LV end-diastolic volume index (mL/m$^2$) | 47.6 ± 16.1 - (21) | 57.6 ± 17.3 - (17) | 0.90 |
| Diastolic Wall Strain (%) | 34.0 ± 12.0 - (75) | 32.0 ± 9.0 - (72) | 0.23 |
| LV end-systolic volume (mL) | 35.3 ± 16.0 - (60) | 33.5 ± 12.7 - (68) | 0.83 |
| LV end-systolic volume index (ml/m$^2$) | 18.8 ± 8.45 - (20) | 21.8 ± 7.84 - (17) | 0.90 |
| Relative wall thickness (cm) | 0.57 ± 0.16 - (23) | 0.50 ± 0.08 - (16) | 0.97 |
| Left atrial linear dimension (cm) | 4.10 ± 0.64 - (76) | 3.89 ± 0.60 - (77) | 0.03 |
| Mitral peak E velocity (m/s) | 1.09 ± 0.28 - (74) | 1.01 ± 0.26 - (77) | 0.052 |
| Mitral peak A velocity (m/s) | 0.89 ± 0.32 - (73) | 0.79 ± 0.25 - (75) | 0.048 |
| E/A ratio | 1.37 ± 0.60 - (72) | 1.36 ± 0.48 - (73) | 0.68 |
| Ascending aortic root diameter end-diastole (cm | 3.08 ± 0.39 - (75) | 3.04 ± 0.43 - (72) | 0.54 |
| Ascending aortic root diameter end-systole (cm) | 3.31 ± 0.37 - (75) | 3.29 ± 0.42 - (72) | 0.86 |
| Stroke volume (mL) | 81.4 ± 24.5 - (28) | 77.7 ± 17.1 - (38) | 0.82 |
| Stroke volume index (mL/m$^2$) | 41.1 ± 13.3 - (27) | 40.4 ± 10.5 - (38) | 0.74 |
| LV end systolic pressure (mmHg) | 131.4 ± 26.7 - (29) | 126.9 ± 18.9 - (49) | 0.73 |
| Mild Diastolic Dysfunction (%) | 24.7 | 9.1 | 0.04* |
| Moderate Diastolic Dysfunction (%) | 71.4 | 83.1 | |
| Severe Diastolic Dysfunction (%) | 3.9 | 7.8 | |

*Note*: Continuous data expressed as mean ± standard deviation. Categorical variables expressed as percentage. Group size is listed in parentheses
**p*-value calculated using conditional logistic regression with two degrees of freedom

decreased in Group 1 ($n = 17$) compared to Group 2 ($n = 14$; $p = 0.02$). Differences in arterial stiffness and arterial elastance did not reach statistical significance (Table 6).

## Discussion

Our study found that in subjects with asymptomatic diastolic dysfunction, decreased aortic distensibility identified on TTE is associated with an increased risk of developing HFpEF compared to similar subjects with normal aortic distensibility on TTE. These findings extend to the diabetic population with asymptomatic diastolic dysfunction, in which both decreased aortic distensibility and aortic strain were shown to precede the development of HFpEF.

Our findings can be explained by the following pathophysiologic model, initially proposed by Massie in 2003: as the aorta becomes less elastic in the setting of arteriosclerosis, aging and hypertension, parallel structural changes of hypertrophy and fibrosis occur in the cardiac

**Table 4** Markers of vascular stiffness

| Variable | Group 1: HFpEF ($n = 77$) | Group 2: Diastolic Dysfunction ($n = 77$) | *P*-value |
|---|---|---|---|
| Arterial Stiffness (mmHg/mL/m$^2$) | 2.0 ± 0.69 - (22) | 1.7 ± 0.52 – (30) | 0.49 |
| Arterial Elastance (mmHg/mL) | 1.7 ± 0.50 - (22) | 1.7 ± 0.40 – (30) | 0.80 |
| Aortic Strain (%) | 7.5 ± 3.6 – (75) | 8.6 ± 4.2 – (72) | 0.22 |
| Aortic Distensibility (cm$^2$dyne$^{-1}$10$^{-3}$) | 1.9 ± 1.0 – (29) | 2.8 ± 1.8 – (48) | 0.01 |

*Note*: All data expressed as mean ± standard deviation. Group size is listed in parentheses

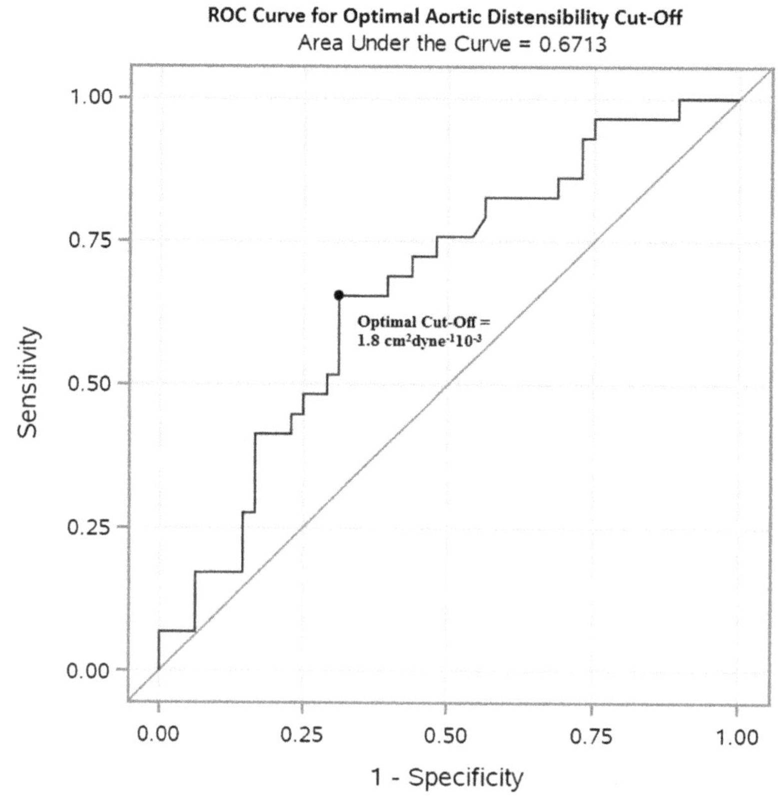


**Fig. 3** ROC curve for optimal aortic distensibility cut-off. ROC curve showing optimal aortic distensibility cut-off of 1.8 $cm^2dyne^{-1}10^{-3}$, with 62.1% sensitivity and 68.8% specificity. The AUC of the ROC curve is 0.671

myocardium because of increased vascular load, leading to decreased myocardial compliance, impaired relaxation and left ventricular diastolic dysfunction. Over time, chronically elevated diastolic pressures in the left ventricle lead to the development of symptomatic heart failure [19]. Gillebert highlighted the concept of load-dependent diastolic dysfunction, a physiologic process by which afterload that crosses a particular threshold causes slow and incomplete myocardial relaxation, resulting in elevated filling pressures and ultimately congestive heart failure [20]. In 2011, Borlaug and Kass further refined the model by incorporating the concept of ventricular-arterial coupling into the pathophysiological development of HFpEF. In brief, the net interaction between ventricular and arterial stiffness impacts cardiac function and dictates the development of symptoms due to a greater dependence on systolic pressure for coronary flow and increased ischemia for a given drop in systolic blood pressure, which is exacerbated by exercise in patients with HFpEF [21]. In support, Ikonomidis et al. found that impaired left ventricular untwisting is associated with increased arterial stiffness, increased markers of collagen turnover and decreased coronary flow reserve in subjects with hypertensive heart disease, suggesting that impaired ventricular-arterial coupling precedes the development of HFpEF [22]. While brachial pulse pressure has historically been used as a crude surrogate for arterial stiffness, Naka et al. suggested in 2015 that the prognostic role of central aortic pressure, a potentially more robust marker of risk in heart failure, needs to be further investigated [23].

Chirinos et al. also demonstrated the concept of pulsatile load, which suggests that wave reflections that arise in peripheral arteries and return to the proximal aorta during mid-to-late systole are important contributors to left ventricular afterload. Their study demonstrated that increased arterial wave reflections during mid-to-late systole are associated with an increased risk for cardiovascular events and the development of heart failure symptoms [24]. Thus, it is possible that increased pulsatile load over time results in chronically elevated pressures in the ascending aorta, resulting in increased aortic stiffness and left ventricular afterload, and ultimately the development of HFpEF by inducing structural and functional changes in the left ventricular myocardium as described in the literature above.

When measuring proximal aortic stiffness, it is important to account for the dynamic effect of pulsatile load on the compliance of the aorta [25]. The equation used to measure proximal aortic distensibility includes pulse

**Table 5** Baseline characteristics for diabetic subset

| Variable | Group 1: Diabetic HFpEF ($n = 43$) | Group 2: Diabetic Diastolic Dysfunction ($n = 21$) | p-value |
|---|---|---|---|
| Age (years) | 66.0 ± 9.40 | 66.9 ± 10.2 | 0.73 |
| Gender (% Female) | 65.1 | 71.4 | 0.61 |
| Race (% African American) | 34.9 | 28.6 | 0.61 |
| Body Surface Area ($m^2$) | 2.0 ± 0.3 | 2.0 ± 0.2 | 0.19 |
| Tobacco Use (%) | 65.9 | 66.7 | 0.95 |
| Alcohol Use (%) | 37.5 | 57.1 | 0.14 |
| Hypertension (%) | 95.3 | 85.7 | 0.18 |
| Coronary Artery Disease (%) | 72.1 | 47.6 | 0.06 |
| Atrial Fibrillation (%) | 30.2 | 14.3 | 0.17 |
| Beta Blockers (%) | 79.1 | 57.1 | 0.07 |
| Calcium Channel Blockers (%) | 32.6 | 23.8 | 0.47 |
| ACE Inhibitors (%) | 27.9 | 14.3 | 0.23 |
| Angiotensin Receptor Blockers (%) | 27.9 | 28.6 | 0.96 |
| Mild Diastolic Dysfunction (%) | 23.3 | 9.5 | 0.16* |
| Moderate Diastolic Dysfunction (%) | 76.7 | 85.7 | |
| Severe Diastolic Dysfunction (%) | 0.0 | 4.8 | |

*Note*: Continuous data expressed as mean ± standard deviation. Categorical variables expressed as percentage
*p-value calculated using Fisher's Exact Test for a 2x3 contingency table

pressure as well as aortic strain; therefore, it accounts for a more physiologic and continuous measurement of aortic stiffness [12]. Even though other reliable non-invasive methods such as brachial-ankle pulse wave velocities take into account the peripheral vascular bed [26], the advantage of measuring proximal aortic stiffness from TTE is that it can still be assessed at the same time diastolic dysfunction is discovered in an individual subject without the need for additional testing.

**Table 6** Echocardiographic markers of vascular stiffness for diabetic subset

| Variable | Group 1: Diabetic HFpEF ($n = 43$) | Group 2: Diabetic Diastolic Dysfunction ($n = 21$) | p-value |
|---|---|---|---|
| Arterial Stiffness ($mmHg/mL/m^2$) | 2.2 ± 0.6 - (14) | 1.7 ± 0.6 - (9) | 0.051 |
| Arterial Elastance ± mmHg/mL) | 1.9 ± 0.4 - (14) | 1.7 ± 0.3 - (9) | 0.098 |
| Aortic Strain (%) | 6.9 ± 3.3 - (43) | 9.7 ± 5.6 - (9) | 0.02 |
| Aortic Distensibility ($cm^2dyne^{-1}10^{-3}$) | 1.8 ± 1.0 - (17) | 3.5 ± 2.6 - (14) | 0.02 |

*Note*: All data expressed as mean ± standard deviation. Group size is listed in parentheses

Increased arterial stiffness has previously been correlated with diastolic dysfunction [27–29]. Namba et al. showed evidence in a cross-sectional study that cardio-ankle vascular index was independently associated with LV diastolic dysfunction in subjects with cardiovascular disease [27]. The study findings reported by Seeland et al. and Alba et al. support the significant associations between pathologic pulse wave velocities and the prevalence of diastolic dysfunction in women [28, 29]. Therefore, the increased correlation between arterial stiffness and asymptomatic diastolic dysfunction in subjects may also account for the lack of statistical significance between the two groups, each with diastolic dysfunction in our study. However, the statistically significant difference in aortic distensibility found between the two groups in our study suggests that even though increased peripheral arterial stiffness is associated with asymptomatic diastolic dysfunction, the additional contribution of increased proximal aortic stiffness may be required for the progression from asymptomatic diastolic dysfunction to HFpEF. In other words, it may be that the increased stiffness of the ascending aorta rather than the peripheral vasculature is the pathologic mechanism which drives the progression from diastolic dysfunction to HFpEF. Prospective studies are needed to further investigate the contribution of proximal aortic stiffness to the development of HFpEF.

### Strengths

The strengths of our analysis included the longitudinal nature of the study, which allowed us to investigate whether increased vascular stiffness precedes the development of HFpEF in patients with asymptomatic diastolic dysfunction. In addition, our matched cohort design allowed us to control for confounding variables including age, race and gender, all of which are known to be associated with vascular stiffness [28, 30, 31]. Subjects were also matched for BSA because BSA is a key determinant of aortic root and arch dimension [32]. In addition, matching allowed us to use a smaller sample size as compared to an unmatched study. Furthermore, our calculated values for aortic distensibility and aortic strain were similar to those published in previous literature, particularly for hypertensive and diabetic patients [18].

### Limitations

The number of subjects and retrospective design are important limitations of the study and any associations discussed should be considered in this context. Our sample size was further limited due to missing data in the analyzed TTE reports. For instance, 48/77 subjects in Group 1 and 28/77 subjects in Group 2 did not have blood pressure recordings at the time of their echocardiogram, rendering it impossible to calculate all the indices of vascular stiffness for these subjects. We did counter this limitation by including aortic strain as part of our analysis, so that at minimum we could assess proximal aortic stiffness in the absence of blood pressure recordings in all subjects. Despite this, arterial stiffness, arterial elastance and aortic strain were not significantly correlated with the development of HFpEF. A larger sample size may be needed to demonstrate statistically significant results, particularly in the diabetic sub-group.

Since 2003, the guidelines for assessing and grading diastolic dysfunction have been updated twice, most recently in 2016 [33]. Therefore, it is possible that some echocardiograms interpreted as having diastolic dysfunction or that some studies that were assumed to have normal diastolic function in 2003 would no longer receive the same classification under the new guidelines. However, incorporating peak E and A-wave velocities and E/A ratio into the determination of diastolic function has not changed since 2002.

Subjects were not matched for co-morbidities commonly seen in HFpEF such as hypertension, DM and CKD because we wanted to confirm the validity of our data set by reproducing the previously demonstrated association between the development of HFpEF and these co-morbidities. These covariates were adjusted for in the multiple logistic regression analysis to eliminate the effect of these variables on HFpEF development.

## Conclusions

This study confirmed the previously demonstrated association between the development of HFpEF and the presence of hypertension, DM, CAD, CKD and AF [5, 11–13]. However, the presence of decreased aortic distensibility on TTE in patients with diastolic dysfunction prior to the development of HFpEF is a novel finding.

In summary, these data support the conclusion that incorporating the simple measurements and calculations of proximal aortic stiffness, including distensibility and strain, when diastolic dysfunction is first identified on TTE may help to identify higher risk patients prior to the development of HFpEF. Larger prospective studies are needed to further investigate this relationship and to determine whether early interventions to control blood pressure and diabetes can alter the outcome in these patients.

### Abbreviations

AF: Atrial fibrillation; ANOVA: Analysis of variance; ASE: American Society of Echocardiography; AUC: Area under curve; BP: Blood pressure; BSA: Body surface area; CAD: Coronary artery disease; CHF: Congestive heart failure; CKD: Chronic kidney disease; d.f.: Degrees of freedom; DM: Diabetes mellitus; DWS: Diastolic wall strain; EACVI: European Association of Cardiovascular Imaging; EF: Ejection fraction; EHR: Electronic health record; ESP: End systolic pressure; FMLH: Froedtert Memorial Lutheran Hospital; FS: Fractional shortening; GFR: Glomerular filtration rate; HFpEF: Heart failure with preserved ejection fraction; ICD-9: International Classification of Diseases, 9th Edition; LV: Left ventricular; LVEDV: Left ventricular end diastolic volume; LVEF: Left ventricular ejection fraction; LVESV: Left ventricular end systolic volume; LVIDd: Left ventricular internal diameter at end-diastole; LVIDs: Left ventricular internal diameter at end-systole; LVPWd: Left ventricular posterior wall thickness at end-diastole; LVPWs: Left ventricular posterior wall thickness at end-systole; MRI: Magnetic resonance imaging; NT-proBNP: N-terminal pro-hormone brain natriuretic peptide; PP: Pulse pressure; ROC: Receiver operating characteristic; RWT: Relative wall thickness; SAS: Statistical Analysis System; SV: Stroke volume; SV: Stroke volume; SVI: Stroke volume index; TR: Triscuspid regurgitant; TTE: Transthoracic echocardiogram

### Acknowledgments

The authors would like to acknowledge the contributions of Joshua Meskin, MD (Medical College of Wisconsin, Department of Cardiology) and Tammy O'Toole (Clinical Database Specialist) for their assistance in building the database used to complete this study. No compensation was received for these contributions.

### Funding

This work was supported by the National Institutes of Health K08 Grant Number HL111148 (J.L.S.) and the Clinical and Translational Science Institute grant (8UL1TR000055). The National Institute of Health did not play a role in the design of the study, the collection, the analysis or interpretation of data, nor in the writing of the manuscript.

### Authors' contributions

IK carried out the retrospective review of the clinical and echocardiographic data, manually performed the echocardiographic measurements, and drafted the manuscript. OA assisted with the review and extraction of clinical data. RS performed the statistical analysis. JLS conceived of the study, and participated in its design, coordination and interpretation. All authors read and approved the final manuscript.

### Competing interests

The authors declare that they have no competing interests, financial or otherwise.

### Author details

[1]Department of Medicine, Medical College of Wisconsin, 9200 Wisconsin Ave, Milwaukee, WI 53226, USA. [2]Division of Biostatistics, Medical College of Wisconsin, Milwaukee, WI, USA. [3]Division of Cardiovascular Medicine, Medical College of Wisconsin, Milwaukee, WI, USA.

### References

1. Borlaug BA, Paulus WJ. Heart failure with preserved ejection fraction: pathophysiology, diagnosis, and treatment. Eur Heart J. 2011;32(6):670–9.
2. Kawaguchi M, Hay I, Fetics B, Kass DA. Combined ventricular systolic and arterial stiffening in patients with heart failure and preserved ejection fraction: implications for systolic and diastolic reserve limitations. Circulation. 2003;107(5):714–20.
3. Bell V, Mitchell GF. Influence of vascular function and pulsatile hemodynamics on cardiac function. Curr Hypertens Rep. 2015;17(9):580.

4. Hundley WG, Kitzman DW, Morgan TM, Hamilton CA, Darty SN, Stewart KP, et al. Cardiac cycle-dependent changes in aortic area and distensibility are reduced in older patients with isolated diastolic heart failure and correlate with exercise intolerance. J Am Coll Cardiol. 2001;38(3):796–802.
5. Ul Haq MA, Wong C, Hare DL. Heart failure with preserved ejection fraction: an insight into its prevalence, predictors, and implications of early detection. Rev Cardiovasc Med. 2015;16(1):20–7.
6. Owan TE, Hodge DO, Herges RM, Jacobsen SJ, Roger VL, Redfield MM. Trends in prevalence and outcome of heart failure with preserved ejection fraction. N Engl J Med. 2006;355(3):251–9.
7. Fonarow GC, Stough WG, Abraham WT, Albert NM, Gheorghiade M, Greenberg BH, et al. Characteristics, treatments, and outcomes of patients with preserved systolic function hospitalized for heart failure: a report from the OPTIMIZE-HF Registry. J Am Coll Cardiol. 2007;50(8):768–77.
8. Shah SJ, Heitner JF, Sweitzer NK, Anand IS, Kim HY, Harty B, et al. Baseline characteristics of patients in the treatment of preserved cardiac function heart failure with an aldosterone antagonist (TOPCAT) trial. Circ Heart Fail. 2012;6(2):184–92.
9. Chow B, Rabkin SW. The relationship between arterial stiffness and heart failure with preserved ejection fraction: a systemic meta-analysis. Heart Fail Rev. 2015;20(3):291–303.
10. MacDonald MR, Petrie MC, Varyani F, Ostergren J, Michelson EL, Young JB, et al. Impact of diabetes on outcomes in patients with low and preserved ejection fraction heart failure: an analysis of the Candesartan in Heart failure: Assessment of Reduction in Mortality and morbidity (CHARM) programme. Eur Heart J. 2008;29(11):1377–85.
11. Fang ZY, Prins JB, Marwick TH. Diabetic cardiomyopathy: evidence, mechanisms, and therapeutic implications. Endocr Rev. 2004;25(4):543–67.
12. Cavalcante JL, Lima JA, Redheuil A, Al-Mallah MH. Aortic stiffness: current understanding and future directions. J Am Coll Cardiol. 2011;57(14):1511–22.
13. Stefanadis C, Stratos C, Boudoulas H, Kourouklis C, Toutouzas P. Distensibility of the ascending aorta: comparison of invasive and non-invasive techniques in healthy men and in men with coronary artery disease. Eur Heart J. 1990;11(11):990–6.
14. Lang RM, Badano LP, Mor-Avi V, Afilalo J, Armstrong A, Ernande L, et al. Recommendations for cardiac chamber quantification by echocardiography in adults: an update from the American Society of Echocardiography and the European Association of Cardiovascular Imaging. J Am Soc Echocardiogr. 2015;28(1):1–39.e14.
15. Quiñones MA, Otto CM, Stoddard M, Waggoner A, Zoghbi WA. Recommendations for quantification of Doppler echocardiography: a report from the Doppler Quantification Task Force of the Nomenclature and Standards Committee of the American Society of Echocardiography. J Am Soc Echocardiogr. 2002;15(2):167–84.
16. Nagueh SF, Appleton CP, Gillebert TC, Marino PN, Oh JK, et al. Recommendations for the evaluation of left ventricular diastolic function by echocardiography. J Am Soc Echocardiogr. 2009;22(2): 107–33.
17. Levey AS, Stevens LA, Schmid CH, Zhang YL, Castro 3rd AF, et al. A new equation to estimate glomerular filtration rate. Ann Intern Med. 2009;150(9):604–12.
18. Eren M, Gorgulu S, Uslu N, Celik S, Dagdeviren B, Tezel T. Relation between aortic stiffness and left ventricular diastolic function in patients with hypertension, diabetes, or both. Heart. 2004;90(1):37–43.
19. Massie BM. Natriuretic peptide measurements for the diagnosis of "nonsystolic" heart failure: good news and bad. J Am Coll Cardiol. 2003; 41(11):2018–21.
20. Gillebert TC, Leite-Moreira AF, De Hert SG. Load dependent diastolic dysfunction in heart failure. Heart Fail Rev. 2000;5(4):345–55.
21. Borlaug BA, Kass DA. Ventricular-vascular interaction in heart failure. Cardiol Clin. 2011;29(3):447–59.
22. Ikonomidis I, Tzortzis S, Triantafyllidi H, Parissis J, Papadopoulos C, et al. Association of impaired left ventricular twisting-untwisting with vascular dysfunction, neurohumoral activation and impaired exercise capacity in hypertensive heart disease. Eur J Heart Fail. 2015;17(12):1240–51.
23. Naka KK, Ikonomidis I. Brachial pulse pressure in heart failure: simple to measure but complex to interpret. Eur Heart J. 2015.
24. Chirinos JA, Kips JG, Jacobs Jr DR, Brumback L, Duprez DA, Kronmal R, et al. Arterial wave reflections and incident cardiovascular events and heart failure: MESA (Multiethnic Study of Atherosclerosis). J Am Coll Cardiol. 2012; 60(21):2170-7.
25. Chirinos JA, Segers P. Noninvasive evaluation of left ventricular afterload: part 1: pressure and flow measurements and basic principles of wave conduction and reflection. Hypertension. 2010;56(4):555–62.
26. Asmar R, Benetos A, Topouchian J, Laurent P, Pannier B, et al. Assessment of arterial distensibility by automatic pulse wave velocity measurement Validation and clinical application studies. Hypertension. 1995;26(3):485–90.
27. Namba T, Masaki N, Matsuo Y, Sato A, Kimura T, et al. Arterial stiffness is significantly associated with left ventricular diastolic dysfunction in patients with cardiovascular disease. Int Heart J. 2016;57(6):729–35.
28. Seeland U, Brecht A, Nauman AT, Oertelt-Prigione S, Ruecke M, et al. Prevalence of arterial stiffness and the risk of myocardial diastolic dysfunction in women. Biosci Rep. 2016;36(5):e00400.
29. Albu A, Fodor D, Bondor C, Poantă L. Arterial stiffness, carotid atherosclerosis and left ventricular diastolic dysfunction in postmenopausal women. Eur J Intern Med. 2013;24(3):250–4.
30. Redheuil A, Yu WC, Wu CO, Mousseaux E, de Cesare A, et al. Reduced ascending aortic strain and distensibility: earliest manifestations of vascular aging in humans. Hypertension. 2010;55(2):319–26.
31. Goel A, Maroules CD, Mitchell GF, Peshock R, Ayers C, et al. Ethnic Difference in Proximal Aortic Stiffness: An Observation From the Dallas Heart Study. JACC Cardiovasc Imaging. 2016.
32. Wang YL, Wang QL, Wang L, Wu YB, Wang ZB, et al. Body surface area as a key determinant of aortic root and arch dimensions in a population-based study. Exp Ther Med. 2013;5(2):406-410.
33. Nagueh SF, Smiseth OA, Appleton CP, Byrd 3rd BF, Dokainish H, et al. Recommendations for the evaluation of left ventricular diastolic function by echocardiography: an update from the american society of echocardiography and the european association of cardiovascular imaging. J Am Soc Echocardiogr. 2016;29(4):277–314.
34. Ohtani T, Mohammed SF, Yamamoto K, Dunlay SM, Weston SA, Sakata Y, et al. Diastolic stiffness as assessed by diastolic wall strain is associated with adverse remodelling and poor outcomes in heart failure with preserved ejection fraction. Eur Heart J. 2012;33(14):1742–9.
35. Mohammed SF, Borlaug BA, Roger VL, Mirzoyev SA, Rodeheffer RJ, Chirinos JA, et al. Comorbidity and ventricular and vascular structure and function in heart failure with preserved ejection fraction: a community-based study. Circ Heart Fail. 2012;5(6):710–9.
36. Palmieri V, Russo C, Pezzullo S, Di Minno MN, Celentano A. Relation of flow-mediated dilation to global arterial load: impact of hypertension and additional cardiovascular risk factors. Int J Cardiol. 2011;152(2):225–30.
37. Muntinga HJ, Gosselink AT, Blanksma PK, De Kam PJ, Van Der Wall EE, Crijns HJ. Left ventricular beat to beat performance in atrial fibrillation: dependence on contractility, preload, and afterload. Heart. 1999;82(5):575–80.

# 23

# Therapy optimization in patients with heart failure: the role of the wearable cardioverter-defibrillator in a real-world setting

Susanne Röger[1,2*], Stefanie L. Rosenkaimer[1,2], Anna Hohneck[1,2], Siegfried Lang[1,2], Ibrahim El-Battrawy[1,2], Boris Rudic[1,2], Erol Tülümen[1,2], Ksenija Stach[1,2], Jürgen Kuschyk[1,2], Ibrahim Akin[1,2] and Martin Borggrefe[1,2]

## Abstract

**Background:** The wearable cardioverter-defibrillator (WCD) has emerged as a valuable tool to temporarily protect patients at risk for sudden cardiac death (SCD). The aim of this study was to determine the value of the WCD for therapy optimization of heart failure patients.

**Methods:** One hundred five consecutive patients that received WCD between 4/2012 and 9/2016 were included in the study. All patients were followed for clinical outcome and echocardiographic parameters during WCD therapy and had continued follow-up after WCD therapy, irrespective of subsequent implantable cardioverter-defibrillator (ICD) implantation.

**Results:** The most common indication for WCD were newly diagnosed ischemic (ICM) or non-ischemic cardiomyopathy (NICM) with left ventricular ejection fraction (LVEF) ≤35%. Mean WCD wear time was 68.8 ± 50.4 days with a mean daily use of 21.5 ± 3.5 h. Five patients (4.8%) received a total of five appropriate WCD shocks.

During WCD wear, patients with ICM and NICM showed significant improvement in LVEF, reducing the proportion of patients with a need for primary preventive ICD implantation to 54.8% (ICM) and 48.8% (NICM). An ICD was finally implanted in 51.4% of the study patients (24 trans-venous ICDs, 30 subcutaneous ICDs).

After discontinuation of WCD therapy, all patients were followed for a mean of 18.6 ± 12.3 months. 5.6% of patients with implanted ICDs received appropriate therapies. No patient with subcutaneous ICD needed change to a trans-venous device. None of the patients without an implanted ICD suffered from ventricular tachyarrhythmias and no patient died suddenly.

In patients with NICM a significant LVEF improvement was observed during long-term follow-up (from 34.8 ± 11.1% to 41.0 ± 10.2%).

**Conclusions:** WCD therapy successfully bridged all patients to either LVEF recovery or ICD implantation. Following WCD, ICD implantation could be avoided in almost half of the patients. In selected patients, prolongation of WCD therapy beyond 3 months might further prevent unnecessary ICD implantation. The WCD as an external monitoring system contributed important information to optimize device selection in patients that needed ICD implantation.

**Keywords:** Heart failure, Ischemic cardiomyopathy, Non-ischemic cardiomyopathy, Subcutaneous ICD, Sudden cardiac death, Wearable cardioverter-defibrillator

* Correspondence: susanroeger@hotmail.com
[1]First Department of Medicine, University Medical Centre Mannheim (UMM), Faculty of Medicine Mannheim, University of Heidelberg, Theodor-Kutzer-Ufer 1-3, 68167 Mannheim, Germany
[2]German Centre for Cardiovascular Research (DZHK), Partner Site Heidelberg/ Mannheim, Mannheim, Germany

## Background

Sudden cardiac death (SCD) causes about 13% of deaths in the overall population and about 36% of deaths in heart failure patients [1]. Clinical trials have shown the benefit of the implantable cardioverter-defibrillator (ICD) for treatment of SCD in both patients with ischemic (ICM) and non-ischemic cardiomyopathies (NICM) [2, 3].

Risk stratification for SCD is mainly based on left ventricular ejection fraction (LVEF) [4]. However, in patients with newly diagnosed heart failure, prior to medical therapy or in patients soon after myocardial infarction (MI) LVEF may improve with medical treatment obviating the indication for ICD. In the VALIANT trial patients with impaired LVEF were at highest risk for SCD in the first 30 days after MI [5]. Despite this risk, ICDs do not improve overall survival early after MI; lower rates of arrhythmic deaths appear counterbalanced by more non-arrhythmic deaths [6]. Current heart failure guidelines recommend optimal medical treatment (OMT) for at least 3 months before ICD implantation in both patients with ICM and NICM [4]. Recent data suggest that even longer waiting periods are appropriate in patients with newly diagnosed NICM [7]. This creates a window of susceptibility of several months when the propensity for malignant arrhythmias is high and no prophylactic therapy is provided.

The wearable cardioverter-defibrillator (WCD) provides a non-invasive temporary therapeutic option for patients during a period when the risk of SCD is changing or unclear.

Data from large registries have demonstrated safety and efficacy of WCD [8–10]. Episodes of sustained ventricular arrhythmias were recorded in about 1–3% of the patients during approximately 3 months of WCD use depending on WCD indication [8–10]. In the 2015 ESC Guidelines for the management of patients with ventricular arrhythmias and the prevention of SCD, it was stated that the WCD may be considered for adult patients with poor LV systolic function who are at risk of SCD for a limited period, but are not candidates for an ICD (e.g. bridge to transplant, bridge to trans-venous implant, peripartum cardiomyopathy, active myocarditis and arrhythmias in the early phase post-myocardial infarction) [11].

Currently, there is a paucity of data on the long-term outcome of patients after termination of WCD therapy. To our knowledge, this is one of the first studies providing continued clinical and echocardiographic follow-up data after WCD therapy, irrespective of subsequent ICD implantation. Furthermore, we evaluated whether the WCD, as an external monitoring system with an integrated bradycardia alarm, can contribute to the optimization of device selection in patients who need ICD implantation after wearing a WCD.

## Methods

### Patient recruitment

This observational cohort study included all patients receiving a WCD at our tertiary care University Center between 2012 and September 2016. All patients were fitted with a ZOLL Life Vest™ system (Pittsburgh, USA).

All patients received OMT. Each subject provided consent for the de-identified analysis of standard clinical data. The study was approved by the local ethics committee and conforms to the 1975 Declaration of Helsinki.

### The wearable cardioverter-defibrillator

The WCD ZOLL Life Vest™ system (Pittsburgh, USA) has been described previously [8]. The WCD programming was individually adapted to the patient's underlying heart disease and electrocardiographic patterns. In general, for older patients the ventricular tachycardia (VT) zone was programmed at a heart rate of 150 bpm with a VT response time of 60 s and the ventricular fibrillation (VF) zone at a rate of 200 bpm with a VF response time of 25 s. For younger and more active patients the VT zone was programmed at a heart rate of 180 bpm. First shock energy was set at maximum output (150 J) in all patients. Any arrhythmia episode was considered as a separate episode when occurring with a minimum delay of 3 min from the previous one. Each individual episode was reviewed and classified into the following categories: sustained VT (lasting 30 s or longer) or VF with WCD shock therapy, non-sustained VT (lasting less than 30 s), bradycardia of 30 beats per minute or less or asystole. Inappropriate WCD therapy was classified as a non-VT/– VF episode treated by WCD shock.

### Follow-up and data collection

Data were prospectively collected from the time of the initial hospitalization with WCD implementation. Baseline data included the indication for WCD, co-morbidities, baseline medications, ECG data, and echocardiographic results. LVEF was calculated using Simpsons's method. WCD was generally prescribed for 3 months irrespective of the underlying WCD indication. Data on arrhythmias during follow-up were prospectively collected clinically and simultaneously retrieved from the ZOLL LifeVest Network™.

In patients with primary preventive indication follow-up visits were scheduled 2 months after diagnosis. If LVEF had increased beyond 35% after 2 months, WCD therapy was terminated early. If LVEF had not increased above the 35% threshold, echocardiography was repeated 1 month later. If LVEF remained below 35% on OMT patients received primary prophylactic ICD implantation.

If a patient with primary preventive WCD indication was incompliant and returned the device earlier than planned while LVEF was still below 35%, the patient received normal clinical and echocardiographic controls. An ICD was implanted if LVEF remained below 35% after 3 months on OMT.

If patients had an appropriate WCD shock, a secondary prophylactic ICD was implanted within the following few days. In patients with an indication for cardiac resynchronization therapy (CRT), a cardiac resynchronization therapy defibrillator (CRT-D) was implanted according to current guidelines [4]. Patients with previously explanted ICDs were followed according to clinical indications.

Patients suspected of or demonstrated to have sinus bradycardia, asystole or intermittent AV-block (Mobitz II) or third-degree AV-block received a 2-chamber ICD. Patients with no suspected or reported bradycardia received an S-ICD or a 1-chamber ICD.

Long-term follow-up was counted from the day on which the patient returned the WCD. During long-term follow-up, all study patients irrespective of the duration of WCD therapy or subsequent ICD implantation received clinical and echocardiographic assessments every 6 months and when clinically indicated.

Heart failure medication consisted of angiotensin converting-enzyme inhibitor/angiotensin receptor blocker (ACE-I/ARB), betablocker and mineralocorticoid receptor antagonist (MRA) according to current heart failure guidelines [4]. Procoralan was prescribed in selected cases. Medication doses were adjusted during each follow-up visit. Since January 2016 selected patients received angiotensin receptor-neprilysin inhibitor instead of ACE-I or ARB. Furthermore, all patients were screened for iron deficiency in heart failure. Intravenous iron substitution was performed if required [4].

For missing data, particularly in cases of missed follow-up visits, the patient or other treating physicians were contacted.

### Statistical analysis

GraphPad PRISM Version 7.0a was used for data analysis. Data are presented as mean ± standard deviation or median (range) for continuous variables or as number of cases for categorical variables. Baseline characteristics were compared by t-test for parametric continuous variables and by Fishers exact test (4 groups) or $\chi 2$ test (more than 4 groups) for categorical variables. For analysis of longitudinal evolution and more than 2 groups with paired nonparametric data the Friedman test with Dunn's multiple comparisons post-test was used. A two-tailed $P$ value < 0.050 was considered statistically significant.

## Results

### Patient's baseline data

Between April 2012 and September 2016 114 patients were prescribed a WCD. Eight patients returned their WCD during the first hours after initiation because of unwillingness or inability to handle it. One patient was lost to follow-up. 105 patients had complete data sets of baseline and follow-up during and after WCD use and were included in the data analysis.

Patients were classified according to WCD indication: The most common indication for WCD (in 84 of 105 patients) was primary preventive therapy in patients with heart failure symptoms and newly diagnosed ICM or NICM with baseline LVEF ≤35% (Fig. 1, Table 1). These patients received the WCD to bridge the duration of implementing OMT to monitor whether LVEF rose above 35%. Further indications are shown in Fig. 1.

Median patient age of the whole patient population was 60 years with a male predominance (82%). Further details of the patients' baseline data are presented in Table 1.

Comparing baseline data of patients with newly diagnosed ICM and NICM, patients with ICM were older (ICM versus NICM, median (range): 62 (43–78) versus

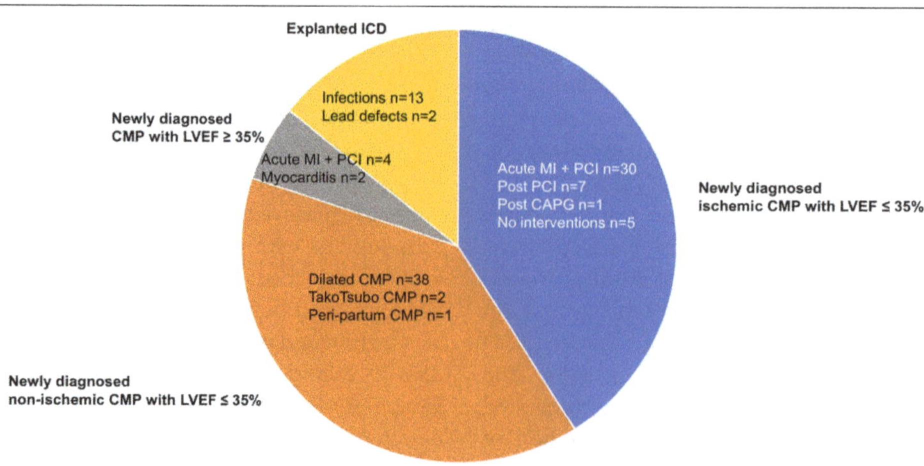


**Fig. 1** WCD indications of the 105 patients

**Table 1** Patient's baseline data at prescription of WCD

| Total number of patients | All patients | Newly diagnosed ICM LVEF ≤ 35% | Newly diagnosed NICM LVEF ≤ 35% | ICD explant | Newly diagnosed CMP LVEF ≥ 35% |
|---|---|---|---|---|---|
| | *n* = 105 | *n* = 43 | *n* = 41 | *n* = 15 | *n* = 6 |
| Age, years, median (range) | 60 (26–79) | 62 (43–78) | 54 (30–78) | 62 (29–79) | 53 (26–63) |
| Male sex, n (%) | 82 (78.1) | 35 (81.4) | 28 (68.3) | 14 (93.3) | 5 (83.3) |
| BMI kg/ m², mean ± SD | 28.6 ± 6.6 | 28.2 ± 6.2 | 29.8 ± 7.1 | 28.7 ± 6.7 | 23.5 ± 3.6 |
| Arrhythmias before WCD | | | | | |
| Atrial flutter or fibrillation, n (%) | 34 (32.4) | 10 (23.3) | 15 (36.6) | 8 (53.3) | 1 (16.7) |
| Previous VT/VF/SCD, n (%) | 21 (20.0) | 6 (14.0) | 2 (4.9) | 8 (53.3) | 5 (83.3) |
| Conduction Disorders | | | | | |
| LBBB, n (%) | 19 (18.1) | 3 (7.0) | 10 (24.4) | 6 (40.0) | 0 (0) |
| Cardiovascular risk factors | | | | | |
| Diabetes, n (%) | 29 (27.6) | 14 (32.6) | 10 (24.4) | 4 (26.7) | 1 (16.7) |
| Hypertension, n (%) | 71 (67.6) | 38 (88.4) | 16 (6.6) | 13 (86.7) | 4 (66.6) |
| Hyperlipidemia, n (%) | 62 (59.0) | 31 (72.1) | 17 (41.5) | 12 (80.0) | 2 (33.3) |
| Concomitant diseases | | | | | |
| Kidney Dysfunction, n (%) | 20 (19.0) | 10 (23.3) | 6 (14.6) | 3 (20.0) | 1 (16.7) |
| COPD, n (%) | 9 (8.6) | 3 (7.0) | 3 (7.3) | 2 (13.3) | 1 (16.7) |
| NYHA, mean ± SD | 2.7 ± 1.2 | 2.7 ± 1.3 | 3.0 ± 1.0 | 2.5 ± 0.9 | 1.3 ± 0.5 |
| LVEF baseline, mean % ± SD | 28.3 ± 9.8 | 28.9 ± 6.0 | 23.3 ± 6.9 | 32.2 ± 13.3 | 49.0 ± 7.5 |
| Medication | | | | | |
| Betablocker, n (%) | 102 (97.1) | 41 (95.3) | 40 (97.6) | 15 (100.0) | 6 (100.0) |
| ACE-I/ARB, n (%) | 97 (92.4) | 42 (97.7) | 39 (95.1) | 11 (73.3) | 5 (83.3) |
| MRA, n (%) | 67 (63.8) | 25 (58.1) | 35 (85.4) | 5 (33.3) | 2 (33.3) |
| ARNI, n (%) | 1 (1.0) | 0 (0) | 1 (2.4) | 0 (0) | 0 (0) |
| Procoralan, n (%) | 6 (5.7) | 0 (0) | 5 (12.2) | 1 (6.7) | 0 (0) |
| Diuretic, n (%) | 71 (67.6) | 26 (60.5) | 31 (75.6) | 12 (80.0) | 2 (33.3) |
| Amiodarone, n (%) | 12 (11.4) | 1 (2.3) | 5 (12.2) | 6 (40.0) | 0 (0) |

*ACE-I* = angiotensin converting-enzyme inhibitor, *ARB* = Angiotensin receptor blocker, *ARNI* = angiotensin receptor-neprilysin inhibitor, *BMI* = Body mass index, *CABG* = coronary artery bypass graft, *CMP* = cardiomyopathy, *COPD* = chronic obstructive pulmonary disease, *ICD* = implantable cardioverter-defibrillator, *ICM* = ischemic cardiomyopathy, *LBBB* = left bundle branch block, *LVEF* = left ventricular ejection fraction, *MRA* = mineralocorticoid receptor antagonist, *n* = number of patients, *NICM* = non-ischemic cardiomyopathy, *PCI* = percutaneous coronary intervention, *RBBB* = right bundle branch block, *SCD* = sudden cardiac death, *SD* = standard deviation, *VT* = ventricular tachycardia, *VF* = ventricular fibrillation, *WCD* = wearable cardioverter-defibrillator

54 (30–78)) ($p = 0.0008$) and had a lower prevalence of left bundle branch block ($p = 0.03$) than patients with NICM. They were more likely to suffer from arterial hypertension ($p < 0.0001$) and hyperlipidemia ($p = 0.005$) than patients with NICM and were less often treated with mineralocorticoid-receptor antagonists ($p = 0.008$). LVEF was significantly higher in ICM patients than in NICM patients ($p = 0.0002$).

### WCD data

The mean WCD wear time of all 105 patients was 68.8 ± 50.4 days with a mean daily use of 21.5 ± 3.5 h (Table 2).

Of the 84 patients with primary preventive indication, 37 returned their WCD earlier than the prescribed 3 months due to early LVEF improvement (21 of 37 patients), non-compliance (12 of 37 patients), early ICD-implantation due to an appropriate WCD shock (3 of 37 patients) and non-cardiac death (1 of 37 patients).

Mean WCD wear time was 57.8 ± 42.6 days in patients with newly diagnosed ICM with LVEF ≤ 35% and 69.2 ± 39.6 days in patients with newly diagnosed NICM with LVEF ≤ 35% ($p$ = n.s.).

Patients with a previous explanted trans-venous ICD had a mean WCD wear time of 92.5 ± 87.0 days.

Patients with previous explanted ICDs had a higher mean daily use (23.1 ± 1.1 h/day) than did patients in the other patient groups (Table 2). This was caused by the higher risk awareness in this patient group.

Five of the 105 patients (4.8%) received appropriate WCD shocks. Characteristics of these patients are

**Table 2** Follow-up during and after WCD use

| Total number of patients | All patients<br>n = 105 | Newly diagnosed ICM LVEF ≤ 35%<br>n = 43 | Newly diagnosed NICM LVEF ≤ 35%<br>n = 41 | ICD explant<br>n = 15 | Newly diagnosed CMP LVEF ≥ 35%<br>n = 6 |
|---|---|---|---|---|---|
| Wearing days, mean ± SD | 68.8 ± 50.4 | 57.8 ± 42.6 | 69.2 ± 39.6 | 92.5 ± 87.0 | 70.2 ± 31.2 |
| Wearing hours/day, mean ± SD | 21.5 ± 3.5 | 21.0 ± 3.8 | 21.3 ± 3.5 | 23.1 ± 1.1 | 22.4 ± 1.7 |
| LVEF % baseline, mean ± SD | 28.3 ± 9.8 | 28.9 ± 6.0 | 23.3 ± 6.9 | 32.2 ± 13.3 | 49.0 ± 7.5 |
| LVEF % end of WCD use, mean ± SD | 36.1 ± 11.5 | 36.3 ± 10.3 | 34.8 ± 11.1 | 32.9 ± 13.0 | 50.8 ± 8.6 |
| ($p$ value of LVEF baseline versus end of WCD use) | ($p < 0.001$) | ($p < 0.001$) | ($p < 0.001$) | ($p$ = n.s.) | ($p$ = n.s.) |
| ICD implanted | | | | | |
| Total n (%) | 54 (51.4) | 21 (48.8) | 18 (43.9) | 13 (86.7) | 2 (33.3) |
| Days WCD start to ICD implantation, mean ± SD | 103.8 ± 73.7 | 127.7 ± 84.1 | 90.0 ± 36.8 | 94.7 ± 90.3 | 37.0 ± 18.4 |
| Single-chamber ICD, n (%) | 8 (7.6) | 3 (7.0) | 4 (9.8) | 0 (0) | 1 (16.7) |
| Dual-chamber ICD, n (%) | 4 (3.8) | 1 (2.3) | 0 (0) | 2 (13.3) | 1 (16.7) |
| CRT-D, n (%) | 12 (11.4) | 3 (7.0) | 5 (12.2) | 4 (26.7) | 0 (0) |
| S-ICD, n (%) | 30 (28.6) | 14 (32.6) | 9 (22.0) | 7 (46.7) | 0 (0) |
| No ICD implanted | | | | | |
| Total, n (%) | 51 (48.6) | 22 (51.2) | 23 (56.1) | 2 (13.3) | 4 (66.7) |
| LVEF recovery to > 35%, n (%) | 40 (38.1) | 19 (44.2) | 21 (51.2) | 0 (0) | 0 (0) |
| Transient WCD indication, n (%) | 4 (3.8) | 0 (0) | 0 (0) | 0 (0) | 4 (33.3) |
| Patient refused ICD, n (%) | 5 (4.8) | 2 (4.7) | 2 (4.9) | 1 (6.7) | 0 (0) |
| Death during WCD wear, n (%) | 2 (1.9) | 1 (2.3) | 0 (0) | 1 (6.7) | 0 (0) |
| Arrhythmic death during WCD wear, n (%) | 0 (0) | 0 (0) | 0 (0) | 0 (0) | 0 (0) |

*CRT-D* = cardiac resynchronization therapy with defibrillator, *ICM* = ischemic cardiomyopathy, *ICD* = implantable cardioverter-defibrillator, *LVEF* = left ventricular ejection fraction, *n* = number of patients, *NICM* = non-ischemic cardiomyopathy, *SD* = standard deviation, *S-ICD* = subcutaneous ICD, *WCD* = wearable cardioverter-defibrillator

presented in Table 3. Four patients had WCD shock because of VF, one patient experienced WCD shock because of VT. In all five patients VT or VF was successfully terminated with the first WCD shock. In each of the five patients WCD shocks occurred after discharge from hospital between 3 to 154 days after initiation of WCD.

The single patient who received an appropriate WCD shock after 154 days of WCD wear was a 71-year-old man with ICM. He received prolonged WCD therapy due to persistent bacterial infection triggered by his knee prosthesis. The WCD shock was delivered because of sustained VT with ventricular heart rate of 180/min.

**Table 3** Characteristics of patients with appropriate WCD shocks

| Patient, Age | Indication for WCD | Baseline LVEF | Shock days from start of WCD | Type of arrhythmia | 1.Shock successful | Time to shock |
|---|---|---|---|---|---|---|
| Male, 64 | ICM<br>STEMI, PCI RCA | 35% | 72 | VF | yes | 54 s |
| Male, 50 | ICM<br>STEMI, PCI LAD | 25% | 3 | VF | yes | 46 s |
| Male, 45 | Dilated CMP<br>Previous explant of primary preventive trans-venous ICD | 30% | 67 | VF | yes | 49 s |
| Male, 71 | ICM<br>WCD because of systemic infection that precluded ICD implant | 20% | 154 | VT with heart rate 180/min | yes | 69 s |
| Female, 26 | Myocarditis | 53% | 38 | VF | yes | 63 s |

*WCD* = wearable cardioverter-defibrillator, *PCI* = percutaneous coronary intervention, *VT* = ventricular tachycardia, *VF* = ventricular fibrillation, *LVEF* = left ventricular ejection fraction, *ICM* = ischemic cardiomyopathy, *sec* = seconds

Then, an S-ICD was successfully implanted within the following days.

One patient had asymptomatic non-sustained VT that was detected via the ZOLL LifeVest Network™. Furthermore, one patient had an asystole of 10s during sleep that was detected via the ZOLL LifeVest Network™.

One 74-year-old female patient with mild cognitive defects and newly diagnosed ICM received an inappropriate WCD shock on day 3. This was triggered by artifactual voltage fluctuations misinterpreted by the WCD as ventricular arrhythmia. The patient had ignored both tactile and audible alarms and failed to press the response button of her WCD.

None of the 21 patients with early LVEF improvement and none of the 12 patients who returned their WCD early due to non-compliance showed signs of ventricular tachyarrhythmias during the missed WCD time period.

**Changes in LVEF and ICD implantations after WCD wear**

***LVEF assessment***

At the end of WCD wear mean LVEF of all 105 patients had improved from 28.3 ± 9.8% at baseline to 36.1 ± 11.5% ($p < 0.001$) (Table 2).

The 43 patients with newly diagnosed ICM with LVEF ≤35% showed a significant improvement of mean LVEF from 28.9 ± 6.0% to 36.3 ± 10.3% ($p < 0.001$) (Fig. 2a). 19 of the 43 patients (44.2%) showed improvement of LVEF beyond 35% and surpassed the threshold for ICD implantation (Fig. 2b). 54.8% of the patients alive had persistent primary prophylactic ICD indication.

The 41 patients with newly diagnosed NICM with LVEF ≤35% also showed significant improvement of mean LVEF from 23.3 ± 6.9% to 34.8 ± 11.1% ($p < 0.001$) (Fig. 3a). 21 of the 41 patients (51.2%) showed improvement of LVEF beyond 35% (Fig. 3b). 48.8% had persistent primary prophylactic ICD indication.

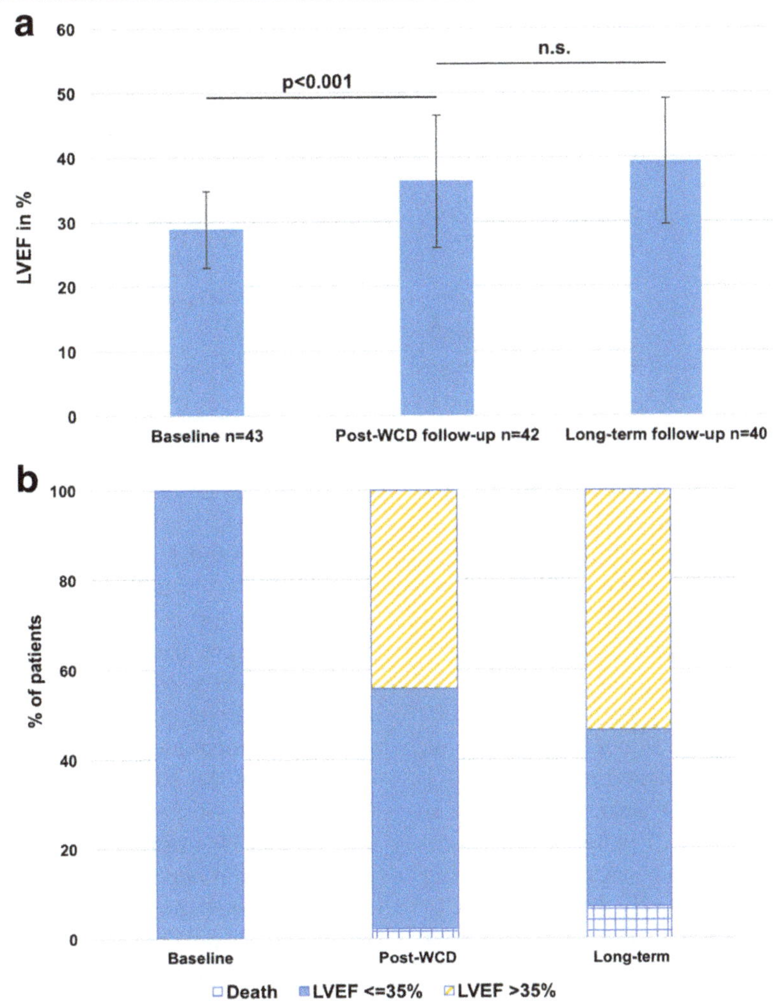


**Fig. 2** **a** Evolution of LVEF during follow-up in patients with newly diagnosed ICM with LVEF ≤35% (mean ± SD). **b** Evolution of LVEF/ICD indication in patients with newly diagnosed ICM with LVEF ≤ 35%

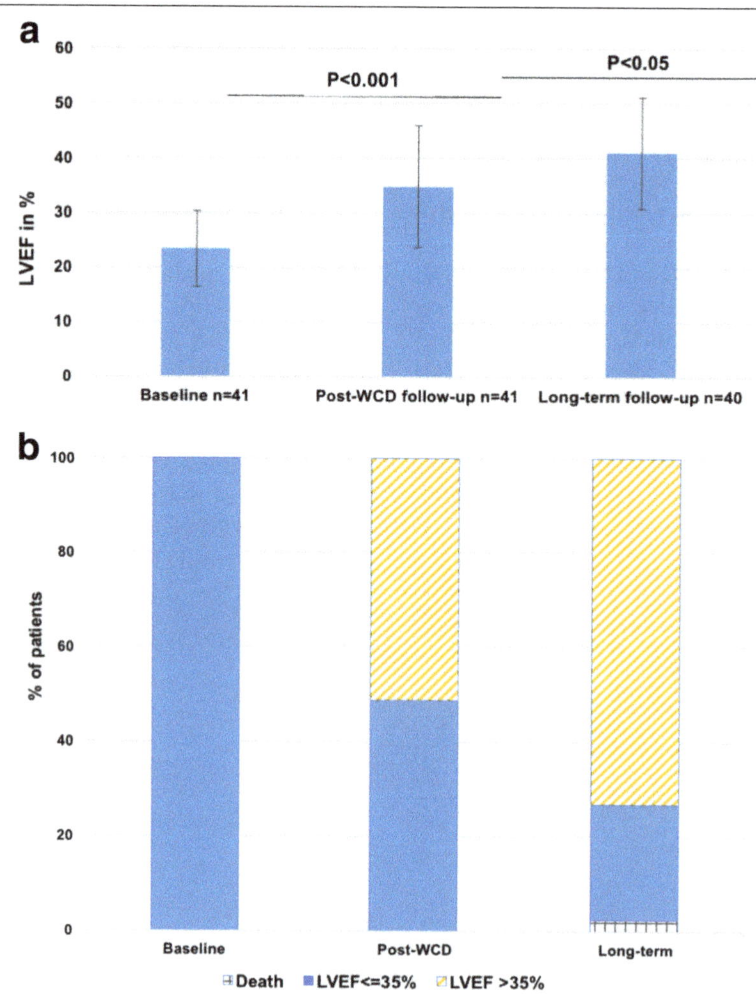


**Fig. 3 a** Evolution of LVEF during follow-up in patients with newly diagnosed NICM with LVEF ≤35% (mean ± SD). **b** Evolution of LVEF/ICD indication in patients with newly diagnosed NICM with LVEF ≤ 35%

Patients with explanted ICDs showed no significant changes in LVEF (32.2 ± 13.3% at baseline to 32.9 ± 13.0% at the end of WCD wear) ($p$ = n.s.). Furthermore, patients with newly diagnosed CMP and LVEF ≥ 35% had no significant changes in LVEF (49.0 ± 7.5% at baseline to 50.8 ± 8.6% at the end of WCD wear) ($p$ = n.s.).

### *ICD implantations*

An ICD was implanted in 54 (51.4%) out of 105 patients (Table 2). Mean time to ICD implantation was 103.8 ± 73.7 days from the start of WCD wear. In the patient group with newly diagnosed ICM 21 patients (48.8%) received an ICD after 127.7 ± 84.1 days from starting WCD. In the patient group with newly diagnosed NICM 18 patients (43.9%) received an ICD after 90 ± 36.8 days from starting WCD. ICD implantation rate was highest in patients with a previous explanted ICD (86.7%).

The five patients with appropriate WCD shocks all received secondary prophylactic ICD. The patient that had asystole detected by the WCD received a 2-chamber ICD.

Figure 4 provides an overview of the patients' arrhythmias and distribution of implanted devices. In total, eight of the 54 patients with ICD received a single-chamber ICD, 4 patients received a dual-chamber ICD, and 12 patients received a CRT-D. Furthermore, 30 patients without prior evidence of bradyarrhythmias received a subcutaneous ICD (S-ICD).

Fifty-one of the 105 patients (48.6%) did not receive an ICD (Table 2): 40 patients with ICM/ NICM and LVEF < 35% had LVEF improvement beyond 35%, five patients refused recommended ICD implantation and in four patients with newly diagnosed CMP and LVEF > 35% WCD indication was only transient. Two patients had died while wearing the WCD. The cause of death was endocarditis followed by septic shock in one patient and pulseless electrical activity and pumping failure after hemodialysis in the other. Neither clinical observation nor the ZOLL

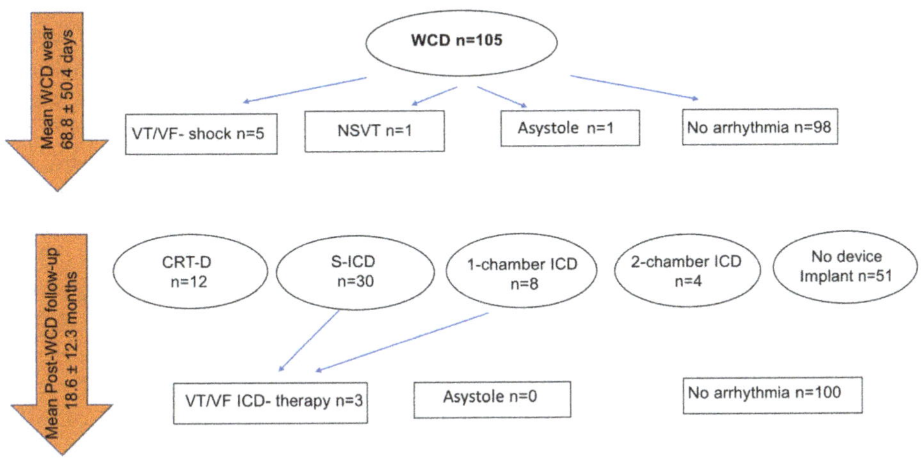


**Fig. 4** Overview arrhythmias and devices

LifeVest Network™ showed evidence of tachyarrhythmia or bradyarrhythmia in either patient.

#### Long-term follow-up after discontinuation of WCD

After end of WCD use all 103 patients alive were followed for a mean period of 18.6 ± 12.3 months- irrespective if they had received an ICD or not.

##### *LVEF during long-term follow-up*

Mean LVEF of all patients further improved from 36.1 ± 11.5% at end of WCD wear to 40.7 ± 11.0% at last follow-up ($p < 0.001$).

In the patient group with newly diagnosed ICM mean LVEF changed not significantly from 36.3 ± 10.3% at end of WCD wear to 39.3 ± 9.8% at last follow-up ($p$ = n.s.; Fig. 2a). Mean change of LVEF from baseline to last follow-up was 9.4 ± 1.8%. 4 of the 43 patients (9.3%) with newly diagnosed ICM showed late LVEF recovery to > 35%. During long-term follow-up, the proportion of patients with LVEF beyond 35% increased not significantly from 44.2% at end of WCD wear to 53.5% (p = n.s.; Fig. 2b). At last follow-up 42.5% of the patients alive had persistent LVEF ≤ 35%.

In the patient group with newly diagnosed NICM mean LVEF significantly improved from 34.8 ± 11.1% at end of WCD wear to 41.0 ± 10.2% at last follow-up ($p < 0.05$; Fig. 3a). Mean change of LVEF from baseline to last follow-up was 17.7 ± 1.9%. Nine patients (22.0%) showed late recovery of LVEF to > 35%. The proportion of patients with LVEF ≥35% significantly increased from 51.2% at end of WCD wear to 73.2% ($p = 0.038$; Fig. 3b). At last follow-up only 25.0% of the patients alive had LVEF ≤35%.

##### *Arrhythmias during long-term follow-up*

During long-term follow-up three of the 54 patients (5.6%) with implanted ICDs received a total of 16 appropriate ICD treatments (Table 4). One patient received one S-ICD shock because of VT. Another patient received 13 ATPs from his single-chamber ICD because of a recurrent monomorphic VT that was subsequently ablated. Both of them had ICM with LVEF < 35% that did not improve throughout the study.

Another patient who had already received an appropriate WCD shock for VF received two appropriate shocks of his single-chamber ICD for VF. He was subsequently treated with amiodarone. His WCD indication was newly diagnosed ICM and baseline LVEF < 35%. His LVEF did not change during WCD wear but improved during long-term follow-up and the appropriate ICD shocks occurred while LVEF was 42%.

None of the patients that had no ventricular tachyarrhythmias during WCD wear and who showed late LVEF improvement beyond 35% had ventricular tachyarrhythmias throughout the study.

None of the 30 patients implanted with an S-ICD showed evidence of bradycardia and none of these patients needed subsequent implantation of a pacemaker or device change to a trans-venous ICD system.

**Table 4** Long-term follow-up after discontinuation of WCD

| | ICD implanted $n = 54$ | No ICD implanted $n = 49$ |
|---|---|---|
| Sustained VT/VF, n (%) | 3 (5.6) | 0 (0) |
| Appropriate ICD therapy, n (%) | 3 (5.6) | – |
| Inappropriate ICD therapy, n (%) | 2 (3.7) | – |
| Asystole, n (%) | 0 (0) | 0 (0) |
| Death, n (%) | 1 (1.9) | 2 (4.1) |
| Arrhythmic death, n (%) | 0 (0) | 0 (0) |
| Non-arrhythmic death, n (%) | 1 (1.9) | 2 (4.1) |

*ICD* = implantable cardioverter-defibrillator, *n* = number of patients, *VT* = ventricular tachycardia, *VF* = ventricular fibrillation, *WCD* = wearable cardioverter-defibrillator

Furthermore, none of the 51 patients who had not received an ICD showed evidence of ventricular tachyarrhythmias.

#### *Inappropriate shocks during long-term follow-up*

Two out of the 54 patients (3.7%) with ICD had inappropriate shocks (Table 4): one patient had one inappropriate shock within hours after S-ICD implantation that was caused by residual air in the vicinity of the newly implanted sensing electrode which led to a decrease of the S-ICD signal amplitude and abrupt baseline shift. The trapped air dissolved spontaneously and no further sensing abnormalities were observed during follow-up. Furthermore, one patient who was implanted with a single-chamber ICD had one inappropriate shock because of atrial fibrillation.

#### *Deaths during long-term follow-up*

Three patients died during long-term follow-up (Table 4), and all three died because of non-arrhythmic reasons. Two patients without permanent ICD died because of septic shock. One patient who had received an S-ICD died of lung empyema 14 months later. Postmortem ICD interrogation showed no evidence of ventricular arrhythmia. No patient died from SCD.

## Discussion

The major findings of our study were as follows

1. WCD therapy proved to be safe and effective. All patients, independent of WCD indication, were successfully bridged to either LVEF recovery or ICD implantation.
2. Both patient groups with newly diagnosed ICM and with NICM showed significant LVEF improvement during WCD wear. Following WCD treatment, ICD implantation could be avoided in almost half of the patients. During long-term follow-up, further significant LVEF improvement was observed in patients with NICM.
3. The WCD, as an external monitoring system for detecting asystole or bradycardia, contributed important information for device selection in patients who needed ICD implantation after WCD wear. During long-term follow-up, no patient with S-ICD needed change to a trans-venous device. Furthermore, none of the patients without an implanted ICD showed any signs of ventricular tachyarrhythmias.

### WCD efficacy and safety

Several observational studies have shown WCD to successfully identify and interrupt VT and VF with shock efficacy rates of 99–100% [8–10, 12]. The present study confirmed effectiveness and safety of the WCD therapy. 4.8% of the patients had sustained VT/VF, and all episodes were successfully terminated by WCD shock.

The percentage of VT/VF was slightly higher than in multi-center registries reporting appropriate WCD shocks in 1.1 to 2.1% of the patients [8–10]. Other single center data showed similar results to our patients with appropriate shocks in 3.9 to 7% of patients [13–16].

Several publications have reported higher WCD shock rates in patients with newly diagnosed ICM than in patients with newly diagnosed NICM [9, 16, 17]. Sing et al. even questioned the utility of the WCD in patients with NICM [17]. Nevertheless, Duncker et al. found an incidence of VT in the early stage of NICM of 38.7 of 100 person-years, reflecting the relevant arrhythmogenic risk in patients with NICM and non-optimized heart failure medication [18]. High rates of appropriate WCD shocks have been described in several publications evaluating patients with explanted ICDs [8, 10]. As a result, WCD prescription is now generally accepted in this patient group [11].

In our study, the majority of rescued patients had new onset ICM. However, one patient with NICM and LVEF < 35% whose primary prophylactic ICD had to be explanted and another patient with myocarditis also received lifesaving WCD shocks because of VF. The numbers of patients in the four groups in our study (especially in the patient group with explanted ICDs and myocarditis) were too small to permit interesting conclusions about predictive factors for arrhythmias. Nevertheless, our data confirm the usefulness of WCD in both patients with ICM and NICM and support its application in patients with a wide range of indications.

One of the problems associated with WCD therapy is incorrect use [19] which caused inappropriate shock in one patient. However, rates of inappropriate WCD shocks were low (0.4–3.0%) [8–10, 12]. Importantly, no death has been attributed to WCD technical failure since its introduction [20].

Another common problem [19] we faced in the study was that several patients were reluctant to wear the WCD or returned the device earlier than planned. Poor compliance or inappropriate use of the WCD may have catastrophic consequences [19]. Patient education on how to properly wear the device, change the battery and disable shock delivery is crucial. Furthermore, patients should understand their cardiac disease and the potential benefits associated with the use of the WCD. Patients should be selected carefully and the device should not be deployed in patients unfit or unwilling to properly manage it. Because WCD use may be monitored online, detection of incorrect use of the device is possible and should be used to provide prompt feedback and motivation to a non-compliant patient. In non-compliant patients who are at high risk for ventricular tachyarrhythmias, other forms of monitoring or therapy should be discussed (patient monitoring in-hospital, early ICD implantation, etc.)

**LVEF improvement**

ICD implantation rate in the whole patient cohort was 54%. This parallels other studies with similar patient collectives that reported implantation rates of 34 to 57% [9, 14, 16, 21, 22]. Naturally, ICD implantation rate was highest in the patient group with a prior explanted transvenous ICD. Following WCD, ICD implantation could be avoided in almost half of the patients with ICM and NICM. LVEF improvement was the most common reason not to implant an ICD.

Current heart failure guidelines recommend primary preventive ICD implantation in both patients with ICM and NICM with LVEF ≤35% despite at least 3 months of OMT [4]. OMT is currently defined as combination of high dose betablocker and high dose angiotensin converting-enzyme inhibitor, with the addition of a mineralocorticoid receptor antagonist in patients with persistent symptoms of heart failure [4]. As a result, ICD implantation 3 months after diagnosis might be too early in many patients because patients would be assumed to be on OMT already at the moment of diagnosis.

A previous study including patients with acute myocardial infarction who were treated with modern therapies including early revascularization, showed greatest LVEF improvement within the first month. Nevertheless, a smaller part of patients showed LVEF improvement beyond the initial 40 days after acute myocardial infarction [23].

On the other hand, recent studies including patients with NICM reported late LVEF improvement after implantation of a primary preventive ICD [24, 25]. Verma et al. reported LVEF improvement to > 35% in 12% of patients [24]. Grimm et al. found LVEF improvement in 24% of patients with NICM after ICD implantation reducing incidence of appropriate ICD therapies to ~1% per year in patients with improved LVEF [25]. In both studies, multivariate analysis identified no other significant predictor for LVEF improvement after ICD implantation than a short time from diagnosis to device implant. Consistent with the data of Varma and Grimm, 22.0% of our patients with NICM showed late LVEF improvement beyond 35%. It should be noted that approximately half of the NICM patients in our study who had late LVEF improvement had received a CRT-D device (12.2%). The CRT is known to have an important effect on LVEF recovery.

In patients with ICM we observed a trend towards late LVEF improvement. 9.3% of ICM patients skipped the ICD threshold during long-term follow-up and developed LVEF > 35% while 7.0% had received CRT-D.

Patients in our study received optimization of medical therapy not only during WCD period but were seen every 6 months in our heart failure outpatient clinic where doses of medication were adjusted. Our study overlapped the debut of newer heart failure therapies such as sacubitril/valsartan which may have played a role in improving LVEF. Sacubitril/valsartan has been shown to improve morbidity and mortality in heart failure [1]. Furthermore, this medication has also been shown to reduce the incidence of VT and arrhythmogenic deaths which might contribute to the low rate of shocks delivered to patients who received an ICD [26].

A recently published study by Duncker et al. which included 156 patients with newly diagnosed NICM or ICM (with a majority of NICM) showed 11 ± 11% improvement in LVEF during 3 months of OMT and WCD use [15]. Even in patients without CRT-D implant they demonstrated improvement of LVEF to > 35% in 33% of their patients during a prolonged period of OMT beyond 3 months [15]. Nevertheless, patients had a relevant risk for life-threatening VT as long as LVEF was ≤35%. Therefore, they proposed a prolonged regimen of WCD use beyond 3 months in patients with one of the three indications: improvement of LVEF to 30–35% or Δ LVEF ≥5% during the first 3 months of WCD wear or insufficient optimization of medical dosages (especially MRA).

Duncker et al. did not stratify subjects by etiology of heart failure (ICM vs NICM) which might have improved their ability to personalize indications for WCD use. Conversely the smaller numbers of subjects in the present study preclude further subanalysis of specific patient subgroups who might benefit from prolonged use of WCD or ICD implantation reduction.

The recently published DANISH trial confirmed the risk of life-threatening ventricular arrhythmias in the chronic phase of NICM, during which primary preventive ICD implantation did not reduce overall mortality [27]. Given that primary preventive ICD implantation in NICM has become debatable, a prolonged WCD regimen might offer prevention from SCD during careful optimization of heart failure therapy and may avoid too early or even not mortality reducing ICD implantation in patients with NICM.

In general, the potential for LVEF improvement indicates a more favorable outcome in both patients with ICM and NICM [28]. Nevertheless, existing guidelines, especially for patients with dilated cardiomyopathy, lack sensitivity and specificity in the selection of patients who need primary- prevention ICD implantation. There is a need for a more precise risk stratification algorithm that considers new markers other than LVEF to provide a more comprehensive system for disease phenotyping. Such new promising markers include the extent or pattern of myocardial replacement fibrosis detected by late gadolinium enhancement cardiac magnetic resonance imaging, cardiac autonomic dysfunction detected by $^{123}$I-meta-iodobenzylguanidine myocardial scintigraphy, several ECG-derived markers and genetic testing [29, 30]. Future ICD studies should also consider the antiarrhythmic effects of modern heart failure therapies such as sacubitril/valsartan.

### ICD implantations

Next to its function to detect and terminate VT/VF the WCD also acts as an external monitoring system to identify bradycardias and asystole. Asymptomatic asystole was identified in one patient who subsequently received a 2-chamber ICD. Currently the WCD only records bradycardias with heart rates less than 10/min. Recording of less severe bradycardia might help to better identify patients at risk for symptomatic bradycardia.

In our study 30 patients were transitioned to S-ICD after wearing the WCD. The S-ICD, like the WCD, is an innovative device without the need to implant trans-venous ICD leads avoiding lead related complications. The S-ICD, similar to the WCD, has no permanent pacing functions and is therefore not indicated in patients who need bradycardia support, cardiac resynchronization or antitachycardiac pacing [11]. During post WCD long-term follow-up, both trans-venous ICDs and S-ICDs successfully terminated VT/VF. Importantly, none of the S-ICD patients needed implantation of a pacemaker or device change to a trans-venous ICD system. In the literature, changes from S-ICD to trans-venous ICD due to the need for ATP have been described in about 0.5% to 0.8% of patients [31, 32]. Changes from S-ICD to resynchronization therapy have been described in 0.4% of patients [32]. Furthermore, several cases have been described where a pacemaker was added to S-ICD for ventricular pacing [33, 34]. In our patients, the monitoring function of the WCD helped to optimize patient selection for S-ICD implantation.

### Deaths

Five patients died, primarily because of fatal infection, and no patient died from SCD during the study period. Four of the five patients treated with the WCD had VF as a first arrhythmic event and would likely have died without the WCD therapy. Patients who had received appropriate WCD shocks and patients whose LVEF did not improve beyond 35% were implanted with a permanent ICD. In the other patients, the vulnerable phase until recovery of LVEF was safely bridged with the WCD. None of the patients with recovered LVEF and no ventricular tachyarrhythmia event during WCD wear showed late signs of tachyarrhythmia. Therefore, with the use of the WCD all study patients could be provided a comprehensive safety net avoiding SCD.

### *Limitations of the study*

This was a single center study including a variety of patient conditions. It was non-randomized but selection bias was minimized by evaluating all eligible subjects prospectively. Moreover, patients presenting in our department were consecutively included representing a real-world heart failure population. Furthermore, the decision if a 1-chamber ICD or an S-ICD was implanted was made by the operator and not in a randomized manner. It has to be emphasized that the WCD diagnoses bradycardia/ asystole only during wear time. As highgrade AV block was described to occur in about 1% to 2% of heart failure patients per year future need for cardiac pacing cannot be excluded.

## Conclusions

The WCD was confirmed to be safe and effective in protecting patients against arrhythmic death. Patients were successfully bridged to either LVEF recovery or ICD implantation. Future studies are warranted to examine if a prolonged WCD regimen in certain patient groups can minimize risks and costs of permanent ICD implantation while allowing left ventricular reverse remodeling during intensified drug therapy.

It was shown for the first time that the use of the WCD as an external monitoring system can provide important information for an easier decision regarding which kind of ICD should be used for device treatment.

#### Abbreviations

ACE-I: Angiotensin converting-enzyme inhibitor; ARB: Angiotensin receptor blocker; ARNI: Angiotensin receptor-neprilysin inhibitor; BMI: Body mass index; CABG: Coronary artery bypass graft; CMP: cardiomyopathy; COPD: Chronic obstructive pulmonary disease; CRT: Cardiac resynchronization therapy; ICD: Implantable cardioverter-defibrillator; ICM: Ischemic cardiomyopathy; J: Joule; LBBB: Left bundle branch block; LVEF: Left ventricular ejection fraction; MI: Myocardial infarction; MRA: Mineralocorticoid receptor antagonist; NICM: Non-ischemic cardiomyopathy; OMT: Optimal medical treatment; PCI: Percutaneous coronary intervention; RBBB: Right bundle branch block; SCD: Sudden cardiac death; SD: Standard deviation; sec: Seconds; S-ICD: Subcutaneous implantable cardioverter-defibrillator; VT: Ventricular tachycardia; WCD: Wearable cardioverter-defibrillator

#### Acknowledgements

Not applicable.

#### Funding

No funding was received for this study.

#### Authors' contributions

SUR designed and coordinated the study, participated in data analysis and wrote the draft of manuscript. STR, AH, BR, KS and JK cared for the patients in the inpatient and outpatient clinic and collected the study data. SL performed data analysis and assisted in modifying the manuscript. IE-B and ET assisted in data analysis and interpretation, and made critical revision of the manuscript for important intellectual content. IA and MB assisted in design and coordination of the study and made critical revision of the manuscript for important intellectual content. All authors read and approved the final manuscript.

**Competing interests**

The authors declare that they have no competing interests.

**References**

1. Desai AS, McMurray JJ, Packer M, Swedberg K, Rouleau JL, Chen F, Gong J, Rizkala AR, Brahimi A, Claggett B, et al. Effect of the angiotensin-receptor-neprilysin inhibitor LCZ696 compared with enalapril on mode of death in heart failure patients. Eur Heart J. 2015;36(30):1990–7.
2. Bardy GH, Lee KL, Mark DB, Poole JE, Packer DL, Boineau R, Domanski M, Troutman C, Anderson J, Johnson G, et al. Amiodarone or an implantable cardioverter-defibrillator for congestive heart failure. N Engl J Med. 2005; 352(3):225–37.
3. Moss AJ, Zareba W, Hall WJ, Klein H, Wilber DJ, Cannom DS, Daubert JP, Higgins SL, Brown MW, Andrews ML, et al. Prophylactic implantation of a defibrillator in patients with myocardial infarction and reduced ejection fraction. N Engl J Med. 2002;346(12):877–83.
4. Ponikowski P, Voors AA, Anker SD, Bueno H, Cleland JG, Coats AJ, Falk V, Gonzalez-Juanatey JR, Harjola VP, Jankowska EA, et al. 2016 ESC guidelines for the diagnosis and treatment of acute and chronic heart failure: the task force for the diagnosis and treatment of acute and chronic heart failure of the European Society of Cardiology (ESC)developed with the special contribution of the heart failure association (HFA) of the ESC. Eur Heart J. 2016;37(27):2129–200.
5. Solomon SD, Zelenkofske S, McMurray JJ, Finn PV, Velazquez E, Ertl G, Harsanyi A, Rouleau JL, Maggioni A, Kober L, et al. Sudden death in patients with myocardial infarction and left ventricular dysfunction, heart failure, or both. N Engl J Med. 2005;352(25):2581–8.
6. Steinbeck G, Andresen D, Seidl K, Brachmann J, Hoffmann E, Wojciechowski D, Kornacewicz-Jach Z, Sredniawa B, Lupkovics G, Hofgartner F, et al. Defibrillator implantation early after myocardial infarction. N Engl J Med. 2009;361(15):1427–36.
7. Sheppard R, Mather PJ, Alexis JD, Starling RC, Boehmer JP, Thohan V, Pauly DF, Markham DW, Zucker M, Kip KE, et al. Implantable cardiac defibrillators and sudden death in recent onset nonischemic cardiomyopathy: results from IMAC2. J Card Fail. 2012;18(9):675–81.
8. Chung MK, Szymkiewicz SJ, Shao M, Zishiri E, Niebauer MJ, Lindsay BD, Tchou PJ. Aggregate national experience with the wearable cardioverter-defibrillator: event rates, compliance, and survival. J Am Coll Cardiol. 2010; 56(3):194–203.
9. Kutyifa V, Moss AJ, Klein H, Biton Y, McNitt S, MacKecknie B, Zareba W, Goldenberg I. Use of the wearable cardioverter defibrillator in high-risk cardiac patients: data from the prospective registry of patients using the wearable cardioverter defibrillator (WEARIT-II registry). Circulation. 2015; 132(17):1613–9.
10. Wassnig NK, Gunther M, Quick S, Pfluecke C, Rottstadt F, Szymkiewicz SJ, Ringquist S, Strasser RH, Speiser U. Experience with the wearable cardioverter-defibrillator in patients at high risk for sudden cardiac death. Circulation. 2016;134(9):635–43.
11. Priori SG, Blomstrom-Lundqvist C, Mazzanti A, Blom N, Borggrefe M, Camm J, Elliott PM, Fitzsimons D, Hatala R, Hindricks G, et al. 2015 ESC guidelines for the management of patients with ventricular arrhythmias and the prevention of sudden cardiac death: the task force for the management of patients with ventricular arrhythmias and the prevention of sudden cardiac death of the European Society of Cardiology (ESC). Endorsed by: Association for European Paediatric and Congenital Cardiology (AEPC). Eur Heart J. 2015;36(41):2793–867.
12. Epstein AE, Abraham WT, Bianco NR, Kern KB, Mirro M, Rao SV, Rhee EK, Solomon SD, Szymkiewicz SJ. Wearable cardioverter-defibrillator use in patients perceived to be at high risk early post-myocardial infarction. J Am Coll Cardiol. 2013;62(21):2000–7.
13. Salehi N, Nasiri M, Bianco NR, Opreanu M, Singh V, Satija V, Jhand AS, Karapetyan L, Safadi AR, Surapaneni P, et al. The wearable cardioverter defibrillator in Nonischemic cardiomyopathy: a US National Database Analysis. Can J Cardiol. 2016;32(10):1247. e1241-7 e1246
14. Erath JW, Vamos M, Sirat AS, Hohnloser SH. The wearable cardioverter-defibrillator in a real-world clinical setting: experience in 102 consecutive patients. Clin Res Cardiol. 2017;106(4):300–6.
15. Duncker D, Konig T, Hohmann S, Bauersachs J, Veltmann C. Avoiding untimely implantable cardioverter/defibrillator implantation by intensified heart failure therapy optimization supported by the wearable cardioverter/defibrillator-the PROLONG study. J Am Heart Assoc. 2017;6(1) https://doi.org/10.1161/JAHA.116.004512.
16. Beiert T, Malotki R, Kraemer N, Stockigt F, Linhart M, Nickenig G, Schrickel JW, Andrie RP. A real world wearable cardioverter defibrillator experience - very high appropriate shock rate in ischemic cardiomyopathy patients at a European single-center. J Electrocardiol. 2017;50(5):603–9.
17. Singh M, Wang NC, Jain S, Voigt AH, Saba S, Adelstein EC. Utility of the wearable cardioverter-defibrillator in patients with newly diagnosed cardiomyopathy: a decade-long single-center experience. J Am Coll Cardiol. 2015;66(23):2607–13.
18. Duncker D, Konig T, Hohmann S, Bauersachs J, Veltmann C. Ventricular arrhythmias in patients with newly diagnosed nonischemic cardiomyopathy: insights from the PROLONG study. Clin Cardiol. 2017;40(8):586–90.
19. Lenarczyk R, Potpara TS, Haugaa KH, Hernandez-Madrid A, Sciaraffia E, Dagres N. Scientific initiatives committee EHRA. The use of wearable cardioverter-defibrillators in Europe: results of the European heart rhythm association survey. Europace. 2016;18(1):146–50.
20. Barraud J, Cautela J, Orabona M, Pinto J, Missenard O, Laine M, Thuny F, Paganelli F, Bonello L, Peyrol M. Wearable cardioverter defibrillator: bridge or alternative to implantation? World J Cardiol. 2017;9(6):531–8.
21. Quast A, van Dijk VF, Wilde AAM, Knops RE, Boersma LVA. Outpatient treatment with the wearable cardioverter defibrillator: clinical experience in two Dutch centres. Neth Heart J. 2017;25(5):312–7.
22. Kao AC, Krause SW, Handa R, Karia D, Reyes G, Bianco NR, Szymkiewicz SJ. Wearable defibrillator use in heart failure I: wearable defibrillator use in heart failure (WIF): results of a prospective registry. BMC Cardiovasc Disord. 2012;12:123.
23. Sjoblom J, Muhrbeck J, Witt N, Alam M, Frykman-Kull V. Evolution of left ventricular ejection fraction after acute myocardial infarction: implications for implantable cardioverter-defibrillator eligibility. Circulation. 2014;130(9):743–8.
24. Verma A, Wulffhart Z, Lakkireddy D, Khaykin Y, Kaplan A, Sarak B, Biria M, Pillarisetti J, Bhat P, Di Biase L, et al. Incidence of left ventricular function improvement after primary prevention ICD implantation for non-ischaemic dilated cardiomyopathy: a multicentre experience. Heart. 2010;96(7):510–5.
25. Grimm W, Timmesfeld N, Efimova E. Left ventricular function improvement after prophylactic implantable cardioverter-defibrillator implantation in patients with non-ischaemic dilated cardiomyopathy. Europace. 2013;15(11):1594–600.
26. de Diego C, Gonzalez-Torres L, Nunez JM, Centurion Inda R, Martin-Langerwerf DA, Sangio AD, Chochowski P, Casasnovas P, Blazquez JC, Almendral J. Effects of angiotensin-neprilysin inhibition compared to angiotensin inhibition on ventricular arrhythmias in reduced ejection fraction patients under continuous remote monitoring of implantable defibrillator devices. Heart Rhythm. 2017; https://doi.org/10.1016/j.hrthm.2017.11.012.
27. Kober L, Thune JJ, Nielsen JC, Haarbo J, Videbaek L, Korup E, Jensen G, Hildebrandt P, Steffensen FH, Bruun NE, et al. Defibrillator implantation in patients with Nonischemic systolic heart failure. N Engl J Med. 2016;375(13):1221–30.
28. Kalogeropoulos AP, Fonarow GC, Georgiopoulou V, Burkman G, Siwamogsatham S, Patel A, Li S, Papadimitriou L, Butler J. Characteristics and outcomes of adult outpatients with heart failure and improved or recovered ejection fraction. JAMA Cardiol. 2016;1(5):510–8.
29. Halliday BP, Cleland JGF, Goldberger JJ, Prasad SK. Personalizing risk stratification for sudden death in dilated cardiomyopathy: the past, present, and future. Circulation. 2017;136(2):215–31.
30. Pontone G, Guaricci AI, Andreini D, Solbiati A, Guglielmo M, Mushtaq S, Baggiano A, Beltrama V, Fusini L, Rota C, et al. Prognostic benefit of cardiac magnetic resonance over transthoracic echocardiography for the assessment of ischemic and Nonischemic dilated cardiomyopathy patients referred for the evaluation of primary prevention implantable cardioverter-defibrillator therapy. Circ Cardiovasc Imaging. 2016;9(10). https://doi.org/10.1161/CIRCIMAGING.115.004956.
31. Olde Nordkamp LR, Dabiri Abkenari L, Boersma LV, Maass AH, de Groot JR, van Oostrom AJ, Theuns DA, Jordaens LJ, Wilde AA, Knops RE. The entirely subcutaneous implantable cardioverter-defibrillator: initial clinical experience in a large Dutch cohort. J Am Coll Cardiol. 2012;60(19):1933–9.
32. Boersma L, Barr C, Knops R, Theuns D, Eckardt L, Neuzil P, Scholten M, Hood M, Kuschyk J, Jones P, et al. Implant and midterm outcomes of the subcutaneous implantable cardioverter-defibrillator registry: the EFFORTLESS study. J Am Coll Cardiol. 2017;70(7):830–41.
33. Kuschyk J, Stach K, Tulumen E, Rudic B, Liebe V, Schimpf R, Borggrefe M, Roger S. Subcutaneous implantable cardioverter-defibrillator: first single-center experience with other cardiac implantable electronic devices. Heart Rhythm. 2015;12(11):2230–8.

# Impaired chronotropic response to physical activities in heart failure patients

Hong Shen[1†], Jianrong Zhao[2†], Xiaohong Zhou[3], Jingbo Li[1*], Qing Wan[1], Jing Huang[1], Hui Li[2], Liqun Wu[4], Shungang Yang[3,5] and Ping Wang[3,5]

**Abstract**

**Background:** While exercise-based cardiac rehabilitation has a beneficial effect on heart failure hospitalization and mortality, it is limited by the presence of chronotropic incompetence (CI) in some patients. This study explored the feasibility of using wearable devices to assess impaired chronotropic response in heart failure patients.

**Methods:** Forty patients with heart failure (left ventricular ejection fraction, LVEF: 44.6 ± 5.8; age: 54.4 ± 11.7) received ECG Holter and accelerometer to monitor heart rate (HR) and physical activities during symptom-limited treadmill exercise testing, 6-min hall walk (6MHW), and 24-h daily living. CI was defined as maximal HR during peak exercise testing failing to reach 70% of age-predicted maximal HR (APMHR, 220 – age). The correlation between HR and physical activities in Holter-accelerometer recording was analyzed.

**Results:** Of 40 enrolled patients, 26 were able to perform treadmill exercise testing. Based on exercise test reports, 13 (50%) of 26 patients did not achieve at least 70% of APMHR (CI patients). CI patients achieved a lower % APMHR (62.0 ± 6.3%) than non-CI patients who achieved 72.0 ± 1.2% of APMHR ($P < 0.0001$). When Holter-accelerometer recording was used to assess chronotropic response, the percent APMHR achieved during 6MHW and physical activities was significantly lower in CI patients than in non-CI patients. CI patients had a significantly shorter 6MHW distance and less physical activity intensity than non-CI patients.

**Conclusion:** The study found impaired chronotropic response in 50% of heart failure patients who took treadmill exercise testing. The wearable Holter-accelerometer recording could help to identify impaired chronotropic response to physical activities in heart failure patients.

**Keywords:** Chronotropic incompetence, Heart rate, Heart failure rehabilitation, Treadmill exercise testing, 6 min hall walk

## Background

Heart failure patients experience a variety of symptoms, of which the most frequently presenting symptoms are exertional breathlessness, fatigue, and intolerance to physical activities, leading to poor quality of life. While, historically, patients with heart failure were suggested to avoid exertion, exercise-based cardiac rehabilitation has now been recognized as having a beneficial effect on heart failure hospitalization and mortality [1–4]. Currently, exercise prescription is commonly based on heart rate. However, exercise level or target intensity that depends on achievable maximal heart rate can be significantly limited in heart failure patients with chronotropic incompetence (CI) [3, 4].

In response to physical exercise that increases oxygen demand, heart rate (HR), via enhanced sympathetic activity and/or withdrawal of parasympathetic activity, increases to meet the body's metabolic demand. CI is a condition when HR increases inadequately in response to increased metabolic demand [5–8]. Patients with CI often show exercise intolerance and hence have impaired quality of life. Furthermore, studies have also demonstrated that CI is an independent risk factor for major cardiovascular adverse events including overall mortality [9–12]. The

* Correspondence: jbli@medmail.com.cn
†Equal contributors
[1]Department of Cardiology, Shanghai Sixth People's Hospital, Shanghai Jiao Tong University, Shanghai, China
Full list of author information is available at the end of the article

prevalence of CI in patients with heart failure has been reported to vary from 25% to 65% [8, 9, 13, 14].

At present, the method that clinically assesses CI is dynamic incremental exercise testing or exercise tolerance testing during which cardiac chronotropic capacity is measured [6–12]. CI is believed to be present if maximal HR during the peak of exercise testing cannot reach a certain percentage of the age-predicted maximal heart rate value (APMHR, usually 220 – age), such as 80%, or even 70% [6–8, 12]. The magnitude of the change in HR during exercise testing is also used to detect impaired chronotropic incompetence, e.g., the HR reserve (the difference between maximal HR during peak exercise and resting HR prior to exercise testing) [8, 9, 11, 12].

While exercise-based cardiac rehabilitation has been recommended for heart failure patients, the adoption of the guidelines is negatively impacted by CI. In other words, if CI is assessed and better managed, target intensity and exercise formula can be better prescribed. The purpose of the present study was to investigate a method of heart rate and physical activity recording to assess chronotropic response during treadmill exercise testing and daily physical activities in patients with heart failure.

## Methods

The study was conducted in two centers and the study protocol was approved by both hospitals' Institutional Review Boards and in compliance with the Declaration of Helsinki. All patients completed written informed consent.

### Selection of patients

Forty patients were enrolled between June 2014 and April 2015. The inclusion criteria included: (1) patients had heart failure based on ESC 2012 heart failure guidelines; (2) patients' NYHA classification was ranged from I to III and left ventricular ejection fraction (LVEF) was more than 35%; (3) patients were capable of performing moderate exercise. Patients were excluded if they (1) received a pacemaker, implantable cardioverter-defibrillator or cardiac resynchronization therapy device; (2) had persistent or permanent atrial fibrillation; (3) were incapable of exercise due to angina, heart failure decompensation, ST deviation >2 mm, or active pericarditis and myocarditis; (4) had acute myocardial infarction <45 days; (5) had uncontrolled hypertension; or (6) had other medical issues that would compound the present study.

### Study procedures

All enrolled patients received 24-h Holter ECG (NorthEast Monitoring, Inc., Maynard, MA, USA) for HR and ActiGraph GT3 accelerometer (ActiGraph, Shalimer, FL, USA) monitoring for determining the magnitude of physical activities. The clinically validated Actigraph accelerometer determined counts of 10-s acceleration activities in X-, Y-, and Z- vectors with each count equal to 16 m-g per second where the g is 9.825 $m{\bullet}s^{-2}$ [15–17]. The vector magnitude (VM) was calculated as the square root of the sum of the second power of X-, Y-, and Z-vector counts. Once the Holter-Actigraph monitoring was in place, patients underwent a 6 min hall walk (6MHW) and a symptom-limited treadmill exercise test. Some patients, based on physicians' clinical judgment and patients' willingness, did not participate in treadmill exercise testing. All enrolled patients received stable medication and there was no requirement to withhold any medication. Patients' demographic information, echocardiography, blood pro-NT-BNP, and medications were collected at enrollment.

The symptom-limited maximal treadmill exercise test adopted the modified Naughton-Balke method [18]. Briefly, the total time of treadmill exercise testing was 14 min with two minutes at base speed with slope 0 (no inclination), two minutes at slope 1 level and speed 2, and two minutes at each of next five slopes with no change in speed. During exercise testing, 12-lead electrocardiogram and blood pressure were recorded in addition to Holter-Actigraph recording.

### Assessment of chronotropic incompetence

The assessment of chronotropic incompetence was based on the achieved maximal HR during peak treadmill exercise. CI is defined as maximal HR at peak treadmill exercise that fails to reach an arbitrary percentage of APMHR, for which 70% was chosen as the criterion for diagnosis of CI in heart failure patients [12, 19, 20]. In the present study, as most patients took beta-blockers, a newly proposed equation based on HR reserve for determining chronotropic impairment was also used to assess CI, e.g., chronotropic index for patients with beta blockers (called chronotropic index-β) = (HR at peak exercise – resting HR) / (119 + (resting HR / 2) – (age / 2) – resting HR) [11].

Chronotropic response during daily living was assessed by 24-h Holter-Actigraph recording. An event of physical activity was defined once Actigraph recording reported 10 or more than 10 s of activities. Maximal Actigraph VM value in counts and HR were determined for each physical activity. Resting HR was determined by averaging HR values in the time window from 10 min after the previous activity event to the time right before the incoming activity. Thus, for each physical activity, three parameters, e.g., resting HR, maximal HR and maximal Actigraph VM, were obtained. The regression between HR values and corresponding Actigraph activity levels was performed for 24-h daily living. The overall intensity of daily physical activities was expressed as the averaged maximal VM of all physical activities during the recording window.

### Statistical analysis

Continuous variables are expressed with mean ± standard deviation. The categorical variables are used for number of patients. Comparisons for continuous variables were made using *t* test whenever appropriate. Categorical variables were compared using the Chi square test. The correlation between the CI values by exercise test reports and those by Holter-Actigraph recording was determined using Pearson correlation coefficients with corresponding correlation equations. The simple linear regression between HR and physical activities for 24-h Holter-Actigraph recording was performed. To minimize the impact of variations among individuals on regression analysis results, HR was taken as a function of the percentage of the maximal daily physical activity. Binary logistic regression was used to detect the effect of variables in patient characteristics (age, weight, gender, coronary heart disease, cardiomyopathy, LVEF, NYHA, β-blockers) on the results (CI or no-CI) of treadmill exercise testing. A two-tailed $P$ value of ≤0.05 was considered significant. The statistical tool SPSS was used for the statistical analyses.

## Results

### Treadmill exercise testing

All 40 enrolled patients (median age: 57.5 years old, range 30–70) were diagnosed with heart dysfunction with LVEF 44.6 ± 5.8% and symptoms of exertion-associated dyspnea, asthenia and fatigue. Most patients (60%) were in NYHA class II. The clinical characteristics of patients are presented in Table 1. Of the 40 enrolled patients, 26 patients underwent treadmill exercise testing and the remaining 14 patients declined treadmill exercise testing. There was no significant difference in clinical characteristics between patients taking treadmill exercise testing and those not taking (Table 2). In 13 of 26 patients (50%) who underwent treadmill exercise testing, maximal heart rate at peak exercise did not reach at least 70% of APMHR (CI patients) while in the remaining 13 patients (50%) maximal heart rate did reach ≥70% of APMHR (non-CI patients). Of 5 patients with NYHA III, maximal heart rate in 2 patients reached ≥70% of APMHR but not in other 3 patients. The binary logistic regression analysis showed only gender affected the CI results of treadmill exercise testing with an odd ratio 0.04 (for male), 0.002–0.805 95% CI and $P$ value = 0.036.

**Table 1** Patient characteristics and results of treadmill exercise testing

| | All patients (*N* = 40) | ≥70% APMHR (*N* = 13) | <70% APMHR (*N* = 13) | *P* value |
|---|---|---|---|---|
| Age (years) | 54.4 ± 11.7 | 53.1 ± 10.9 | 52.5 ± 13.8 | 0.905 |
| Weight (Kg) | 74.8 ± 17.6 | 78.2 ± 19.3 | 74.4 ± 19.4 | 0.634 |
| Male, N (%) | 30 (75) | 13 (92.3) | 7 (53.8) | 0.005 |
| NYHA class | 2.2 ± 0.6 | 1.9 ± 0.6 | 2.2 ± 0.4 | 0.166 |
| LVEF (%) | 44.6 ± 5.8 | 45.8 ± 5.5 | 42.0 ± 5.2 | 0.090 |
| LVESD (mm) | 45.9 ± 7.6 | 45.2 ± 7.1 | 49.9 ± 4.8 | 0.066 |
| LVEDD (mm) | 59.4 ± 7.7 | 58.2 ± 7.8 | 62.8 ± 4.5 | 0.084 |
| 6MHW (m) | 413.8 ± 86.9 | 486.2 ± 62.0 | 416.7 ± 37.1 | 0.003 |
| SBP (mmHg) | 125.6 ± 18.1 | 126.6 ± 20.1 | 126.8 ± 17.4 | 0.987 |
| DBP (mmHg) | 76.8 ± 9.9 | 79.2 ± 10.0 | 76.2 ± 11.4 | 0.528 |
| BNP (pg/mL) | 147.5 ± 225.8 | 114.7 ± 96.8 | 124.0 ± 145.9 | 0.855 |
| CAD, N (%) | 15 (37.5) | 4 (33.3) | 5 (35.7) | 0.680 |
| Cardiomyopathy, N (%) | 35 (87.5) | 11 (84.6) | 12 (92.3) | 0.539 |
| B-blocker, N (%) | 38 (95.0) | 12 (92.3) | 13 (100.0) | 0.308 |
| ACE inhibitor, N (%) | 16 (40.0) | 6 (46.2) | 8 (61.5) | 0.431 |
| Diuretics, N (%) | 20 (50.0) | 7 (53.8) | 7 (53.8) | 1.000 |
| Digoxin, N (%) | 10 (25.0) | 2 (15.4) | 6 (46.2) | 0.089 |
| Patients taking treadmill exercise testing (*N* = 26) | | | | |
| Rest HR (bpm) | 78.2 ± 10.9 | 80.1 ± 10.1 | 76.2 ± 11.8 | 0.373 |
| Maximum HR (bpm) | 112.0 ± 14.8 | 120.1 ± 8.8 | 103.9 ± 15.4 | 0.003 |
| HR reserve (bpm) | 33.9 ± 11.9 | 40.0 ± 10.5 | 27.2 ± 10.2 | 0.006 |
| APMHR | 167.6 ± 12.5 | 166.8 ± 11.4 | 168.4 ± 14.0 | 0.775 |
| Achieved %APMHR | 67.0 ± 6.8 | 72.0 ± 1.2 | 62.0 ± 6.3 | <0.0001 |
| C index-β (%) | 62.7 ± 19.6 | 75.3 ± 12.9 | 46.4 ± 15.3 | <0.0001 |

**Table 2** Baseline characteristics in patients with or without treadmill exercise testing

| | TET (*N* = 26) | No TET (*N* = 14) | *P* value |
|---|---|---|---|
| Age (years) | 52.8 ± 12.4 | 57.5 ± 9.4 | 0.233 |
| Weight (Kg) | 76.3 ± 19.4 | 72.0 ± 13.0 | 0.471 |
| Male, N (%) | 20 (76.9) | 10 (71.4) | 0.702 |
| LVEF (%) | 43.9 ± 5.7 | 45.8 ± 5.9 | 0.346 |
| NYHA class | 2.1 ± 0.5 | 2.3 ± 0.7 | 0.318 |
| LVESD (mm) | 47.5 ± 6.5 | 42.8 ± 8.5 | 0.062 |
| LVEDD (mm) | 60.5 ± 6.8 | 57.2 ± 8.8 | 0.208 |
| 6MHW (m) | 451.4 ± 61.8 | 344.1 ± 83.9 | <0.001 |
| BNP (pg/mL) | 119.4 ± 123.8 | 119.8 ± 336.1 | 0.294 |
| CAD, *N* (%) | 9 (34.6) | 5 (35.7) | 0.945 |
| Cardiomyopathy, *N* (%) | 23 (88.5) | 12 (85.7) | 0.802 |
| Β-blocker, *N* (%) | 25 (96.2%) | 13 (92.9) | 0.648 |

*TET* treadmill exercise testing

When β-blocker use was taken into account in the analysis using chronotropic index-β, 38.5% patients (10 / 26) failed to achieve 60% chronotropic index-β. While there were no significant differences in age and corresponding APMHR between CI and non-CI patients, CI patients achieved significantly lower maximal HR, HR reserve, and chronotropic index-β than non-CI patients (Table 1).

Figure 1a shows an example of HR and physical activity levels recorded by the Holter-Actigraph devices during treadmill exercise testing in a patient. There was a significant correlation between HR and activity levels, e.g., HR = (0.0629 × VM) + 80.999 ($R$ = 0.7322, $P$ < 0.0001, Fig. 1b), demonstrating an increase in HR in response to the increase in physical activity levels. The magnitude of physical activity level (VM) during peak exercise appeared lower in CI patients (VM: 380.3 ± 194.5 unit counts) than in non-CI patients (VM: 475.5 ± 142.0 unit counts, $P$ = 0.183 vs. the CI patients).

### HR analysis during 24-h daily living

An example of the relationship between HR and the VM of physical activities from a patient is presented in Fig. 2a, showing chronotropic response. The overall relationship between HR and all physical activities over the 24-h time window in all patients is presented in Fig. 2b, in which HR is significantly correlated with VM levels of physical activities. The correlation coefficients were at the same level between non-CI patients (Fig. 2c) and CI patients (Fig. 2d). However, the frequency of HR over 100 bpm during activity events was significantly higher ($P$ = 0.0006) in non-CI patients (20% of all activity events, Fig. 2c) than in CI patients (8.8% of all activity events, Fig. 2d).

Maximal HR achieved during daily physical activities was 106.7 ± 11.8 bpm (equal to 63.9 ± 6.8% APMHR) in CI patients, which was lower than 121.8 ± 17.3 bpm (73.0 ± 9.6% APMHR) in non-CI patients ($P$ = 0.020 vs. CI patients). The maximal HR reserve achieved during the 24-h window was 31.9 ± 7.0 bpm in CI patients, significantly smaller than that in non-CI patients (40.9 ± 12.2 bpm $P$ = 0.035 vs. CI patients). The overall intensity (VM) of daily maximal physical activities was 333.2 ± 87.6 counts in CI patients, which was smaller than in non-CI patients (390.0 ± 118.8 counts, $P$ = 0.178 vs. CI patients).

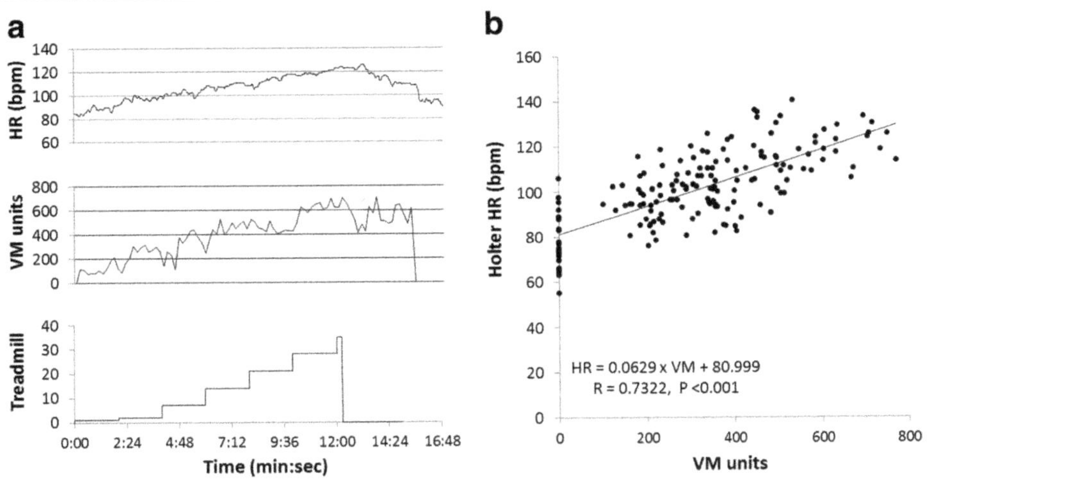


**Fig. 1** Heart rate and Actigraph VM recording during treadmill exercise testing. **a** Holter heart rate (*top*) and Actigraph activity in VM (*middle*) recording during 7 levels of treadmill exercise testing (*bottom*) in one patient. **b** the correlation between Holter heart rate and levels of VM during treadmill exercise testing in all 26 patients. Each dot represents the measurement of a maximal VM value in one of 7 levels of treadmill exercise testing

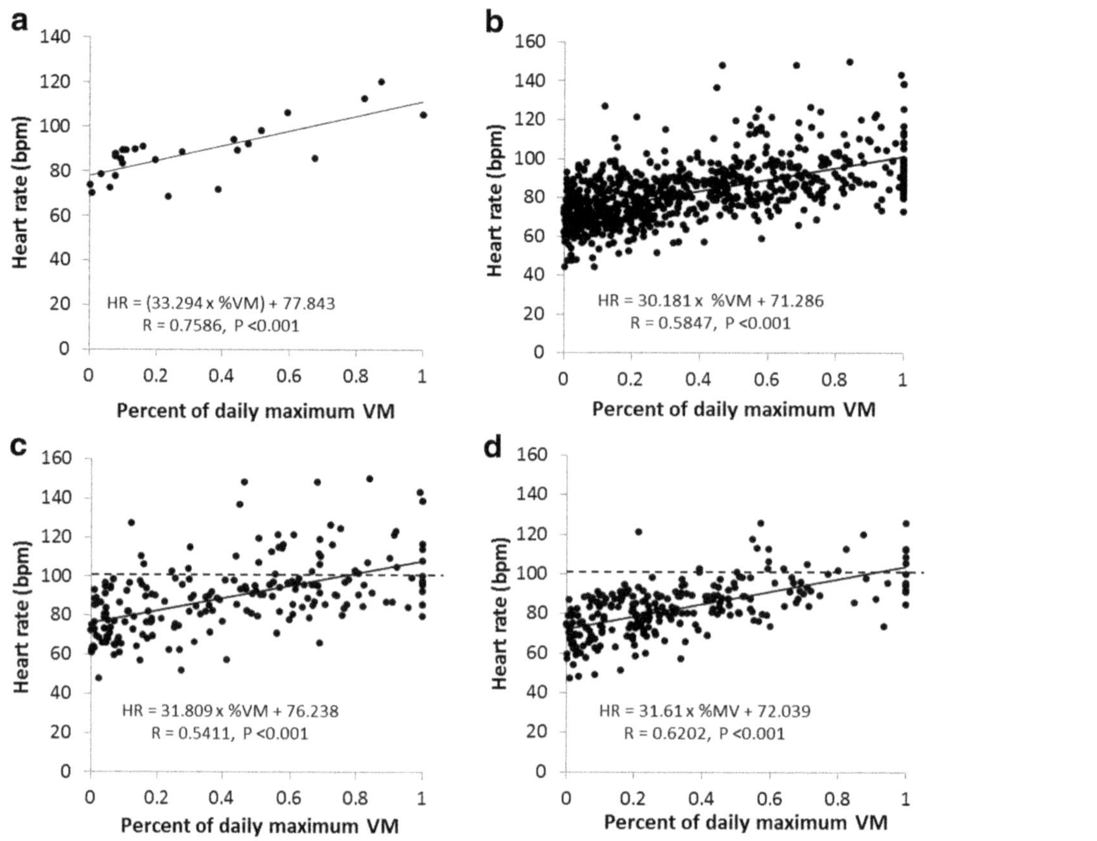


**Fig. 2** Correlation between heart rate and physical activities during daily living. **a** the correlation between heart rate (bpm, the ordinate) and the percentage of each maximal daily physical activity over the greatest maximal daily physical activity (the abscissa) in one patient; **b** the correlation for all 40 patients; **c** the correlation for 13 non-CI patients; **d** the correlation for 13 CI patients. Dashed line in (**c** and **d**) represents the maximal HR above 100 bpm during physical activity events

### HR analysis during 6-min hall walk

Maximal HR achieved during 6MHW (100.1 ± 19.6 bpm) was significantly lower than maximal HR achieved during the peak of treadmill exercise testing (112.0 ± 14.8 bpm, $P = 0.012$). However, there was a significant correlation between the 6MHW distance and the corresponding percent APMHR achieved during treadmill exercise testing (Distance = 571.7 × %APMHR + 68.6, $R = 0.615$, $P = 0.001$). The percent APMHR achieved during 6MHW was 57.5 ± 6.3% in CI patients which was significantly smaller than that in non-CI patients (63.5 ± 6.9%, $P = 0.038$ vs. CI patients) and the 6MHW distance was significantly shorter in CI patients (416.7 ± 37.1 m) than in non-CI patients (486.2 ± 62.0 m, $P = 0.003$, Table 1).

### CI assessment in patients without treadmill exercise testing

Fourteen patients did not take treadmill exercise testing based on patients' willingness and physicians' clinical judgment. In these 14 patients, the achieved percent APMHR was 60 ± 6.3% during daily physical activities and 56.4 ± 7.9% during 6MHW, both values of the percent APMHR were significantly lower than in non-CI patients (73.0 ± 9.6% APMHR during daily activities and 63.5 ± 6.9% during 6MHW, both $P$ values <0.05 vs. corresponding values in 14 patients), but comparable to the values of the percent APMHR in CI patients (63.9 ± 6.8% APMHR during daily activities and 57.5 ± 6.3% during 6MHW, both $P$ values >0.05 vs. the corresponding values in 14 patients). Moreover, the overall intensity (VM) of daily maximal physical activities was 315.5 ± 107.8 counts in VM, which appeared lower than in non-CI patients (390.0 ± 118.8 counts, $P = 0.101$) but not significantly different compared with CI patients (333.2 ± 87.6 counts, $P > 0.05$).

## Discussion

The present study used two methods to assess impaired chronotropic response to physical activities in patients with heart failure. The method of traditional treadmill exercise testing identified 50% of patients whose maximal HR during peak exercise failed to reach at least 70% of APMHR, a criterion for CI diagnosis in heart failure patients [12, 19, 20]. Holter-Actigraph recording and corresponding measurements showed a high concordance with the results of exercise testing. Furthermore, in the 24-h recording of HR and physical activities by the Holter-Actigraph system, the assessment of chronotropic response during 6-MHW and daily living found worse chronotropic response in CI patients than in non-CI patients, demonstrating the feasibility of assessment of impaired chronotropic response in heart failure patients by this method.

In the present study, maximal HR during peak exercise failed to reach at least 70% of APMHR in 50% of tested patients, thus CI was diagnosed accordingly for these patients. When HR reserve and chronotropic index-β were used to assess CI, 21 (80.8%) of 26 patients who took exercise testing failed to attain ≥80% of HR reserve and 10 (38.5%) patients failed to attain ≥60% of the chronotropic index-β. Thus, the CI incidence in heart failure population depends on the methods used for diagnosis [8]. The criterion of 70% APMHR was used in the present study, based on which the study found that (1) patients who met the CI diagnosis criterion had a significantly lower HR reserve and chronotropic index-β than those who did not meet the CI diagnosis criterion, and (2) HR changes in response to daily physical activities and the 6MHW distance were significantly smaller in patients who met the CI criterion than those who did not. When compared to the general population who have no heart failure and can reach the target heart rate during exercise testing (e.g., ≥85% APMHR) [7, 8], the heart failure patients in the present study whose heart rate during exercise testing could reach ≥70% APMHR, but still less than 85% might have reduced chronotropic response even though the CI could not be definitively diagnosed.

The present study applied a wearable recording system (Holter-Actigraph) during treadmill exercise testing in heart failure patients and assessed the correlation between treadmill exercise test results and measurements by Holter-Actigraph recording. The rationale to adopt Holter-Actigraph recording was to validate an ease-of-use tool that can be used to screen for and assess CI without the need of special infrastructure like a treadmill exercise test laboratory. The uniqueness of the present study was to use Holter-Actigraph recording to determine HR during physical activities during daily living including 6MHW and thus evaluate chronotropic capacity. The analysis of HR and physical activities based on Holter-Actigraph recording revealed a significant correlation between heart rate and physical activity levels, e.g., chronotropic response. Furthermore, the study found a significant correlation between the 6MHW distance and the percent APMHR achieved during exercise testing and reduced physical activity intensity in patients with impaired chronotropic incompetence. Thus, the Holter-Actigraph system can potentially be used to screen for CI and assess impaired chronotropic response in heart failure patients.

Exercise intolerance and symptoms of dyspnea and fatigue on effort are clinical manifestations in patients with heart failure. It is assumed that the appearance of these symptoms is more likely due to heart failure if rapid heart rate occurs in response to a moderate activity rather than the cause of CI in which there is a lack of a significant increase in heart rate. Thus, heart rate changes in response to a physical activity can be used to distinguish whether symptoms are caused by CI or not.

**Clinical perspectives**

Recent studies have demonstrated a high incidence of CI in the heart failure population and CI has been recognized as an independent risk factor for cardiovascular morbidity and mortality. Daily exercise is recommended for patients with chronic heart failure. However, the exercise intensity in terms of magnitude and time interval still remains uncertain and the intensity of exercise is significantly influenced by the capability of chronotropic response. Furthermore, use of β-blockers complicates chronotropic response, leading to a reduced chronotropic response [8, 9, 11, 21–23]. On the other hand, β-blockers have been a standard therapy that prolongs survival of heart failure patients in several clinical trials [24–26]. There are approximately 5.8 million patients with heart failure in the United States and 23 million worldwide [27]. It can be assumed that the majority of heart failure patients would not receive an assessment of their chronotropic response. As shown in the present study, of 40 heart failure patients, 14 (35%) patients who declined treadmill exercise testing did have low %APMHR achieved during 6MHW and daily physical activities. Thus, if a simple, ease-of-use tool can be used to screen for CI and assess impaired chronotropic response in heart failure population, more patients with impaired chronotropic response could be identified and better managed during heart failure treatment including exercise-based cardiac rehabilitation and treatment with β-blockers. Rate-responsive pacing is an effective method to relieve symptoms caused by CI [8, 28]. However, such a therapy may be underutilized in the heart failure population because exercise intolerance-related symptoms are more often recognized as heart failure symptoms instead CI-caused symptoms. Exertional dyspnea and weakness-asthenia are common symptoms in both chronic heart failure and CI. If drug therapy, such as loop diuretics, does not effectively relieve exertion-related symptoms in heart failure patients with CI, rate-responsive pacing can be considered. In addition, CI can be a manifestation of sick sinus dysfunction whose symptoms include dyspnea, asthenia, fatigue, frequent dizziness, and possible fainting or syncope with the potential of precipitating or aggravating a state of heart failure [29]. Thus, rate-responsive pacing can be used if these patients receive a pacemaker. The present study clinically not only confirmed a high CI incidence in heart failure patients, but also investigated the feasibility of using Holter-Actigraph recording as an alternate and simpler tool to identify heart failure patients with CI and impaired chronotropic response. Prospective studies are needed to evaluate clinical benefits that can be provided by the assessment of chronotropic impairment with the use of tools as the Holter-Actigraph recording.

### Limitations

The present study used the symptom-limited maximal exercise test that did not have respiratory monitoring or measurement of peak oxygen consumption. Thus, the present study did not incorporate the information of metabolic and oxygen demand during exercise. Second, the present study had a relatively small sample size and enrolled heart failure patients with LVEF ranging from 35% to 53%. Moreover, exercise intolerance is one of the clinical manifestations of heart failure and use of β-blockers further complicates chronotropic response [8, 11, 21–23]. Thus, the variables for determining CI or chronotropic impairment derived from the present study need to be further confirmed in a clinical study with a large population including patients with all levels of LVEF and different medications.

## Conclusions

The present study found 50% of tested patients whose maximal HR during peak exercise failed to reach at least 70% of APMHR, a criterion for CI diagnosis in heart failure patients. Use of the HR-activity recording system identified worse chronotropic response and lower physical activity intensity in CI patients than in non-CI patients, demonstrating the feasibility of assessment of impaired chronotropic response in heart failure patients by this simple method. Clinical utility of non-invasive monitoring tools as the Holter-Actigraph system in diagnosing and treating CI should be investigated in a larger heart failure population.

#### Abbreviations

6MHW: 6 min hall walk; APMHR: Age-predicted maximal heart rate value; CI: Chronotropic incompetence; ECG: Electrocardiography; HR: Heart rate; LVEF: Left ventricular ejection fraction; VM: Vector magnitude

#### Acknowledgements

The authors wish to thank Dr. Hongyang Lu, a scientist at Medtronic Shanghai Innovation Center, for his assistance in the discussions and revisions of the manuscript.

#### Funding

No funding was received.

#### Authors' contributions

All authors helped to draft the manuscript. In addition, JL, JZ and XZ contributed to conception, study design, result interpretation and manuscript writing. HS and HL contributed to data acquisition, analysis, and interpretation. QW, JH and LW contributed to result interpretation and revised manuscript. SY and PW contributed to data acquisition and analysis. All authors read and approved the final manuscript.

#### Competing interests

Xiaohong Zhou, Shungang Yang and Ping Wang are Medtronic employees. To the best of authors' knowledge, Medtronic holds no stocks or shares in NorthEast Monitoring Inc. or ActiGraph. Medtronic may use the content of this manuscript as a reference for patent applications.

#### Author details

[1]Department of Cardiology, Shanghai Sixth People's Hospital, Shanghai Jiao Tong University, Shanghai, China. [2]Department of Cardiology, Ruijin Hospital Luwan Branch, Shanghai Jiao Tong University School of Medicine, Shanghai, China. [3]Cardiac Rhythm and Heart Failure, Research and Technology, Medtronic plc, Mounds View, MN, USA. [4]Department of Cardiology, Ruijin Hospital, Shanghai Jiao Tong University School of Medicine, Shanghai, China. [5]Medtronic Shanghai Innovation Center, Medtronic (Shanghai) Ltd., Shanghai, China.

#### References

1. http://www.heart.org/HEARTORG/HealthyLiving/PhysicalActivity/FitnessBasics/American-Heart-Association-Recommendations-for-Physical-Activity-in-Adults_UCM_307976_Article.jsp.
2. Achttien RJ, Staal JB, van der Voort S, et al. Exercise-based cardiac rehabilitation in patients with chronic heart failure: a Dutch practice guideline. Nath Heart J. 2015;23:6–17.
3. Sagar VA, Davies EJ, Briscoe S, et al. Exercise-based rehabilitation for heart failure: systematic review and meta-analysis. Open Heart. 2015;2:e000163.
4. Carvalho VO, Mezzani A. Aerobic exercise training intensity in patients with chronic heart failure: principles of assessment and prescription. Eur J Cardiovasc Prev Rehabil. 2011;18:5–14.
5. Camm AJ, Lu F. Chronotropic incompetence –clinical implications. Clin Cardiol. 1996;19:503–8.
6. Tanaka H, Monahan KD, Seals DR. Age-predicted maximal heart rate revisited. J Am Coll Cardiol. 2001;37:153–6.
7. Brubaker PH, Kitzman DW. Prevalence and management of chronotropic incompetence in heart failure. Current Cardiol Rep. 2007;9:229–35.
8. Brubaker PH, Kitzman DW. Chronotropic incompetence: causes, consequences, and management. Circulation. 2011;123:1010–20.
9. Khan MN, Pothier CE, Lauer MS. Chronotropic incompetence as a predictor of death among patients with normal electrograms taking beta blockers (*Metoprolol* or *Atenolol*). Am J Cardiol. 2005;96:1328–33.
10. Savonen KP, Kiviniemi V, Laukkanen JA, et al. Chronotropic incompetence and mortality in middle-aged men with known or suspected coronary heart disease. Eur Heart Journal. 2008;29:1896–902.
11. Dobre D, Zannad F, Keteyian SJ, et al. Association between resting heart rate, chronotropic index, and long-term outcomes in patients with heart failure receiving b-blocker therapy: data from the HF-ACTION trial. Eur Heart Journal. 2013;34:2271–80.
12. Magrì D, Corrà U, Lenarda AD, et al. Cardiovascular mortality and chronotropic incompetence in systolic heart failure: the importance of a reappraisal of current cut-off criteria. Eur J of Heart Failure. 2014;16:201–9.
13. Clark AL, Coats AJS. Chronotropic incompetence in chronic heart failure. International J Cardiol. 1995;49:225–31.
14. Roche F, Pichot V, Da Costa A. Chronotropic incompetence response to exercise in congestive heart failure, relationship with autonomic status. Clin Physiol. 2001;21:335–42.
15. Silva DA, Lima AC, Vargas FT, et al. Association between physical activity measurements and key parameters of cardiopulmonary exercise testing in patients with heart failure. J Cardiac Fail. 2013;19:635–40.

16. Garcia-Ortiz L, Recio-Rodriguez JI, Puig-Ribera A, et al. Blood pressure circadian pattern and physical exercise assessment by accelerometer and 7-day physical activity recall scale. Am J Hypertension. 2014;27:665–73.
17. García-Ortiz L, Recio-Rodríguez JI, Schmidt-Trucksäss A, et al. Relationship between objectively measured physical activity and cardiovascular aging in the general population – the EVIDENT trial. Atherosclerosis. 2014;233:434–40.
18. Patterson JA, Naughton J, Pietras RJ, et al. Treadmill exercise in assessment of the functional capacity of patients with cardiac disease. Am J Cardiol. 1972;30:757–62.
19. Meyer TE, Day JD, Merkel S, et al. Predictors of Chronotropic incompetence in heart Failure patients. J Card Fail. 2006;12:S18. (abstr)
20. Martin DO, Day JD, Murphy A, et al. Does Chronotropic incompetence limit the functional status of heart failure patients? J Card Fail. 2008;14:S67. (Abstr)
21. Witte KKA, Cleland JGF, Clark AL. Chronic heart failure, chronotropic incompetence, and the effects of β blockade. Heart. 2006;92:481–6.
22. Gauri AJ, Raxwal VK, Roux L, et al. Effects of chronotropic incompetence and β-blocker use on the exercise treadmill test in men. Am Heart J. 2001;142:136–41.
23. Magri D, Palermo P, Cauti FM, et al. Chronotropic Incompentence and functional capacity in chronic heart failure: no role of *β*-blockers and *β*-blocker dose. Cardiovasc Ther. 2012;30:100–8.
24. Packer M, Bristow MR, Cohn JN, et al. The effect of Carvedilol on morbidity and mortality in patients with chronic heart failure. N Engl J Med. 1996;334:1349–55.
25. The RESOLVD Investigators. Effects of Metoprolol CR in patients with ischemic and dilated Cardiomyopathy. Circulation. 2000;101:378–84.
26. MERIT-HF Study Group. Effect of metoprolol CR/XL in chronic heart failure: Metoprolol CR/XL randomised intervention trial in congestive heart failure (MERIT-HF). Lancet. 1999 Jun 12;353(9169):2001–7.
27. Bui AL, Horwich TB, Fonarow GC. Epidemiology and risk profile of heart failure. Nat Rev Cardiol. 2011;8:30–41.
28. Tse HF, Siu CW, Lee KLF, et al. The incremental benefit of rate-adaptive pacing on exercise performance during cardiac resynchronization therapy. J Am Coll Cardiol. 2005;46:2292–7.
29. Semelka M, Gera J. Sick sinus syndrome: a review. Am Fam Physician. 2013;87(10):691–6.

# A moderate 500-m treadmill walk for estimating peak oxygen uptake in men with NYHA class I-II heart failure and reduced left ventricular ejection fraction

Gianni Mazzoni[1,2], Biagio Sassone[3], Giovanni Pasanisi[4], Jonathan Myers[5,6], Simona Mandini[7*], Stefano Volpato[8], Francesco Conconi[7], Giorgio Chiaranda[9] and Giovanni Grazzi[1,2]

**Abstract**

**Background:** Maximal cardiopulmonary exercise testing (CPX) is the gold-standard for cardiorespiratory fitness assessment in chronic heart failure (CHF) patients. However, high costs, required medical supervision, and safety concerns make maximal exercise testing impractical for evaluating mobility-impaired adults. Thus, several submaximal walking protocols have been developed and currently used to estimate peak oxygen consumption ($VO_2$peak) in CHF patients. However, these tests have to be performed at close to maximum exercise intensity. The aim of this study was to examine the validity of a 500-m treadmill-walking test carried out at moderate intensity for estimating $VO_2$peak in community-dwelling adult and elderly patients with CHF and reduced left ventricular ejection fraction (HFrEF).

**Methods:** Forty-three clinically stable men with HFrEF (age 67.7 ± 9.2 years, and left ventricular ejection fraction, LVEF 38% ± 6%) underwent exercise testing during an outpatient cardiac rehabilitation/secondary prevention program. Each patients completed a CPX, and a moderate and self-paced (11–13/20 on the Borg scale) 500-m treadmill-walking test. Age, weight, height, walk time, and heart rate during the 500-m test were entered into prediction equations previously validated for $VO_2$peak estimation from a 1000-m walking test in patients with cardiovascular disease and preserved LVEF.

**Results:** Directly measured and estimated $VO_2$peak values were not different (21.6 ± 4.9 vs 21.7 ± 4.6 mL/kg/min). The comparison between measured and estimated $VO_2$peak values yielded a correlation of $R = 0.97$ (SEE = 0.7 mL/kg/min, $P < 0.0001$). The slope and the intercept coincided with the line of identity (Passing and Bablock analysis, $P = 0.50$). Residuals were normally distributed, and the examination of the Bland-Altman analysis do not show systematic or proportional error.

**Conclusions:** A moderate and self-regulated 500-m treadmill-walking test is a valid tool for $VO_2$peak estimation in patients with HFrEF. These findings may have practical implications in the context of transitioning from clinically based programs to fitness facilities or self-guided exercise programs in adults and elderly men with HFrEF.

**Keywords:** Heart failure, Left ventricular dysfunction, Cardiorespiratory fitness, Walking test

* Correspondence: simona.mandini@unife.it
[7]Center of Biomedical Studies Applied to Sport, University of Ferrara, via Gramicia 35 -, 44123 Ferrara, Italy
Full list of author information is available at the end of the article

## Background

Chronic heart failure (CHF) is an increasingly important health problem because of the aging population, improved survival rate after acute cardiovascular events, and the escalating costs attributable to symptoms and associated repeated hospitalizations, despite optimal medical therapy [1]. Cardiorespiratory fitness (CRF), usually best reflected by peak exercise oxygen consumption ($VO_2$peak), has been shown to be a powerful and independent prognostic marker in patients with CHF [2, 3], and is strongly related to walking speed [4, 5].

Walking tests of varying distance and times are commonly used to assess exercise tolerance in various clinical conditions (including CHF). These tests have to be performed at an intensity close to maximum. In fact, the participants are instructed to *"cover as much ground as you possibly can"* during a certain time [6] or *"to walk as fast as possible"* for a certain distance [7, 8].

However, daily activities rarely require maximal effort, and thus the ability to perform sustained submaximal exercise is an important component of health-related fitness assessment. In this respect, examination of submaximal exercise capacity can be useful not only to functionally evaluate patients but also for developing appropriate exercise prescriptions, adjusting the medical regimen, and identifying the need for further diagnostic interventions [9].

Submaximal walking tests for CRF assessment may be useful for measuring improvements not captured by $VO_2$peak such as the capacity to perform activities of daily living, particularly for populations whose health limits their ability to exercise at maximal effort [10]. Slow walking in older adults reflects disease severity and underlying frailty, and has significant consequences for the individual, and the public health system [11]. In addition, the need of using simple exercise tests to improve the admission on cardiac rehabilitation/secondary prevention programs has been recently emphasized, particularly for low-resource settings [12].

The moderate speed maintained during a 1-km treadmill walk (1 k-TWT) has been demonstrated to be a valid and simple tool for CRF estimation [13, 14], and is inversely related to survival [15, 16], and hospitalization [17] in outpatients with cardiovascular disease (CVD) and preserved left ventricular ejection fraction (LVEF). However, the 1 k-TWT can be time-consuming, particularly when performed by functionally limited patients. A shorter test providing similar functional information while limiting physical demands of patients and taking less time could be valuable. Thus, the aim of this study was to examine the validity of a 500-m treadmill-walking test carried out at moderate intensity for estimating peak oxygen consumption ($VO_2$peak) in community-dwelling adult and elderly patients with CHF and reduced left ventricular ejection fraction (HFrEF).

## Methods

### Participants

43 consecutive medically stable male outpatients with HFrEF (LVEF ≤45%), aged 35 to 83 yrs. (67% over 65 yrs), classified as NYHA class I-II are included in the study. Each subject completed a clinical evaluation including personal and family history and a medical examination. Left ventricular ejection fraction was derived from recent echocardiographic evaluation. Standard blood chemistry analyses previously performed were recorded. Weight and height were measured and used to calculate body mass index (BMI). Blood pressure (BP) was measured, and hypertension was defined as systolic BP ≥ 140 mmHg, diastolic BP ≥ 90 mmHg, or use of antihypertensive agents. All patients performed a maximal cardiopulmonary exercise test (CPX) for direct $VO_2$peak determination, and a 500-m moderate treadmill-walking test for $VO_2$peak estimation. Patients were instructed not to change dietary habits, not to consume any food or beverages except water for ≥2 h before testing, and not to engage in any type of physical activity for two days before testing. All were evaluated while receiving their usual medications and were on a stable medical regimen for at least three months before testing. 37 (86%) subjects were receiving β-blockers as follows: bisoprolol ($n$ = 19, 6 ± 3 mg/d), carvedilol ($n$ = 11, 31 ± 19 mg/d), and metoprolol ($n$ = 7, 135 ± 42 mg/d).

### Exercise testing procedures

#### *Cardiopulmonary exercise testing*

$VO_2$peak was determined using a treadmill ramp protocol beginning at speed of 1.5 mph (2.4 km/h) and 1.5% grade with subsequent increments of 0.1 mph and 0.5% grade every thirty seconds [18]. Patients performed the maximal test until subjective exhaustion, exertional chest pain or other untoward findings that would necessitate termination. Exercise was considered adequate if it was limited by dyspnea or muscle fatigue (Rate of perceived exertion, RPE ≥ 18/20), and by the attainment of at least two of the three following criteria: heart rate value ≥85% of the age-predicted maximum, $VO_2$ plateau approaching maximal exertion, and a respiratory exchange ratio ≥ 1.05 [19, 20]. Tight gripping of the handrails was not permitted; finger or palm placement on the handrails was allowed for balance only when necessary. Standard 12-lead electrocardiograms were continuously monitored and recorded during the test (Quark T12x, Cosmed, Rome, Italy). Gas-exchange measurements were performed using a metabolic cart (Omnia 1.5, Cosmed, Rome, Italy). Calibration of the system was performed before each test using a three-liter syringe to calibrate the flowmeter and by using gases with known oxygen, carbon dioxide and nitrogen concentrations to calibrate the gas analyzers. $VO_2$ and carbon dioxide output were acquired breath-by-breath and averaged over 15 s intervals. $VO_2$peak was defined as the highest level of $VO_2$ achieved during the test.

#### *500-m treadmill-walking test*

Within one week from the CPX, each patient performed a 500-m treadmill-walking test. Each patients were informed to adopt a comfortable walking pace sustainable for 10 to 20 min. Participants were educated to maintain a moderate perceived exercise intensity using the Borg 6–20 scale. The test was performed on the level, and began with a preliminary phase at 2.0 km/h, with subsequent increases of 0.3 km/h every 30 s up to a walking speed corresponding to a perceived exertion of 11–13 on the Borg scale. The 500-m walk was then started and the rate of perceived exertion acquired every 2 min. Walking speed was adjusted by the operator following the patient's perceived intensity. In this way, the exercise intensity was individualized and maintained at moderate perceived exertion.

Heart rate was monitored continuously during the test using a Polar RS100 heart rate monitor (Polar Electro, Kempele, Finland). Blood pressure was monitored before and immediately after the test. Heart rate was averaged every five seconds and mean and maximal values during the test were determined. Age, height, weight, time to walk 500-m multiplied by two, and heart rate were entered into the equations developed to estimate $VO_2$peak by the 1 k-TWT [13]. The two equations were determined using a multivariate forward stepwise regression procedure [13]. A coefficient of determination was calculated for each variable for the $VO_2$peak estimation. After removal of variables that were not significant, the model included age, BMI, walking speed and heart rate. The model was set as follows:

$$Y = \beta_0 - \beta_1 X_1 - \beta_2 X_2 - \beta_3 X_3 - \beta_4 X_4$$

where Y = directly measured $VO_2$peak; $\beta$ = regression coefficient for each of the independent variables; $X_1$ = mean walking speed in km/h; $X_2$ = BMI in weight/height$^2$; $X_3$ = age in years; and $X_4$ = higher heart rate in beats per minute (bpm). The resulting predictive equations were:

$$[33.42 + 2.79\ (\text{walking speed}) - 0.49\ (\text{BMI}) - 0.14\ (\text{age})]$$

and

$$[46.11 + 4.41\ (\text{walking speed}) - 0.40\ (\text{BMI}) - 0.30\ (\text{age}) - 0.11\ (\text{heart rate})]$$

for patients taking and not taking $\beta$-blockers, respectively.

#### *Data analysis*

Normal distribution of collected data has been verified by using D'Agostino Pearson test. Therefore, the predicting equations previously developed and validated [13] were applied using Pearson product moment correlations, SEE and paired t-test for comparison of measured and predicted $VO_2$peak. Passing and Bablok regression analysis was used to determine the relationship between measured and predicted values. Agreement between methods has been assessed calculating the Concordance Correlation Coefficient. Appropriateness of the model was assessed using Bland-Altman analysis and normal probability plots of the residuals. The level of statistical significance was set at $P < 0.05$. Statistical analyses were performed using the package Medcalc 16.2 software (Ostende, Belgium).

### Results

Both the CPX and the 500-m treadmill-walking tests were completed by all subjects without complications. Three subjects did not satisfy the criteria for adequate effort. One patient interrupted the test prematurely because of mask intolerance (i.e. claustrophobic). The analysis thus included the results of 39 subjects. Descriptive characteristics of the study population are presented in Table 1. CPX test results are presented in Additional file 1: Table S1.

Average walking speed during the 500-m treadmill-walking test was 4.37 ± 1.08 km/h. Mean heart rate was 90 ± 21 bpm, representing 59% ± 14% of the age-predicted maximal heart rate (based on 220-age).

$VO_2$peak values measured by CPX and predicted from the 500-m treadmill-walking test resulted 21.6 ± 4.9 mL/kg/min and 21.7 ± 4.6 mL/kg/min respectively ($t$ = 0.9, $P$ = 0.37). 500-m test results are presented in Table 2.

The correlation coefficient between measured and predicted $VO_2$peak was 0.97 ($P < 0.0001$), and the SEE was 0. 7 mL/kg/min. The slope and the intercept of the relationship between measured and predicted $VO_2$peak were not significantly different from the line of identity (Passing and Bablock analysis, $P$ = 0.50, Fig. 1). The Concordance Correlation Coefficient resulted 0.97. Residuals were normally distributed with a mean residual value of – 0.1 mL/kg/min. Examination of the Bland-Altman analysis do not show systematic or proportional error (Fig. 2).

### Discussion

The major finding of this study was the $VO_2$peak prediction by a 500-m treadmill-walking test carried out at moderate intensity in subjects with HFrEF. Predicted $VO_2$peak strongly paralleled $VO_2$peak measured directly by CPX. This was supported by the

**Table 1** Descriptive characteristics of the participants

| n | 39 |
|---|---|
| Age (y) | 67.7 (9.2) |
| Body mass index (kg/m²) | 28.8 (3.8) |
| Left ventricular ejection fraction (%) | 38 (6) |
| Ischemic etiology (%) | 72 |
| NYHA functional class I/II (%) | 62/38 |
| Serum sodium (mEq/L) | 140 (2) |
| Cardiovascular risk factors | |
| Family history of CVD (%) | 66 |
| Hypertension (%) | 72 |
| Fasting glucose (mg/dl) | 105 (25) |
| Total cholesterol (mg/dl) | 167 (47) |
| HDL cholesterol (mg/dl) | 42 (9) |
| Triglycerides (mg/dl) | 107 (52) |
| Serum creatinine (mg/dl) | 1.03 (0.2) |
| Current smoking (%) | 6 |
| Medical history (%) | |
| Coronary artery by-pass graft | 41 |
| Myocardial infarction | 39 |
| PTCA | 30 |
| Valvular repair/replacement | 11 |
| Other | 8 |
| Medications (%) | |
| ACE inhibitor or ARB | 89 |
| Aspirin | 80 |
| β-blockers | 89 |
| Calcium antagonists | 14 |
| Diuretics | 81 |
| Statins | 75 |

Data are presented as mean (standard deviation) or percentage. *ACE* angiotensin-converting enzyme, *ARB* angiotensin receptor blocker, *CVD* cardiovascular disease, *NYHA* New York Heart Association, *PTCA* Percutaneous Transluminal Coronary Angioplasty

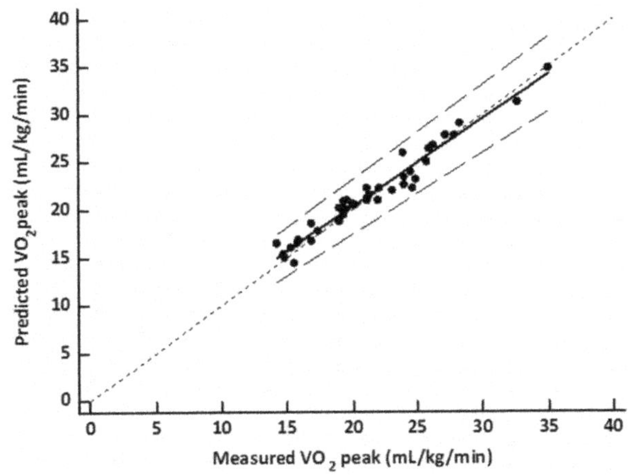


**Fig. 1** Regression of the $VO_{2peak}$ estimated from 500-m moderate treadmill-walking test on the measured $VO_{2peak}$ (y = 2,37 + 0,90×). The diagonal line represents the line of perfect agreement (line of identity), and the dotted lines represent confidence interval lines

high correlation and concordance coefficients, and by the small SEE (0.7 mL/kg/min). These findings suggest that the equations validated for predicting $VO_2$peak using a 1000-m moderate treadmill walk in outpatients with CVD and preserved ejection fraction, are similarly appropriate for predicting $VO_2$peak when using a 500-m moderate treadmill walk in CHF outpatients with mild to moderately reduced ejection fraction.

These results are in agreement with those obtained by others that have attempted to predict $VO_2$peak using submaximal walking protocols, mainly in healthy subjects and in patients with CVD and preserved LVEF [5, 7, 21–24].

In our study, by using population specific-equations developed for men with CVD and preserved LVEF, $VO_2$peak was accurately estimated in adults and elderly subjects with HFrEF by performing a 500-m moderate walk. In addition, the relationship between moderate and perceptually regulated walking and cardiorespiratory fitness in CHF outpatients has not been determined in previous studies. Correlation coefficients observed in our original study [13] and the present results further support the strong association between walking speed and peak $VO_2$ [4].

**Table 2** 500-m treadmill walking test results

| Variable | Mean (SD) |
|---|---|
| Exercise time (min:sec) | 6:51 (2:24) |
| Mean walking speed (km/h) | 4.37 (1.08) |
| Highest walking speed (km/h) | 4.54 (1.06) |
| Mean heart rate (bpm) | 90 (21) |
| Highest heart rate (bpm) | 94 (17) |
| Estimated $VO_2$peak (mL/kg/min) | 21.7 (4.7) |

Data are presented as mean (standard deviation)

The 500-m treadmill-walking test relies on the familiar task of moderate walking, which is the most common activity engaged in by adults. In particular, older adults reported that walking was their preferred form of exercise [25, 26]. The habitual nature of walking reduces the possibility that lack of familiarity with the task reduces the predictive accuracy of the results. This characteristic may also make the 500-m walking test particularly appropriate for less fit patients or for those whom walking is their preferred

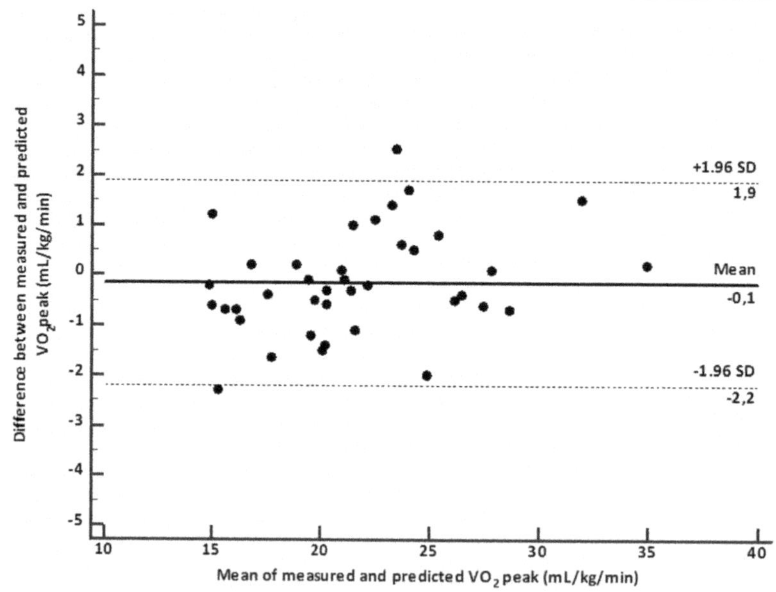


**Fig. 2** Difference compared to the mean of $VO_2$ measured by CPX and estimated from 500-m walk (Bland and Altman plot)

form of physical activity. This reduces the influence that lack of familiarity with the task might have on the accuracy of the test. Various walking tests have also been proposed as functional tools s for patients with CHF; thus, we felt that a submaximal test such as the 500-m treadmill-walking test would be valuable in this population, particularly for low-resource settings [12].

An advantage of the 500-m treadmill-walking test is the fact that it is performed at an individualized and patient-determined moderate intensity (11 to 13 on the RPE scale). This was confirmed by the average 59% of the age-predicted maximal heart rate value in the present study, which falls within current recommended limits (55% to 69%) for moderate intensity [27]. Moreover, the average heart rate during the 500-m test was close and well correlated with the heart rate value at ventilatory threshold during CPX (90 ± 21 bpm vs 93 ± 16 bpm, $R = 0.83$, $P < 0.0001$).

As such, the test may also serve as a learning trial for proper intensity for an exercise prescription. In fact, the exercise intensity at an RPE value between 11 and 13/20 has been associated with the lactate threshold, independent of training state [28]. Aerobic conditioning at such an intensity has been demonstrated to be safe and optimal to enhance cardiorespiratory function in patients with chronic disease [28].

The 500-m treadmill-walking test is a simple test that could be applied to stable mild-to-moderate CHF subjects, accurately reflecting activities of daily living. The current results provide insights into the underlying characteristics and treatment of CHF patients with reduced left ventricular ejection fraction, which may be useful to help quantify CRF improvement or deterioration.

### Study limitations

First, the small number of patients is a limit of this study. Second, our study comprised male participants only: thus, the results may not be generalizable to women. Third, participants were in the mid-range of reduced LVEF, and therefore the results may not apply to patients with more impaired ventricular function. Fourth, these results were obtained from patients with an interest in participating in an exercise-based secondary prevention program. Finally, reproducibility was not assessed in this study. However, we previously demonstrated good cross-validation and reproducibility among cardiac outpatients performing the test over the 1000-m distance [13]. Therefore, external validation of our findings is needed. In particular, future work should focus on the application of the protocol to women with CVD and to subjects with more impaired CRF, as well as to examine the prognostic value of the 500-m moderate walking test, including the determination of clinically meaningful cut-points.

## Conclusions

In outpatients with mild-to-moderate CHF, the determination of submaximal exercise capacity by a moderate and perceptually-regulated the 500-m treadmill-walking test, accurately predicts $VO_2$peak. Since it is important to document functional capacity in heart failure patients over time, the 500-m treadmill-walking test represents a simple and potentially useful tool in the serial evaluation of clinical status or the response to therapeutic interventions including exercise prescription. While the CPX remains the gold-standard for cardiorespiratory fitness assessment in chronic heart failure patients, the 500-m walking test may also provide an inexpensive screening tool in this and other patient groups in which it has been validated.

### Abbreviations

1 k-TWT: 1-km treadmill walking test; BMI: body mass index; BP: blood pressure; CHF: chronic heart failure; CPX: Cardiopulmonary exercise testing; CRF: cardiorespiratory fitness; CVD: cardiovascular disease; HFrEF: heart failure and reduced left ventricular dysfunction; LVEF: left ventricular dysfunction; NYHA: New York Hear Association; RPE: rate of perceived exertion; SEE: standard errors of estimate; $VO_2$peak: peak oxygen uptake; VT: Ventilatory threshold

### Authors' contributions

GM, BS, GP, JM, SM, SV, FC, GC, GG takes responsibility for all aspects of the reliability and freedom from bias of the data presented and their discussed interpretation. All authors made substantial contributions to conception, design, acquisition of data, analysis and interpretation of data. All authors were involved in drafting the manuscript or revising it critically for important intellectual content and given final approval of the version to be published. Each author should have participated sufficiently in the work to take public responsibility for appropriate portions of the content and agreed to be accountable for all aspects of the work in ensuring that questions related to the accuracy and integrity of any part of the work are appropriately investigated and resolved.

### Competing interests

The authors declare that they have no competing interests.

### Author details

[1]Department of Biomedical and Specialty Surgical Sciences, University of Ferrara, Ferrara, Italy. [2]Public Health Department, AUSL Ferrara, Ferrara, Italy. [3]Department of Medicine, Division of Cardiology, Cento Hospital, AUSL Ferrara, Ferrara, Italy. [4]Department of Medicine, Division of Cardiology, "Delta" Hospital, AUSL Ferrara, Ferrara, Italy. [5]Veterans Affairs Palo Alto Health Care System, Palo Alto, CA, USA. [6]Stanford University School of Medicine, Stanford, CA, USA. [7]Center of Biomedical Studies Applied to Sport, University of Ferrara, via Gramicia 35 -, 44123 Ferrara, Italy. [8]Department of Medical Sciences, University of Ferrara, Ferrara, Italy. [9]General Directorship for Public Health and Integration Policy, Emilia-Romagna Region, Bologna, Italy.

### References

1. Ross R, Blair SN, Arena R, *et al.* Importance of assessing cardiorespiratory fitness in clinical practice: A case for fitness as a clinical vital sign. A Scientific Statement from the American Heart Association. Circulation 2016; 134(24):e653–99. https://doi.org/10.1161/CIR.0000000000000461.
2. Corrà U, Mezzani A, Bosimini E, et al. Cardiopulmonary exercise testing and prognosis in chronic heart failure: a prognosticating algorithm for the individual patient. Chest. 2004;126:942–50.
3. Corrà U, Piepoli MF, Carré F, et al. Secondary prevention through cardiac rehabilitation: physical activity counselling and exercise training. Eur Heart J. 2010;31:1967–76.
4. Simonsick EM, Fan E, Fleg JL. Estimating cardiorespiratory fitness in well-functioning older adults: treadmill validation of the long distance corridor walk. J Am Geriatr Soc. 2006;54:127–32.
5. Pober DM, Freedson PS, Kline GM, et al. Development and validation of a one-mile treadmill walk test to predict peak oxygen uptake in healthy adults ages 40 to 79 years. Can J Appl Physiol. 2002;27:575–88.
6. Beatty AL, Schiller NB, Whooley MA. Six-minute walk test as a prognostic tool in stable coronary heart disease. Arch Int Med. 2012;172:1096–102.
7. Kline GM, Porcari JP, Hintermeister R, et al. Estimation of $VO_2$max from a one-mile track walk, gender, age, and body weight. Med Sci Sports Exerc. 1987;19:253–259.
8. Newman AB, Simonsick EM, Naydeck BL, et al. Association of long-distance corridor walk performance with mortality, cardiovascular disease, mobility limitation, and disability. JAMA. 2006;295:2018–26.
9. Morice A, Smithies T. The 100m walk: a simple and reproducible exercise test. Br J Dis Chest. 1984;78:392–4.
10. Clarke J, De Lannoy L, Ross R. Comparison of measures of maximal and submaximal fitness in response to exercise. Med Sci Sports Exerc. 2017;49: 711–6.
11. Best JR, Liu-Ambrose T, Metti AL, et al. Longitudinal associations between walking speed and amount of self-reported time spent walking over a 9-year period in older women and men. J Gerontol Medical Sciences. 2017; https://doi.org/10.1093/gerona/glx129.
12. Grace SL, Turk-Adawic KI, Contractor A, et al. Cardiac RehabilitationDeliveryModel for low-resource settings: an International Council of Cardiovascular Prevention and Rehabilitation Consensus Statement. Prog Cardiovasc Dis. 2016;59:303–22.
13. Chiaranda G, Myers J, Mazzoni G, et al. Peak oxygen uptake prediction from a moderate, perceptually regulated, 1-km treadmill walk in male cardiac patients. J Cardiopulm Rehabil Prev. 2012;32:262–9.
14. Grazzi G, Chiaranda G, Myers J, Pasanisi G, Lordi R, Conconi F, Mazzoni G. Outdoor reproducibility of a 1-km treadmill-walking test to predict peak oxygen consumption in cardiac outpatients. J Cardiopulm Rehab Prev. 2017; 37(5):347–9.
15. Chiaranda G, Bernardi E, Codecà L, et al. Treadmill walking speed and survival prediction in men with cardiovascular disease: a 10-year follow-up study. BMJ Open. 2013;3:e003446.
16. Grazzi G, Myers J, Bernardi E, et al. Association between $VO_2$peak estimated by a 1-km treadmill walk and mortality. A 10-year follow-up study in patients with cardiovascular disease. Int J Cardiol. 2014;173:248–52.
17. Grazzi G, Mazzoni G, Myers J, et al. Improved walking speed is associated with lower hospitalisation rates in patients in an exercise-based secondary prevention programme. Heart. 2016 Dec 1;102(23):1902–8. https://doi.org/10.1136/heartjnl-2015-309126.
18. American Association of Cardiovascular and Pulmonary Rehabilitation. Guidelines for cardiac rehabilitation and secondary prevention programs, 4th ed. Champaign, IL: Human Kinetics; 2004.
19. Balady GJ, Arena R, Sietsema K, et al. Clinician's guide to cardiopulmonary exercise testing in adults. A scientific statement from the American Heart Association. Circulation. 2010;122:191–225.
20. Guazzi M, Adams V, Conraads V, et al. Clinical recommendations for cardiopulmonary exercise testing data assessment in specific patient populations. Circulation. 2012;126:2261–74.
21. American College of Sports Medicine's Guidelines for Exercise Testing and Prescription 8th ed. Philadelphia. PA. In: Lippincot Williams & Wilkins; 2010.
22. Lipkin DP, Scriven AJ, Crake T, et al. Six minute walking test for assessing exercise capacity in chronic heart failure. BMJ. 1988;292:653–5.
23. Vehrs PR, Georgea JA, Fellinghamb GW, et al. Submaximal treadmill exercise test to predict $VO_2$max in fit adults. Meas Phys Educ Exerc Sci. 2007;11(2): 61–72.
24. Widrick J, Ward A, Ebbeling C, et al. Treadmill validation of an over-ground walking test to predict peak oxygen consumption. Eur J Appl Physiol. 1992; 64:304–8.
25. Belza B, Walwick J, Shiu-Thornton S, et al. Older adult perspectives on physical activity and exercise: voices from multiple cultures. Prev Chronic Dis. 2004;1:1–12.
26. Burton E, Lewin G, Boldy D. Physical activity preferences of older home care clients. Int J Older People Nursing. 2015;10:170–8.

# 26

# Does stress perfusion imaging improve the diagnostic accuracy of late gadolinium enhanced cardiac magnetic resonance for establishing the etiology of heart failure?

Gaurav S. Gulsin[1,2*], Abishek Shetye[1,2], Jeffrey Khoo[1,2], Daniel J. Swarbrick[1,2], Eylem Levelt[1,2], Florence Y. Lai[1,2], Iain B. Squire[1,2], Jayanth R. Arnold[1,2] and Gerry P. McCann[1,2]

**Abstract**

**Background:** Late gadolinium enhanced cardiovascular magnetic resonance (LGE-CMR) has excellent specificity, sensitivity and diagnostic accuracy for differentiating between ischemic cardiomyopathy (ICM) and non-ischemic dilated cardiomyopathy (NICM). CMR first-pass myocardial perfusion imaging (perfusion-CMR) may also play role in distinguishing heart failure of ischemic and non-ischemic origins, although the utility of additional of stress perfusion imaging in such patients is unclear. The aim of this retrospective study was to assess whether the addition of adenosine stress perfusion imaging to LGE-CMR is of incremental value for differentiating ICM and NICM in patients with severe left ventricular systolic dysfunction (LVSD) of uncertain etiology.

**Methods:** We retrospectively identified 100 consecutive adult patients (median age 69 years (IQR 59–73)) with severe LVSD (mean LV EF 26.6 ± 7.0%) referred for perfusion-CMR to establish the underlying etiology of heart failure. The cause of heart failure was first determined on examination of CMR cine and LGE images in isolation. Subsequent examination of complete adenosine stress perfusion-CMR studies (cine, LGE and perfusion images) was performed to identify whether this altered the initial diagnosis.

**Results:** On LGE-CMR, 38 patients were diagnosed with ICM, 46 with NICM and 16 with dual pathology. With perfusion-CMR, there were 39 ICM, 44 NICM and 17 dual pathology diagnoses. There was excellent agreement in diagnoses between LGE-CMR and perfusion-CMR ($\kappa$ 0.968, $p<0.001$). The addition of adenosine stress perfusion images to LGE-CMR altered the diagnosis in only two of the 100 patients.

**Conclusion:** The addition of adenosine stress perfusion-CMR to cine and LGE-CMR provides minimal incremental diagnostic yield for determining the etiology of heart failure in patients with severe LVSD.

**Keywords:** Cardiovascular magnetic resonance, Heart failure, Late gadolinium enhancement, Adenosine stress perfusion, Non-ischemic cardiomyopathy

* Correspondence: gg149@leicester.ac.uk
[1]Department of Cardiovascular Sciences, University of Leicester, Glenfield Hospital, Groby Road, Leicester LE3 9QP, UK
[2]The NIHR Leicester Cardiovascular Biomedical Research Unit, Glenfield Hospital, Leicester, UK

## Background

Identifying the etiology of heart failure has important management and prognostic implications [1]. Therapeutic strategies for ischemic cardiomyopathy (ICM) include revascularisation and/or secondary prevention measures such as antiplatelet and lipid lowering therapies. Conversely, the management of non-ischemic dilated cardiomyopathy (NICM) relies predominantly on pharmacological agents and device therapy [2]. Rarer causes of NICM (e.g. sarcoid, amyloid, HIV) require treatment of the underlying condition [3]. Importantly survival rates are poorer in those patients with heart failure of ischemic origin [4]. Clinical guidelines suggest echocardiography as the initial investigation of choice for evaluation of chronic heart failure [1, 5]. In many instances, echocardiography may reliably establish the underlying cause of heart failure. Myocardial regional wall motion abnormalities alone, however, may not distinguish heart failure of ischemic origin from NICM, since segmental wall motion abnormalities may accompany both [6]. Where echocardiography does not clearly identify the etiology of chronic heart failure, cardiac magnetic resonance imaging (CMR) is advantageous [1], owing to its capacity to detect evidence of myocardial infarction and non-ischemic fibrosis and assess ischemia and viability in a single examination [7].

Late gadolinium enhanced CMR (LGE-CMR) has been shown to be non-inferior (and indeed may be superior) to coronary angiography in differentiating heart failure due to coronary artery disease (CAD) from NICM [8, 9]. Subendocardial LGE is present in CAD, whereas patients with NICM have either no LGE or mid-wall late enhancement that does not correspond to a coronary artery territory (Fig. 1) [9]. Patients with heart failure and a history of ischemic heart disease have a high prevalence of LGE visible on CMR (88% in one report) [10]. This suggests a high likelihood that LGE-CMR will yield a diagnosis of ICM by hyperenhancement patterns alone, without the need for additional perfusion imaging. Following myocardial infarction, the presence of LGE affecting ≤50% of the thickness of the myocardium predicts the likelihood of functional recovery in response to revascularisation of the affected coronary territory [11, 12]. In NICM, the presence of mid-wall fibrosis is also of prognostic value, being an independent predictor of cardiovascular and all-cause mortality [13].

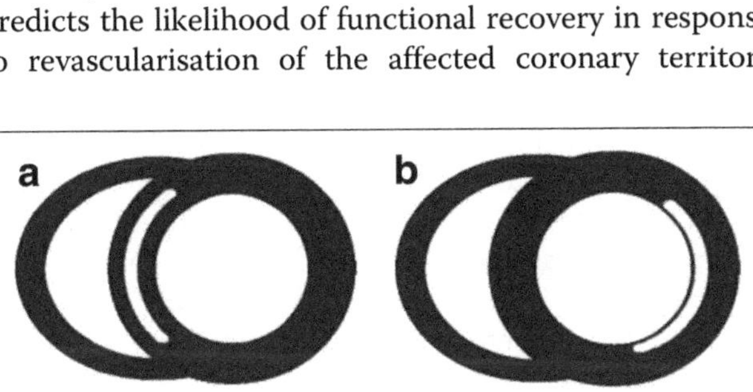


**Fig. 1** Illustration of typical patterns of LGE seen in NICM and ICM. White areas within the myocardium represent LGE. **a** Mid-wall LGE is commonly seen in NICM, whereas **b** a subendocardial distribution of LGE is typical in ICM

CMR first-pass myocardial perfusion imaging (perfusion-CMR) has been shown in several large studies to have excellent sensitivity and specificity for detection of CAD and may thus play a role in distinguishing heart failure of ischemic and non-ischemic origins [14, 15]. However, the added value of adenosine stress perfusion-CMR in subjects with severe left ventricular systolic dysfunction (LVSD) has not been investigated previously. Given that LGE-CMR alone has excellent specificity (96%), sensitivity (100%) and diagnostic accuracy (95%) for differentiating between ICM and NICM [8], the utility of additional of stress perfusion imaging in such patients is questionable.

Adenosine stress perfusion-CMR imaging adds time (approximately 15 min added time for the perfusion-CMR protocol) and expense to the CMR protocol, due to the need for additional electrocardiograms, adenosine preparations, infusion pumps and lines, as well as physician-supervision. Undesirable symptoms and potentially serious complications may occur with adenosine infusion, albeit infrequently [16–19]. These include wheeze secondary to bronchospasm, Mobitz II 2nd or 3rd degree atrioventricular block, and angina requiring sublingual nitrates [17]. Furthermore, in patients with heart failure, there is impairment of adenosine receptor expression and signal-transduction [20], which may diminish the hemodynamic response for stress perfusion assessment, compromising diagnostic confidence.

In our regional cardiac centre, over 1000 clinical perfusion-CMR studies are performed annually. Approximately 10% of these are to identify the cause of heart failure, and despite a lack of evidence of additional benefit, stress perfusion is usually requested and performed.

The aim of this retrospective study was to assess whether the addition of adenosine stress perfusion imaging to LGE-CMR is of incremental value for differentiating ICM and NICM in patients with severe LVSD of uncertain etiology.

## Methods

### Study population

We retrospectively identified 100 consecutive adult patients with severe LVSD on echocardiography, referred for perfusion-CMR to ascertain the underlying etiology of heart failure. Patients were scanned between April 2015 and March 2016. Severe LVSD was defined as a left ventricular ejection fraction (LV EF) ≤35% and was confirmed by CMR volumetric and functional analysis prior to inclusion in the study. Participants' past medical history, medications, electrocardiographic data, resting pulse and blood pressure were recorded at the time of the CMR.

The study was approved as a clinical audit and ethics approval was deemed unnecessary.

***CMR image acquisition***

Clinical perfusion-CMR studies were undertaken on either a 1.5 T (Siemens Avanto, Erlangen, Germany) or 3 T scanner (Siemens Skyra, Erlangen, Germany). Cardiac volumes and function were performed using standard CMR techniques as previously described by our group [21]. For stress perfusion, adenosine (140mcg/kg/min, increased up to a maximum of 210mcg/kg/min to achieve a satisfactory haemodynamic stress response) [18] was infused for 3–5 min. Patients underwent pulse, blood pressure and pulse oximetry monitoring at baseline and at 1-min intervals during adenosine infusion. Symptomatic response to adenosine was documented. During peak stress a bolus of gadolinium-based contrast (Gadoterate meglumine, Dotarem, Guerbet LLC, France) was injected (0.1 mmol/kg at 1.5 T and 0.075 mmol/kg at 3 T), followed by a 20 mL bolus of normal saline, at a rate of 5 mL/s and perfusion images were acquired using a saturation recovery gradient echo pulse sequence. Adenosine infusion was then discontinued and a complete short axis cine stack was performed before rest perfusion images were acquired following administration of a second bolus of gadolinium-based contrast agent (total dose 0.15 mmol/kg). LGE images in 3 long axis views and a complete short axis stack were acquired after a further delay of 5–10 min.

***CMR image analysis***

Scans were anonymized and sent to a separate workstation for analysis which was performed blinded to all patient details, by two specialists in CMR (JRA and JK) as recommended by expert consensus [22]. No clinical information was made available prior to or during image analysis. Definitions for etiology of severe LVSD were predefined as "ischemic", "non-ischemic" or "dual-pathology" (having both ischemic and non-ischemic components and where the extent of infarction and/or ischemia did not explain the degree of LVSD). Image quality was rated as "good", "moderate", "poor" or "not-analyzable" for each modality. A two-stage process was employed for image analysis. The etiology of severe LVSD was determined first determined by consensus between JRA and JK after examination of cine and LGE images. Following this, the perfusion sequences were interpreted with the cine and LGE images and it was recorded whether the etiology of LVSD changed depending on the presence of reversible perfusion defects.

***Invasive coronary angiography***

Coronary angiograms were examined in those patients in the cohort who underwent angiography on clinical grounds. Images were analyzed blinded to patient details and CMR image interpretation results by an experienced cardiologist (GPM). Coronary artery disease was predefined as being present if a coronary artery stenosis of ≥50% the luminal diameter of the artery was observed and was noted as severe if stenosis severity was >70%.

***Statistical analyses***

Normality was assessed using Kolmogorov-Smirnov tests, histograms, and Q-Q plots. Continuous data were expressed as mean ± standard deviation, if normally distributed. Non-parametric variables were expressed as median and interquartile range. One-way analysis of variance (ANOVA) was used to compare normal data and the Independent-Samples Kruskal-Wallis test for non-normal data between groups. The Kappa statistic was used as a measure of agreement between the components of the CMR scans with and without stress perfusion. Statistical analysis was undertaken using SPSS version 20.0 software.

## Results

### Baseline characteristics

The study group consisted of 100 patients referred for clinical stress perfusion-CMR to investigate the etiology of severe LVSD. Demographic characteristics and CMR volumetric and functional data are shown in Table 1. The mean LV EF of the cohort was 26.6 ± 7.0% and there were no significant differences in LV function or volumes between patients with a diagnosis of ICM, NICM or dual pathology (Table 1).

***Etiology of LVSD by combined cine plus LGE-CMR***

Image quality was excellent or good in 98 and poor in 2 studies. Thirty-eight patients were classified as having ischemic, 46 non-ischemic and 16 dual pathology as the cause of LVSD (Table 2). Fifty-three patients had subendocardial or transmural hyperenhancement consistent with previous myocardial infarction. Forty-nine (80%) patients with NICM or dual pathology had evidence of mid-wall hyperenhancement on LGE-CMR; the other 13 had no visible LGE. The vast majority ($n$ = 15, 94%) of patients with dual pathology had a combination of hyperenhancement patterns (subendocardial/transmural and mid-wall).

***Etiology of LVSD by complete stress perfusion-CMR studies***

Image quality for first-pass perfusion was rated as good or excellent in 99 and poor in 1 patient. There were reversible perfusion defects in 23/54 (43%) patients with infarction and in 1 patient with no LGE. There was excellent agreement in diagnoses between LGE-CMR and perfusion-CMR (κ 0.968, $p$=<0.001) (Table 2), yielding a change in diagnosis from LGE-CMR in only 2 cases. In the first of these (78-year-old male, LV EF 26%), the LGE-CMR diagnosis was NICM. There was global LV hypokinesis with basal inferoseptal mid-wall

**Table 1** Baseline characteristics of the 100 study participants

| | All patients ($n$ = 100) | ICM ($n$ = 39) | NICM ($n$ = 44) | Dual pathology ($n$ = 17) | *P*-value |
|---|---|---|---|---|---|
| Median age (years) | 69 (59–73) | 69 (54–84) | 69 (50–88) | 69 (57–81) | 0.984 |
| Gender | 77% M, 33% F | 77% M, 33% F | 70% M, 30% F | 94% M, 6% F | |
| SBP (mmHg) | 134.7 ± 23.7 | 135.9 ± 24.4 | 132.0 ± 19.8 | 134.5 ± 30.7 | 0.715 |
| DBP (mmHg) | 79.9 ± 14.8 | 79.7 ± 13.2 | 80.3 ± 14.5 | 77.6 ± 20.2 | 0.824 |
| Pulse rate (beats/min) | 72.3 ± 14.1 | 69.9 ± 12.4 | 75.1 ± 16.3 | 71.9 ± 11.4 | 0.263 |
| ACEI (%) | 73 | 72 | 71 | 83 | 0.68 |
| ARB (%) | 13 | 19 | 9 | 8 | 0.426 |
| Beta blocker (%) | 82 | 84 | 76 | 92 | 0.419 |
| Loop diuretic (%) | 51 | 50 | 53 | 50 | 0.967 |
| Thiazide diuretic (%) | 1 | 0 | 3 | 0 | 0.519 |
| Aldosterone antagonist (%) | 28 | 38 | 24 | 17 | 0.283 |
| Calcium channel antagonist (%) | 5 | 3 | 3 | 17 | 0.144 |
| Digoxin (%) | 13 | 9 | 15 | 17 | 0.738 |
| Ivabradine (%) | 3 | 0 | 3 | 8 | 0.292 |
| Creatinine (umol/L) | 93 ± 24 | 96 ± 30 | 89 ± 19 | 95 ± 22 | 0.334 |
| LVEF (%) | 26.6 ± 7.0 | 27.2 ± 7.1 | 28.2 ± 6.4 | 23.5 ± 6.5 | 0.095 |
| LVEDVi (mL/m2) | 139 ± 35 | 137.2 ± 33.3 | 135.0 ± 40.5 | 152.0 ± 29.5 | 0.406 |
| LVESVi (mL/m2) | 104 ± 34 | 101.5 ± 33.8 | 97.5 ± 36.1 | 117.6 ± 29.2 | 0.133 |

LGE (Fig. 2a). The perfusion-CMR diagnosis was dual pathology as an inferolateral subendocardial perfusion abnormality was visualised, suggestive of ischemia (Fig. 2b), but not severe enough to account for the degree of LV impairment observed. In the second case (a 77-year-old female), the LGE-CMR diagnosis was NICM: image quality for LGE imaging was rated as poor (though still considered diagnostic), and no enhancement was visualised (Fig. 3a). The diagnosis by perfusion-CMR was ICM with demonstration of a subendocardial basal and mid LV anteroseptal perfusion defect (Fig. 3b). Subsequently coronary angiography revealed a significant LAD stenosis (Fig. 3c) and the patient underwent revascularisation.

### *Angiographic findings*

Thirty-two of the patients underwent coronary angiography after CMR. The vast majority ($n$ = 30, 93.8%) of these showed significant CAD. Both patients who underwent angiography that did not reveal significant CAD had LGE-CMR and perfusion-CMR diagnoses of NICM. LGE-CMR had a sensitivity of 87% for predicting significant CAD in subjects with severe LVSD, identifying ICM or dual pathology in 26/30 patients with significant CAD on angiography. Sensitivity of perfusion-CMR for predicting significant CAD was 90% (27/30 patients with significant CAD identified as having ICM or dual pathology). Only three cases of CAD identified by angiography were not detected by either LGE-CMR or perfusion-CMR (Table 3). In two of these, the degree of coronary disease was not deemed severe enough to alone account for the degree of LV impairment.

**Table 2** Cause of LVSD diagnosed by LGE-CMR and perfusion-CMR

| | LGE-CMR | PERFUSION-CMR | |
|---|---|---|---|
| Cause of LVSD (n) | | | |
| Ischemic | 38 | 39 | K = 0.968, $p < 0.001$ |
| Non-ischemic | 46 | 44 | |
| Dual pathology | 16 | 17 | |

## Discussion

This study is the first to evaluate the incremental value of perfusion-CMR over LGE-CMR in identifying the etiology of heart failure in patients with severe

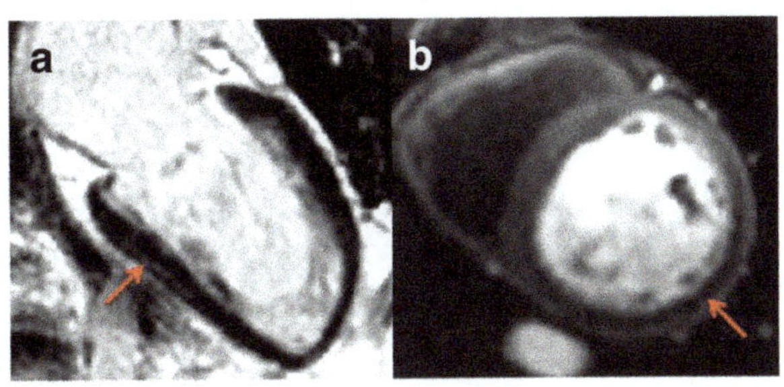


**Fig. 2** **a** Two-chamber LGE image with inferior LV mid-wall hyperenhancement (*arrow*). **b** First-pass perfusion-CMR image demonstrating an inferolateral subendocardial perfusion abnormality (*arrow*)

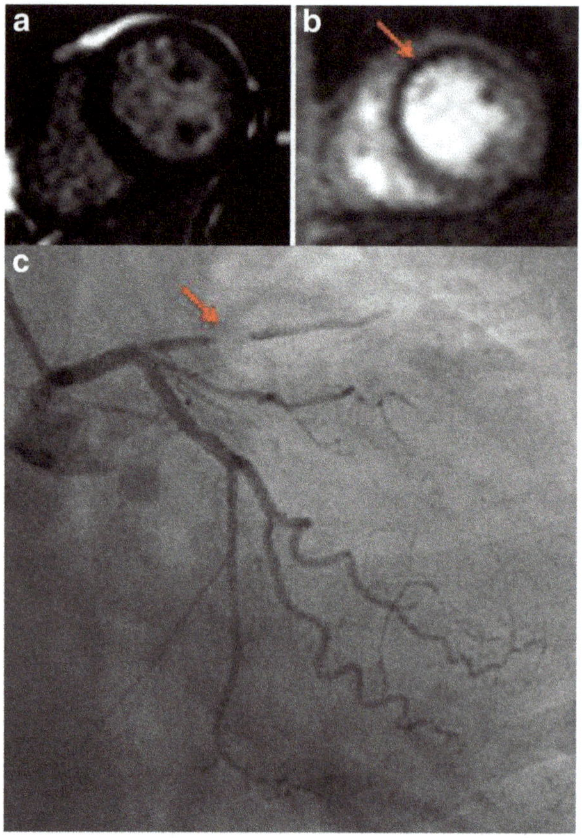


**Fig. 3 a** Mid short-axis LGE window; there is no hyperenhancement to suggest myocardial infarction. **b** First-pass perfusion-CMR image showing a mid LV anteroseptal reversible perfusion defect *(arrow)*. **c** The corresponding coronary angiogram image; there is a chronic total occlusion of the proximal-mid left anterior descending artery *(arrow)*

LVSD. We have shown that the vast majority of patients with LVSD are identified by LGE and that the addition of stress perfusion only identified one additional patient with important ischemia requiring revascularisation.

**LGE-CMR versus perfusion-CMR**

LGE-CMR is a proven technique for determining the etiology of heart failure [9], having been shown in previous studies to accurately differentiate between ICM and NICM [23, 24]. Clinical guidelines advocate the use of LGE-CMR in heart failure, when echocardiography is non-diagnostic [1, 25]. The utilisation of LGE-CMR in this context is known to have significant clinical impact; influencing patient management, clinical decisions and diagnoses in 65% of patients in one study [26]. When mid-wall LGE is present in NICM, this portends a poorer prognosis [13]. A high proportion of our patients with NICM had mid-wall LGE in comparison to the published literature (80 versus 30% in Gulati et al.) [13]. This is probably the result of our study group being older (69 (59–73) versus 51 ± 15 years) and with much poorer LV systolic function (mean LV EF 27.5 ± 6.8% versus 37.2 ± 13.1%) [13].

Perfusion-CMR is highly accurate for identifying myocardial ischemia due to CAD [15, 27, 28]. No published data exist, however, characterising the role of perfusion-CMR in determining the etiology of severe LVSD. Despite this, it is routine in our institution to undertake full adenosine stress perfusion-CMR studies for identifying the cause of heart failure in patients with newly diagnosed severe LVSD. The EuroCMR registry, which includes data on more than 27,000 consecutive CMR studies from over 15 European countries, showed that almost a third (29.3%) of CMR studies include adenosine stress perfusion imaging [16]. Data on the specific indications for perfusion-CMR are not presented in the EuroCMR registry, but it is likely that a significant number of these studies were also performed in subjects with severe LVSD.

Adenosine stress perfusion imaging adds time and expense to the CMR protocol. Seventy five to 100% of all complications associated with CMR occur due to administration of pharmacologic stress agents [16]. There is also evidence to suggest that patients with heart failure

**Table 3** Summary of angiographic and CMR findings in patients with angiographically-determined significant CAD and a diagnosis of NICM on CMR

| Angiogram findings | Non-stress CMR findings | Perfusion-CMR findings | Comments |
|---|---|---|---|
| Moderate (50% stenosis) LCx disease. | Global LV hypokinesis. Severe bi-atrial dilatation with MR and TR.<br>Mid-wall LGE present. | No perfusion abnormality detected. | CAD likely coincident and not main etiological factor. |
| Mild left mainstem (~30%) and severe RCA disease. | Global LVSD and marked intraventricular dyssynchrony.<br>Severely dilated LA. Moderate MR.<br>No LGE. | No perfusion abnormality detected. | CAD likely coincident and not main etiological factor.<br>Patient condition improved with intensive medical therapy (now NYHA class I). |
| Three-vessel coronary disease.<br>Severe LAD and LCx disease, moderate RCA disease. | Severe hypokinesis starting in the midanterior segment, becoming akinetic in the apex.<br>No valve disease.<br>No LGE. | No perfusion abnormality detected. | True false-negative CMR.<br>Patient underwent CABG. |

exhibit a diminished response to adenosine due to down regulation of adenosine receptors in the failing myocardium [16]. Clearly the role of perfusion-CMR in determining the etiology of heart failure should be subject to scrutiny before routine implementation in clinical practice.

We found excellent agreement between the causes of LVSD diagnosed by LGE-CMR and by perfusion-CMR, suggesting that perfusion-CMR is of limited additional benefit over LGE-CMR for the specific indication of identifying the etiology of heart failure. In only two of our 100 patients did perfusion-CMR alter the diagnosis established by LGE-CMR (and led to a meaningful change in patient management, i.e. revascularisation, in only one patient). Perfusion-CMR did, however, identify reversible ischemia in 43% of patients with a non-stress-CMR diagnosis of ICM/dual pathology. Whilst this did not alter the diagnosis in these patients it may have implications on clinical management. Generally both LGE-CMR and perfusion-CMR had excellent sensitivity for detection of CAD. Importantly these analyses were made entirely blinded to patient details and medical history, which in clinical practice would ordinarily guide risk stratification and decision-making and raise suspicion of CAD.

### Clinical implications

Our study demonstrates that stress perfusion-CMR is of minimal incremental benefit in diagnosing the cause of severe LVSD. It is therefore contentious whether stress testing should be routinely performed in this context. Patients with severe LVSD attributed to previous infarction on LGE-CMR with a likelihood of functional recovery often undergo coronary angiography and revascularisation. However the role of revascularization in patients with ICM in the absence of symptoms is controversial. In the STITCH trial, there was no significant difference in outcomes when patients with heart failure and coronary artery disease underwent surgical revascularization versus medical therapy alone [29]. In such instances perfusion-CMR is therefore of limited added benefit. In cases of severe LVSD where LGE-CMR excludes ICM by patterns of hyperenhancement specific to NICM, exposing the patient to risks of invasive angiography could be unwarranted as the likelihood of identifying significant coronary disease is low. On the other hand, we found that perfusion-CMR identified additional ischemia in half our patients diagnosed with ICM. In these cases, perfusion-CMR may influence subsequent management, although the benefit of routine revascularisation in the absence of angina over medical management is far from clear [29].

The present study challenges the incremental role of perfusion-CMR over LGE-CMR for diagnosing the etiology of heart failure in severe LVSD. Clinical guidelines do not specifically recommend perfusion-CMR for this purpose [1, 5]. However, observations from our own clinical practice and EuroCMR registry data suggest that perfusion-CMR is routinely utilised to determine the cause of severe LVSD when echocardiography is non-diagnostic [16]. Exposing patients in these cases to the added risks of adenosine infusion, together with increasing MR scanning times and expense are probably unjustified at present.

### Limitations

The retrospective and single-centre design limits the strength of this study, as does the relatively small sample size. Coronary angiography, as the reference standard for CAD, was not performed on all subjects in the cohort to exclude CAD. Computed tomography coronary angiography can be used to reliably exclude the presence of CAD but will be difficult to interpret in high risk patients with coronary calcium and does not provide prognostic information related to LGE [30].

## Conclusions

Adenosine stress perfusion-CMR is of minimal additional benefit to cine and LGE-CMR for determining the etiology of heart failure in patients with severe LVSD. Prospective studies are required to define the role of perfusion-CMR in heart failure and identify those patients most likely to benefit from the addition of perfusion imaging to LGE-CMR.

#### Abbreviations

CAD: Coronary artery disease; CMR: Cardiac magnetic resonance; ICM: Ischemic cardiomyopathy; LGE: Late gadolinium enhancement; LVEF: Left ventricular ejection fraction; LVSD: Left ventricular systolic dysfunction; NICM: Non-ischemic cardiomyopathy

#### Acknowledgements

None.

#### Funding

None.

#### Authors' contributions

GSG, GPM, JRA and IS conceived the idea for the study and developed the initial protocol. GSG, AS, EL and DJS developed study documents, retrospectively identified patients and managed the study. JRA and JK performed the CMR analyses. GPM performed the coronary angiography analysis. GSG and FL performed statistical analysis. GSG wrote the paper, which all authors critically reviewed. All authors read and approved the final manuscript.

#### Competing interests

The authors declare that they have no competing interests.

## References


1. Ponikowski P, Voors AA, Anker SD, Bueno H, Cleland JG, Coats AJ, et al. 2016 ESC Guidelines for the diagnosis and treatment of acute and chronic heart failure: The Task Force for the diagnosis and treatment of acute and chronic heart failure of the European Society of Cardiology (ESC) Developed with the special contribution of the Heart Failure Association (HFA) of the ESC. Eur Heart J. 2016.
2. Wu AH. Management of patients with non-ischaemic cardiomyopathy. Heart. 2007;93(3):403–8.
3. Cerrato E, D'Ascenzo F, Biondi-Zoccai G, Calcagno A, Frea S, Grosso Marra W, et al. Cardiac dysfunction in pauci symptomatic human immunodeficiency virus patients: a meta-analysis in the highly active antiretroviral therapy era. Eur Heart J. 2013;34(19):1432–6.
4. Bart BA, Shaw LK, McCants Jr CB, Fortin DF, Lee KL, Califf RM, et al. Clinical determinants of mortality in patients with angiographically diagnosed ischemic or nonischemic cardiomyopathy. J Am Coll Cardiol. 1997;30(4):1002–8.
5. Yancy CW, Jessup M, Bozkurt B, Butler J, Casey Jr DE, Drazner MH, et al. 2013 ACCF/AHA guideline for the management of heart failure: executive summary: a report of the American College of Cardiology Foundation/ American Heart Association task force on practice guidelines. Circulation. 2013;128(16):1810–52.
6. Wallis DE, O'Connell JB, Henkin RE, Costanzo-Nordin MR, Scanlon PJ. Segmental wall motion abnormalities in dilated cardiomyopathy: a common finding and good prognostic sign. J Am Coll Cardiol. 1984;4(4):674–9.
7. Karamitsos TD, Neubauer S. Cardiovascular magnetic resonance in heart failure. Curr Cardiol Rep. 2011;13(3):210–9.
8. Assomull RG, Shakespeare C, Kalra PR, Lloyd G, Gulati A, Strange J, et al. Role of cardiovascular magnetic resonance as a gatekeeper to invasive coronary angiography in patients presenting with heart failure of unknown etiology. Circulation. 2011;124(12):1351–60.
9. McCrohon JA, Moon JC, Prasad SK, McKenna WJ, Lorenz CH, Coats AJ, et al. Differentiation of heart failure related to dilated cardiomyopathy and coronary artery disease using gadolinium-enhanced cardiovascular magnetic resonance. Circulation. 2003;108(1):54–9.
10. Bourantas CV, Nikitin NP, Loh HP, Lukaschuk EI, Sherwi N, de Silva R, et al. Prevalence of scarred and dysfunctional myocardium in patients with heart failure of ischaemic origin: a cardiovascular magnetic resonance study. J Cardiovasc Magn Reson. 2011;13:53.
11. Kim RJ, Wu E, Rafael A, Chen EL, Parker MA, Simonetti O, et al. The use of contrast-enhanced magnetic resonance imaging to identify reversible myocardial dysfunction. N Engl J Med. 2000;343(20):1445–53.
12. Selvanayagam JB, Kardos A, Francis JM, Wiesmann F, Petersen SE, Taggart DP, et al. Value of delayed-enhancement cardiovascular magnetic resonance imaging in predicting myocardial viability after surgical revascularization. Circulation. 2004;110(12):1535–41.
13. Gulati A, Jabbour A, Ismail TF, Guha K, Khwaja J, Raza S, et al. Association of fibrosis with mortality and sudden cardiac death in patients with nonischemic dilated cardiomyopathy. JAMA. 2013;309(9):896–908.
14. Greenwood JP, Motwani M, Maredia N, Brown JM, Everett CC, Nixon J, et al. Comparison of cardiovascular magnetic resonance and single-photon emission computed tomography in women with suspected coronary artery disease from the clinical evaluation of magnetic resonance imaging in coronary heart disease (CE-MARC) trial. Circulation. 2014;129(10):1129–38.
15. Schwitter J, Wacker CM, van Rossum AC, Lombardi M, Al-Saadi N, Ahlstrom H, et al. MR-IMPACT: comparison of perfusion-cardiac magnetic resonance with single-photon emission computed tomography for the detection of coronary artery disease in a multicentre, multivendor, randomized trial. Eur Heart J. 2008;29(4):480–9.
16. Bruder O, Wagner A, Lombardi M, Schwitter J, van Rossum A, Pilz G, et al. European cardiovascular magnetic resonance (EuroCMR) registry–multi national results from 57 centers in 15 countries. J Cardiovasc Magn Reson. 2013;15:9.
17. Karamitsos TD, Arnold JR, Pegg TJ, Cheng AS, van Gaal WJ, Francis JM, et al. Tolerance and safety of adenosine stress perfusion cardiovascular magnetic resonance imaging in patients with severe coronary artery disease. Int J Cardiovasc Imaging. 2009;25(3):277–83.
18. Karamitsos TD, Ntusi NA, Francis JM, Holloway CJ, Myerson SG, Neubauer S. Feasibility and safety of high-dose adenosine perfusion cardiovascular magnetic resonance. J Cardiovasc Magn Reson. 2010;12:66.
19. Khoo JP, Grundy BJ, Steadman CD, Sonnex EP, Coulden RA, McCann GP. Stress cardiovascular MR in routine clinical practice: referral patterns, accuracy, tolerance, safety and incidental findings. Br J Radiol. 2012;85(1018):e851–7.
20. Asakura M, Asanuma H, Kim J, Liao Y, Nakamaru K, Fujita M, et al. Impact of adenosine receptor signaling and metabolism on pathophysiology in patients with chronic heart failure. Hypertens Res. 2007;30(9):781–7.
21. Steadman CD, Jerosch-Herold M, Grundy B, Rafelt S, Ng LL, Squire IB, et al. Determinants and functional significance of myocardial perfusion reserve in severe aortic stenosis. JACC Cardiovasc Imaging. 2012;5(2):182–9.
22. Schulz-Menger J, Bluemke DA, Bremerich J, Flamm SD, Fogel MA, Friedrich MG, et al. Standardized image interpretation and post processing in cardiovascular magnetic resonance: Society for Cardiovascular Magnetic Resonance (SCMR) board of trustees task force on standardized post processing. J Cardiovasc Magn Reson. 2013;15:35.
23. Casolo G, Minneci S, Manta R, Sulla A, Del Meglio J, Rega L, et al. Identification of the ischemic etiology of heart failure by cardiovascular magnetic resonance imaging: diagnostic accuracy of late gadolinium enhancement. Am Heart J. 2006;151(1):101–8.
24. Soriano CJ, Ridocci F, Estornell J, Jimenez J, Martinez V, De Velasco JA. Noninvasive diagnosis of coronary artery disease in patients with heart failure and systolic dysfunction of uncertain etiology, using late gadolinium-enhanced cardiovascular magnetic resonance. J Am Coll Cardiol. 2005;45(5):743–8.
25. NICE. Chronic heart failure: management of chronic heart failure in adults in primary and secondary care. 2010.
26. Abbasi SA, Ertel A, Shah RV, Dandekar V, Chung J, Bhat G, et al. Impact of cardiovascular magnetic resonance on management and clinical decision-making in heart failure patients. J Cardiovasc Magn Reson. 2013;15:89.
27. Greenwood JP, Maredia N, Younger JF, Brown JM, Nixon J, Everett CC, et al. Cardiovascular magnetic resonance and single-photon emission computed tomography for diagnosis of coronary heart disease (CE-MARC): a prospective trial. Lancet. 2012;379(9814):453–60.
28. Nandalur KR, Dwamena BA, Choudhri AF, Nandalur MR, Carlos RC. Diagnostic performance of stress cardiac magnetic resonance imaging in the detection of coronary artery disease: a meta-analysis. J Am Coll Cardiol. 2007;50(14):1343–53.
29. Velazquez EJ, Lee KL, Jones RH, Al-Khalidi HR, Hill JA, Panza JA, et al. Coronary-artery bypass surgery in patients with ischemic Cardiomyopathy. N Engl J Med. 2016;374(16):1511–20.
30. Vavere AL, Arbab-Zadeh A, Rochitte CE, Dewey M, Niinuma H, Gottlieb I, et al. Coronary artery stenoses: accuracy of 64-detector row CT angiography in segments with mild, moderate, or severe calcification–a subanalysis of the CORE-64 trial. Radiology. 2011;261(1):100–8.

# Does improvement in self-management skills predict improvement in quality of life and depressive symptoms? A prospective study in patients with heart failure up to one year after self-management education

Gunda Musekamp[1*], Michael Schuler[1], Bettina Seekatz[1], Jürgen Bengel[2], Hermann Faller[1] and Karin Meng[1]

**Abstract**

**Background:** Heart failure (HF) patient education aims to foster patients' self-management skills. These are assumed to bring about, in turn, improvements in distal outcomes such as quality of life. The purpose of this study was to test the hypothesis that change in self-reported self-management skills observed after participation in self-management education predicts changes in physical and mental quality of life and depressive symptoms up to one year thereafter.

**Methods:** The sample comprised 342 patients with chronic heart failure, treated in inpatient rehabilitation clinics, who received a heart failure self-management education program. Latent change modelling was used to analyze relationships between both short-term (during inpatient rehabilitation) and intermediate-term (after six months) changes in self-reported self-management skills and both intermediate-term and long-term (after twelve months) changes in physical and mental quality of life and depressive symptoms.

**Results:** Short-term changes in self-reported self-management skills predicted intermediate-term changes in mental quality of life and long-term changes in physical quality of life. Intermediate-term changes in self-reported self-management skills predicted long-term changes in all outcomes.

**Conclusions:** These findings support the assumption that improvements in self-management skills may foster improvements in distal outcomes.

**Keywords:** Chronic heart failure, Self-management, Quality of life, Latent change, Cardiac rehabilitation, Patient education

## Background

Chronic heart failure (HF) is a common, disabling and fatal medical condition [1]. In view of the aging population it will affect even more people in the future [2]. It requires multidisciplinary management programs including patient education concerning self-care/self-management [3–5]. Self-management includes management of symptoms, treatment, consequences and lifestyle changes implicated by HF and aims to maintain quality of life [6]. For patients with HF, self-monitoring and responding to changes in symptoms are central components of self-management. The situation-specific theory of heart failure self-care [7, 8] states that self-care is a decision-making process, which involves maintenance (treatment adherence and healthy behavior), symptom perception and management (response to symptoms). Self-management interventions proved to be effective with regard to knowledge, self-efficacy, self-management behavior, quality of life, hospitalization, and mortality [9–11]. Thus, self-management is considered the central outcome of such programs and a means to achieve other important outcomes [5, 12]. Self-management can

* Correspondence: gunda.musekamp@uni-wuerzburg.de
[1]Department of Medical Psychology and Psychotherapy, Medical Sociology and Rehabilitation Sciences, University of Würzburg, Klinikstr. 3, D-97070 Würzburg, Germany
Full list of author information is available at the end of the article

be conceived of as an important proximal outcome of patient education that is a necessary (but not sufficient) prerequisite for the achievement of more distal goals as course of disease, quality of life or social participation [13]. Furthermore, in addition to improving self-management skills during treatment, it is important for patients to sustain and apply the acquired skills after treatment.

Studies have shown that quality of life in HF patients is reduced compared to the general population or patients with other chronic conditions [14–16]. Furthermore, depression is common among patients with HF and worsens the prognosis [17–19]. Therefore, both quality of life and depressive symptoms are considered important distal outcomes in patients with HF.

However, the relations between proximal and distal outcomes of self-management programs have rarely been studied so far. For example, there is no evidence yet that in patients with HF improvement in self-management is actually associated with subsequent improvement in quality of life. Most studies only report separate effects on different proximal and distal outcomes without relating them to each other [10, 11, 20], e. g., without examining whether improvements in knowledge or self-care lead to improvements in quality of life. Two cross-sectional studies showed that self-care behavior (in contrast to self-care confidence) was not associated with higher quality of life in patients with HF [21, 22]. However, these studies did not take into account changes in self-care or quality of life. According to the situation-specific theory of heart failure self-care [7, 8], one study tested whether there were different patterns of change in HF self-care management and whether these were associated with different patterns of change in quality of life over six months [23]. Results show that those who improved in self-care management over time also improved in quality of life. However, the study did not include an intervention and investigated concurrent rather than subsequent changes in outcome variables. In a previous study in patients with different chronic disorders, we showed that short-term changes (before/after inpatient rehabilitation including patient education) in self-reported self-management skills predicted 3-months changes in quality of life and depressive symptoms [24]. The purpose of the present study was to examine whether similar relationships are found in patients with HF and to extend the follow-up period. Particularly, this study investigated whether patients with HF who report an increase in self-reported self-management skills both directly after inpatient rehabilitation including self-management education and after six months show a subsequent increase in quality of life and a decrease in depressive symptoms after both six and twelve months. We hypothesized (1) that the difference of self-reported self-management skills between start and *end of rehabilitation* (duration 3 weeks) predicts the difference of both quality of life and depressive symptoms between start of rehabilitation and follow-up measurements six and twelve months later. We further hypothesized (2) that the difference of self-reported self-management skills between start of rehabilitation and *follow-up after six months* predicts the difference of both quality of life and depressive symptoms between start of rehabilitation and follow-up after twelve months.

## Methods

### Participants and procedure

This is a secondary analysis based on data from a study that evaluated a self-management patient education program for patients with chronic heart failure in inpatient cardiac rehabilitation [25] the results of which were presented elsewhere [26]. A cluster-randomized trial of patients with HF was conducted in four rehabilitation clinics. All participants received a 3-week multidisciplinary inpatient rehabilitation including medical treatment, exercise therapy/physical training, health education, psychological support, relaxation and social counselling as well as a self-management patient education program of different lengths: Patients in the intervention group received a new self-management educational program consisting of five interactive sessions of at least 60 min each provided in small groups. A physician, a nurse, a psychologist and a physiotherapist, respectively, held the interdisciplinary program. Contents were disease and treatment knowledge, self-management behaviors, medication, promotion of physical activity, illness related problems in everyday life, emotional distress and coping strategies. Patients in the control group received a short lecture-based educational program (one lecture of 60 min held by a physician). Contents were disease information and self-management recommendations.

Patients were consecutively included if they had a diagnosis of chronic systolic heart failure (ICD-10: I50) with left ventricular ejection fraction (LVEF) of $\leq 40$ and New York Heart Association (NYHA) functional classification II or III. Exclusion criteria were acute events of decompensation, cognitive impairment, insufficient German language ability and severe visual or hearing impairment. Patients completed several standardized patient reported questionnaires at the start (T1) and end (T2) of inpatient rehabilitation as well as after six (T3) and twelve months (T4). Participation in the study was voluntary and all participants provided written informed consent. The study complied with the Declaration of Helsinki and was approved by the ethical review committee of the Faculty of

Medicine, University of Würzburg (reference number: 60/11). Detailed information about this trial is presented elsewhere [26]. Of 517 eligible patients 475 comprised the initial study sample. The present analyses are based on those $n = 342$ patients (72%) with data at all four measurement points.

The data of both intervention group ($n = 178$) and control group ($n = 164$) patients were analyzed together, because all received a patient self-management education program. This study does not investigate differences between different education programs but relationships in changes after education programs.

### Measures

We used latent constructs, with selected items from standardized questionnaires serving as indicators.

*Self-management skills* were assessed with the *Skill and technique acquisition* subscale of the Health Education Impact Questionnaire (heiQ$^{TM}$) [27, 28]. It asks for the subjective appraisal of skills and techniques that help manage a chronic disease and related problems (item example: "When I have symptoms, I have skills that help me cope"). It proved to be reliable (Raykov's Composite Reliability Coefficient = 0.77), uni-dimensional and measurement invariant over time [27, 29]. The items are assessed on a 1-to-4 point Likert scale with higher scores indicating higher skills. All 4 items were used as single indicators for the latent construct *Self-management skills*.

*Quality of life* was assessed using the Kansas City Cardiomyopathy Questionnaire (KCCQ) [30, 31], a disease-specific quality of life measure which proved to be reliable, valid and sensitive to clinical change. The 3 items of the subscale (mental) quality of life (item example: "Over the past 2 weeks, how much has your heart failure limited your enjoyment of life?") were used as indicators of the latent construct *Mental quality of life*. For the latent construct *Physical quality of life*, 3 (out of 6) items of the physical limitation subscale representing moderate physical activity were chosen as indicators. This subscale measures impairment of everyday activities by HF and thus captures an important aspect of physical quality of life. An item example is: "Please indicate how much you are limited by heart failure (shortness of breath or fatigue) in your ability to do the following activities over the past 2 weeks: Climbing a flight of stairs without stopping". We did not chose the items covering light physical activity (e.g., dressing or bathing) because we supposed that they might be too "easy" for this sample. All items are scaled from 1 to 5, with higher scores indicating a higher level of quality of life. For the items covering *Physical quality of life*, the response format included a possibility to indicate that the activity was limited or not done for other reasons. Due to this, the sample for the analyses concerning *Physical quality of life* was limited to those $n = 214$ patients who did not indicate this response option in one of these items at any measurement point. The patients who were excluded did not differ from the remaining patients with respect to age, sex, living with a partner, educational level, working status, New York Heart Association (NYHA) class and mean left ventricular ejection fraction (LVEF), respectively (data not shown).

*Depressive symptoms* were assessed with the 2-item-version of the depression module of the Patient Health Questionnaire, PHQ-2 [32]. This reliable ($\alpha = 0.83$) and valid measure contains two main criteria of depression, diminished interest or pleasure and depressed mood ("Over the past 2 weeks, how often have you been bothered by any of the following problems? Little interest or pleasure in doing things"; "Feeling down, depressed or hopeless"). Items are scaled from 1 to 4, with higher scores indicating higher levels of depressive symptoms. Both items were used as single indicators of the latent construct *Depressive symptoms*.

### Statistical analyses

Statistical analyses were performed similar to Musekamp et al. [24], and detailed description of analytical procedures can be found there. Structural equation modeling techniques were used to investigate the hypotheses.

All models were computed using Mplus version 7.11 [33]. Full information maximum likelihood (FIML) algorithm [34] was used to handle missing data. Proportion of missing data was low (≤7%) for all variables. All models were estimated using a maximum likelihood estimator with robust standard errors [35]. Model fit was assessed based on Chi-square goodness of fit test, Comparative Fit Index (CFI) and Root Mean Square Error of Approximation (RMSEA), with CFI close to or higher than 0.95 and RMSEA close to or lower than 0.06 indicating good model fit [36]. Alpha was set to 0.05 for all analyses.

As preliminary analyses, confirmatory factor analyses (CFA) were applied to test measurement invariance (scalar invariance) over time [37, 38].

Then, to examine the hypotheses, changes in self-reported *Self-management skills* and changes in *Quality of life* and *Depressive symptoms* were modelled applying Latent True Change Modeling [39–42]. This approach allows modelling *inter*individual differences in *intra*individual change in a structural equation framework. Thus, latent ("true") change can be analysed without measurement error. For judging the size of changes, standardized effect sizes ($SES = Mean/SD_1$) were computed for all latent change variables. Standardized estimates for path coefficients are reported for assessment of relations among latent variables. Separate models for the three outcomes (*Physical quality of life, Mental quality of life, Depressive* *symptoms*) were tested. For identifying the models, the loading of the first item of each factor was fixed to 1, and the first intercept of each factor was fixed to 0. To model indicator-specific effects, correlations between the same indicators (items) at different measurement points were allowed [43]. Two types of models were estimated for all outcomes. The models of the first type use all four measurement points. They predict that changes in self-reported *Self-management skills* between T1 and T2 predict changes in *Physical quality of life* (model A1), *Mental quality of life* (model B1) and *Depressive symptoms* (model C1) between T1 and T3 and between T1 and T4, respectively (subsequent changes). They further assume the prediction of changes in these outcomes between T1 and T2 (concurrent changes). The models of the second type use the measurement points T1, T3 and T4. These models predict that changes in self-reported *Self-management skills* between T1 and T3 predict changes in the three outcomes (*Physical quality of life*: model A2, *Mental quality of life*: model B2, *Depressive symptoms*: model C2) between T1 and T4 (subsequent changes), in addition to the prediction of changes between T1 and T3 (concurrent changes).

## Results

### Sample

The sample comprises 342 patients with HF. Table 1 presents the sociodemographic and clinical characteristics. Mean age was 62.0 years (SD = 10.7), 76% were male, and 71% were living with a partner. Educational level was vocational training for most (68%). Most participants were retired (43%) or employed (42%). New York Heart Association (NYHA) class was II for 58%, mean left ventricular ejection fraction (LVEF) was 32.3 (SD = 6.7).

**Table 1** Sample characteristics ($n = 342$)

| | n | % |
|---|---|---|
| Male sex | 261 | 76,3 |
| Living with a partner[a] | 244 | 71,3 |
| Educational level[b] | | |
| Vocational training | 232 | 67,8 |
| Technical college | 38 | 11,1 |
| University | 19 | 5,6 |
| Other | 40 | 11,7 |
| Working status[c] | | |
| Employed | 143 | 41,8 |
| Retirement | 147 | 43,0 |
| Unemployed | 27 | 7,9 |
| Other | 24 | 7,0 |
| NYHA II[d] | 197 | 57,6 |
| | M | SD |
| Age | 62,0 | 10,7 |
| LVEF[c] | 32,3 | 6,7 |

*NYHA* New York Heart Association class, *LVEF* left ventricular ejection fraction;[a] missing: $n = 3$.[b] missing: $n = 13$.[c] missing: $n = 1$.[d] missing: $n = 7$

### Preliminary analyses

CFAs testing for configural invariance over time showed good model fit for all variables (CFI > 0.99, RMSEA < 0.05). Metric and scalar invariance models still showed good model fit for all variables (CFI > 0.96, RMSEA < 0.08). There were no misspecifications of parameters as shown by EPC and modification indices. Thus, the assumption of scalar measurement invariance over time was met.

### Latent true change models

#### *Model fit*

All latent change models yielded good fit with CFI > 0.96 and RMSEA > 0.05 (Table 2). Although the Chi-quare test was significant in some cases, the other fit indices indicated a good approximate fit of the models.

#### *Model parameters and effect sizes*

Table 3 shows the unstandardized intercepts and factor loadings for the six latent change models. All indicators of one factor have comparable factor loadings, are thus rather homogenous and contribute similarly to the latent constructs.

The means, variances and effect sizes (standardized effect size, SES) of latent change variables for all models are shown in table 4. All means of all latent change variables were significantly different from zero, which indicates change in these variables over measurement points. In addition, all variances of all latent change variables were significantly different from zero, indicating interindividual differences in intraindividual change.

**Table 2** Goodness of fit summary for latent change models

| Outcome | $\chi^2$ | df | $p$ | CFI | RMSEA |
|---|---|---|---|---|---|
| Model A1: Physical quality of life | | | | | |
| (T1 throughT4) | 174.40 | 151 | 0.093 | 0.99 | 0.03 |
| Model B1: Mental quality of life | | | | | |
| (T1 throughT4) | 263.44 | 151 | <0.001 | 0.97 | 0.05 |
| Model C1: Depressive symptoms | | | | | |
| (T1 throughT4) | 98.24 | 85 | 0.155 | 0.99 | 0.02 |
| Model A2: Physical quality of life | | | | | |
| (T1, T3, T4) | 118.10 | 110 | 0.282 | 1.00 | 0.02 |
| Model B2: Mental quality of life | | | | | |
| (T1, T3, T4) | 150.59 | 110 | 0.006 | 0.99 | 0.03 |
| Model C2: Depressive symptoms | | | | | |
| (T1, T3, T4) | 82.61 | 67 | 0.095 | 0.99 | 0.03 |

*CFI* comparative fit index, *RMSEA* root mean square error of approximation

**Table 3** Estimated intercepts and unstandardized factor loadings for the latent change models

| Model | Item | 1: measurement points T1 through T4 | | 2: measurement points T1, T3, T4 | |
|---|---|---|---|---|---|
| | | Intercept | Unstandardized factor loading (SE) | Intercept | Unstandardized factor loading (SE) |
| A | SM1 | 0.00* | 1.00* (–) | 0.00* | 1.00* (–) |
| | SM2 | −0.12 | 1.13 (0.09) | −0.07 | 1.09 (0.09) |
| | SM3 | −0.19 | 1.16 (0.10) | 0.01 | 1.07 (0.09) |
| | SM4 | 0.82 | 0.89 (0.09) | 1.00 | 0.81 (0.08) |
| | pQL1 | 0.00* | 1.00* (–) | 0.00* | 1.00* (–) |
| | pQL2 | −0.37 | 1.08 (0.04) | −0.37 | 1.08 (0.05) |
| | pQL3 | −0.93 | 1.06 (0.05) | −0.89 | 1.06 (0.05) |
| B | SM1 | 0.00* | 1.00* (–) | 0.00* | 1.00* (–) |
| | SM2 | −0.23 | 1.16 (0.06) | −0.20 | 1.14 (0.06) |
| | SM3 | −0.11 | 1.11 (0.07) | −0.15 | 1.12 (0.07) |
| | SM4 | 0.97 | 0.83 (0.06) | 0.89 | 0.84 (0.06) |
| | mQL1 | 0.00* | 1.00* (–) | 0.00* | 1.00* (–) |
| | mQL2 | −0.41 | 0.96 (0.04) | −0.43 | 0.98 (0.04) |
| | mQL3 | 0.46 | 0.89 (0.03) | 0.49 | 0.89 (0.03) |
| C | SM1 | 0.00* | 1.00* (–) | 0.00* | 1.00* (–) |
| | SM2 | −0.26 | 1.17 (0.06) | −0.22 | 1.14 (0.06) |
| | SM3 | −0.15 | 1.13 (0.07) | −0.16 | 1.12 (0.07) |
| | SM4 | 0.94 | 0.84 (0.06) | 0.90 | 0.84 (0.06) |
| | D1 | 0.00* | 1.00* (–) | 0.00* | 1.00* (–) |
| | D2 | −0.04 | 0.83 (0.09) | −0.06 | 0.85 (0.06) |

Fixed parameters are marked with an asterisk. Intercepts and unstandardized factor loadings of same indicators were set equal over measurement points. SM1 to SM4 = Indicators for Self-management skills, pQL1 to pQL3 = Indicators for Physical quality of life, mQL1 to mQL4 = Indicators for Mental quality of life, D1 and D2 = Indicators for Depressive symptoms. SE = standard error

Effect sizes show that changes in *Self-management skills* are of medium size, changes in *Physical quality of life* and *Depressive symptoms* are small to medium and changes in *Mental quality of life* are medium to large.

### *Path coefficients*

Figure 1 shows the standardized path coefficients for the structural models A1, B1 and C1 with measurement points T1 through T4. In model A1, interindividual differences in intraindividual change in *Physical quality of life* between T1 and T4 were significantly predicted by change in *Self-management skills* between T1 and T2 in such a way that increases of *Self-management skills* predicted increases in *Physical quality of life* ($\beta = 0.23$). Changes in *Self-management skills* did not predict changes in *Physical quality of life* between T1 and T2 or T1 and T3, respectively. In model B1, increases in *Self-management skills* predicted increases in *Mental quality of life* between T1 and T2 ($\beta = 0.36$) and between T1 and T3 ($\beta = 0.24$), respectively, but not between T1 and T4. In model C1, increases in *Self-management skills* predicted decreases in *Depressive symptoms* between T1 and T2 ($\beta = -0.29$), but not at the later occasions. Additionally, the baseline level of *Self-management skills* predicted changes in both *Mental quality of life* and *Depressive Symptoms* between T1 and T4.

The standardized path coefficients in models A2, B2 and C2 with measurement points T1, T3 and T4 are shown in Fig. 2. In all three models, changes in *Self-management skills* between T1 and T3 predict changes in distal outcomes between T1 and T4. Increases in *Self-management skills* predict increases in *Physical quality of life* ($\beta = 0.39$), increases in *Mental quality of life* ($\beta = 0.22$), and decreases in *Depressive symptoms* ($\beta = -0.20$). Additionally, changes between T1 and T3 in all three outcomes were also predicted by changes in *Self-management skills* ($\beta = 0.32$, $\beta = 0.38$ and $\beta = -0.34$, respectively). Furthermore, the baseline level of *Self-management skills* predicted changes in *Depressive symptoms* between T1 and T4.

## Discussion

To our knowledge, this is the first study that examined the associations between change in self-reported self-management skills and subsequent change in quality of life and depressive symptoms in patients with HF undergoing inpatient rehabilitation including

**Table 4** Unstandardized means and variances and effect sizes of latent change variables

| LCV | Model | Mean | Variance | SES |
|---|---|---|---|---|
| $\Delta SM_2 - SM_1$ | A1 | 0.26* | 0.23* | 0.48 |
| | B1, C1 | 0.29* | 0.25* | 0.50 |
| $\Delta SM_3 - SM_1$ | A2 | 0.27* | 0.28* | 0.47 |
| | B2, C2 | 0.31* | 0.26* | 0.53 |
| $\Delta pQL_2 - pQL_1$ | A1 | 0.23* | 0.80* | 0.23 |
| $\Delta pQL_3 - pQL_1$ | A1 | 0.36* | 0.97* | 0.37 |
| | A2 | 0.35* | 0.96* | 0.36 |
| $\Delta pQL_4 - pQL_1$ | A1 | 0.37* | 0.91* | 0.37 |
| | A2 | 0.37* | 0.91* | 0.37 |
| $\Delta mQL_2 - mQL_1$ | B1 | 0.52* | 0.31* | 0.58 |
| $\Delta mQL_3 - mQL_1$ | B1 | 0.63* | 0.73* | 0.71 |
| | B2 | 0.65* | 0.73* | 0.72 |
| $\Delta mQL_4 - mQL_1$ | B1 | 0.71* | 0.78* | 0.80 |
| | B2 | 0.73* | 0.78* | 0.81 |
| $\Delta D_2 - D_1$ | C1 | −0.29* | 0.24* | −0.38 |
| $\Delta D_3 - D_1$ | C1 | −0.28* | 0.49* | −0.36 |
| | C2 | −0.28* | 0.50* | −0.35 |
| $\Delta D_4 - D_1$ | C1 | −0.30* | 0.61* | −0.38 |
| | C2 | −0.30* | 0.61* | −0.38 |

*LCV* Δ = latent change variable, *SM* Self-management skills, *pQL* Physical quality of life, *mQL* Mental quality of life, *D* Depressive symptoms, *SES* Standardized effect size. Subscripted figures represent measurement points
* $p < .05$

self-management patient education. Results show that changes in self-management skills predict changes in these distal outcomes. Concerning hypothesis 1, results differ between outcomes. Short-term change in self-reported self-management skills (between start and end of rehabilitation) predicted long-term change in physical quality of life (between start of rehabilitation and follow-up twelve months later), but not intermediate-term change (after six months). By contrast, it predicted intermediate-term, but not long-term, change in mental quality of life. Finally, it did neither predict intermediate nor long-term change in depressive symptoms. Thus, hypothesis 1 was only partly confirmed. Regarding hypothesis 2, the picture is consistent: Intermediate-term change in self-reported self-management skills (between start of rehabilitation and follow-up after six months) predicted long-term changes in all three outcomes (between start of rehabilitation and follow-up after twelve months). Thus, hypothesis 2 was confirmed.

The results are in line with Musekamp et al. [24], but not only confirm the prior findings in a HF sample but also expand them with regard to the follow-up period. Although there may be differences in concrete self-management activities between different conditions, increase in self-reported self-management skills is associated with subsequent increase in quality of life and decrease in depressive symptoms regardless of condition. These results are consistent with definitions of self-management and models of patient education in patients with chronic conditions in general suggesting such relationships between self-management skills and quality of life [6, 13]. They are also consistent with the propositions of the situation specific theory of heart failure self-care [8]. Together, they support the importance of self-management in HF patient education [4, 5].

Our results suggest that, in patients with HF, the acquirement of self-management skills during self-management education may have a long-term influence on physical quality of life and an intermediate-term influence on mental quality of life. Thus, improved self-management skills may influence mental quality of life more directly, because they immediately convey a sense of exerting control. Physical quality of life may be influenced in a delayed (but more sustainable) fashion, however, because it takes more time to influence physical conditions. For example, it takes some time until the appropriate reaction to HF symptoms affects the physical condition and the individual takes notice of this improvement. For the long-term changes in mental quality of life and depressive symptoms the baseline level of self-management skills seems a better predictor than the short-term change in self-management skills.

Changes in self-reported self-management skills were not only observed immediately after rehabilitation, but also after six months, with medium effect sizes. Thus, the aim of rehabilitation and self-management patient education to sustain self-management skills in everyday life was reached. Interestingly, change of self-management skills up to six months after rehabilitation seems to influence further change in distal outcomes. Thus, it is not only important to increase self-management skills during self-management education, but also to sustain them afterwards. This emphasizes the importance of fostering self-management skills that can be applied and sustained after treatment. Self-management programs should therefore have a strong focus on everyday life and implement aftercare plans.

However, it remains unclear, whether changes in distal outcomes are initiated by self-management education alone or also by other processes or events coming into effect during the follow-up period. This might for example include events like job changes or retirement.

Further studies should investigate treatment mechanisms of self-management patient education, as they are still unclear [44]. The causal pathway between self-management skills and quality of life needs

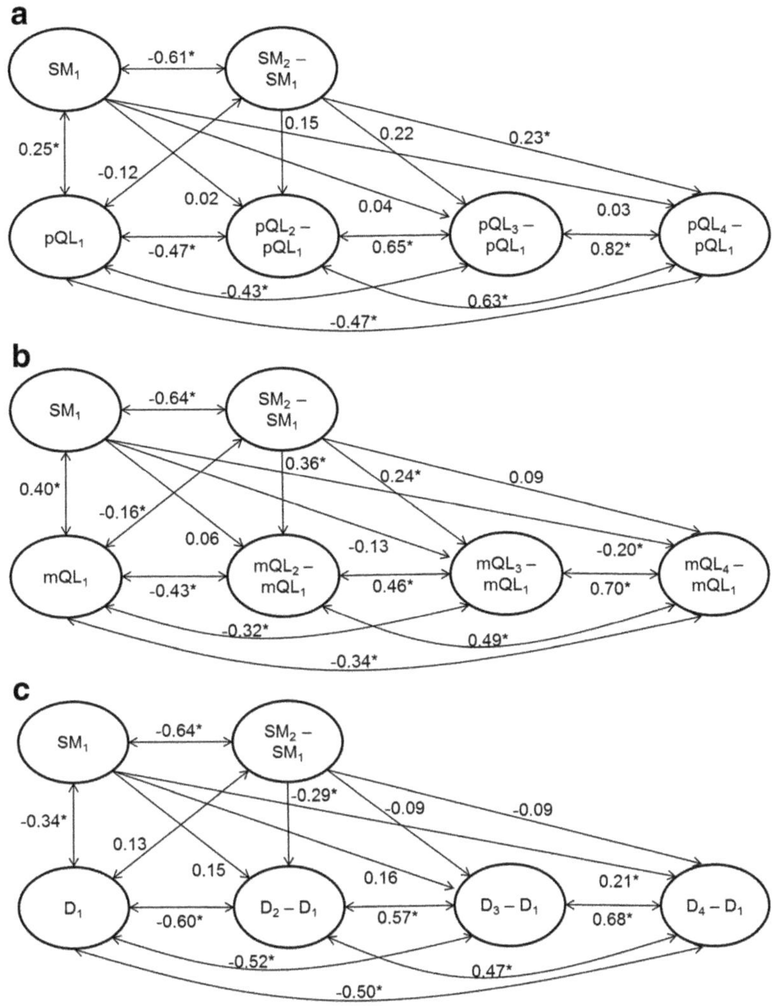


**Fig. 1** Latent change model (*structural model*) with standardized path coefficients. Predictor Self-management skills (SM), measurement points T1 throughT4. A1: Outcome Physical quality of life (pQL). B1: Outcome Mental quality of life (mQL). C1: Outcome Depressive symptoms (D). Circles represent latent variables, single-headed arrows show the impact of one variable on another, double arrows show correlations allowed between variables. Subscripted figures represent measurement points. $^*p < 0.05$

further examination. It should be examined whether the influence of self-management skills is mediated by actual self-management/self-care behaviors, such as symptom monitoring and responding to symptoms or health behaviors, such as adherence to medication or moderate physical activity [4, 8]. These variables should be included in future models to clarify the effects of self-management skills and other potential predictor variables. Others [45] have investigated the effect of improvement in knowledge after a nurse-led education session on clinical outcomes and found associations with reduced hospital readmissions. On the other hand, knowledge alone may not be sufficient to establish adequate self-care [46]. Therefore, it should be investigated how knowledge and skills work together in establishing adequate self-management behavior and quality of life.

#### Limitations

There are some limitations that should be considered. First, while longitudinal associations were examined, causality cannot be proved due to the non-experimental design of our study.

Second, the scale used to assess self-management skills is generic in nature and possibly does not cover all self-management skills important for patients with HF as symptom-monitoring [3]. Thus, our scale might not be specific enough to cover more than general expectations about self-management. Further studies should explore whether specific measures of self-management skills in HF add to prediction of distal outcomes. Third, it was based on self-report and thus susceptible to bias. However, it is difficult to implement objective measures of self-management. Fourth, possibly confounding factors influencing the course of

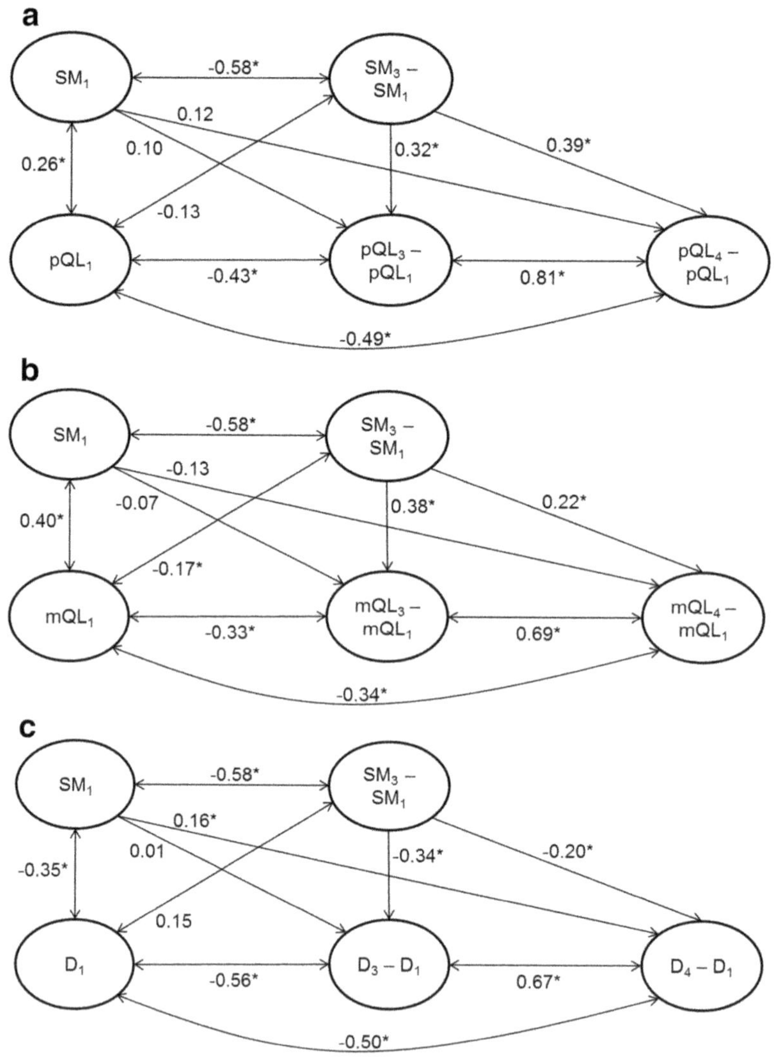


**Fig. 2** Latent change model (*structural model*) with standardized path coefficients. Predictor Self-management skills (SM), measurement points T1, T3, and T4. A2: Outcome Physical quality of life (pQL). B2: Outcome Mental quality of life (mQL). C2: Outcome Depressive symptoms (D). Circles represent latent variables, single-headed arrows show the impact of one variable on another, double arrows show correlations allowed between variables. Subscripted figures represent measurement points. $^{*}p < 0.05$

both quality of life and depressive symptoms after self-management education were not taken into account in this study. For example, trait factors like dispositional optimism might influence assessment of both self-management skills and quality of life [47].

## Conclusion

This study adds to previous evidence in that it supports the assumption that self-management skills improved during short- and intermediate-term are associated with intermediate and long-term improvements in both quality of life and depressive symptoms in patients with HF. Thus, relationships between an important proximal outcome of self-management patient education and various important distal outcomes could be demonstrated. The results support the conclusion that patient education interventions for patients with HF should target self-management skills. These should be addressed with a focus on sustainability and suitability in everyday life as some changes became evident only several months after the completion of the educational program. Further studies should investigate additional predictor variables as self-care behavior as well as treatment mechanisms of self-management programs.

#### Abbreviations

CFA: Confirmatory factor analysis; CFI: Comparative fit index; D: Depressive symptoms; FIML: Full information maximum likelihood; heiQ: Health education impact questionnaire; HF: Heart failure; KCCQ: Kansas city cardiomyopathy questionnaire; LVEF: Left ventricular ejection fraction; M: Mean; mQL: Mental quality of life; NYHA: New York Heart Association; PHQ-2: Patient health questionnaire depression module 2-item version; pQL: Physical quality of life;

RMSEA: Root mean square error of approximation; SD: Standard deviation; SE: Standard error; SES: Standardized effect size; SM: Self-management skills

**Acknowledgements**

The authors wish to thank the participating rehabilitation clinics: Rehabilitation Hospital Kirchberg-Klinik (Dr. Ernst Knoglinger), Rehabilitation Hospital Möhnesee (Dr. Rainer Schubmann), Rehabilitation Hospital Wetterau (Dr. Ulrich Kiwus), Segeberger Kliniken GmbH, Rehabilitation Hospital (Dr. Ronja Westphal), which supported the evaluation of the program.

**Funding**

This study was funded by the German Statutory Pension Insurance Scheme (Deutsche Rentenversicherung Bund; grant number: 8011 – 106 – 31/31.93.1). This publication was funded by the German Research Foundation (DFG) and the University of Wuerzburg in the funding programme Open Access Publishing.

**Authors' contributions**

GM is the principal investigator, developed the research question, undertook guidance of data collection, performed the statistical analyses and is the main author of the manuscript. MS gave statistical advice, contributed to the design of the study and drafted the manuscript. BS undertook guidance of data collection and helped draft the manuscript. JB and HF contributed to the design of the study and helped draft the manuscript. KM developed the primary study, contributed to the design of the study and drafted the manuscript. All authors read and approved the final manuscript.

**Competing interests**

The authors declare that they have no competing interests.

**Author details**

[1]Department of Medical Psychology and Psychotherapy, Medical Sociology and Rehabilitation Sciences, University of Würzburg, Klinikstr. 3, D-97070 Würzburg, Germany. [2]Institute of Psychology, Department of Rehabilitation Psychology and Psychotherapy, University of Freiburg, Engelbergerstraße 41, D-79085 Freiburg, Germany.

**References**

1. McMurray JJV, Pfeffer MA. Heart failure. Lancet. 2005;365:1877–89.
2. Stewart S, MacIntyre K, Capewell S, McMurray JJ. Heart failure and the aging population: an increasing burden in the 21st century? Heart. 2003;89:49–53.
3. McMurray JJV, Adamopoulos S, Anker SD, Auricchio A, Böhm M, Dickstein K, et al. ESC guidelines for the diagnosis and treatment of acute and chronic heart failure 2012. Eur J Heart Fail. 2012;14:803–69.
4. Lainscak M, Blue L, Clark AL, Dahlström U, Dickstein K, Ekman I, et al. Self-care management of heart failure: practical recommendations from the Patient Care Committee of the Heart Failure Association of the European Society of Cardiology. Eur J Heart Fail. 2011;13:115–26.
5. Strömberg A. The crucial role of patient education in heart failure. Eur J Heart Fail. 2005;7:363–9.
6. Barlow J, Wright C, Sheasby J, Turner A, Hainsworth J. Self-management approaches for people with chronic conditions: a review. Patient Educ Couns. 2002;48:177–87.
7. Riegel B, Dickson W. A situation-specific theory of heart failure self-care. J Cardiovasc Nurs. 2008;23:190–6.
8. Riegel B, Dickson W, Faulkner KM. The situation-specific theory of heart failure self-care: revised and updated. J Cardiovasc Nurs. 2015. doi:10.1097/JCN.0000000000000244.
9. Ditewig JB, Blok H, Havers J, van Veenendaal H. Effectiveness of self-management interventions on mortality, hospital readmissions, chronic heart failure hospitalization rate and quality of life in patients with chronic heart failure: a systematic review. Patient Educ Couns. 2010;78:297–315.
10. Jovicic A, Holroyd-Leduc JM, Straus SE. Effects of self-management intervention on health outcomes of patients with heart failure: a systematic review of randomized controlled trials. BMC Cardiovasc Disord. 2006;6:43.
11. Barnason S, Zimmerman L, Young L. An integrative review of interventions promoting self-care of patients with heart failure. J Clin Nurs. 2012;21:448–75.
12. Deaton C. Outcomes measurement. J Cardiovasc Nurs. 2000;14:116–8.
13. Faller H, Reusch A, Meng K. DGRW-Update: Patientenschulung. Rehabilitation. 2011;50:284–91.
14. Juenger J, Schellberg D, Kraemer S, Haunstetter A, Zugck C, Herzog W, et al. Health related quality of life in patients with congestive heart failure: comparison with other chronic diseases and relation to functional variables. Heart. 2002;87:235–41.
15. Hobbs FD, Kenkre JE, Roalfe AK, Davis RC, Hare R, Davies MK. Impact of heart failure and left ventricular systolic dysfunction on quality of life: a cross-sectional study comparing common chronic cardiac and medical disorders and a representative adult population. Eur Heart J. 2002;23:1867–76.
16. Calvert MJ, Freemantle N, Cleland JG. The impact of chronic heart failure on health-related quality of life data acquired in the baseline phase of the CARE-HF study. Eur J Heart Fail. 2005;7:243–51.
17. Rutledge T, Reis VA, Linke SE, Greenberg BH, Mills PJ. Depression in heart failure: a meta-analytic review of prevalence, intervention effects, and associations with clinical outcomes. J Am Coll Cardiol. 2006;48:1527–37.
18. Jiang W, Kuchibhatla M, Clary GL, Cuffe MS, Christopher EJ, Alexander JD, et al. Relationship between depressive symptoms and long-term mortality in patients with heart failure. Am Heart J. 2007;154:102–8.
19. Faller H, Störk S, Schowalter M, Steinbüchel T, Wollner V, Ertl G, et al. Depression and survival in chronic heart failure: does gender play a role? Eur J Heart Fail. 2007;9:1018–23.
20. Grady KL. Self-care and quality of life outcomes in heart failure patients. J Cardiovasc Nurs. 2008;23:285–92.
21. Buck HG, Lee CS, Moser DK, Albert NM, Lennie T, Bentley B, et al. Relationship between self-care and health-related quality of life in older adults with moderate to advanced heart failure. J Cardiovasc Nurs. 2012;27:8–15.
22. Seto E, Leonard KJ, Cafazzo JA, Masino C, Barnsley J, Ross HJ. Self-care and quality of life of heart failure patients at a multidisciplinary heart function clinic. J Cardiovasc Nurs. 2011;26:377–85.
23. Lee CS, Mudd JO, Hiatt SO, Gelow JM, Chien C, Riegel B. Trajectories of heart failure self-care management and changes in quality of life. Eur J Cardiovasc Nurs. 2015;14:486–94.
24. Musekamp G, Schuler M, Bengel J, Faller H. Improved self-management skills predict improvements in quality of life and depression in patients with chronic disorders. Patient Educ Couns. 2016;99:1355–1361. doi:10.1016/j.pec.2016.03.022.
25. Meng K, Musekamp G, Seekatz B, Glatz J, Karger G, Kiwus U, et al. Evaluation of a self-management patient education program for patients with chronic heart failure undergoing inpatient cardiac rehabilitation: study protocol of a cluster randomized controlled trial. BMC Cardiovasc Disord. 2013;13:60.
26. Meng K, Musekamp G, Schuler M, Seekatz B, Glatz J, Karger G, et al. The impact of a self-management patient education program for patients with chronic heart failure undergoing inpatient cardiac rehabilitation. Patient Educ Couns. 2016;99:1190–1197. doi:10.1016/j.pec.2016.02.010.
27. Schuler M, Musekamp G, Faller H, Ehlebracht-König I, Gutenbrunner C, Kirchhof R, et al. Assessment of proximal outcomes of self-management programs: translation and psychometric evaluation of a German version of the Health Education Impact Questionnaire (heiQTM). Qual Life Res. 2013;22:1391–403.
28. Osborne RH, Elsworth GR, Whitfield K. The Health Education Impact Questionnaire (heiQ): An outcomes and evaluation measure for patient education and self-management interventions for people with chronic conditions. Patient Educ Couns. 2007;66:192–201.
29. Schuler M, Musekamp G, Bengel J, Schwarze M, Spanier K, Gutenbrunner C, et al. Measurement of stable changes of self-management skills after rehabilitation: a latent state-trait analysis of the Health Education Impact Questionnaire (heiQTM). Qual Life Res. 2014;23:2531–43.
30. Faller H, Steinbüchel T, Schowalter M, Spertus JA, Störk S, Angermann CE. Der Kansas City Cardiomyopathy Questionnaire (KCCQ) - ein neues krankheitsspezifisches Messinstrument zur Erfassung der Lebensqualität bei chronischer Herzinsuffizienz. Psychometrische Prüfung der deutschen Version. Psychoth, Psychosom Med Psychol. 2005;55:200–8.

31. Green CP, Porter CB, Bresnahan DR, Spertus JA. Development and evaluation of the Kansas City Cardiomyopathy Questionnaire: a new health status measure for heart failure. J Am Coll Cardiol. 2000;35:1245–55.
32. Löwe B, Kroenke K, Gräfe K. Detecting and monitoring depression with a two-item questionnaire (PHQ-2). J Psychosom Res. 2005;58:163–71.
33. Muthén LK, Muthén BO. Mplus user's guide. 6th ed. Muthén & Muthén: Los Angeles, CA; 2010.
34. Enders CK. The impcat of nonnormality on full information maximum-likelihood estimation for structural equation models with missing data. Psychol Methods. 2001;6:352–70.
35. Weston R, Gore PA. A brief guide to structural equation modeling. Couns Psychol. 2006;34:719–51.
36. Hu L, Bentler PM. Cutoff criteria for fit indexes in covariance structure analysis: conventional criteria versus new alternatives. Struct Equ Model. 1999;6:1–55.
37. Millsap RE. Statistical approaches to measurement invariance. New York: Psychology Press; 2011.
38. Meredith W. Measurement invariance, factor analysis and factioral invariance. Psychom. 1993;58:525–43.
39. Geiser C, Eid M, Nussbeck FW, Courvoisier DS, Cole DA. Analyzing true change in longitudinal multitrait-multimethod-studies: application of a multimethod change model to depression and anxiety in children. Dev Psychol. 2010;46:29–45.
40. Reuter T, Ziegelmann JP, Wiedemann AU, Geiser C, Lippke S, Schüz B, et al. Changes in intentions, planning, and self-efficacy predict changes in behaviors. J Health Psychol. 2010;15:935–47.
41. Steyer R, Eid M, Schwenkmezger P. Modeling true intraindividual change: true change as a latent variable. Methods Psychol Res Online. 1997;2:21–33.
42. McArdle JJ. Latent variable modeling of differences and changes with longitudinal data. Annu Rev Psychol. 2009;60:577–605.
43. Cole DA, Maxwell SE. Testing mediational models with longitudinal data: questions and tips in the use of structural equation modeling. J Abnorm Psychol. 2003;112:558–77.
44. Jonkman NH, Schuurmans MJ, Groenwold RH, Hoes AW, Trappenburg JC. Identifying components of self-management interventions that improve health-related quality of life in chronically ill patients: Systematic review and meta-regression analysis. Patient Educ Couns. 2016;99:1087–1098. doi: 10.1016/j.pec.2016.01.022.
45. Kommuri NVA, Johnson ML, Koelling TM. Relationship between improvements in heart failure patient disease specific knowledge and clinical events as part of a randomized controlled trial. Patient Educ Couns. 2012;86:233–8.
46. Dickson W, Riegel B. Are we teaching what patients need to know? Building skills in heart failure self-care. Heart Lung. 2009;38:253–61.
47. Kostka T, Jachimowicz V. Relationship of quality of life to dispositional optimism, health locus of control and self-efficacy in older subjects living in different environments. Qual Life Res. 2010;19:351–61.

# Permissions

All chapters in this book were first published in CD, by BioMed Central; hereby published with permission under the Creative Commons Attribution License or equivalent. Every chapter published in this book has been scrutinized by our experts. Their significance has been extensively debated. The topics covered herein carry significant findings which will fuel the growth of the discipline. They may even be implemented as practical applications or may be referred to as a beginning point for another development.

The contributors of this book come from diverse backgrounds, making this book a truly international effort. This book will bring forth new frontiers with its revolutionizing research information and detailed analysis of the nascent developments around the world.

We would like to thank all the contributing authors for lending their expertise to make the book truly unique. They have played a crucial role in the development of this book. Without their invaluable contributions this book wouldn't have been possible. They have made vital efforts to compile up to date information on the varied aspects of this subject to make this book a valuable addition to the collection of many professionals and students.

This book was conceptualized with the vision of imparting up-to-date information and advanced data in this field. To ensure the same, a matchless editorial board was set up. Every individual on the board went through rigorous rounds of assessment to prove their worth. After which they invested a large part of their time researching and compiling the most relevant data for our readers.

The editorial board has been involved in producing this book since its inception. They have spent rigorous hours researching and exploring the diverse topics which have resulted in the successful publishing of this book. They have passed on their knowledge of decades through this book. To expedite this challenging task, the publisher supported the team at every step. A small team of assistant editors was also appointed to further simplify the editing procedure and attain best results for the readers.

Apart from the editorial board, the designing team has also invested a significant amount of their time in understanding the subject and creating the most relevant covers. They scrutinized every image to scout for the most suitable representation of the subject and create an appropriate cover for the book.

The publishing team has been an ardent support to the editorial, designing and production team. Their endless efforts to recruit the best for this project, has resulted in the accomplishment of this book. They are a veteran in the field of academics and their pool of knowledge is as vast as their experience in printing. Their expertise and guidance has proved useful at every step. Their uncompromising quality standards have made this book an exceptional effort. Their encouragement from time to time has been an inspiration for everyone.

The publisher and the editorial board hope that this book will prove to be a valuable piece of knowledge for researchers, students, practitioners and scholars across the globe.

# List of Contributors


**Evelien ES van Riet, Arno W Hoes, Marcel AJ Landman and Frans H Rutten**
Julius Center for Health Sciences and Primary care, University Medical Center Utrecht, 3508 AB, Utrecht, The Netherlands

**Alexander Limburg**
Diakonessenhuis Zeist, Zeist, The Netherlands

**Berhe W. Sahle, Alice J. Owen, Henry Krum and Christopher M. Reid**
Centre of Cardiovascular Research and Education in Therapeutics, Department of Epidemiology and Preventive Medicine, Monash University, 99 Commercial Road, Melbourne, Vic 3004, Australia

**Berhe W. Sahle**
School of Public Health, Mekelle University, Mekelle, Ethiopia

**Mutsa P. Mutowo**
School of Public Health, Department of Epidemiology and Preventive Medicine, Monash University, Melbourne, Australia

**Christopher M. Reid**
School of Public Health, Curtin University, Perth, Australia

**Rachel R Huxley**
Epidemiology & Biostatistics Division, School of Population Health, University of Queensland, Brisbane, Australia

**Federica Barzi and Mark Woodward**
The George Institute for Global Health, University of Sydney, Sydney, Australia

**Jean Woo**
Department of Medicine and Therapeutics, Faculty of Medicine, The Chinese University of Hong Kong, Hong Kong, China

**Graham Giles**
Cancer Epidemiology Centre, The Cancer Council Victoria, Melbourne, Australia

**Tai Hing Lam**
School of Public Health/Department of Community Medicine, The University of Hong Kong, Hong Kong, China

**Kazem Rahimi**
George Centre for Healthcare Innovation, University of Oxford, Oxford, UK
Department of Cardiovascular Medicine, University of Oxford, Oxford, UK

**Suma Konety**
Division of Epidemiology and Community Health, School of Public Health, University of Minnesota, Minneapolis, Minnesota, USA

**Takayoshi Ohkubo**
Department of Health Science, Shiga University of Medical Science, Shiga, Japan

**Sun Ha Jee**
Institute for Health Promotion, Graduate School of Public Health, Yonsei University, Seoul, Korea

**Xianghua Fang**
Department of Epidemiology and Social Medicine, Xuanwu Hospital, Capital Medical University, Beijing, China

**Mark Woodward**
Division of Epidemiology, Johns Hopkins University, Baltimore, USA

**Simona Kirbiš and Andreja Sinkovič**
Department of intensive care unit, University Clinical Center Maribor, Ljubljanska 5, Maribor, SI 2000, Slovenia

**Maksimiljan Gorenjak**
Department of laboratory diagnostics, University Clinical Center Maribor, Maribor, Slovenia

**F Gaborit, K Iversen, T Kümler and M Schou**
Department of Cardiology, Herlev University Hospital, DK-2730 Herlev, Denmark

**H Bosselmann and N Tønder**
Department of Internal Medicine KNEA, North Zealand University Hospital, DK-3400 Hillerod, Denmark

**C Kistorp**
Department of Internal Medicine O, Herlev University Hospital, DK-2730 Herlev, Denmark

**G Sölétormos**
Department of Clinical Biochemistry, North Zealand University Hospital, DK-3400 Hillerod, Denmark

**J P. Goetze**
Department of Clinical Biochemistry, Rigshospitalet, DK-2100 Copenhagen, Denmark

**Hai-Yan Pan, Jian-Hua Zhu, Yong Gu, Xiao-Hong Yu and Min Pan**
Department of Cardiology, Affiliated Hospital of Nantong University and Institute of Cardiovascular Research, Nantong University, Jiangsu 226001, China

**Hong-Yin Niu**
Department of Echocardiography, Affiliated Hospital of Nantong University, Jiangsu, China

**Patric Karlström**
Department of Medicine, Division of Cardiology, County Hospital Ryhov, Jönköping, Sweden

**Peter Johansson, Ulf Dahlström and Urban Alehagen**
Department of Cardiology and Department of Medical and Health Sciences, Linköping University, Linköping, Sweden

**Kurt Boman**
Research unit Skellefteå Department of Medicine, Institution of Public Health and Clinical Medicine, Umeå University, Umeå, Sweden

**Ruud F. Spee, Victor M. Niemeijer and Hareld M.C. Kemps**
Department of Cardiology, Máxima Medical Centre, De Run 4600, Veldhoven 5500 MB, The Netherlands

**Bart Wessels**
Department of Biomedical Engineering, Eindhoven University of Technology, Eindhoven, The Netherlands

**Jasper P. Jansen and Pieter F. F. Wijn**
Department of Clinical Physics and Clinical Informatics, Máxima Medical Centre Veldhoven, Veldhoven, The Netherlands

**Pieter F. F. Wijn**
Department of Applied Physics, Eindhoven University of Technology, Eindhoven, The Netherlands

**Pieter A. F. M. Doevendans**
Department of Cardiology, University Medical Centre Utrecht, Utrecht, The Netherlands

**Hareld M. C. Kemps**
Department of Medical Informatics, Academic Medical Centre, University of Amsterdam, Amsterdam, The Netherlands

**Amer H. S. Aljundi, Shaban F. K. Mohammed and Jassim Al Suwaidi**
Department of Clinical Pharmacology, Heart Hospital, Hamad Medical Corporation, Doha, Qatar

**Rajvir Singh**
Cardiovascular Research, Heart Hospital, Hamad Medical Corporation, Doha, Qatar

**Ashfaq Patel, Abdulrahman Arabi and Hajar A. AlBinali**
Cardiology and Cardiovascular Surgery, Heart Hospital, Hamad Medical Corporation, Doha, Qatar

**Freja Stoltze Gaborit, Kasper Iversen, Thomas Kumler and Morten Schou**
Department of Cardiology, Herlev University Hospital, Herlev, Denmark

**Helle Bosselmann**
Department of Internal Medicine KNEA, North Zealand University Hospital, Hillerod, Denmark

**Caroline Kistorp**
Department of Internal Medicine, Endocrinology Unit, Herlev University Hospital, Herlev, Denmark

**Finn Gustafsson and Helle Bosselmann**
Department of Cardiology, Rigshospitalet, Copenhagen, Denmark

**Jens P. Goetze**
Department of Clinical Biochemistry, Rigshospitalet, Copenhagen, Denmark

**György Sölétormos**
Department of Clinical Biochemistry, North Zealand University Hospital, Hillerod, Denmark

**Freja Stoltze Gaborit, Caroline Kistorp, Kasper Iversen and Morten Schou**
Department of Clinical Medicine, University of Copenhagen, Copenhagen, Denmark

**Christine D Jones, Darren A DeWalt, Crystal W Cene and Michael Pignone**
Division of General Medicine and Clinical Epidemiology, University of North Carolina at Chapel Hill, Chapel Hill, NC, USA

**Christine D Jones, George M Holmes, Darren A DeWalt, Brian Erman, Crystal W Cene, Victoria Hawk, Kimberly Broucksou and Michael Pignone**
The Cecil G. Sheps Center for Health Services Research, University of North Carolina at Chapel Hill, Chapel Hill, NC, USA

**George M Holmes**
Department of Health Policy and Management, University of North Carolina at Chapel Hill, Chapel Hill, NC, USA

**Jia-Rong Wu**
School of Nursing, University of North Carolina at Chapel Hill, Chapel Hill, NC, USA

**David W Baker and Bernice Ruo**
Division of General Internal Medicine, Feinberg School of Medicine, Northwestern University, Chicago, IL, USA

**Dean Schillinger and Kirsten Bibbins-Domingo**
Division of General Internal Medicine and Center for Vulnerable Populations, Department of Medicine at San Francisco General Hospital, University of California San Francisco, San Francisco, CA, USA

**Aurelia Macabasco-O'Connell**
Olive View-UCLA Medical Center, UCLA School of Nursing, University of California, Los Angeles, CA, USA

**Christine D Jones**
NRSA Primary Care Fellowship, Division of General Medicine and Clinical Epidemiology, University of North Carolina at Chapel Hill, 5034 Old Clinic Building, CB# 7110, Chapel Hill, NC 27599, USA

**Anna Ledakowicz-Polak and Marzenna Zielińska**
Intensive Cardiac Therapy Clinic, Department of Cardiology and Cardiosurgery, Medical University, Pomorska 251, 92-213 Lodz, Poland

**Jarosław Bartodziej**
Department of Anaesthesiology and Intensive Care, Jonscher Municipal Hospital, Lodz, Poland

**Agata Majos**
Department of Radiology, Medical University, Lodz, Poland

**Ursula Hoffmann, Florian Espeter, Siegfried Lang, Ibrahim Akin, Martin Borggrefe and Michael Behnes**
First Department of Medicine, University Medical Centre Mannheim (UMM), Faculty of Medicine Mannheim, University of Heidelberg, Theodor-Kutzer-Ufer 1-3, 68167 Mannheim, Germany

**Christel Weiß**
Department of Statistical Analysis, Faculty of Medicine Mannheim, University of Heidelberg, Mannheim, Germany

**Parviz Ahmad-Nejad**
Institute for Microbiology and Laboratory Medicine, HELIOS Klinikum Wuppertal, University of Witten/Herdecke, Wuppertal, Germany

**Martina Brueckmann**
Boehringer Ingelheim GmbH & Co. KG, Ingelheim am Rhein, Germany
Faculty of Medicine Mannheim, University of Heidelberg, Mannheim, Germany

**Michael Neumaier**
Institute for Clinical Chemistry, University Medical Centre Mannheim (UMM), Faculty of Medicine Mannheim, University of Heidelberg, Mannheim, Germany

**Kuo-Tzu Sung, Charles Jia-Yin Hou and Chung-Lieh Hung**
Division of Cardiology, Department of Internal Medicine, Mackay Memorial Hospital, Taipei, Taiwan

**Chun-Ho Yun**
Department of Radiology, Mackay Memorial Hospital, Taipei, Taiwan

**Chun-Ho Yun, Charles Jia-Yin Hou and Chung-Lieh Hung**
Department of Medicine, Mackay Medical College and Mackay Medicine, Nursing and Management College, Taipei, Taiwan

**Chung-Lieh Hung**
Cardiovascular Medicine, Mackay Memorial Hospital, No. 92, Section 2, Chung Shan North Road, Taipei, Taiwan

**Meng-Die Chen, Si-Si Dong, Meng-Di Fan, Su-Ping Gu, Jin-Jue Zheng, Hai-Min Yin, Xin-He Zhou, Liang-Xue Wang, Chun-Ying Li and Chao Zheng**
Diabetes Center and Department of Endocrinology, The Second Affiliated Hospital of Wenzhou Medical University, No. 109 West Xueyuan Road, 325027, Wenzhou, Zhejiang, China

**Ning-Yu Cai**
Department of Orthopedics, The Second Affiliated Hospital of Wenzhou Medical University, 325027, Wenzhou, Zhejiang, China

**De-Chun Yin, Zhao-Jun Wang, Shuai Guo, Hong-Yu Xie, Lin Sun, Wei Feng, Wei Qiu and Xiu-Fen Qu**
Department of Cardiology, The First Affiliated Hospital of Harbin Medical University, Harbin 150001, P.R. China

**Xiu-Fen Qu**
Department of Cardiology, The First Affiliated Hospital of Harbin Medical University, Dazhi Street No.199, Nangang District, Harbin 150001, P.R. China

**Pernille Holmager, Jens Faber and Caroline Kistorp**
Department of Medicine, Endocrine Unit, Herlev University Hospital, Herlev, Denmark

**Pernille Holmager, Morten Schou, Jens Faber and Caroline Kistorp**
Faculty of Health and Medical Sciences, Copenhagen University, Copenhagen, Denmark

**Michael Egstrup**
Department of Cardiology, Rigshospitalet, Copenhagen, Denmark

**Ida Gustafsson**
Department of Cardiology, Hvidovre University Hospital, Hvidovre, Denmark

**Morten Schou**
Department of Cardiology, Herlev University Hospital, Herlev, Denmark

**Jordi S. Dahl**
Department of Cardiology and Cardiothoracic Surgery, Odense University Hospital, Odense, Denmark

**Lars Melholt Rasmussen**
Department of Clinical Biochemistry and Pharmacology, Odense University Hospital, Odense, Denmark
Centre of Individualized Medicine in Arterial Diseases, Odense University Hospital, Odense, Denmark

**Jacob E. Møller**
Department of Cardiology, Odense University Hospital, Odense, Denmark

**Christian Tuxen**
Department of Cardiology, Bispebjerg University Hospital, Copenhagen, Denmark

**Pernille Holmager**
Department of Endocrinology, Herlev Hospital, Herlev, Denmark

**Joana Pereira, Ana Ribeiro, João Ferreira-Coimbra and Patrícia Lourenço**
Department of Internal Medicine, São João Hospital, Porto, Portugal

**Isaac Barroso**
Department of Biochemistry, São João Hospital, Porto, Portugal

**João-Tiago Guimarães**
Department of Clinical Pathology, São João Hospital, Porto, Portugal

**João-Tiago Guimarães, Paulo Bettencourt and Patrícia Lourenço**
Unidade de Investigação e Desenvolvimento Cardiovascular do Porto, Faculty of Medicine of University of Porto, Porto, Portugal

**Paulo Bettencourt**
Hospital da CUF, Porto, Portugal

**Joana Pereira**
Serviço de Medicina Interna, Hospital S. João, Alameda Professor Hernâni Monteiro, 4202-451 Porto, Portugal

**Pedro Pallangyo, Smita Bhalia, Paulina Nicholaus, Peter Kisenge and Mohamed Janabi**
Department of Cardiovascular Medicine, Jakaya Kikwete Cardiac Institute, Dar es Salaam, Tanzania

**Francis Fredrick, Benjamin Mtinangi and Stephen Humphrey**
Muhimbili University of Health and Allied Sciences, Dar es Salaam, Tanzania

**Brent A. Williams**
Geisinger Health System, 100 N. Academy Avenue, Danville, PA 17822, USA

**Grunde Gjesdal, Oscar Ö. Braun, J. Gustav Smith, Fredrik Scherstén and Patrik Tydén**
Department of Cardiology, Clinical Sciences, Lund University and Skåne University Hospital, SE-221 81 Lund, Sweden

**Ilya Karagodin, Omer Aba-Omer and Jennifer L. Strande**
Department of Medicine, Medical College of Wisconsin, 9200 Wisconsin Ave, Milwaukee, WI 53226, USA

**Rodney Sparapani**
Division of Biostatistics, Medical College of Wisconsin, Milwaukee, WI, USA

**Jennifer L. Strande**
Division of Cardiovascular Medicine, Medical College of Wisconsin, Milwaukee, WI, USA

**Susanne Röger, Stefanie L. Rosenkaimer, Anna Hohneck, Siegfried Lang, Ibrahim El-Battrawy, Boris Rudic, Erol Tülümen, Ksenija Stach, Jürgen Kuschyk, Ibrahim Akin and Martin Borggrefe**
First Department of Medicine, University Medical Centre Mannheim (UMM), Faculty of Medicine Mannheim, University of Heidelberg, Theodor-Kutzer-Ufer 1-3, 68167 Mannheim, Germany
German Centre for Cardiovascular Research (DZHK), Partner Site Heidelberg/ Mannheim, Mannheim, Germany

**Hong Shen, Jingbo Li, Qing Wan and Jing Huang**
Department of Cardiology, Shanghai Sixth People's Hospital, Shanghai Jiao Tong University, Shanghai, China

**Jianrong Zhao**
Department of Cardiology, Ruijin Hospital Luwan Branch, Shanghai Jiao Tong University School of Medicine, Shanghai, China

**Xiaohong Zhou, Shungang Yang and Ping Wang**
Cardiac Rhythm and Heart Failure, Research and Technology, Medtronic plc, Mounds View, MN, USA

**Liqun Wu**
Department of Cardiology, Ruijin Hospital, Shanghai Jiao Tong University School of Medicine, Shanghai, China

**Shungang Yang and Ping Wang**
Medtronic Shanghai Innovation Center, Medtronic (Shanghai) Ltd., Shanghai, China

**Gianni Mazzon and Giovanni Grazzi**
Department of Biomedical and Specialty Surgical Sciences, University of Ferrara, Ferrara, Italy

**Gianni Mazzoni**
Public Health Department, AUSL Ferrara, Ferrara, Italy

**Biagio Sassone**
Department of Medicine, Division of Cardiology, Cento Hospital, AUSL Ferrara, Ferrara, Italy

**Giovanni Pasanisi**
Department of Medicine, Division of Cardiology, "Delta" Hospital, AUSL Ferrara, Ferrara, Italy

**Jonathan Myers**
Veterans Affairs Palo Alto Health Care System, Palo Alto, CA, USA
Stanford University School of Medicine, Stanford, CA, USA

**Simona Mandini**
Center of Biomedical Studies Applied to Sport, University of Ferrara, via Gramicia 35, 44123 Ferrara, Italy

**Stefano Volpato**
Department of Medical Sciences, University of Ferrara, Ferrara, Italy

**Giorgio Chiaranda**
General Directorship for Public Health and Integration Policy, Emilia-Romagna Region, Bologna, Italy

**Gaurav S. Gulsin, Abishek Shetye, Jeffrey Khoo, Daniel J. Swarbrick, Eylem Levelt, Florence Y. Lai, Iain B. Squire, Jayanth R. Arnold and Gerry P. McCann**
Department of Cardiovascular Sciences, University of Leicester, Glenfield Hospital, Groby Road, Leicester LE3 9QP, UK
The NIHR Leicester Cardiovascular Biomedical Research Unit, Glenfield Hospital, Leicester, UK

**Gunda Musekamp, Michael Schuler, Bettina Seekatz, Hermann Faller and Karin Meng**
Department of Medical Psychology and Psychotherapy, Medical Sociology and Rehabilitation Sciences, University of Würzburg, Klinikstr. 3, D-97070 Würzburg, Germany

**Jürgen Bengel**
Institute of Psychology, Department of Rehabilitation Psychology and Psychotherapy, University of Freiburg, Engelbergerstraße 41, D-79085 Freiburg, Germany

# Index

CPSIA information can be obtained
at www.ICGtesting.com
Printed in the USA
LVHW060857030122
707669LV00002B/219

9 781639 270286